GLENCOE
HEALTH

About the Author

Mary H. Bronson, Ph.D., has taught health education in grades K–12, as well as health education methods classes at the undergraduate and graduate levels. As health education specialist for the Dallas School District, Dr. Bronson developed and implemented a district-wide health education program, *Skills for Living*, which was used as a model by the state education agency. She has assisted school districts throughout the country in developing local health education programs. She is also the author of Glencoe's *Teen Health* textbook series.

Cover image: McGraw-Hill Education

my.mheducation.com

Send all inquiries to:
McGraw-Hill Education
8787 Orion Place
Columbus, OH 43240

Glencoe Health, Student Edition:
ISBN: 978-1-26-432021-9
MHID: 1-26-432021-3

Printed in the United States of America.

8 9 10 11 12 LWI 27 26 25 24 23

HEALTH AND EDUCATIONAL CONSULTANTS

Lisa M. Carlson, MPH, C.H.E.S.
Academic Program Director
Emory Transplant Center
Atlanta, Georgia

Betty M. Hubbard, Ed.D., C.H.E.S.
Professor of Health Education
Department of Health Sciences
University of Central Arkansas
Conway, Arkansas

Deborah L. Tackmann, M.E.P.D.
Health Education Instructor
North High School
Eau Claire, Wisconsin

Rani Desai, Ph.D., M.P.H.
Associate Professor
Yale University
New Haven, Connecticut

Jili English
Health Education and Evaluation
Consultant
Orange, California

Roberta Duyff, R.D., C.F.C.S.
Food and Nutrition Education
Consultant
St. Louis, Missouri

Don L. Rainey
Lecturer and Director
Physical Fitness and Wellness
Program
Texas State University
San Marcos, Texas

Dyan Campbell, R.N., M.P.H.
Campbell Consulting L.L.C.
Parksville, New York

Susan Giarratano Russell, Ed.D., M.S.P.H., C.H.E.S.
Health Education and Evaluation
Consultant
Valencia, California

Jeanne Title
Coordinator, Prevention Education
Napa County Office of Education
and Napa Valley Unified School
District Napa, California

Donna Breitenstein
Health Educator
Boone, North Carolina

Ismael Nuño, M.D.
Chief, Cardiac Surgery
LAC+USC Medical Center
Los Angeles, California

Kelly Cartwright
College of Lake County
Department of Biological and
Health Sciences
Grayslake, Illinois

Greg Stockton
American Red Cross
Washington, DC

TEACHER REVIEWERS

TABLE OF CONTENTS

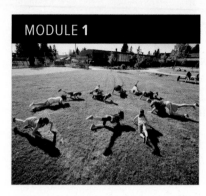

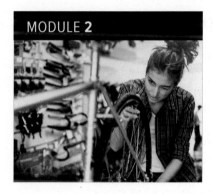

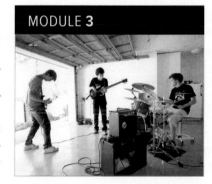

(t)Thomas Barwick/Getty Images, (c)Todor Tsvetkov/Getty Images, (b)Juice Images/Alamy Stock Photo

TABLE OF CONTENTS

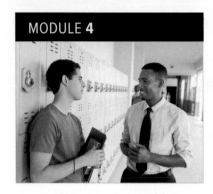
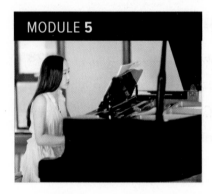
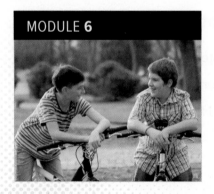

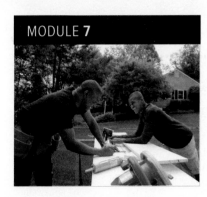

MODULE **7**

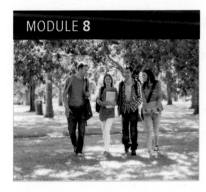

MODULE **8**

TABLE OF CONTENTS

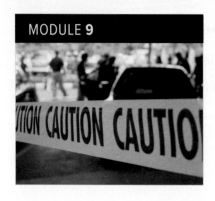
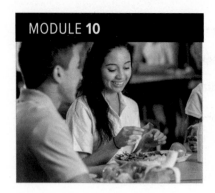
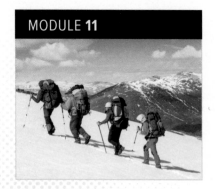

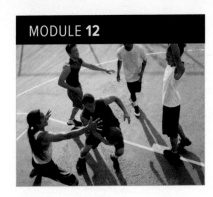

MODULE 12

Physical Activity and Fitness 278

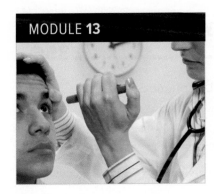

MODULE 13

Personal Health Care 310

(t)Sam Edwards/Glow Images, (b)Paul Burns/Getty Images

TABLE OF CONTENTS

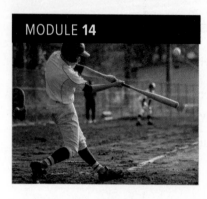

MODULE 14

Skeletal, Muscular, and Nervous Systems 332

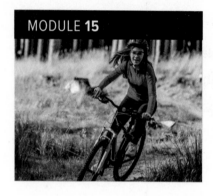

MODULE 15

Cardiovascular, Respiratory, and Digestive Systems 356

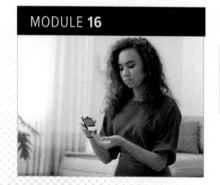

MODULE 16

Endocrine and Reproductive Health 388

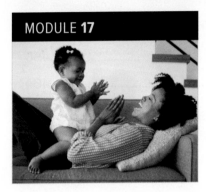

MODULE 17

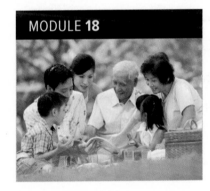

MODULE 18

(t)monkeybusinessimages/Getty Images, (b)Floresco Productions/age fotostock

TABLE OF CONTENTS

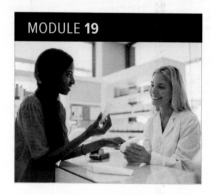
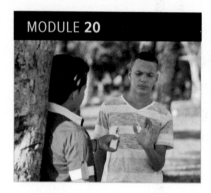
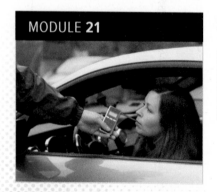

TABLE OF CONTENTS

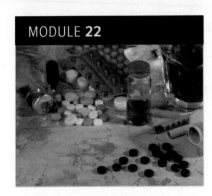
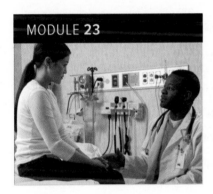

TABLE OF CONTENTS

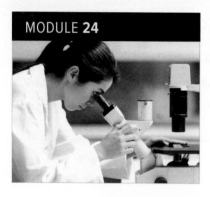

MODULE 24

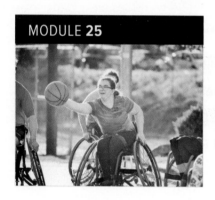

MODULE 25

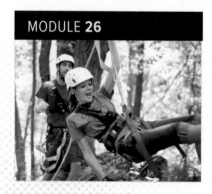

MODULE 26

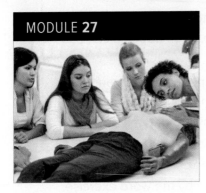
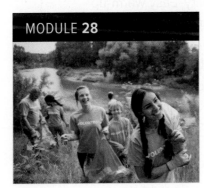

FITNESS HANDBOOK

Physical fitness is for everyone, regardless of a person's skill level. Non-athletes who choose not to join organized sports can develop a personal fitness plan to stay in shape. Even athletes can use some of the tips to cross train for their favorite sport.

Planning a Routine: The Fitness Handbook helps you plan a fitness routine that helps your body adjust slowly to activity. Over time, you will increase both the length of time you spend and the number of times that you are physically active each week. Teens should aim to get at least one hour of physical activity each day. These periods of physical activity can be divided into shorter segments, such as three 20-minute segments each day.

Before You Start Exercising: Before we begin, let's explain what we mean by the word exercise. Exercise can include any physical activity, such as completing a fitness program, playing individual or group sports, or even helping clean at home. The key is to keep your body moving.

Every activity session should begin with a warm-up to prepare your body for exercise. Warm-ups raise your body temperature and get your muscles ready for physical activity. Easy warm-up activities include walking, marching, and jogging, as well as basic calisthenics or stretches. A warm-up can also be an easier version of the exercise you have chosen. For example, if you have decided to run five miles, as a warm-up you may choose to jog for the first 10 minutes.

As you increase the time you spend doing a fitness activity, you should increase the time you spend warming up. Check the Sample Physical Fitness Plan to see how much time you should dedicate to warm-ups and fitness activities. For additional fitness activities, visit the Fitness Zone section within the Glencoe Health digital experience.

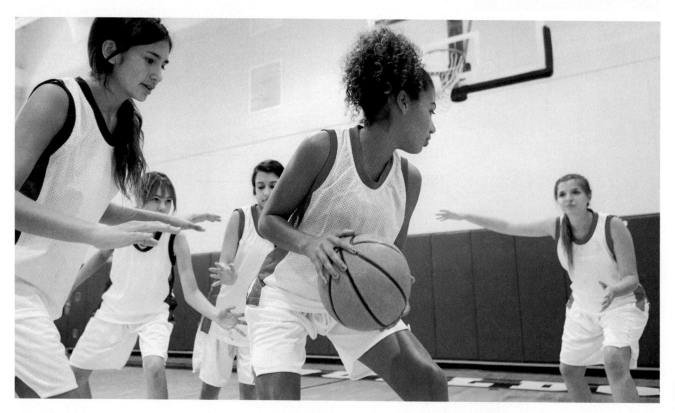

The Five Elements of Fitness

When developing a fitness plan, it's helpful to have a goal. Maybe your goal is to comfortably run three miles each day to stay in shape, or maybe you want to run in a marathon in the future. Regardless of the reasons why you develop a fitness plan, focusing on the five elements of fitness, or health-related fitness, will help you achieve overall physical fitness.
The five elements are:

1. Cardiorespiratory Endurance

The ability of your heart, lungs, and blood vessels to send fuel and oxygen to your tissues during long periods of moderate to vigorous activity. Examples are jogging, walking, bike riding, and swimming.

2. Muscular Endurance

The ability of your muscles to perform physical tasks over a period of time without tiring. Many activities that build cardiovascular endurance also build muscle endurance, such as jogging, walking, and bike riding.

3. Muscular Strength

The amount of force your muscles can exert. Activities that can help build muscular endurance include push-ups, pull-ups, lifting weights, and running stairs.

4. Flexibility

The ability to move your body parts through their full range of motion. You can improve your flexibility by stretching before and after exercise.

5. Body Composition

The ratio of fat to lean tissue in your body. A healthy body is made up of more lean tissue and less fat. Body composition is a result of diet, exercise, and heredity.

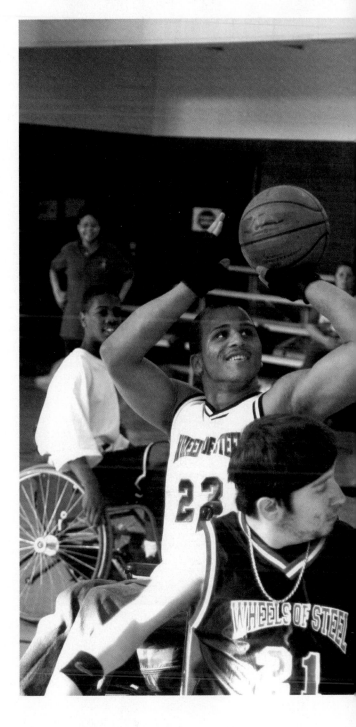

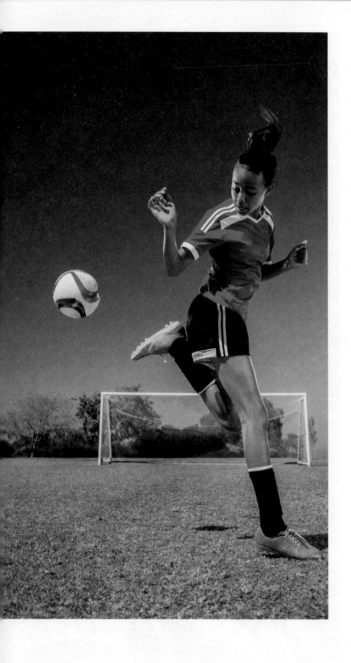

Skill-Related Fitness

Skill-related fitness can enhance your ability to complete daily tasks unrelated to exercise. For health-related and skill-related fitness activities, visit the Fitness Zone section within the Glencoe Health digital experience. Skill-related fitness requires that you consider six elements. These include:

1. Agility

The ability to change and control the direction and position of the body while maintaining a constant, rapid motion. Sports that require a high level of agility include football, soccer, basketball, baseball, and softball.

2. Balance

The ability to control or stabilize the body while standing or moving. Examples of sports that require balance include gymnastics, golf, and ice skating.

3. Coordination

The ability to use the senses to determine and direct the movement of your limbs and head. Gymnastics, cheerleading, and juggling demand a high level of coordination.

4. Speed

The ability to move your body, or parts of it, swiftly. Foot speed is measured over a short and straight distance, usually less than 200 meters. Other speed evaluations might include hand and arm speed. The baseball pitcher, boxer, sprinter, and volleyball spiker all require specific kinds of speed.

5. Power

The ability to move the body parts swiftly while simultaneously applying the maximum force of your muscles. The long jump, power lifting, and swimming all require high levels of power.

6. Reaction Time

The ability to react or respond quickly to what you hear, see, or feel. Good reaction time is important to sprinters and swimmers, who must react to starts. The tennis player, boxer, and hockey goalie all require quick reaction times as well.

Creating a Fitness Plan

When planning a personal activity program, choose activities that you enjoy and that you can realistically do. For example, think about what type of activity can realistically fit into your schedule. If your schedule is already full of after-school activities will you be tempted to skip workouts?

Another factor to consider when choosing a type of exercise is whether or not the exercise will help the social and mental/emotional sides of your health triangle. If meeting new people is one of your goals, will playing the sport help you meet people with whom you share interests? Also, your cultural background may impact your choices. In the U.S., football, basketball, and baseball are all popular sports. In most of the world, soccer is the most popular sport. You may choose to play soccer because it is a popular sport in the country of your ancestors, and you want to learn more about their lifestyle. Learning about a sport that commonly played in another country may help you learn more about that culture through the sport.

Most importantly, pick an activity that you enjoy. If you do not enjoy the activity, chances are you will find excuses not to exercise. The list below offers other factors may affect your activity choices:

- **Cost.** Some activities require expensive equipment. It may make sense to borrow or rent equipment, rather than buying it, when you try a new sport.
- **Where you live.** Is your local area flat or hilly? What is the climate like? Factors like these will affect the activities that you can do close to home.
- **Your schedule.** If you like to sleep late, planning to jog every morning will probably fail. Choose activities that fi t your schedule and habits.
- **Your health and fitness level.** Do you have a health condition that may affect your exercise plan, such as asthma? If so, talk to your doctor before starting a new activity.
- **Personal safety.** When choosing activities, make sure that you have a safe environment to perform them in. For instance, you should not go running on busy streets with no sidewalks.

Sample Physical Fitness Plan

WEEK	MONDAY Warm Up	MONDAY Activity	TUESDAY Warm Up	TUESDAY Activity	WEDNESDAY Warm Up	WEDNESDAY Activity	THURSDAY Warm Up	THURSDAY Activity	FRIDAY Warm Up	FRIDAY Activity
1	5 min	5 min	–	–	5 min	5 min	–	–	5 min	5 min
2	5 min	5 min	–	–	5 min	5 min	–	–	5 min	5 min
3	5 min	5 min	–	–	5 min	5 min	–	–	5 min	5 min
4	5 min	5 min	–	–	5 min	5 min	–	–	5 min	5 min
5	7 min	7 min	–	–	7 min	7 min	–	–	7 min	7 min
6	7 min	7 min	–	–	7 min	7 min	–	–	7 min	7 min
7	10 min	10 min	–	–	10 min	20 min	–	–	10 min	20 min
8	10 min	10 min	10 min	20 min	10 min	20 min	–	–	10 min	20 min
9	10 min	10 min	10 min	20 min	10 min	20 min	10 min	20 min	10 min	20 min

ACTIVITIES AND SPORTS

Fitness Circuit

Many public parks have Fitness Circuits (sometimes called Par Courses) with exercise stations located throughout a park. You walk or run between stations as part of your workout. You may also consider creating your own par course at home. Fitness Circuits can be adapted to a person's individual skill level and ability.

What Will I Need?

- Access to a public park or a home-made Fitness Circuit course.
- Comfortable workout clothes that wick away perspiration.
- Athletic shoes.
- Stopwatch (optional).
- Jump rope, dumbbells, elastic exercise bands, or check out the Fitness Zone Clipboard Energizer Activity Cards, Circuit Training for ideas.

How Do I Start?

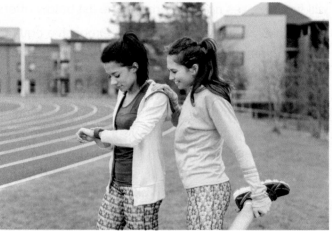

- Warm-up with a 5-minute walk and stretching
- Read the instructions at each exercise station and perform the exercises as shown. Use the correct form. Try to do as many repetitions as you can for 30 seconds.
- After you finish the exercise, walk or run to the next station and complete that exercise.
- Check your heart rate to see how intensely you exercised at the end of the Fitness Circuit.
- Cool-down by walking, standing in place and moving your feet up and down, or jogging slowly. End your cool-down with 3 to five minutes of stretching.
- Every month or so, consider adding a new exercise.

How Can I Stay Safe?

- Be alert to your surroundings in a public park. It is best to have a friend with you and it makes exercising even more fun.
- Leave enough room between stations at home to allow you to move and exercise freely. Avoid clutter in your exercise area.
- Perform the exercises correctly and at your own pace.

For more circuit training ideas, visit the Fitness Zone section within the Glencoe Health digital experience.

Walking

By walking for as little as 30 minutes each day you can reduce your risk of heart disease, manage your weight, and even reduce stress. Walking requires very little equipment and you can do it almost anywhere. Walking is also something you can do by yourself or with friends and family.

What Will I Need?

- Running or walking shoes. Many athletic shoe stores sell both.
- Loose comfortable clothes that wick away perspiration. Layering is also a good idea. Consider adding a hat, sunglasses, and sunscreen if needed.
- Stopwatch and water bottle unless there are water fountains on your route.
- A pedometer or GPS to track your distance.

How Do I Start?

- Warm-up for 10 minutes by walking slowly and stretching.
- Walk upright with good posture. Do not exaggerate your stride or swing your arms across your body.
- Build your time and distance slowly. One mile or 20 minutes every other day may be enough for the first couple weeks. Eventually you will want to walk at least 30–60 minutes five days a week.
- End your walk with a 5-minute cool-down to stretch your muscles.

How Can I Stay Safe?

- Let your parents know where you will be walking and how long you will be gone.
- Avoid wearing headphones if by yourself or if walking on a road or street.

For more information about using a pedometer, visit the Fitness Zone section within the Glencoe Health digital experience.

ACTIVITIES AND SPORTS

Running

Running uses the large muscles of the legs thereby burning lots of calories and also gives your heart and lungs a good workout in a shorter amount of time. Running also helps get you into condition to play team sports like basketball, football, or soccer. Running can be done on your schedule although it's also fun to run with a friend or two.

What Will I Need?

- A good pair of running shoes. Ask your physical education teacher or an employee at a specialist running shop to help you choose the right pair.
- Socks made of cotton or another type of material that wicks away perspiration.
- Bright colored or reflective clothing.
- A stopwatch or watch with a second hand to time your runs or track your distance.
- Optional equipment might include a jacket or other layer depending on the weather, sunscreen, and sunglasses.

How Do I Start?

Your ultimate goal is to run at least 20 to 30 minutes at least 3 days a week. Use the training schedule shown below. Start by walking and gradually increasing the amount of time you run during each exercise session. Starting slowly will help your muscles and tendons adjust to the increased workload. Try spacing the three runs over an entire week so that you have one day in-between runs to recover. Here is a plan to get you started as a runner:

- Start each run with a brisk 3- to 5-minute walk to warm-up.
- Take some time to slowly stretch the muscles and areas of the body involved in running. Avoid "bouncing" when stretching or try to force a muscle or tendon to stretch when you start to feel tightness.
- Begin slowly and gradually increase your distance and speed. The running plan included in this section can give you some tips on how to train for a 5K run.
- Use the "talk test." Can you talk in complete sentences during your training runs? If not, you are running too fast.

For more information about the talk test, visit the Fitness Zone section within the Glencoe Health digital experience.

Training Schedule

M W F	Split Schedule	Duration
Week 1	Brisk 5 min. walk Walk: 60–90 seconds Run: 60 seconds	Repeat for 20 minutes
Week 2 and 3	Brisk 5 min. walk Walk: 60 seconds Run: 60–90 seconds	Repeat for 20 minutes
Week 4	Brisk 5 min. walk Walk: 60 seconds Run: 3–5 minutes	Repeat for 20 minutes
Week 5+	Brisk 5 min. walk Run: 20–30 minutes	

Preparing for Sports and Other Activities

Are you are thinking about playing a sport? If so, think about developing a fitness plan for that sport. Some of the questions to ask yourself are: Does the sport require anaerobic activity, like running and jumping hurdles? Does the sport require aerobic fitness, like cross-country running? Other sports, such as football and track require muscular strength. Sports like basketball require special skills like dribbling, passing, and shot making. A workout plan for that sport will help you get into shape before organized practice and competition begins.

What Will I Need?

Talk to a coach or physical education teacher about how to get ready for your sport. You can also conduct online research to learn what type of equipment you will need, such as:

- Proper footwear and workout clothes for a specific sport.
- What facilities are available for training and practice, such as a running track, tennis court, football or soccer field, or other safe open area.
- Where you can access weights and others form of resistance training as part of your training program.

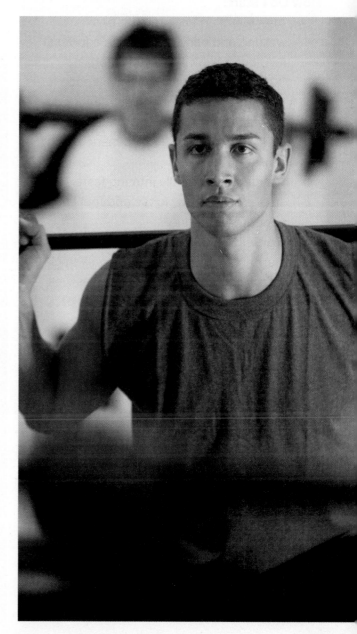

How Do I Start?

Now that your research is done, you can create your fitness plan. Include the type of exercises you will do each training day. Use the Sample Physical Fitness plan on page xix to create your plan.

- Include a warm-up in your plan.
- List the duration of time that you will work out.
- Plan to exercise 3–5 days a week doing at least one kind of exercise each day. Remember to include stretching before every workout.

How Can I Stay Safe?

- Get instruction on how to use free weights and machines.
- Make sure you start every exercise activity with a warm-up.
- Ease into your Fitness Plan gradually so you do not pull a muscle or do too much too soon.
- Practice good nutrition and drink plenty of water to stay hydrated.

For more individual and team sport ideas, visit the Fitness Zone section within the Glencoe Health digital experience.

Comstock/Getty Images

Interval Training

Interval training consists of a mix of activities. First you do a few minutes of intense exercise. Next, you do easier, less-intense activity that enables your body to recover. Interval training can improve your cardiovascular endurance. It also helps develop speed and quickness. Intervals are typically done as part of a running program. However, intervals can also be done riding a bicycle or while swimming. On a bicycle, alternate fast pedaling with easier riding. In a pool, swim two fast laps followed by slower, easier laps.

What Will I Need?

- A running track or other flat area with marked distances like a football or soccer field.
- If at a park, 5–8 cones or flags to mark off distances of 30 to 100 yards.
- A training partner to help you push yourself (optional).

How Do I Start?

- After warming up, alternate brisk walking and easy jogging. On a football field or track, walk 30 yards, jog 30 yards, and then run at a fast pace for 30 yards. Rest for one minute and repeat this circuit several times. If at a park, use cones or flags to mark off similar distances.
- Accelerate gradually into the faster strides so you stay loose and feel in control of the pace.
- If possible, alternate running up stadium steps instead of fast running on a track. This will help your coordination as well as your speed. Running uphill in a park would have similar benefits.

How Can I Stay Safe?

- Interval training should only be done once or twice a week with a day off between workouts.
- Check with your doctor first if you have any medical condition like high blood pressure or asthma.

For more interval training ideas, visit the Fitness Zone section within the Glencoe Health digital experience.

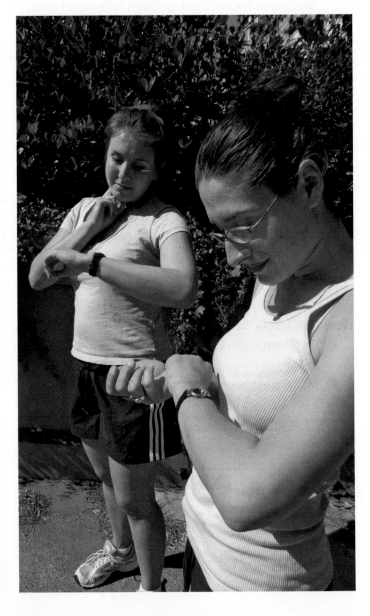

John Flournoy/McGraw-Hill Education

Preventing Injuries

While you may be ready to jump right into a fitness program, it is important to take proper caution to avoid injury. To prevent or safely treat injuries, follow these guidelines:

- Pay attention to your body. If you feel unusually sore or fatigued, postpone activity or exercise until you feel better.
- Include a proper warm-up and cool-down in your personal fitness program.
- Monitor the frequency, intensity, time, and type of your exercise closely. Progress slowly but steadily.
- If you run or walk along busy streets, always face oncoming traffic.
- Wear reflective clothing during night physical activities or exercise, such as walking or jogging.
- Use proper safety equipment for activities with a higher injury risk, such as skateboarding, snowboarding, and cycling.
- Always seek medical attention when you have an injury.

Being a Good Sport

What does it mean to be a good sport? Sportsmanship means you play fairly and follow the rules, respect your opponents, and show polite behavior to coaches, officials, teammates, and opponents. Practicing good sportsmanship also means using appropriate language and not trash-talking your opponents. Supporting your team is a great idea and can add to the fun. However, using insulting and cruel references to another team or individual does not show good sportsmanship. Participating in sports can be exciting and emotions can be strong, however remember to take a deep breath and think before you say something out of anger. Whether you win or lose, remember that everyone deserves to be treated fairly.

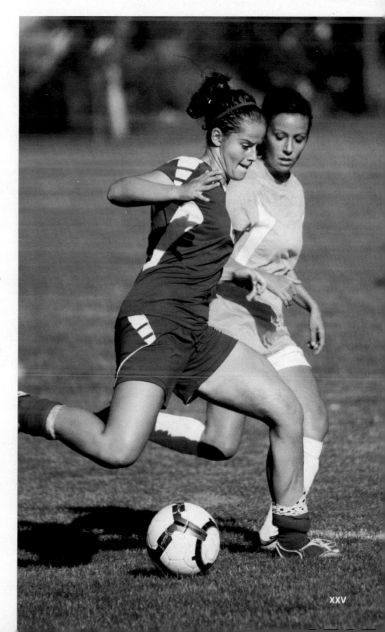

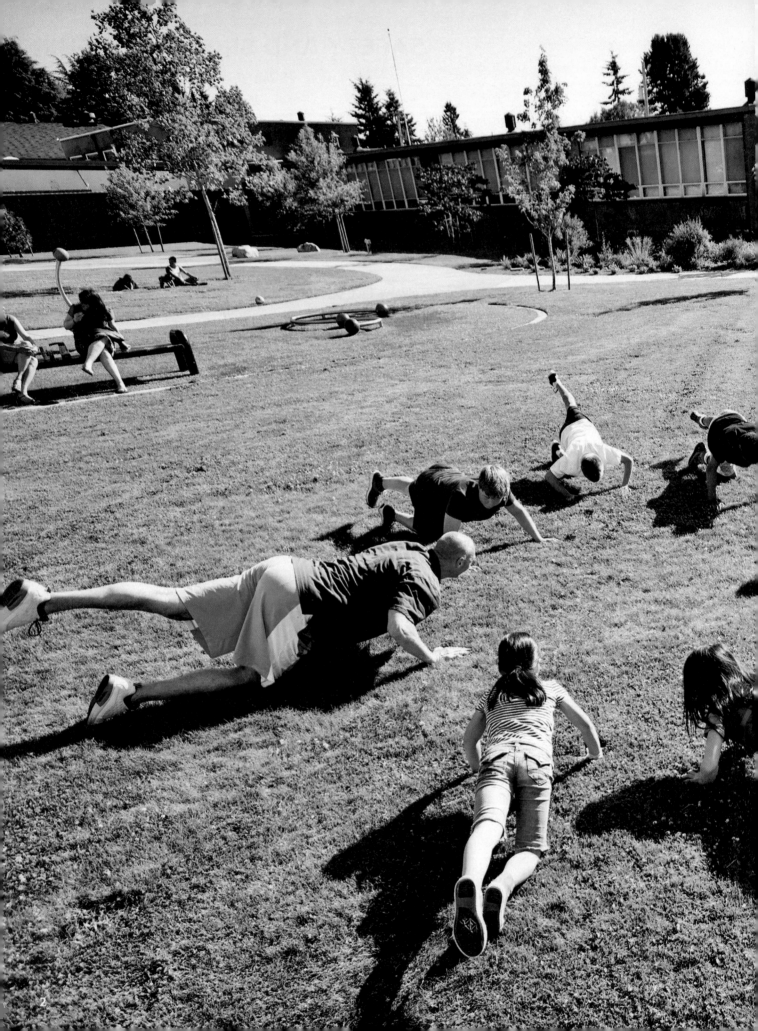

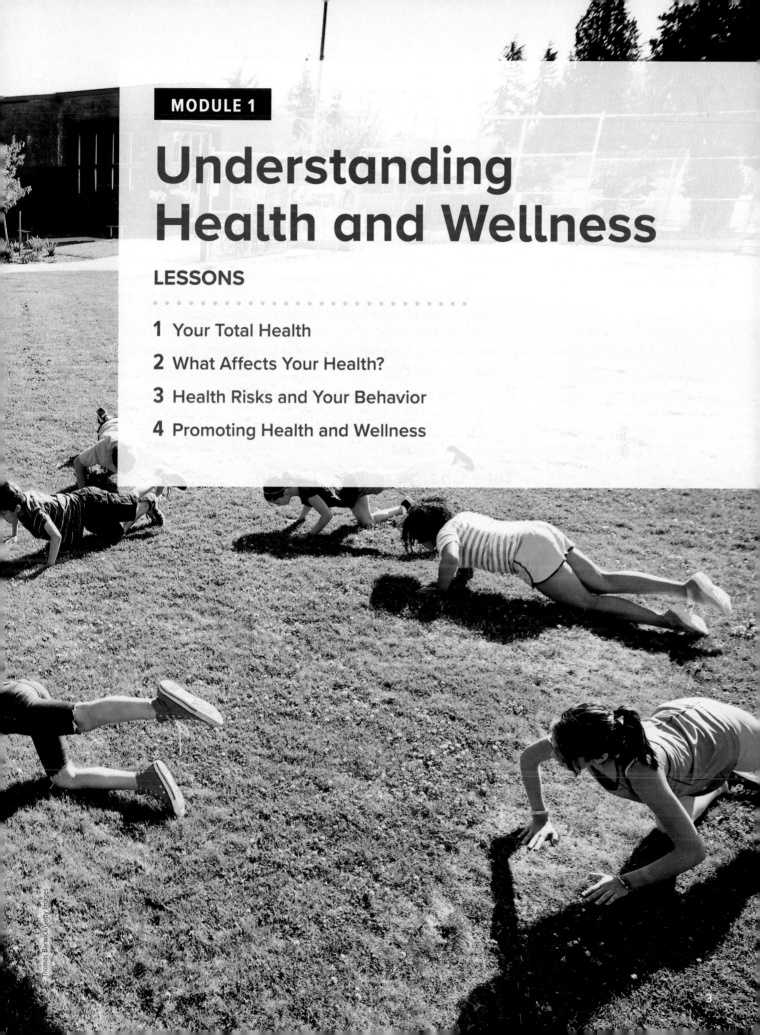

MODULE 1

Understanding Health and Wellness

LESSONS

3

Your Total Health

BEFORE YOU READ

Create a Cluster Chart. Draw a circle and label it "Health." Use surrounding circles to define and describe this term. As you read, continue filling in the chart with more details.

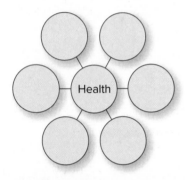

Vocabulary

health
spiritual health
wellness
chronic disease

BIG IDEA A lifetime of good health involves making healthy choices and practicing healthful behaviors.

REAL LIFE ISSUES

Being Healthy. On the first day of spring semester, Keisha comes home thinking about the question her health teacher asked during class: What does health mean to you and your future? Keisha opens her notebook and pauses. There are so many things to write about. She starts thinking about what she wants to accomplish in life and about the role that good health will play in helping her achieve her goals. *Write Keisha's journal entry for this day.*

After completing the lesson, review and analyze your response to the Real Life Issues question.

Take Charge of Your Health

MAIN IDEA You are responsible for your own health.

Close your eyes and try to picture a healthy person. Do you see someone who is physically active and involved in sports? Do you think that a healthy individual gets along well with others and generally feels good about himself or herself? These images are all part of the "big picture" of **health**. Health is the combination of physical, mental/emotional, and social well-being. When you are in good health, you have the energy to enjoy life and pursue your dreams.

Every day, you make decisions that shape your health. Some choices, such as what to eat for lunch, may seem fairly small, but over time they can add up to have a big effect on your total health. That's why it's important to develop the knowledge and skills you need to make healthy choices and take charge of your health for a lifetime. Giving you that knowledge is what these lessons are all about.

Your Health Triangle

MAIN IDEA It's important to balance your physical, mental/emotional, and social health.

What can you do to stay healthy? The first step is to understand the three areas of health. These are:

- physical health

- mental/emotional health

- social health

The health triangle is show as having three sides, one representing each of the three areas of health. It's important to pay attention to all three areas of your health triangle. Balancing all three side of the health triangle means that your physical, mental/emotional, and social health is in balance. If you concentrate too much or too little on one area, the triangle can become unbalanced.

Physical Health

Physical health is all about how well your body functions. Having a high level of physical health means having enough energy to perform your daily activities, deal with everyday stresses, and avoid injury.

What does it take to get and keep a healthy body? Here are five important actions you can take:

- Get eight to ten hours of sleep each night.
- Eat healthful foods and drink plenty of fluids.
- Make time for 30 to 60 minutes of physical activity every day.
- Avoid the use of tobacco, alcohol, and other drugs.
- Bathe daily, and brush and floss your teeth every day.

Mental/Emotional Health

Mental and emotional health is about your feelings and thoughts. It's a reflection of how you feel about yourself, how you meet the demands of your daily life, and how you cope with problems. People who are mentally and emotionally healthy

- enjoy challenges that help them grow.
- accept responsibility for their actions.
- have a sense of control over their lives.
- can express their emotions in **appropriate** ways.
- can deal with most of life's stresses and frustrations.
- generally have a positive outlook.
- make thoughtful and responsible decisions.

Fitness Zone

I hear that we should try to walk 10,000 steps every day. So, my best friend and I wear pedometers and walk as much as possible. Instead of taking a bus, we walk. We also use the stairs rather than an escalator or elevator. We've been doing this for three months now, and we feel great! For more physical activity ideas, visit the Fitness Zone online.

ACADEMIC VOCABULARY

appropriate (adjective): proper or fitting

Your health triangle is made up of three equally important areas. **What do you do to stay in good health?**

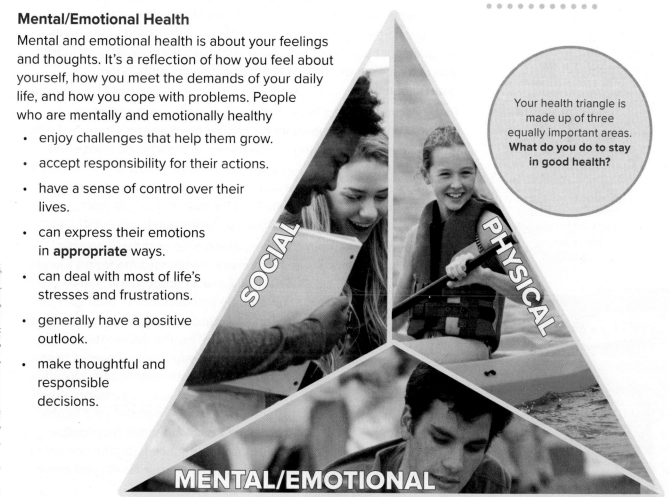

SOCIAL

PHYSICAL

MENTAL/EMOTIONAL

Spiritual Health. Mental/emotional health also includes **spiritual health**. Spiritual health is a deep-seated sense of meaning and purpose in life. Being spiritually healthy does not necessarily mean that you belong to a religious group, although having a spiritual community can be a part of it. Spiritual health also includes having a sense of your values and a feeling of purpose in your life.

Social Health

Your social health, or how well you get along with others, is as important a part of your total health as having a fit body and mind. Your social network includes your family, friends, teachers, and other members of your community. You don't need to have lots of friends to have good social health. Sometimes just having a few people to share your thoughts and feelings with is enough. Maintaining healthy relationships is one way of caring for your social health. This involves:

- seeking and lending support when needed.
- communicating clearly and listening to others.
- showing respect and care for yourself and others.

Keeping a Balance

When your health triangle is balanced, you have a high degree of **wellness**, which is an overall state of wellbeing or total health. Wellness comes from making the right decisions about your health—decisions that are based on sound knowledge and healthy attitudes. Maintaining wellness means keeping a balance among the three aspects of health.

To understand why balance is important, think about someone whose friends are the most important part of her life. She loves to go out with them or stay up late talking on the phone. Although she always has a great time, she doesn't always get the rest she needs. She often feels tired and has a hard time concentrating on her schoolwork. She pays more attention to her social health at the expense of her mental/emotional health. The result is that her health triangle is out of balance.

To take another example, consider a teen who spends all his time working out. He's always in the gym and never has time for his friends. Physically, he's in great shape, but he often feels lonely and depressed. This teen pays too much attention to his physical health at the expense of his mental/emotional and social health. If you ignore any area of your health triangle, your total health will suffer. To keep a balance, you need to pay equal attention to all three parts of your health. You will learn how to make responsible decisions and practice healthful behaviors that help you keep your health in balance and maintain your wellness.

Reading Check

Identify List the three components of health.

When you feel your best, you perform at your best. **Which areas of this teen's health triangle are receiving attention?**

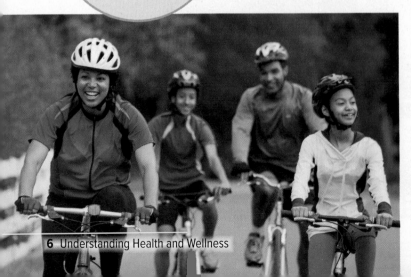

Ariel Skelley/Blend Images/Getty Images

The Health Continuum

MAIN IDEA Healthful behaviors will promote your wellness.

Your health and wellness are always changing. For instance, you may feel great one day and catch a cold the next. Your health at any moment can be seen as a point along a *continuum,* or sliding scale. The continuum spans the complete range of health, from a lack of health and wellness at one end to a high level of wellness at the other.

Reading Check

Explain What is a continuum?

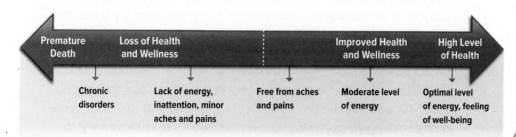

As you grow older, your position on the continuum will continue to change. Many Americans, unfortunately, start moving toward the lower end of the continuum as they age. One-half of all Americans live with a **chronic disease**, which is an ongoing condition or illness such as heart disease, obesity, or cancer. There are many factors that can increase your risk of developing a chronic disease. The leading ones are smoking, lack of physical activity, poor nutrition, being overweight, and lack of health screenings. Fortunately, most of these are risks that you can avoid. By making a lifelong commitment now to take the best possible care of your health, you will be more likely to stay at the higher end of the continuum your whole life.

Your health can be measured on a sliding scale. **Where would you place your health along the continuum right now?**

Lesson 1 Review

Facts and Vocabulary

1. Define the word *health.*

2. List important steps you can take to promote your physical health.

3. Describe the purpose of the health continuum? What do the continuum's endpoints represent?

Thinking Critically

4. **Relate.** Describe how poor mental/emotional health can affect physical health.

5. **Predict.** How might your behaviors today affect your health now? How might they affect your health in the future?

Applying Health Skills

6. **Communication Skills.** Create a poster that explains the three areas of health to fourth or fifth graders.

Writing Critically

7. **Persuasive.** Write an editorial for the school newspaper about why each person is responsible for his own health, and why this is important.

What Affects Your Health?

. . . .

BEFORE YOU READ

Create a K-W-L Chart. Make a three-column chart. In the first column, list what you **k**now about influences on your health. In the second column, list what you **w**ant to know about this topic. As you read use the third column to summarize what you **l**earned.

K	W	L

Vocabulary

heredity
environment
peers
culture
media
technology

. . . .

BIG IDEA Understanding how heredity, environment, and other factors that affect your health can help you make healthy decisions.

REAL LIFE ISSUES

Too Much Sun. Jason enjoys being outdoors, and he spends a lot of time in the sun as a member of the cross-country team. He always uses sunscreen. During the summer months, he and his friends enjoy swimming and boating at the lake. He has invited his cousin Sean to come to the lake for a week. The first day, when Jason offers Sean some sunscreen, Sean says no. He tells Jason he doesn't like the sticky feeling it leaves on his skin. *Write a brief dialogue between Jason and Sean. Have Jason try to persuade Sean to protect his health by using sunscreen.*

After completing the lesson, review and analyze your response to the Real Life Issues question.

Influences on Your Health

MAIN IDEA Heredity, environment, attitude, behavior, media, and technology can all influence your health.

It is your responsibility to make healthy decisions and take actions to ensure your well-being. Factors such as heredity, environment, attitude, behavior, media, and technology can influence how you live. Understanding these influences will help you make informed decisions about your health.

Your physical environment influences your health in several ways. **Identify some positive and negative influences in your physical environment. How do you use the positive influences to protect your health? How can you overcome the negative influences?**

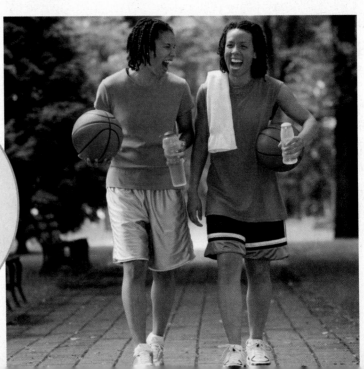

David Buffington/Blend Images/Getty Images

Heredity

Your **heredity** refers to all the traits that were biologically passed on to you from your parents. Heredity can affect your life in many ways. For example, LaToya inherited her black hair, brown eyes, and tall body type from her parents. She also inherited genes that put her at risk for diabetes, a serious disorder that prevents the body from converting food into energy. Both of LaToya's parents have diabetes. They have taken steps to control their diet and started an after-dinner walking program to keep their condition from getting worse.

By watching her parents, LaToya has learned to eat healthfully, maintain a normal weight, get adequate rest, and stay active. She and her parents spend a half hour each week planning their meals for the next week. Her parents' example has taught her that these healthful behaviors may help her avoid getting diabetes herself.

It's important to understand the ways heredity influences your health. Ask your parents or grandparents questions about what health conditions and diseases run in your family. Knowing this information can help you take the right steps to stay well and healthy.

Environment

When you hear the word **environment**, you may instantly think of the physical place where you live. However, your environment also includes the people you see every day and the culture in which you live. Your environment is the sum of your surroundings. All of these can have an impact on your health.

Physical Environment. You may not have much control over your physical environment at this time in your life. However, it's still important to recognize how your physical environment can influence all aspects of your health. Some environmental factors that can affect your health include

- neighborhood and school safety.
- air and water quality.
- availability of parks, recreational facilities, and libraries.
- access to medical care.

There are some parts of your environment that are under your control. For instance, you can keep your room clean and help reduce litter at your school. Think of some other ways that you can improve your physical environment.

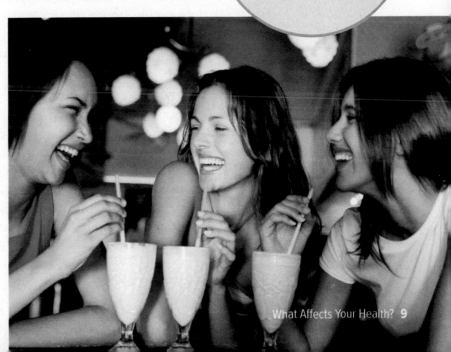

These teens are being influenced by their physical and social environments. **What are some environmental influences that affect you physically? What are some that affect you socially?**

Social Environment. Your social environment is made up of all the people around you, including your family, friends, and **peers**. Your peers are people of the same age who share similar interests, and also include your friends. All these people can influence your behavior in positive or negative ways. For example, Brandon promised his dad that he wouldn't use alcohol. Spending time with peers who do use alcohol, though, made it hard to keep that promise. In the end, Brandon decided to honor his commitment to his dad. As part of that commitment, he found a new group of friends who do not pressure him to do things that are against his personal values. In Brandon's case, his father was a positive influence on his health, while his peers were a negative influence. In other cases, however, peers can affect your health in positive ways. For instance, if your friends are involved in community service, such as a tutoring program for younger kids, you're more likely to join in these activities.

Culture. To what **culture** do you belong? Culture refers to the collective beliefs, customs, and behaviors of a group. Your answer might relate to your ethnic group, your community, your country, or the country where your ancestors were born. Your culture can affect every side of your health triangle. Culture may include the language you speak, the foods you eat, your spiritual beliefs, and the traditions you practice. All of these **factors** can have an influence on your physical, mental/emotional, and social health. For instance, many cultures have traditional foods that are eaten during celebrations. Some cultures may favor a diet based on vegetables, fruits, grains, and very little meat, while others choose only one or two types of meat.

Attitude

Your attitude, or the way you view situations, can have a big impact on your health. If you believe that adopting healthful habits will make your life better, then you're more likely to make the decision to practice them. In addition, optimists—people who view the world more favorably—are usually in better health than pessimists, who adopt an unfavorable stance on circumstances around them. Even if you have a natural tendency toward feeling gloomy, you can make the effort to look at challenging situations in a more upbeat way.

Behavior

Although you can't change your heredity and may have only limited control over your environment, you have total control over your own behaviors. You can take many steps every day to avoid high-risk behaviors and choose more healthful ones. Two examples include choosing low-fat, nutritious foods and getting some physical activity every day. When you consistently make healthy choices on a daily basis, they add up to have a strong, positive impact on your health.

ACADEMIC VOCABULARY

factor *(noun):* an element that contributes to a particular result

Reading Check

Analyze Why is it important to understand the influences on your health?

Media and Technology

Every day you encounter one of the most powerful influences on your health—the **media**. Media are the various methods for communicating information. Media content can be delivered through **technology,** such as phones, computers, radio, and television. It can also be delivered through print media, such as newspapers and magazines. The presence of media messages has a significant influence on your decisions.

For example, think for a moment about some of your favorite celebrities, such as athletes or TV stars. Do you admire these people? Do you wish you could be like them? Media personalities get a lot of attention. Sometimes they are praised for positive achievements, such as excelling at sports or contributing time and money to help others in need. Sometimes, however, these superstars are actually setting a bad example for others. For example, some actors or models may keep themselves extremely thin by eating far less food than they need to stay healthy. You have probably also heard about athletes who take drugs to help them perform better. In addition, characters in movies or TV programs often take part in all kinds of risky behavior. They may drive dangerously, use alcohol, smoke, use illegal drugs, or engage in sexual activity—without ever seeming to face any consequences. When you see these behaviors in the media, you may get the false idea that they are normal and harmless.

Even more powerful and far-reaching than radio, television, newspapers, and magazines is the Internet. Today, the Internet surpasses all other forms of media as an information source. Thousands of pages of health information from all over the world are available online. Unfortunately, not all health messages and sources deliver valid information. Some websites are sponsored by advertisers who want you to buy a product. For valid health information, choose websites that end in *.gov,* such as the Centers for Disease Control and Prevention (CDC). Another good choice is to search for information on sites maintained by professional health organizations that end in .org, such as the American Medical Association (AMA). Sites ending with .edu are maintained by educational institutions, such as colleges and high schools. These sites may also provide good information. However, when doing research on a site ending with .gov, .org, or .edu, make sure that the information on the page has been checked by the government site, organization, or school. Schools, for example, post student pages, and this information may not be checked to make sure it is valid.

One way to tell whether a website has reliable information is to look for the HONcode logo. This is the symbol of the Health on the Net Foundation, which is dedicated to improving the quality of health information. Websites certified by HONcode must follow a strict code of conduct.

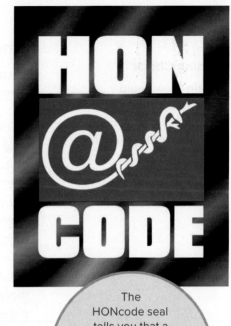

The HONcode seal tells you that a website's information is of high quality. **Why is it important to know whether media messages are trustworthy?**

Myths & Reality

All websites with *.edu* at the end of the address provide reliable information.

Myth: You can trust everything you read on a website ending with .edu.

Reality: A website ending with *.edu* is maintained by an educational institution. However, you still need to check the validity of the information on that site. Determine if the page you're reading was developed by staff at the school, or by a student. Some schools host student pages, and do not check the accuracy of information on those pages.

Reading Check

Explain How could understanding the influence of media and technology make a difference in your health?

Understanding Your Influences

MAIN IDEA You can take control of your health by understanding the factors that influence it.

Think about all the factors that influence your health. These include your heredity, your physical and social environment, your culture, your attitudes, your behaviors, and the media. Take a minute to consider how each one of these might affect your health in positive or negative ways. For instance, if you inherited very pale skin from your parents, that might increase your risk for skin cancer. On the other hand, if your neighborhood offers many safe places for exercise, such as parks and bike paths, that might increase the chances that you will be physically active. The better you understand all the influences on your health, the more you can do to support them if they are positive, or to counter them if they are negative. This is the first step toward taking charge of your health.

In this course, you will learn more about risks and behaviors that are harmful to your health. You will gain the knowledge and skills you need to avoid these risks and commit to a healthy lifestyle. Learning health skills and useful facts will help you take responsibility for your own health and maintain wellness. You will also learn about ways to promote the health of others.

Lesson 2 Review

Facts and Vocabulary

1. What does *heredity* mean?

2. Define *environment*. Identify three types of environment.

3. Evaluate two ways that media and technology may influence your health.

Thinking Critically

4. **Evaluate.** How does the environment in which you live affect your health?

5. **Synthesize.** Oliver's family has a history of heart disease. What steps might he take to protect his health?

Applying Health Skills

6. **Communication Skills.** With a classmate, script or role-play a scenario in which a teen tries to persuade a friend to adopt a positive health behavior.

Writing Critically

7. **Narrative.** Write a short story about Jesse, who just moved from a small town to a large city. Choose one of the possible influences on his health and describe how his well-being might be affected by this influence.

Health Risks and Your Behavior

BIG IDEA Risk behaviors can harm your health, but there are steps you can take to avoid or reduce these risks.

REAL LIFE ISSUES

Worrying About a Friend. Jenna and her best friend, Madison, are discussing their plans for the weekend. Jenna is excited because Jackson, a classmate, has invited her to a party on Saturday night. The party is at the home of another classmate whose parents will be away. Madison suspects there will be alcohol at the party and no adult supervision. Jackson has a reputation for being wild, and Madison is worried for Jenna. *Write a dialogue in which Madison discusses with Jenna the potential dangers of going to the party.*

After completing the lesson, review and analyze your response to the Real Life Issues question.

Identifying Health Risks

MAIN IDEA Engaging in risk behaviors can harm your health.

Every day you are faced with some amount of risk. Even simple events, such as crossing a street or using an electrical appliance, carry a little bit of risk. Some risks are not under your control; they are just a part of life. However, you can control **risk behaviors**. These are actions that can potentially threaten your health or the health of others. Examples of risk behaviors include riding in a car without wearing a seat belt, exercising outdoors without sunscreen, or using tobacco. Understanding the dangers of certain behaviors can help steer you away from risk behaviors. It can lead toward safer, more healthful behaviors. It helps you actively protect your health by making safe, responsible decisions.

Recognizing Risk Behaviors

The CDC has identified six risk behaviors. These account for most of the deaths and disability among young people under age 24. Some of the behaviors pose an immediate risk of illness, injury, or **infection**, which is a condition that occurs when pathogens in the body multiply and damage body cells. Others are dangerous because they can lead to heart disease, cancer, and other serious problems later in life.

BEFORE YOU READ

Create a Cluster Chart. Draw a circle and label it "Health Risks." Use surrounding circles to define and describe this term. As you read, continue filling in the chart with ways to reduce these risks.

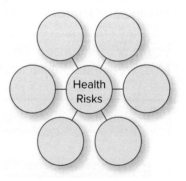

Vocabulary

risk behaviors
infection
cumulative risks
prevention
abstinence
lifestyle factors

The six top risk behaviors are:

- Tobacco use.

- Unhealthy eating.

- Inadequate physical activity.

- Alcohol and other drug use.

- High-risk sexual behaviors (which can result in sexually transmitted diseases and unintended pregnancies)

- Safety risks (which can lead to unintentional injuries and violence)

REAL WORLD CONNECTION

Teen Risk Taking

To track patterns of risk taking among teens, the CDC developed the Youth Risk Behavior Survey (YRBS). It is administered every two years to a sample of high school students across the country. The information gathered in this survey is used in a variety of ways to influence change and improve the health and well-being of teens. Some of the major risk behaviors, with key findings in each category, appear in the graph below. When you analyze the data, you may be surprised. Despite the headlines, most teens are not drinking or using drugs. Most wear automobile safety belts, and two-thirds are physically active.

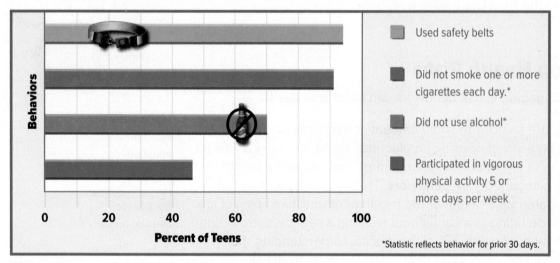

Source: Centers for Disease Control and Prevention, Youth Risk Behavior Surveillance Survey (YRBSS), 2018.

Activity - Mathematics

Use the graph to answer these questions.

1. Approximately what percent of teens did not participate in vigorous physical activity three or more days per week?

2. Which risk behaviors did 90 percent of teens avoid?

3. Write a paragraph explaining how you think these statistics can be used to promote teens' health and well-being.

CONCEPT Measurement and Data: Data Analysis A bar graph represents data using shaded bars to show each value. The legend explains what each shade represents.

Risks and Consequences

Risk behaviors can have a serious impact on your health. In other words, these behaviors carry major negative consequences. They can damage your health and well-being both in the short term and over the long term. For example, smoking can have an immediate impact on health, causing problems such as bad breath, yellow teeth, and headaches. If a person continues to smoke, the long-term consequences of this behavior can be far more serious. The person might develop lung cancer, heart disease, or emphysema as a result of a smoking habit.

Risks can also add up over time. For example, eating an occasional high-fat meal at a fast-food restaurant probably won't have a permanent effect on your overall health. If you regularly eat high-fat meals, though, the negative effects accumulate over time and may lead to serious health problems. That's why it's important to evaluate the consequences of any behavior, not only by itself, but also in terms of its **cumulative risk**. Cumulative risks are related risks that increase in effect with each added risk.

Cumulative risks also increase when several risk factors are combined. For example, speeding in a car increases the risk of getting into an accident. Using a cell phone while driving increases the risk as well. If a person speeds *and* uses a cell phone at the same time, the chance of getting into a car accident becomes even greater. The more risk behaviors you engage in, the more likely you are to face harmful consequences as a result.

How to Avoid or Reduce Risks

MAIN IDEA You can take action to reduce your exposure to health risks.

You can protect your health and lower health risks by practicing positive health behaviors. Many of behaviors you already perform are safety behaviors. Positive health behaviors include fastening your safety belt when you get into a car, checking the depth of water before diving, or putting on a helmet when riding a bike. Another way to reduce health risks is through **prevention**. This means taking steps to keep something from happening or getting worse. One example of prevention is getting regular medical and dental checkups. Checkups can detect health problems early and prevent them from getting worse.

Reading Check

Evaluate Why is it important to understand risk behaviors?

Avoiding high-risk behaviors and choosing friends who do so is one of the best ways to achieve and maintain wellness. **How might friends help you avoid risk behaviors?**

Dmitry Shironosov/iStock/360/Getty Images

Abstaining from High-Risk Behaviors

One of the most effective strategies for promoting your health is to practice **abstinence**. The term abstinence means a deliberate decision to avoid high-risk behaviors, including sexual activity and the use of tobacco, alcohol, and misuse of drugs.

Choosing to abstain from high-risk behaviors improves all areas of your health triangle. For instance, when you avoid tobacco, alcohol, and other drugs, you protect yourself from the chronic diseases associated with using these substances. You can also feel good about yourself because you are taking responsibility for your health. Showing that you value your well-being can also boost your self-esteem in another way: it gets you in the habit of thinking that you, and your health, are worth protecting. This, in turn, strengthens your mental/emotional health and your social relationships.

ACADEMIC VOCABULARY

affect *(verb)*: to produce an effect upon

Participating in positive health behaviors benefits all three sides of your health triangle. **What are some positive health behaviors you and your friends enjoy?**

Promoting Your Health

MAIN IDEA Regularly participating in health-promoting behaviors will help you reach a high level of wellness.

Every day you make decisions, large and small, that **affect** your health. For example, if you choose to play a sport after school, you are likely to have fun and feel good as a result. If you choose to play video games instead, you may end up feeling sluggish and lazy because you were inactive all day. Understanding the impact your decisions have on your health can inspire you to choose healthful behaviors that promote wellness and prevent disease.

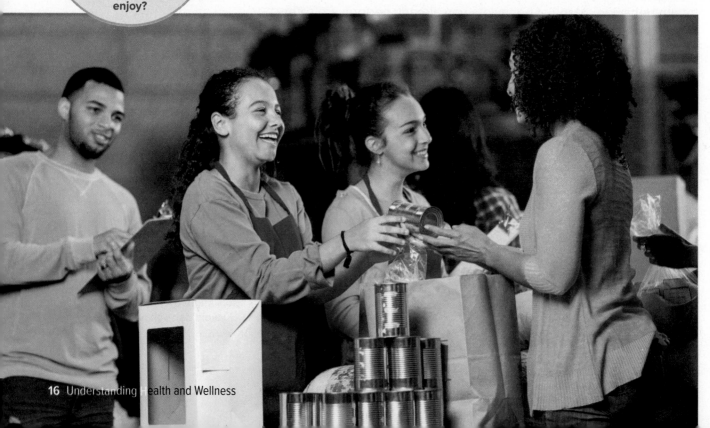

Steve Debenport/E+/Getty Images

Lifestyle Factors

Scientists have found that many **lifestyle factors** can make a difference in people's overall health, happiness, and longevity. Lifestyle factors are the personal habits or behaviors related to the way a person lives. In other words, people who practice positive health habits regularly tend to be healthier and live longer. Lifestyle factors that can improve your health include:

- getting eight hours of sleep each night.
- starting each day with a healthy breakfast.
- eating a variety of nutritious foods each day.
- being physically active for 30 to 60 minutes most days of the week.
- maintaining a healthy weight.
- abstaining from smoking or using other tobacco products.
- abstaining from the use of alcohol and other drugs.

Think about your daily habits. Are the lifestyle factors listed above a regular part of your life? Can you think of ways to incorporate more of these behaviors into your daily routine? Remember, while you cannot avoid all risks in life, you can control your lifestyle. By making the best possible decisions for yourself, you can achieve a high level of wellness now and into adulthood.

Myths & Reality

You may think you're a health expert, but do you know the truth about this health myth?

Myth: Bicycle helmets are just for young children.

Reality: Not wearing a bicycle helmet is a major cause of unintentional injury in children and teens. Bicycle helmets should be worn by riders of all ages. Bicycle helmet use results in a 74 percent to 85 percent reduction in serious brain injuries.

Reading Check

Identify List three lifestyle factors that can promote good health.

Lesson 3 Review

Facts and Vocabulary

1. Define the term *risk behavior*.

2. Why is cumulative risk a serious concern?

3. How might changes in lifestyle factors influence your health in positive ways?

Thinking Critically

4. **Explain.** How might monitoring risk behaviors affect the well-being of teens?

5. **Synthesize.** Consider a risk behavior teens are exposed to, and predict how lifestyle factors can positively influence teens to avoid that risk.

Applying Health Skills

6. **Accessing Information.** Research organizations that offer after-school programs to help teens avoid risk behaviors. Write a short description of one such organization in your community.

Writing Critically

7. **Expository.** Using the data shown in the Real World Connection activity for this lesson, write an article about the results of recent research on how many teens avoid risk behaviors.

Promoting Health and Wellness

Create Vocabulary Cards. Write each new vocabulary term on a separate note card. For each term, write a definition based on your current knowledge. As you read, fill in additional information related to each term.

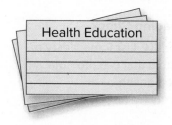

Health Education

Vocabulary

health education
Healthy People
health disparities
health literacy
self-directed

BIG IDEA Staying healthy requires knowledge, a plan, and practicing healthful behaviors.

> **REAL LIFE ISSUES**
>
> **Learning from Experience.** Taylor is taking an elective class called Intergenerations. Students in this class are paired with older adults. Taylor's "classmate" is an active 89-year-old man named Harry. Harry remembers riding in a horse-drawn cart from his family farm to church on Sunday mornings. He also remembers growing up without a television and eating what his family grew on the farm. Taylor's assignment is to interview Harry about his secrets to a long, healthy, and happy life. *Write a short questionnaire listing what Taylor might ask Harry. Cover all the factors you think might contribute to a long, healthy life.*
>
> After completing the lesson, review and analyze your response to the Real Life Issues question.

The Importance of Health Education

MAIN IDEA Individual, family, community, and national health require planning and responsible behavior on everyone's part.

Achieving a high level of wellness can help you remain healthy throughout your lifetime. However, achieving good health is not just a goal for individuals. Promoting health is also an important goal for the nation as a whole. Making the public healthier is one way to provide a higher quality of life for all Americans.

Maintaining good health is also a good investment. In 2018, the cost of U.S. healthcare reached $3.6 trillion a year, or $11,172 per person. Much of that expense could be avoided if people made healthier decisions. Some of the ways to make healthier decisions include adopting health-promoting habits, and taking responsibility for maintaining wellness. Health-promoting habits can include choices such as scheduling 30 to 60 minutes of exercise each day or selecting healthful foods. Maintaining wellness might mean that you continue taking medications if prescribed by a doctor, brushing your teeth after meals, and scheduling regular medical and dental visits. **Health education** is the key to creating a healthier nation. Health education includes providing accurate health information and teaching health skills to help people make healthy decisions. Understanding health information and improving health skills can empower people to live better, more healthful lives.

The Nation's Health Goals

Good health is so important that the federal government has established a set of national health goals and objectives. This plan, called **Healthy People**, is revised every ten years. Planning is still underway for *Healthy People 2030*. The current plan, *Healthy People 2020,* has objectives for the year 2020. One of the goals of *Healthy People 2020* is to reduce the overweight and obesity rates in America.

Healthy People provides a common plan for everyone to follow. National, state, and local health agencies across the country carry out programs based on the plan's goals to promote health and prevent disease. The government tracks health behaviors and outcomes to measure the success of these programs in achieving national health goals.

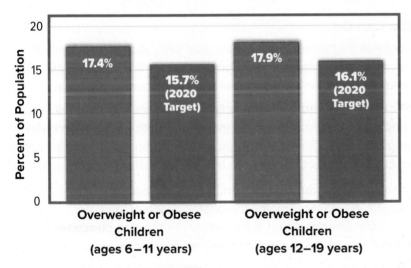

Source: CDC | NCHS, National Health and Nutrition Examination Survey (NHANES) 2007–2008.

Overweight and obesity rates from 2005 through 2008 were 17.4 percent for all children aged 6–11 and 17.9 percent for adolescents ages 12–19. Healthy People set goals to reduce these percentages by more than 10 percent by 2020. **Why do you think health is important enough to set national health goals?**

Goals of *Healthy People*. Healthy People 2020 has established two general goals for the future. The first is to increase the quality and length of a healthy life for all Americans. The second is to remove differences in health outcomes that result from factors such as gender, race, education, disability, and location. These differences in health outcomes among groups are called **health disparities**. Working toward these two goals will help more people enjoy the benefits of a healthy life. *Healthy People 2020* is the blueprint that will shape the nation's health priorities over the next several years. The health goals that guided the development of *Healthy People 2020* include the following:

- Help Americans live long, high-quality lives.

- Put an end to preventable illness, injury, disability, and premature death.

- Close the gaps in health across different groups.

- Promote healthy behaviors for people of all ages and stages of life.

- Create healthy physical and social environments.

Reading Check

List What are some of the goals for *Healthy People 2020?*

Becoming Health Literate

MAIN IDEA A health-literate person knows how to find and use reliable health information.

Every day, people all across the country have to make important decisions that affect their health. To make sound health decisions, you need to develop **health literacy**. This means knowing how to:

- find health information.

- determine whether the information is trustworthy.

- assess the risks and benefits of treatment.

- figure out how much medicine to take.

- understand test results.

What You Can Do

Experts believe that health literacy is a vital skill. A person's level of health literacy has a greater impact on overall health than age, income, or education. The list below describes a health-literate individual.

- **A critical thinker and problem solver.** If you are a critical thinker, you know what criteria to use to evaluate health information before making decisions. Being a problem solver means that you can apply these criteria in practical ways to make responsible, healthy choices.

- **A responsible, productive citizen.** If you are a responsible citizen, you act in a way that promotes the overall health of the community. You choose safe, healthful, and legal behaviors that are **consistent** with your family's guidelines and that show respect for yourself and others.

ACADEMIC VOCABULARY

consistent *(adjective):* free from variation or contradiction

People who are informed know how to interpret the information they need to make good health decisions.
Where do you find information to make your daily health decisions?

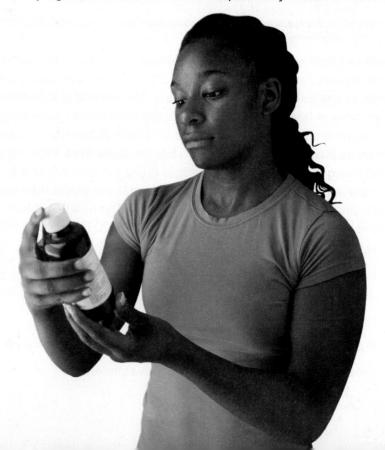

- **A self-directed learner.** As a self-directed learner, you search for health information to make health-related decisions. You know how to evaluate health information to determine if it is reliable, accurate, and up to date. Valid health information is available in print media, on television and radio, on the Internet, and from health care professionals.

- **An effective communicator.** Being an effective communicator means that you can express health knowledge in a variety of ways. These might include talking to friends, writing letters to the school paper, and providing a good example for others through your behavior.

People who are informed know how to find and interpret information to make good health decisions.

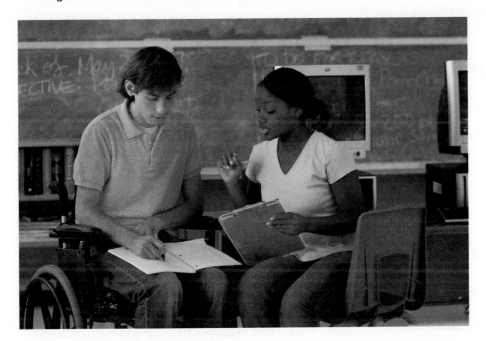

Lesson 4 Review

Facts and Vocabulary

1. Why is health education important?

2. What are *health disparities?*

3. List three criteria that are needed for an individual to make sound health decisions.

Thinking Critically

4. **Analyze.** How does *Healthy People* hope to help the United States become a healthier country?

5. **Synthesize.** What are some steps you can take to become a health-literate individual?

Applying Health Skills

6. **Accessing Information.** Work with classmates to compile a list of resources in your community that supports healthy lifestyle behaviors. Examples might include parks, libraries, and health organizations.

Writing Critically

7. **Expository.** Write an essay explaining what individuals, families, and communities can do to promote wellness.

LESSON 1

Vocabulary Review

Use the correct vocabulary term to complete the following statements.

1. _____ is the combination of physical, mental/emotional, and social well-being.

2. _____ provides people with a deep-seated sense of meaning and purpose in life.

3. A person with a balanced health triangle is said to have a high degree of _____.

Understanding Key Concepts

After reading the question or statement, select the correct answer.

4. Which of the following is not an aspect of physical health?
   a. Eating well and drinking water
   b. Making and keeping friends
   c. Being physically active
   d. Getting enough sleep

5. Which statement is true about a person who is in good social health?
   a. She spends a lot of time alone.
   b. She has few friends at school.
   c. She may not be in good physical health.
   d. She gets along with others.

6. You are likely to move in a negative direction on the health continuum if
   a. you engage in physical activity daily.
   b. you accept responsibility for your health.
   c. you fail to practice healthful behaviors.
   d. you regularly eat a healthful diet.

Thinking Critically

After reading the question or statement, write a short answer using complete sentences.

7. **Describe.** What are some characteristics of a person with good mental/emotional health?

8. **Explain.** How can your health triangle become unbalanced, and how can this imbalance affect your health?

9. **Identify.** List specific actions that teens can take to improve their wellness.

10. **Explain.** How do your health behaviors affect your position on the health continuum?

LESSON 2

Vocabulary Review

Correct the sentences below by replacing the italicized term with the correct vocabulary term.

11. Your *environment* consists of traits that are biologically passed on to you by your parents.

12. A person's ethnicity, religion, and language are part of her *peers.*

13. *Technology* personalities may become our role models for how to behave.

Understanding Key Concepts

After reading the question or statement, select the correct answer.

14. What technique can you use to locate valid health information on the Internet?
    a. Find sites that are the most popular.
    b. Use only sites belonging to manufacturers of health care products.
    c. Locate sites that use .gov or .edu in their addresses.
    d. All of the above

15. Cultural influences on your health include
    a. biologically inherited traits.
    b. beliefs, customs, and behaviors.
    c. the health continuum and triangle.
    d. all of the above.

16. The media is a powerful influence because it
    a. encourages teens to live healthy lives.
    b. is constantly present.
    c. provides healthy role models.
    d. warns the audience of risk behaviors.

Thinking Critically

After reading the question or statement, write a short answer using complete sentences.

17. **Describe.** What are some ways that peers can influence your health both positively and negatively?

18. **Analyze.** Think about your own culture, including your ethnic background, spirituality, language, and community. What are some practices within your culture that influence your health?

19. **Describe.** What are some ways that your attitudes influence your health?

LESSON 3

Vocabulary Review

Choose the correct term in the sentences below.

20. *Risk behaviors/Prevention* means taking steps to keep something from happening or getting worse.

21. *Resiliency/Abstinence* is a deliberate decision to avoid high-risk behaviors.

22. *Cumulative/Serious* risks are risks that add up over time.

Understanding Key Concepts

After reading the question or statement, select the correct answer.

23. Which of the following statements is true?
    a. Risk behaviors are illegal for everyone.
    b. Risk behaviors can harm your health.
    c. Most teens engage in risk behaviors.
    d. There is no way to avoid risk behaviors.

24. A person who practices multiple risk behaviors at the same time is likely to
    a. be unaware of what he is doing.
    b. be a role model for his friends.
    c. face more negative consequences.
    d. show sound judgment.

25. Personal habits and behaviors that relate to the way a person lives are called
    a. negative consequences.
    b. risk participation.
    c. health promotion.
    d. lifestyle factors.

Thinking Critically

After reading the question or statement, write a short answer using complete sentences.

26. **Identify.** What are two risk behaviors that pose a threat to the health of teens today?

27. **Discuss.** How are teens' perceptions of risk behaviors influenced by what they believe others are doing?

28. **Synthesize.** What is abstinence, and what are the effects of practicing abstinence?

LESSON 4

Vocabulary Review

Use the correct vocabulary term to complete the following statements.

29. _____ empowers people to live healthfully and improve their quality of life.

30. Health goals for the United States may be found in _____.

31. A person who lacks _____ finds it difficult to obtain, understand, and use valid health information.

Understanding Key Concepts

After reading the question or statement, select the correct answer.

32. Health education provides
    a. medical health coverage.
    b. accurate health information.
    c. a wellness guarantee.
    d. none of the above.

33. Experts think that poor health literacy influences a person's health more than
    a. critical thinking and problem solving.
    b. attitude, environment, and income.
    c. education, income, and attitude.
    d. age, income, and education.

Thinking Critically

After reading the question or statement, write a short answer using complete sentences.

34. **Explain.** Why is it a good investment for the United States to keep its citizens healthy?

35. **Evaluate.** What role does the individual play in helping the nation achieve the goals of Healthy People?

36. **Describe.** How can health education help the nation achieve the Healthy People goals?

37. **Analyze.** How does being a self-directed learner affect a person's health literacy?

PROJECT-BASED ASSESSMENT

A Health Initiative

BACKGROUND

Healthy People is an initiative set forth by the Department of Health and Human Services. The initiative establishes guidelines and goals that various people, states, communities, and professional organizations can use to improve the health of all Americans.

TASK

Conduct an online search for the goals and guidelines of the initiative, and prepare a multimedia presentation that applies the guidelines to your school.

AUDIENCE

Students at your school

PURPOSE

Create a set of specific recommendations that can help the students in your school be healthier.

PROCEDURE

1. Review the information in Module 1 regarding general health and wellness.

2. With your group, develop a policy for improving school health. Create an outline of the multimedia presentation.

3. Divide the main task into smaller tasks, including the Internet search, creating the slides, and delivering the presentation. Assign tasks to each group member.

4. After the research is complete, meet as a group to discuss the possible applications of Healthy People in your school.

5. Show your multimedia presentation to the class.

Math Practice

Analyze Geometric Properties Read the passage and use the equilateral triangle ABC to answer the questions.

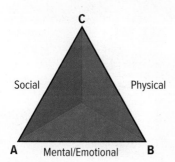

Natalie is doing a report on the health triangle. She sketched a model, but now she needs to make a larger version on poster board so that everyone in the classroom can see it. In her sketch, side AC is 9.5 cm long. Natalie decides to make the triangle on the poster board 3.25 times larger than her scale model.

1. When Natalie finishes drawing the large triangle on the poster board, what will be the approximate measure of side BC? Round to the nearest centimeter.

2. Side AB of the health triangle measures $5x$. Side BC measures $x + 20$. Which of the following statements explains why the equation $5x = x + 20$ can be used to solve for x?
   a. The angle measures of an equilateral triangle are never equal.
   b. Equilateral triangles have unequal sides.
   c. All sides of an equilateral triangle are always equal.
   d. Only two sides of an equilateral triangle are equal.

3. How might Natalie visually represent the health triangle of someone who neglects one or more aspects of health?

Reading/Writing Practice

Understand and Apply Read the passage below, and then answer the questions.

1. Veronica was late for her soccer game. **2.** On her way to the field, she realized she had forgotten to pack her water bottle. **3.** She did not think to get a drink from a nearby water fountain. **4.** Near the end of the first half, Veronica's leg cramped up. **5.** After resting and drinking a bottle of water, she began to feel better. **6.** But her coach told her that she had become dehydrated and refused to let her back into the game. **7.** Veronica hadn't even felt thirsty before she got the cramp. **8.** Veronica didn't recognize you cannot count on thirst for knowing when you need water. **9.** People can become dehydrated without feeling thirsty. **10.** Before playing any sport, make sure you drink plenty of non-carbonated fluids.

1. Which sentence includes details that support the author's point of view?
   a. Sentence 2
   b. Sentence 7
   c. Sentence 9
   d. Sentence 10

2. How does the writer show that the purpose of this essay is to persuade?
   a. The writer emphasizes the use of proper fitting protective gear.
   b. The writer contrasts the different types of soccer gear people use.
   c. The writer explains that soccer's increasing popularity has led to more injuries.
   d. The writer describes what happened to someone who did not drink enough water.

3. Write a paragraph explaining the importance of drinking plenty of water before, during, and after sports activities.

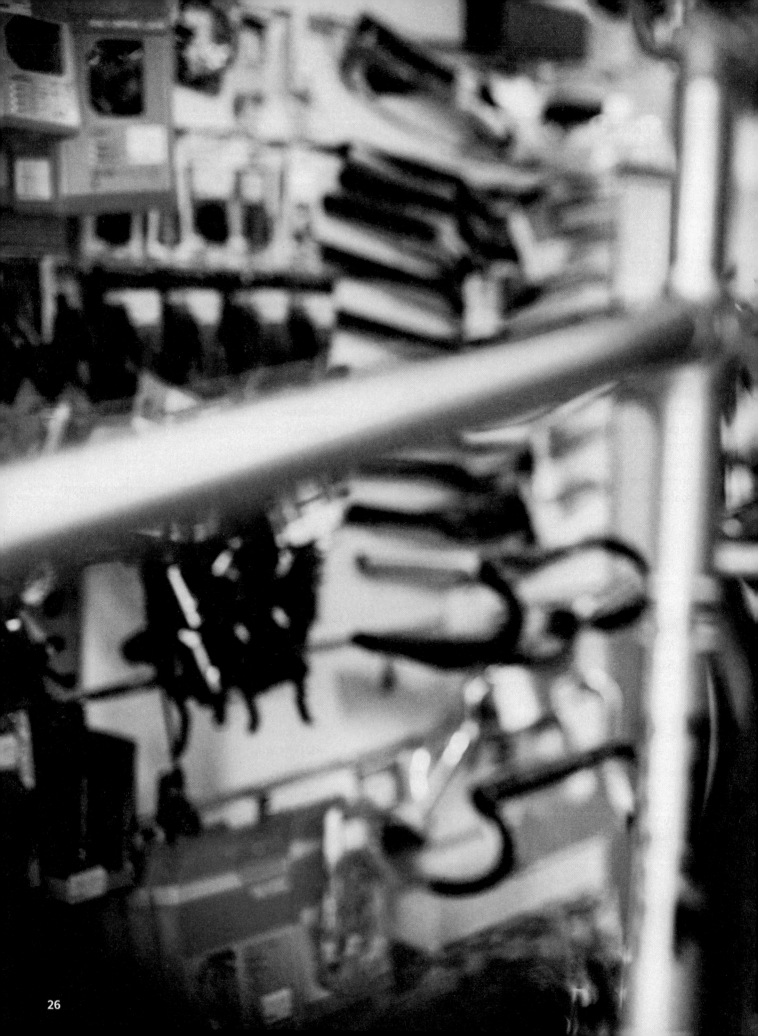

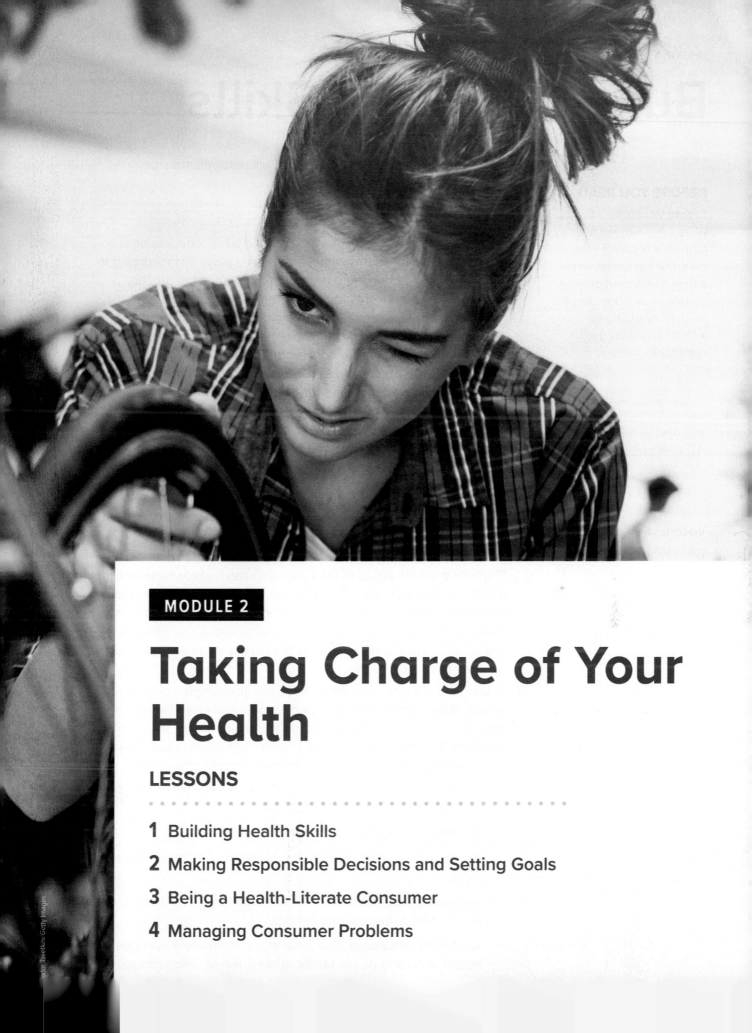

MODULE 2

Taking Charge of Your Health

LESSONS

Building Health Skills

BEFORE YOU READ

Create Vocabulary Cards.
Write each new vocabulary term on a separate note card. For each term, write a definition based on your current knowledge. As you read, fill in additional information related to each term.

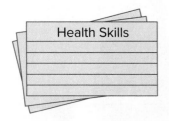

Health Skills

Vocabulary

health skills
interpersonal communication
refusal skills
conflict resolution
stress
stress management skills
advocacy

BIG IDEA You can develop skills that will help you manage your health throughout your life.

REAL LIFE ISSUES

Fitting in Fitness. Alejandro is carrying a full schedule of advanced courses this semester. He also plays an instrument in the school jazz band and has a part-time job at the grocery store. Alejandro wants to begin a regular physical activity program, but finding the time to schedule physical activity in his already busy schedule is difficult. He asks his good friend Phil for suggestions. ***Write a conversation in which Alejandro explains his situation to Phil. Phil should be supportive and offer possible strategies that can help Alejandro add physical activity into his schedule.***

After completing the lesson, review and analyze your response to the Real Life Issues question.

Learning Health Skills

MAIN IDEA Health skills help you manage your health.

Think for a minute about all the things you can do to achieve and maintain a high level of wellness. One important step is to choose healthful behaviors, such as eating right or being physically active. You also need to make good decisions about which behaviors are healthful and which are harmful. In addition, you know how to say no to risk behaviors such as tobacco or alcohol use.

Making the choices described above are all examples of the use of **health skills**. Health skills are specific tools and strategies to maintain, protect, and improve all aspects of your health. There are ten basic health skills you will learn about. Health skills are also known as life skills, because you can use them in every aspect of your life.

- **Communication.** You share your ideas and feelings and listen carefully when others express theirs.

- **Refusal.** You say no to unhealthy behaviors.

- **Conflict Resolution.** You resolve problems with others in healthy ways.

- **Accessing Information.** You locate valid sources of health information, products, and services.

- **Analyzing Influences.** You understand the many influences on your health, including peers, family, culture, media, and technology.

- **Practicing Healthful Behaviors.** You act to reduce risks and protect yourself against illness and injury.
- **Stress Management.** You use healthy strategies to reduce and manage stress in your life.
- **Advocacy.** You work to improve your own health and the health of your family and community.
- **Decision Making.** You use a step-by-step process to evaluate your options and make healthy choices.
- **Goal Setting.** You set goals and develop a plan to achieve them.

Communication Skills

MAIN IDEA Good communication is a vital health skill.

Communication is more than talking to one of your friends about something that interests you both. It involves carefully choosing your words and expressions so that you communicate what you really mean. It also involves listening closely to others. Three health skills show you how to give and receive information. They are: interpersonal communication, refusal skills, and conflict resolution. Good **interpersonal communication**, which is the exchange of thoughts, feelings, and beliefs between two or more people, helps you build strong relationships with others.

Here are a few examples of ways you can strengthen your interpersonal communication skills.

- **Use "I" messages to express your feelings.** If you say, "You never tell me anything," that puts the focus—and the blame—on the other person. Saying, "I feel upset when I'm left out of your plans" focuses on your emotions instead.
- **Communicate with respect and caring.** Keep your voice calm and use a respectful tone when talking to another person.
- **Be an active listener.** Pay attention to what the other person is saying. Let him say what he has to say without interrupting. Try to understand the other person's point of view.

Refusal Skills

Think about a situation in which you need to say no in order to protect your health. One example might be turning down a ride in a car with a driver who has been drinking. Likewise, if you are encouraged to try a cigarette, you would you a refusal skill when saying no. In situations like these, **refusal skills** can help you say no firmly, respectfully, and effectively. Refusal skills are communication strategies that can help you say no when you are urged to take part in behaviors that are unsafe or unhealthful.

Reading Check

Identify Name three communication skills that help protect your health.

The refusal strategies described below can help you when someone tries to persuade you to do something you don't want to do. You can use one or several of these strategies to say no to potentially harmful activities.

- **Say no in a firm voice.** Be calm and polite, but very clear about your refusal. For instance, if someone dares you to ride your bike down a steep, unsafe trail, you could just say, "No thanks, I'd rather not."

- **Explain why.** Tell the other person why the suggested activity or behavior is not acceptable to you. In this case, you could say, "That doesn't look safe to me."

- **Offer alternatives.** Suggest a safe, healthful activity to do instead of the one offered. For instance, you could say, "Why don't we ride over to the lake instead?"

- **Stand your ground.** Make it clear that you don't intend to back down from your position. In this case, if the other person repeats the dare, you can just keep saying, "I really don't want to."

- **Leave if necessary.** If the other person continues to pressure you or won't take no for an answer, simply walk away.

Conflict-Resolution Skills

Think of a recent argument you had. How was it resolved? Was everyone involved satisfied with the outcome? If so, you probably used the skill of **conflict resolution**, or the process of ending a conflict through cooperation and problem solving. This health skill can help people resolve problems in ways that are agreeable to everyone involved.

Conflict-resolution skills include stepping away from an argument, allowing the conflict to subside, using good interpersonal communication, and showing respect for yourself as well as for the other person. This health skill also includes knowing when to compromise in order to resolve the conflict. In a compromise, both parties give up something in order to gain a result that satisfies them both.

Accessing Information

MAIN IDEA Use reliable sources of health information.

Sometimes, to make a decision about your health, you need to obtain information. Knowing how to find and evaluate health information will help you make decisions that support your well-being. To decide whether health information is valid, you need to determine how reliable the source is. Some useful sources of information include:

- health care providers and professionals.
- valid Internet sites, such as those of government agencies that end in .gov and professional health organizations that end in .org.
- trusted adults who are knowledgeable about a particular subject.
- recently published material written by respected, well-known science and health professionals.

Analyzing Influences

MAIN IDEA Understanding what influences you helps you to make more healthful choices.

Do you ever stop and think about just why you do the things you do? Many factors may influence your decisions and actions. The more aware you are of the various influences in your life and how they affect you as an individual, the better you can make informed choices about your health.

INFLUENCES ON YOUR HEALTH	
Personal Values • Things I think are important • Likes and dislikes • Skills and talents	**Your Family and Culture** • Beliefs, behaviors, and habits • Family traditions • Food served at home
Personal Beliefs • Plans for the future • Goals • Hopes and dreams	**Media and Technology** • TV and movies • Magazines • Internet
Perceptions • Behaviors that I think are common or accepted	**Friends and Peers** • Behaviors and opinions of my friends and classmates
Curiosity/Fears • Things I wonder about • Things that scare or frighten me • Things I want to try • Things I never want to try	**School and Community** • Place where I live • School I attend • Air quality • Sources of recreation

Many factors influence your health. **Which sources have the most influence on you?**

Self-Management Skills

MAIN IDEA Practicing healthy habits will help you protect your health.

Self-management means taking charge of your own health. When you manage your behaviors, you act in ways that protect your health and **promote** your own well-being. There are two self-management skills:

- **Practicing healthful behaviors.** You practice healthful behaviors when you make good health habits part of your everyday life.

- **Managing stress.** Do you get nervous before taking a test? Do you get stage fright before performing in front of a large group of people? These are two examples of **stress**. Stress is the reaction of the body and mind to everyday challenges and demands. Stress is a normal part of life, but too much unrelieved stress can lead to illness. That's why it's important to learn **stress management skills**. These are skills that help you reduce and manage stress in your life. Exercise, relaxation, and good time management are some examples of ways to keep your stress levels under control.

ACADEMIC VOCABULARY

promote *(verb)*: to contribute to the growth of

HEALTH BEHAVIORS CHECKLIST

I eat well-balanced meals, including breakfast, and I choose healthful snacks.	I express my emotions in healthy ways.
I get regular daily physical activity and at least eight hours of sleep every night.	I take responsibility for my actions.
I avoid using tobacco, alcohol, and other drugs.	I think of my mistakes as chances to learn.
I floss and brush my teeth regularly.	I relate well to family, friends, and peers.
I wear a safety belt every time I ride in a car.	I have one or more close friends.
I stay within 5 pounds of my healthy weight.	I treat others with respect.
I practice good personal hygiene habits.	I use refusal skills to avoid risk behaviors.
I get regular physical checkups.	I get along with many kinds of people.
I keep a positive attitude.	I can put myself in other people's place and understand their problems.
I wear proper safety equipment.	I volunteer to help others whenever I can.

Myths & Reality

Teens have access to a lot of health information, but really have no control over their health.

Myth: Health is not something individuals have control over.

Reality: Individuals can practice behaviors that promote well-being and enhance health. The choices and decisions people make can have positive or negative impacts on their health.

Advocacy

MAIN IDEA Advocacy lets you share your health knowledge.

When you take part in a community event with other teens, you are engaging in **advocacy**. Advocacy is taking action to influence others to address a health-related concern or to support a health-related belief. Taking part in advocacy activities such as supporting a charitable cause is one way you can encourage others to practice healthful behaviors. Other ways to advocate for better health include:

- Obeying laws that protect community health, such as laws against littering.

- Sharing health information with family and friends. Telling a friend about the risks of riding in a car without a seat belt is one example.

- Sending out health messages—for instance, by wearing an anti-smoking button.

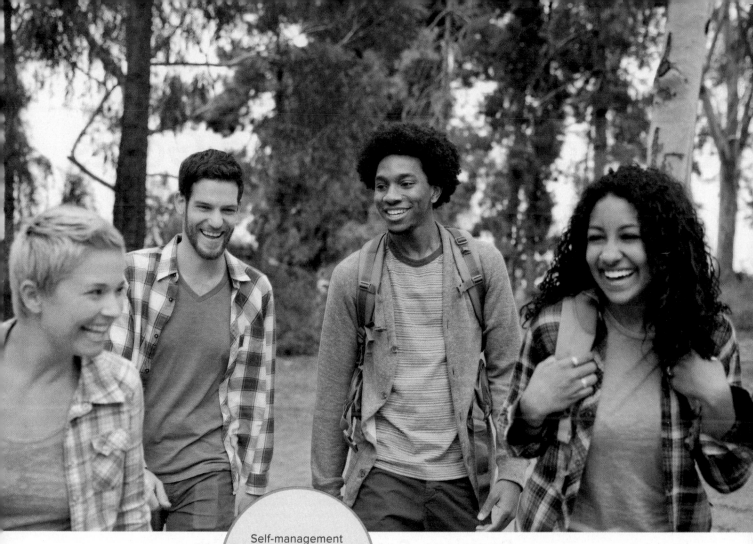

Self-management skills help you stay healthy. **What skill are these teens practicing?**

Lesson 1 Review

Facts and Vocabulary

1. Define the term *health skills*.

2. What are two interpersonal communication skills that can reduce your health risk?

3. What is *advocacy*?

Thinking Critically

4. **Synthesize.** Why is it important to recognize and analyze the various influences on your behavior?

5. **Analyze.** How can advocacy help you with health issues that are important to you?

Applying Health Skills

6. **Stress Management.** List all the healthful strategies you used in the past week to relieve stress. Which ones were most helpful?

Writing Critically

7. **Narrative.** Marcos and Sarah disagree about which movie to see. Write a dialogue in which they resolve their disagreement using effective interpersonal communication strategies.

Making Responsible Decisions and Setting Goals

BEFORE YOU READ

Create a K-W-L Chart. Make a three-column chart. In the first column, list what you know about decision making and goal setting. In the second column, list what you want to know about this topic. As you read, use the third column to summarize what you learned.

K	W	L

Vocabulary

values
decision-making skills
goals
short-term goal
long-term goal
action plan

. . . .

BIG IDEA You can actively promote your well-being by making healthful choices and setting positive goals.

REAL LIFE ISSUES

Making Decisions. Tara has been playing soccer since elementary school. Tryouts for the varsity soccer team are coming up, and she's having trouble deciding whether to try out. Tara loves soccer, but she's not sure she's good enough to make the team. Also, if she does make the team, she might not have enough time to study and do well in school. *Write a conversation in which Tara explains her situation to her school counselor. The counselor should help Tara figure out what the potential outcomes of her choices might be.*

After completing the lesson, review and analyze your response to the Real Life Issues question.

Decisions, Goals, and Your Health

MAIN IDEA Achieving good health begins with making responsible decisions.

Now that you're in high school, do you have more freedom than you did when you were younger? Maybe you're allowed to stay out later on weekends and have more control over your schedule and activities. You may have a wider circle of friends than you did in middle school. Having more freedom is an exciting benefit of growing up.

As you're probably finding out, the freedom that you gain as you grow older comes with more responsibility. For example, having the freedom to choose certain classes in school means you also have to make decisions about what you want to study. These decisions may be related to your long-term goals for your future, such as what job you want to pursue. Making decisions and setting goals are two ways you can take responsibility for the direction you want to go in life.

Decision Making

MAIN IDEA Decision-making skills help you make successful, responsible choices.

Life is filled with decisions. You make plenty of them every day. Some decisions are small, like what to wear to school or what to eat for breakfast.

Other choices may be life changing, such as which college to attend or which job to take. Developing good decision-making skills will help you make responsible choices that contribute to your health and quality of life.

Your Values

The decisions you make reflect your personal **values** and the values of your family. Values are the ideas, beliefs, and attitudes about what is important that help guide the way you live. For example, if you value a strong, healthy body, you are more likely to make decisions that promote good health, such as following a regular exercise plan. If you value your relationships with family and friends, you will make choices that show your caring and respect for them, like making sure to stay in touch if you go away to camp during the summer.

Because you first learned your values from your family, it's often a good idea to talk with family members about a decision that is troubling you. You share important values with them, so they can provide you with helpful feedback.

The Decision-Making Process

Have you ever thought about what actually goes into making a good decision? **Decision-making skills** are steps that enable you to make a healthful decision. These include the following six steps:

- **STEP 1: State the Situation.** Clearly identify the situation. Ask yourself: What decision do I need to make? Who is involved? Am I feeling pressure to make a decision? How much time do I have to decide?

Family members often know you better than anyone else knows you. **Why is it a good idea to talk over important decisions with family members?**

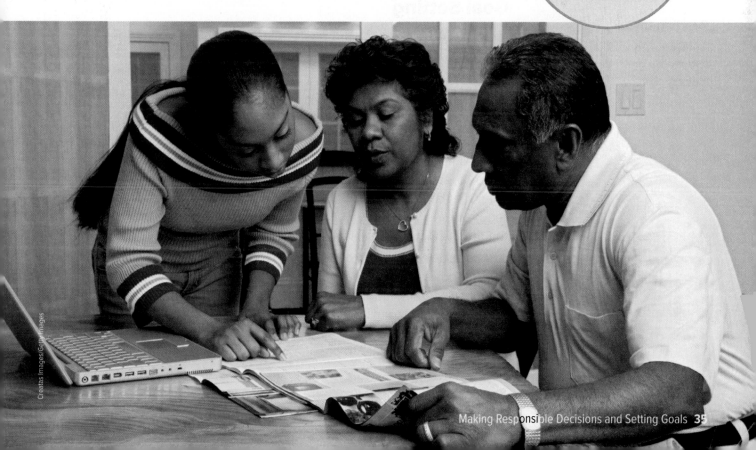

- **STEP 2: List the Options.** What are all the possible choices you could make? Remember that sometimes it is appropriate *not* to take action. Share your options with parents or guardians, siblings, teachers, or friends. Ask for their advice.

- **STEP 3: Weigh the Possible Outcomes.** Weigh the consequences of each option. Use the HELP strategy to guide your choice.

- **STEP 4: Consider Values.** A responsible decision will reflect your values.

- **STEP 5: Make a Decision and Act on It.** Use everything you know at this point to make a responsible decision. You can feel good that you have carefully thought about the situation and your options.

- **STEP 6: Evaluate the Decision.** After you have made the decision and taken action, reflect on what happened. What was the outcome? How did your decision affect your health and the health of those around you? What did you learn? Would you take the same action again? If not, how would your choice differ?

One of the steps involves using the HELP strategy. This strategy includes asking yourself the following questions:

- **H (Healthful)** - Does this choice present any health risks?

- **E (Ethical)** - Does this choice reflect what you value?

- **L (Legal)** - Does this option violate any local, state, or federal laws?

- **P (Parent Approval)** - Would your parents or guardians approve of this choice?

Goal Setting

MAIN IDEA Working toward goals helps you achieve your hopes and dreams.

How do you see yourself in the future? What would you like to accomplish? What are your hopes and dreams? The answers to these questions reflect your **goals** in life. Goals are those things you aim for that take planning and work. Whether you reach your goals—and how successfully you reach them—depends on the plans you make now. For instance, suppose your goal is to go to college. To reach that goal, you'll plan what courses to take in high school so that you meet the entrance requirements of the college you choose. You'll also work hard to earn the grades that will get you in.

Just as you set life goals because you have dreams for the future, you also set goals for your health in order to stay well. For instance, you may set a goal to drink more water and fewer soft drinks. To reach this goal, you need to plan to make water available instead of soda when you're thirsty. You might plan to carry a refillable water bottle in your backpack and to order water instead of soda when you're eating out with friends.

Reading Check

Analyze Why it is important to develop good decision-making skills?

Making Individual or Collaborative Decisions

Many times, you will make decisions for yourself. Some decisions you may face include what to wear to school today, how to respond in a difficult situation, or what college to attend in the future. These are individual decisions. They affect other people, but primarily, they affect you.

Other decisions that you make may affect a group. When this occurs, you may need to make a collaborative decision. Some situations that may require making a collaborative decision include picking a movie to see with your group of friends, deciding with your family where to go on vacation, or deciding with a group of friends whether to attend a party.

Collaborative decision-making requires compromise. Each person in the group should state their opinion and give options. Then the group can decide on a choice. Collaborative decision-making doesn't mean that you should agree to activities that go against your values. For example, a group of friends may decide to attend a party where alcohol will be available. You can make the choice to avoid this high-risk behavior. You can decide not to attend the party. Any decision you make, even collaborative decisions, should align with your values.

• • • • • • • • • • • •

Reading Check

Describe Describe a situation in which you might decide to go against a collaborative decision and make an individual decision.

• • • • • • • • • • • •

Types of Goals

Time is a consideration when you're setting goals. How long do you think it will take to reach your goal? Depending on your answer, the goal you have in mind may be a **short-term goal** or a **long-term goal**. A short-term goal is a goal that you can reach in a short period of time. A long-term goal is a goal that you plan to reach over an extended period of time. Sometimes, short-term goals can be stepping-stones on the way to long-term goals. For example, making a high school sports team can be a stepping-stone to the goal of becoming a professional athlete.

Short-Term Goals. You can accomplish a short-term goal fairly quickly. Let's say your goal is to find and read three articles on an assigned topic over the weekend. On Saturday you search the Internet, locate your articles, and print them out. On Sunday, you read the articles so you're ready to discuss them in class on Monday.

Long-Term Goals. Long-term goals call for more time as well as more planning. If you want to train for a 10K (6.2-mile) race, you know you need to train for several months to build up your endurance and speed. A series of short-term goals can help you achieve this. You can practice running shorter distances until you are able to run a mile in a reasonable time. Then you work up to running 5K (3.1 miles), and finally up to 10K. Working short-term goals into the planning of your long-term goal helps you feel good each week as you run faster and farther.

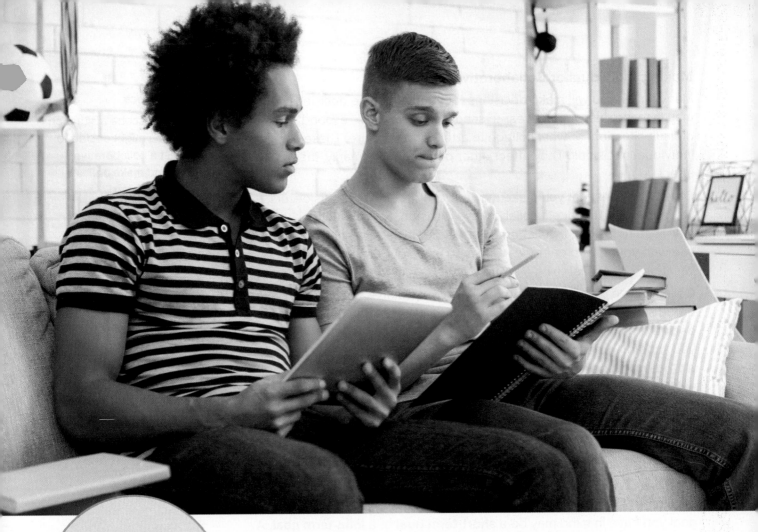

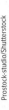

Prostock-studio/Shutterstock

Many teens set health-related goals based on personal assessments of their health. **What steps can you take to improve your health? What strategies could you use?**

Reaching Your Goals

To reach a goal, you need an **action plan**. An action plan is a multistep strategy to identify and achieve your goals and will help you identify the criteria for your goal. The S.M.A.R.T. goal criteria can help you develop your action plan. A S.M.A.R.T. goal is one that is:

- **Specific.** Identify your reasons for wanting to achieve this goal. Ask yourself: What is your goal? Why do you want to achieve this goal? Who can help you reach the goal? How long will it take to reach the goal? When will you begin?

- **Measurable.** Determine how long it will take you to achieve the goal. If it's a long-term goal, should you set short-term goals to identify your progress?

- **Attainable.** Be honest with yourself. Are you capable of attaining the goal? If you're currently about five feet tall, is it realistic to set a goal to grow to six feet in height?

- **Relevant.** Does the goal help you achieve something that is relevant to you? A person who sets a goal to drink more water may prefer soda, but drinking more water will make you healthier. If you choose to be healthier, drinking more water is a relevant goal.

- **Timely.** What is your timeframe for achieving the goal? What is your action plan to meet that deadline? What are the steps in your plan that will help you succeed?

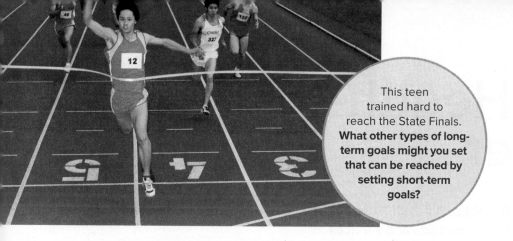

This teen trained hard to reach the State Finals. **What other types of long-term goals might you set that can be reached by setting short-term goals?**

Reading Check

Describe Identify and describe two types of goals.

Fitness Zone

My teacher said that when you set a goal, you need to be specific and choose things that can be measured. Goals like "lose weight" or "gain muscle" are too general. Specific goals are better, like "I want to finish a 5K race," or "I want to eat at least five servings of fruits and vegetables a day." That way you can track your success.

Developing an Action Plan. You can turn your dreams into reality by following these steps to create your action plan:

- **Set a specific, realistic goal and write it down.** You need to have a destination, so you'll know where you're going.

- **List the steps you will take to reach your goal.** Think of short-term goals as the steps that lead you to the long-term goal.

- **Identify sources of help and support.** Who are your team members? They might include friends, family members, teachers, or community leaders.

- **Set a reasonable time frame for achieving your goal.** Write down your time frame next to your goal statement.

- **Evaluate your progress by establishing checkpoints.** Your checkpoints could be particular dates within your time frame, or they could be short-term goals that you plan to accomplish.

- **Reward yourself for achieving your goal.** Celebrate with family and friends when you reach your goal. Plan smaller rewards along the way as you accomplish each short-term goal. This will help keep you motivated.

Lesson 2 Review

Facts and Vocabulary

1. How can decision-making skills improve your health?

2. Why would you set a health goal?

3. Give an example of one short-term and one long-term goal related to improving physical fitness.

Thinking Critically

4. **Evaluate.** What might happen if a teen made a decision that went against her personal values?

5. **Analyze.** How can responsible decision making help you achieve your health goals?

Applying Health Skills

6. **Goal Setting.** Choose a short-term goal that you personally would like to achieve. Write an action plan to accomplish your goal.

Writing Critically

7. **Descriptive.** Recall a time when you had to make a health-related decision. Describe how you made the decision, what happened as a result, and how you might change your decision-making process based on what you learned in this lesson.

Image Source

LESSON 3

Being a Health-Literate Consumer

BEFORE YOU READ

Create a Cluster Chart.
Draw a circle and label it "Health-Literate Consumer." Use surrounding circles to define and describe this term. As you read, continue filling in the chart with more details.

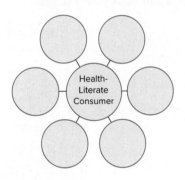

Vocabulary

health consumer
advertising
comparison shopping
warranty

Reading Check

Describe How does advertising influence your decision to buy a health-related product?

BIG IDEA A health-literate consumer carefully evaluates health products and services.

REAL LIFE ISSUES

Analyzing Product Labels. Brad's skin is starting to break out, and he decides to buy an acne cream. In the skin care section at the drugstore, he finds 20 different products. Brad starts to read the package labels. After the fifth label, he feels overwhelmed and doesn't know how to sort out all the information. *If you were Brad, how would you respond to this situation? Write a paragraph explaining which criteria you use to select health products.*

After completing the lesson, review and analyze your response to the Real Life Issues question.

Making Informed Choices

MAIN IDEA You can learn to make good consumer choices.

Are you a smart shopper? Do you try to get a high-quality product at a reasonable price when you shop? Smart shopping is especially important when it comes to making choices about health products and services. It's up to you as a **health consumer** to make informed buying decisions. A health consumer is someone who purchases or uses health products or services.

Probably the most important influence you need to be aware of as a consumer is advertising. Although **advertising** can provide useful information, its main purpose is to get you to buy a product. Advertising is a written or spoken media message designed to interest consumers in purchasing a product or service. Advertisers use various methods and hidden messages to promote their products and services. A health-literate consumer is aware of these messages and knows how to evaluate them.

HIDDEN MESSAGES IN ADVERTISING

Technique	Example	Hidden Message
Bandwagon	Group of people using a product or service	Everyone is using it, and you should too.
Rich and famous	Product displayed in expensive home	It will make you feel rich and famous.
Free gifts	Redeemable coupons for merchandise	It's too good a deal to pass up.
Great outdoors	Scenes of nature	If it's associated with nature, it must be healthy.
Good times	People smiling and laughing	The product will add fun to your life.
Testimonial	People for whom a product has worked	It worked for them, so it will work for you, too.

Evaluating Products

There are two effective ways to develop your consumer skills when buying health products. You should read product labels and comparison shop before buying.

Product Labels. Labels give you important information about what a product contains. Information found on a product label includes:

- the product's name.
- the product's intended use.
- directions for using the product.
- warnings about possible health risks.
- information about the manufacturer, such as the company name and address.
- the amount of a product in the container.

For products such as medicines, you will also find a list of the product's ingredients. In most cases, these are listed by weight in descending order. The active ingredients are the most important. These make the product effective. By comparing the amount of active ingredients in different acne products, for example, you can figure out which one contains most of the active ingredient. You may discover that a less-expensive product contains the same active ingredient as a brand-name product.

Product labels may also include important safety information. They may show that a product has been tested for safety. For example, a label may show the symbol for the Underwriters Laboratory (UL). This group tests and certifies electrical appliances and fire extinguishers. Another group, Snell, and the American National Standards Institute (ANSI), monitor safety standards for helmets and other protective equipment.

Comparison Shopping. Another great tool for health consumers is **comparison shopping**. Comparison shopping helps you choose the most useful products and get the best value for your money. Here are some criteria you can use to judge health products and services:

Recognizing advertising techniques will help you make informed purchasing decisions.

Fitness Zone

My doctor says that a lot of teens don't get the nutrients we need because of poor eating habits. She says that we tend to eat foods that are high in fat, like fast foods. We need to eat more fruits and vegetables and low-fat dairy products.

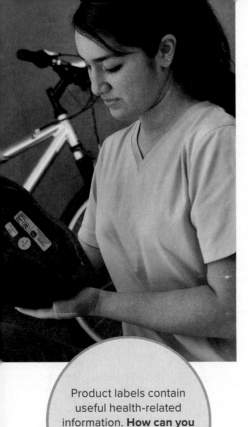

Product labels contain useful health-related information. **How can you tell if a product has been safety tested?**

ACADEMIC VOCABULARY

valid *(adjective)*: well-grounded or justifiable

Reading Check

Explain Why is it important to read product labels and to check the source of information on health products?

- **Cost and quality.** A product's cost does not always reflect its quality. For example, generic medicines may work the same as brand-name products. Compare the quality of lower-cost items, and look for the lowest-priced product that meets your needs.

- **Features.** Figure out which product features are most important to you so that you don't waste money on features you don't want. For instance, if you are buying a water bottle for your bike, you might want one with a sports top that makes it easy to drink from with one hand. However, you might not care whether it comes with a stainless-steel finish.

- **Warranty.** Many products come with a **warranty**. A warranty is a company's or a store's written agreement to repair a product or refund your money if the product doesn't function properly. Ask about warranties before buying expensive products. Read them carefully to make sure you understand what they cover.

- **Safety.** When you are evaluating sports, recreation, and home-safety products, look for the logos of reputable organizations such as UL, ANSI, and Snell.

- **Recommendations.** Listen to the opinions of people you trust who have used the product or service that you are considering. Also, check out ratings of the product from organizations such as Consumer Reports or from online user review sites.

Evaluating Information and Services. Reading product labels and comparison shopping are two useful tools for evaluating products. However, as a health consumer you should apply smart shopping skills to health information and services that you use as well.

When you evaluate health information, remember to look for **valid** sources. These include health care professionals, such as your doctor, nurse, or pharmacist. Publications and websites can also be valid sources of health information, but not all of them are. To evaluate these sources, ask yourself the following questions:

- Who pays for this site or publication? Is it a reputable group, such as a government agency or a professional health organization?

- What is the purpose of the site or publication? Is it simply to provide information, or is it trying to sell a specific product? Sites that are selling something may include only the information that makes the product look good and leave out other important facts.

- Who actually wrote the content? Is the author a respected, well-known science or health professional? Articles that are not written by experts may contain mistakes or misleading information.

You can use similar questions to evaluate health services. For example, does the health service come from a respected provider? Is the person a trained professional? Can you be sure that this person has your best interests at heart? Considering these questions will help you choose reliable health services.

Comparing Products

Teens spend $155 billion each year on clothing, music, personal care items, and other products. As a result, retailers pay close attention to teens' consumer behaviors and promote products directly to them. It's important to look past the glossy advertising and fancy packaging to evaluate a product carefully. One feature to consider is cost and how to get the most for your money. Compare the following products.

PRODUCT	SIZE	PRICE
A. Celebrity-brand purifying gel	5.5 oz.	$25.99
B. Foaming acne cleanser	6 oz.	$6.99
C. Generic-brand acne cleanser	6 oz.	$4.99

Activity: Mathematics

Use the chart to answer these questions.

1. What is the unit price of each cleanser?
2. If you use one bottle of product B every four months, how much will you pay for this product in a year?
3. Write a paragraph describing two or more features you would compare when shopping for a facial cleanser.

CONCEPT Measurement and Data: Unit Price
To calculate unit price, divide the cost of the product by the volume, or total ounces. This will yield the cost per ounce.

Lesson 3 Review

Facts and Vocabulary

1. Who is a *health consumer*?
2. How does comparison shopping make you a smart consumer?
3. Define *warranty*.

Thinking Critically

4. **Synthesize.** Susie wants to buy an expensive pedometer after seeing her favorite actress use it in an ad. The ad says the product is the most accurate on the market. What hidden messages in the ad is Susie responding to?
5. **Analyze.** How does a warranty help you become a smarter consumer?

Applying Health Skills

6. **Accessing Information.** Your friend takes a multivitamin, and you're wondering if you should too. You check a few websites to learn more about multivitamins before you ask your parents for permission to use them. How would you evaluate the validity of the information you find?

Writing Critically

7. **Expository.** Find three ads in a teen magazine. Write a short essay explaining the advertising techniques used in each ad. Refer to "Hidden Messages in Advertising."

Managing Consumer Problems

BEFORE YOU READ

Create Vocabulary Cards.
Write each new vocabulary term on a separate note card. For each term, write a definition based on your current knowledge. As you read, fill in additional information related to each term.

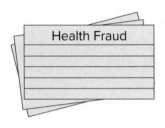
Health Fraud

Vocabulary
consumer advocates
malpractice
health fraud

● ● ● ● ● ● ● ● ● ● ● ●

BIG IDEA Knowing how to handle consumer problems is an important skill to learn.

REAL LIFE ISSUES

Health Fraud Terms. A number of claims and terms are commonly used to sell health products. Some of these health products are legitimate, but others are fraudulent. Claims and terms that may be used with health products to attract customers include: natural, non-toxic, money-back guarantee, scientific breakthrough, testimonials from people who claim amazing results, no-risk, ancient remedy, and miraculous cure. *Think of an advertisement that you have seen that uses one or more of these gimmicks. Write a paragraph describing the product and its potentially false or misleading claims.*

After completing the lesson, review and analyze your response to the Real Life Issues question.

Resolving Consumer Problems

MAIN IDEA You can take action to correct consumer problems.

Have you ever bought a product and been dissatisfied with it after you used it? Maybe the product didn't work the way it should, didn't work at all, or a part was missing or broken. What can you do when this happens?

When searching for a product, find out what the store's return policy is before making a purchase. If the product has a warranty, make sure it's in the package or ask for a copy. After you get home and open the product, save the packaging, along with your receipt and warranty.

If the product comes with instructions, read them carefully. Pay particular attention to the directions for skin and hair care products. Follow all the steps for the product's use or assembly. Make sure you are using the product exactly the way it was designed to be used.

If you are using the product correctly and it still isn't working the way you expected, consult the warranty to learn how you can return it. You may be able to return it to the store where you bought it. However, some manufacturers want the product returned directly to them.

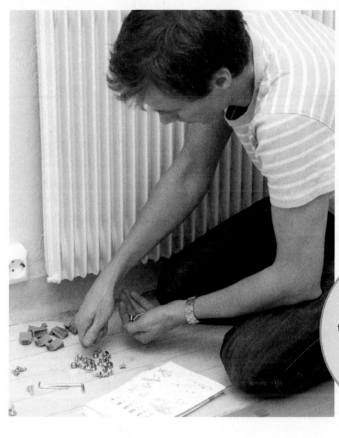

Most products have instructions that tell you how to use them correctly. **What are some products you use that have specific directions to follow?**

Put the product back in its original packaging and follow the manufacturer's return instructions. You may be asked to write a letter explaining the problem and requesting either a replacement or a refund of your money. Date your letter and keep a copy for your files, along with a shipping receipt to prove you returned the product.

Consumer Organizations

Sometimes, even when you follow all the instructions for returning an item properly, the manufacturer doesn't respond. If you try to return a product and are not satisfied with the result, you can seek help from one of the following organizations:

- The Better Business Bureau handles complaints about local merchants. Its basic services are dispute resolution and truth-in-advertising complaints.

- **Consumer advocates** are people or groups whose sole purpose is to take on regional, national, and even international consumer issues. They help consumers in a variety of ways. Groups like Consumer Reports test products and inform the public about potential problems. Others check for consumer concerns about products and services.

- Local, state, and federal government agencies work to protect consumers' rights. The federal agencies most concerned with consumer health issues are the Food and Drug Administration (FDA) and the Consumer Product Safety Commission (CPSC). The FDA ensures that medicines are safe, effective, and correctly labeled. The Consumer Product Safety Commission sends out notices of dangerous products that should be removed from store shelves.

Reading Check

Describe What would you do if you purchased a product that didn't work?

Health Care Problems

Sometimes people have problems with their health care providers. It might be difficult to schedule appointments. Perhaps their health insurance might not cover nontraditional **approaches** such as acupuncture or herbal treatments. Sometimes, the easiest way to resolve a problem with a health care provider is to find a new provider. If an insurance company does not give you a choice of doctors, you may want to choose another insurance company. Also, if you are unsure about a treatment that a doctor has prescribed, think about getting a second opinion from another physician. Many people get a second opinion when they have a major health concern.

Occasionally, health care professionals may not provide adequate treatment. The person may be guilty of **malpractice**, which is failure by a health professional to meet accepted standards. If you experience a serious problem with a health care professional, report your concerns to a state licensing board.

Health Fraud

MAIN IDEA Protect yourself from health fraud.

Have you ever seen an ad on TV or in a magazine that promises an instant cure for a health problem? Did you think the product's claims sounded too good to be true? You were probably right. Such ads are a kind of **health fraud**, or the sale of worthless products or services that claim to prevent disease or cure other health problems. Health fraud is often called *quackery*.

Health clinics that promise "miracle" cures for ailments or offer questionable treatments, such as "microwaving" cancer cells, are also guilty of health fraud. Some fraudulent clinics have been shut down after it was discovered that the people running them were not the doctors they claimed to be; some even had criminal records. These clinics take advantage of people who are very ill and desperate for a cure.

Warning Signs of Health Fraud

Weight-loss and beauty products are two areas in which health fraud is particularly common. That's why it is important to read ads for these products very carefully before deciding to buy. Look out for claims that don't sound realistic. Some "red flag" phrases that can be warning signs of health fraud include:

- "Secret formula"
- "Miracle cure"
- "Overnight results"
- "All natural"
- "Hurry, this offer expires soon"

You can consult a registered pharmacist if you have questions about a product's health claims. **What other reliable sources can you go to for medical advice?**

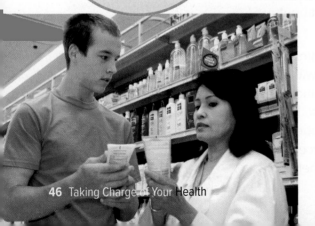

Tim Fuller Photography

Avoiding Health Fraud

If you see an ad with any suspicious phrases listed, you should be very cautious about trying the product. However, some products and services are fraudulent in ways that are harder to detect. To protect yourself from health fraud, you can take the following precautions:

- Seek the opinions of other people who have tried a product to find out whether it works. You can ask family members and friends, or look for reviews online.

- Check out a product's or service's claims with a doctor or other health professional.

- Check with the Better Business Bureau to see if there have been any complaints about the company that offers the product or service.

- Consult professional health organizations to find out whether a product's claims are truthful. The American Diabetes Association, for example, will be familiar with health frauds related to treatments of diabetes.

Remember the phrase, "let the buyer beware." It is usually much easier to avoid buying a fraudulent health product or service in the first place than it is to get your money back if you are unsatisfied. In the end, only you have the power and the responsibility to protect yourself and your well-being.

Reading Check

Describe How can you protect yourself from health fraud when buying a health-related product?

Myths & Reality

Do you believe everything you see on television and the Internet?

Myth: Because of government regulations, all advertising must be accurate.

Reality: Advertisements often use phrases, such as "world's best," that cannot be proven right or wrong. Advertisements also use statistics that may be misleading. For example, an advertisement that includes the phrase "2 out of 3 doctors surveyed" does not give you enough information to determine if this is a valid, scientific result.

Lesson 4 Review

Facts and Vocabulary

1. How do consumer advocates help you to be a better health consumer?

2. What is *malpractice?*

3. Define *health fraud.*

Thinking Critically

4. **Analyze.** Why is it important for health consumers to take an active role if they are dissatisfied with a product or service?

5. **Evaluate.** Review the list of claims that are often associated with health fraud. What do these claims have in common?

Applying Health Skills

6. **Advocacy.** Two of your friends are thinking about purchasing products that promise immediate weight loss. You know these claims are unrealistic and that the products may be unsafe. Create a text message that warns your friends about unrealistic claims in weight-loss products.

Writing Critically

7. **Narrative.** Write a story about a teen who encounters a consumer problem. Your story should describe the problem and demonstrate how the teen handles it.

LESSON 1

Vocabulary Review

Use the correct vocabulary term to complete the following statements.

1. _____ are tools that you can use to maintain all aspects of your health.

2. If you influence another person to adopt a healthful behavior, that's called _____.

3. A person who goes for a brisk walk when feeling overwhelmed by a busy schedule is practicing a health skill called _____.

Understanding Key Concepts

After reading the question or statement, select the correct answer.

4. Sofia is angry that Alisa interrupts her. If Sofia says, "I'm upset because my ideas are not being heard," she is
   a. using an "I" statement to express her feelings.
   b. blaming Alisa for interrupting her.
   c. practicing poor interpersonal communication skills.
   d. all of the above.

5. Joe and Tony are having a heated argument. Tony decides to cool off before continuing the discussion. Tony is practicing a health skill called
   a. advocacy.
   b. conflict resolution.
   c. stress management.
   d. accessing information.

Thinking Critically

After reading the question or statement, write a short answer using complete sentences.

6. **Compare and Contrast.** How are interpersonal communication and conflict-resolution skills similar? How are they different?

7. **Evaluate.** What types of information could you use to evaluate the validity of health information?

8. **Explain.** How does technology influence your health choices?

9. **Analyze.** What does it take to advocate for health?

LESSON 2

Vocabulary Review

Identify which of the following sentences are True and which are False.

10. The decisions you make about your health should reflect your values.

11. Decision making is a random process, depending on your mood.

12. Breaking a long-term goal into several short-term goals can make the long-term goal easier to achieve.

Understanding Key Concepts

After reading the question or statement, select the correct answer.

13. It's a good idea to talk over major decisions with your family because
   a. they always know what is best for you.
   b. they have a right to know everything you do.
   c. they share your values, the basis for making decisions.
   d. they will tell you what you should do.

14. Setting health-related goals
   a. ensures that you will obtain your goals.
   b. helps you plan and safeguard your well-being.
   c. takes a lot of time and creates stress.
   d. is a one-time event when you set healthy goals.

15. An action plan should include
   a. a written statement of your goal.
   b. the steps you will take to accomplish it.
   c. neither a nor b.
   d. both a and b.

Thinking Critically

After reading the question or statement, write a short answer using complete sentences.

16. **Analyze.** Why is decision making a key health skill? How can this skill contribute to your safety and well-being?

17. **Evaluate.** What criteria are important in weighing the possible consequences of your choices?

18. **Analyze.** Why is it important to set health-related goals?

Vocabulary Review

Use the correct vocabulary term to complete the following statements.

19. Each of us is a(n) _____ because we all buy health products and services.

20. Evaluating the features of two similar products is called _____.

21. _____ techniques include bandwagon, rich and famous, free gifts, great outdoors, good times, and testimonial.

Understanding Key Concepts

After reading the question or statement, select the correct answer.

22. To be a critical thinker about advertising,
 a. note how often you see the same ad.
 b. remember product names.
 c. look for hidden messages in ads.
 d. compare ads for similar products.

23. Smart health consumers
 a. read product labels.
 b. listen to infomercials.
 c. write to product manufacturers.
 d. try out different products.

Thinking Critically

After reading the question or statement, write a short answer using complete sentences.

24. **Explain.** What strategies do smart consumers use to protect their health when purchasing health products?

25. **Discuss.** How does an understanding of advertising help you become a smarter consumer?

26. **Evaluate.** What are some effective strategies for evaluating health information and services?

Vocabulary Review

Choose the correct term in the sentences below.

27. Someone who tests products and informs the public about potential problems is a *product expert/consumer advocate*.

28. Selling a worthless weight loss product is an example of *health fraud/trickery*.

29. When a doctor fails to live up to professional standards in medicine, he may be accused of *arrogance/malpractice*.

Understanding Key Concepts

After reading the question or statement, select the correct answer.

30. If you buy a product and are not satisfied with it, you should
 a. read the warranty to find out how to return it.
 b. throw it away.
 c. immediately buy a replacement.
 d. all of the above.

31. Which of the following is *not* a good way to protect yourself from health fraud?
 a. Checking out claims with a health care professional
 b. Trying the product or service for yourself
 c. Talking to others who have used the product or service
 d. Consulting with the Better Business Bureau

Thinking Critically

After reading the question or statement, write a short answer using complete sentences.

32. **Synthesize.** How are consumers empowered to protect their health and well-being?

33. **Explain.** What are the best steps to take if you are dissatisfied with the health-related product that you have purchased?

34. **Analyze.** Why are some people attracted to products that make fraudulent claims?

35. **Discuss.** What criteria would you use to evaluate health services?

PROJECT-BASED ASSESSMENT

Volun-teen

BACKGROUND

Teens can advocate for healthy living on the local, national, and international levels. You can help make a difference by getting involved in this effort too!

TASK

Conduct an online search for volunteer opportunities that promote healthy living and that are available to teens in your community. Write a blog entry or create a web page that describes the volunteer opportunities and encourages teens to get involved. Ask other teens to add information about their favorite volunteer activities.

AUDIENCE

Students in your class and teens in your community

PURPOSE

Inform teens of health-related volunteer opportunities, and encourage their involvement.

PROCEDURE

1. Conduct an online search for volunteer opportunities with several health organizations. Examples include hospitals, the Red Cross, and the American Cancer Society.

2. Gather details about the volunteer opportunities. Find out the type of work involved, the minimum age requirement, the length of the assignment, and any necessary contact information.

3. Review several of the organization's websites to familiarize yourself with their writing style.

4. Write a blog entry or create a web page that describes the volunteer opportunities you researched.

5. The blog or web page should encourage teens to pursue volunteer opportunities.

Math Practice

Interpret Graphs. The graph below shows the percentages of young adults who volunteer each year. Use the graph to answer Questions 1–3.

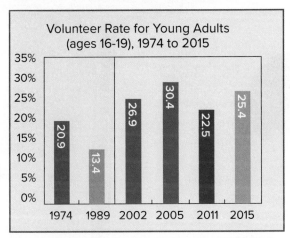

Adapted from "Volunteering in America: 2007 State Trends and Rankings in Civic Life," Corporation for National and Community Service, April 2007.
U.S. Bureau of Labor Statistics, 2016.

1. Which years show an increase from the previous year shown on the graph in the volunteering rate among young adults?
   a. 1974 and 2002
   b. 1989 and 2005
   c. 2005 and 2015
   d. 2002 and 2011

2. Between which two years was there the greatest change in percentage of volunteers?
   a. 2002 and 2005
   b. 2005 and 2011
   c. 2011 and 2015
   d. 1974 and 1989

3. According to the graph, how do volunteering rates in the 2000s compare to rates in the late 1900s?
   a. Fewer young adults volunteer in this century.
   b. More young adults volunteer in this century.
   c. There is no change in the number of young adults who volunteer.
   d. More adults volunteer than young adults during both centuries.

Reading/Writing Practice

Understand and Apply. Read the passage below, and then answer the questions.

Good communication is a skill you can use every day. One way you can demonstrate effective communication skills is to be a good listener. The speaker may think that you are not listening if your eyes wander around the room. Closed body language, such as crossing your arms, conveys that you may not be open to hearing what others have to say. To show that you are listening attentively, make eye contact and let the other person finish what he or she is saying before you speak. Use body language such as nodding your head to show that you are interested in what the person is saying. A good listener makes statements that encourage the speaker to explain his or her views, such as "What do you mean by that?" It can also be helpful to restate what the person tells you to make sure that you understand what is being said.

1. Which of the following is a behavior that characterizes good listening skills?
   a. Crossed arms
   b. Making eye contact
   c. Wandering eyes
   d. Interrupting

2. Which statement best summarizes the main point of the article?
   a. Closed body language is negative.
   b. You can demonstrate effective communication by being a good listener.
   c. Always ask speakers to explain their views.
   d. Never restate what you hear.

3. Describe the effects of attentive listening and poor listening on communication.

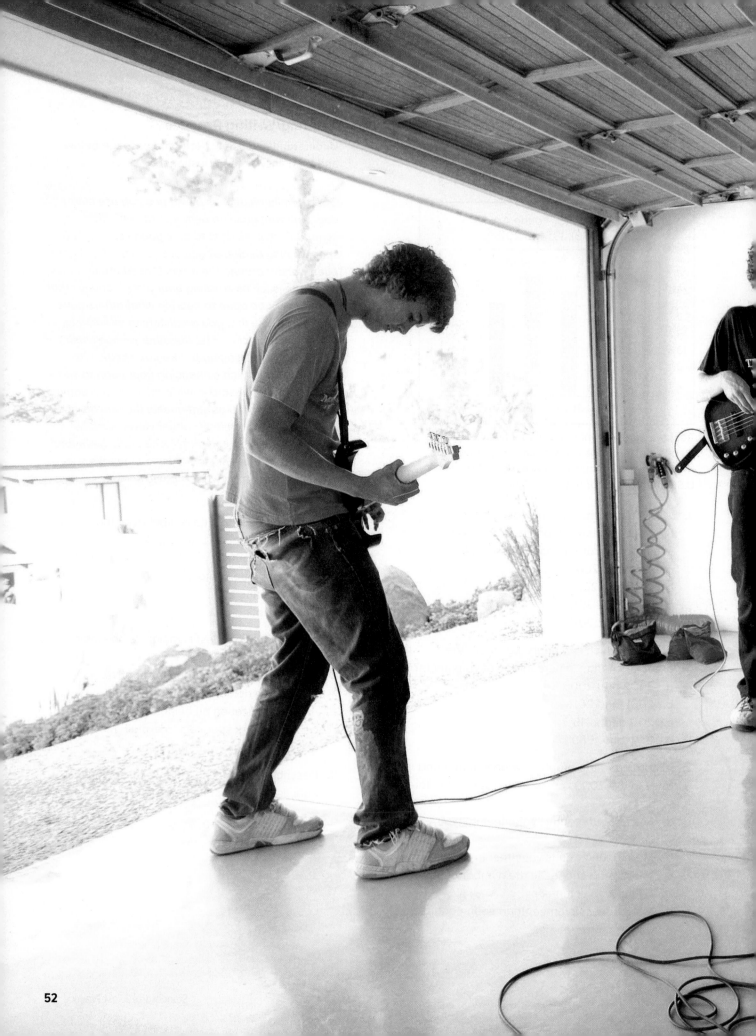

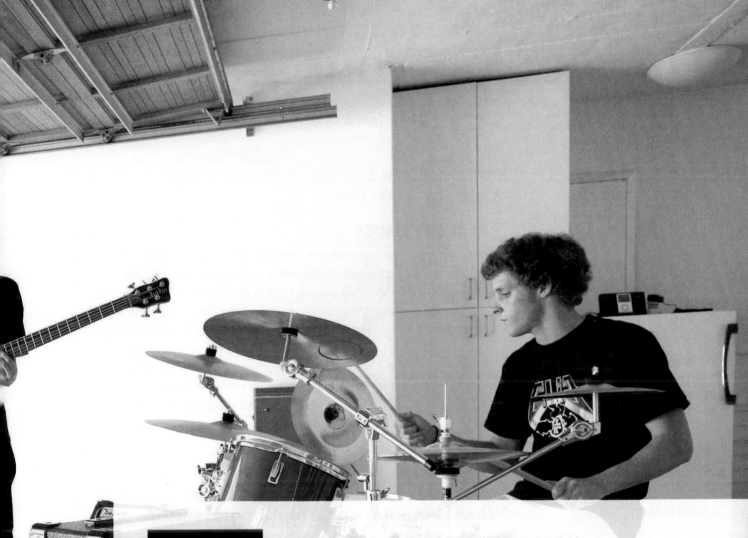

Achieving Mental and Emotional Health

LESSONS

1 Developing Your Self-Esteem

2 Developing Personal Identity and Character

3 Expressing Emotions in Healthful Ways

Developing Your Self-Esteem

BEFORE YOU READ

Create an Outline. Preview this lesson by scanning the pages. Then organize the headings and subheadings into an outline. As you read, fill in your outline with important details.

I.
A.
1.
2.
B.
II.

Vocabulary

mental/emotional health
resilient
self-esteem
competence
hierarchy of needs
self-actualization

ACADEMIC VOCABULARY

mental *(adjective):* of or relating to the mind.

BIG IDEA Good mental and emotional health helps you develop healthy self-esteem.

REAL LIFE ISSUES

Staying Positive. Kevin has been swimming since he was five years old. When he didn't make the swim team this year, he thought there had been a mistake. He did well in swimming competitions throughout elementary school. He even took time to work out every day after school prior to the tryouts. He feels embarrassed about being cut from the team and doesn't know how he can face his friends. *Imagine you are Kevin's close friend. Write a dialogue between yourself and Kevin discussing how he should deal with his disappointment.*

After completing the lesson, review and analyze your response to the Real Life Issues question.

What is Mental and Emotional Health?

MAIN IDEA Mental and emotional health helps you function effectively each day.

Do you see yourself in a positive way? Are you able to handle challenges and setbacks well? Being able to answer "yes" to these questions is one sign of good **mental/emotional health**, which is the ability to accept yourself and others, express and manage emotions, and deal with the demands and challenges you meet in your life. Having good mental and emotional health is an important part of your total health.

The Importance of Mental and Emotional Health

In general, mentally healthy people are happy and enjoy their lives. They feel confident and comfortable spending time alone or with others. They're also flexible and can cope with a wide variety of feelings and situations.

Your **mental** and emotional health influences your physical and social health as well. For example, if you're worried, you might eat an unhealthful diet, not get enough sleep, or stop exercising regularly. If your worries make you irritable, your relationships with friends and others may suffer.

Characteristics of Good Mental and Emotional Health

There are many signs of good mental and emotional health. In general, mentally and emotionally healthy people will share the following characteristics:

- **Sense of belonging.** Mentally and emotionally healthy people feel close to the people in their lives. Their family members, friends, teachers, and others provide them with support.

- **Sense of purpose.** Mentally and emotionally healthy people recognize that they have value and importance as individuals. This knowledge helps them set and reach goals in their lives.

- **Positive outlook.** In general, mentally and emotionally healthy people are able to see the bright side of life. Having a positive outlook reduces stress and increases your chances of success.

- **Self-sufficiency.** Mentally and emotionally healthy people are able to take care of themselves. Their confidence in themselves helps them to make responsible decisions and function independently.

- **Healthy self-esteem.** Finally, mentally and emotionally healthy people have a sense of their own worth. Having healthy self-esteem helps you accept and recover from difficulties and failures.

Having good mental health does *not* mean being happy all the time. Most people have ups and downs throughout their lives. For example, you may feel proud one day because you performed well in a school play, but disappointed the next because you were not chosen for a varsity sports team. Such ups and downs are normal, especially during your teen years when you are adapting to many changes in your life. However, mentally and emotionally healthy people are **resilient** in the face of difficulties. Resilient people have the ability to adapt effectively and recover from disappointment, difficulty, or crisis. They recognize that difficult or stressful situations are a part of life, and they are able to handle them in positive ways.

Reading Check

Name What are the characteristics of good mental/emotional health?

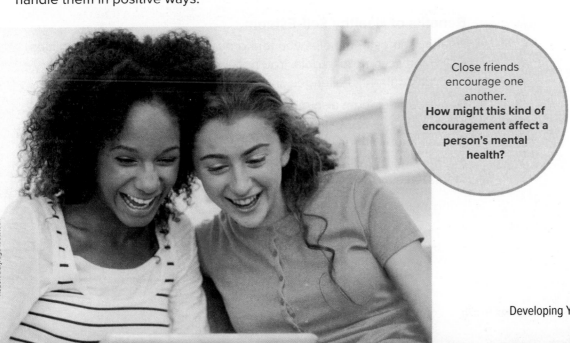

Robert Daly/age footstock

Close friends encourage one another. **How might this kind of encouragement affect a person's mental health?**

Self-Esteem

MAIN IDEA Self-esteem is necessary for good mental/emotional health.

Developing **self-esteem** strengthens the other characteristics of good mental health. This is how much you value, respect, and feel confident about yourself. If you feel valued, loved, and accepted by others—and you also value, love, and accept yourself—your overall attitude and outlook will be good. Having good self-esteem will also affect the health choices you make. A willingness to take healthful risks and try new challenges can raise your self-esteem and your sense of **competence**, or having enough skills to do something.

How You Develop Self-Esteem

You can probably remember a time when your family praised you for doing something well, or reassured you and gave you advice on a task you hadn't yet mastered. Praise for a job well done and reassurance in difficulties both help to promote healthy self-esteem. Your self-esteem also increases when you master new skills. The more challenges you overcome, the more your confidence increases so that you can succeed at other tasks in the future.

Self-talk, the encouragement or criticism that you give yourself, can also affect your self-esteem. Using positive self-talk, such as "I know I can do this," will strengthen your self-esteem. If you find yourself falling victim to negative thoughts, such as "I'm just no good at this," try to replace them with more positive self-talk.

Remember that no one succeeds at new tasks and activities all the time. If you run into difficulties with a new activity, it may help to think about why you may have had problems. Were you adequately prepared for the task? Was it realistic to expect to succeed on your first try? Remember, also, that everyone has unique abilities. You may have to work harder at some particular activities than others, but that does not mean that you cannot succeed if you keep trying.

Benefits of Healthy Self-Esteem

Healthy self-esteem helps you feel proud of yourself and your abilities, skills, and accomplishments. You believe that setbacks are temporary. You can confront challenges and overcome them.

Healthy self-esteem also gives you the confidence to try new things. It can encourage you to take up a new sport, join a club at school, or even take on a job with new responsibilities. People with healthy self-esteem accept that they will not be good at everything, and they don't see themselves as failures if they don't succeed all the time.

Reading Check

Describe Identify several benefits of healthy self-esteem

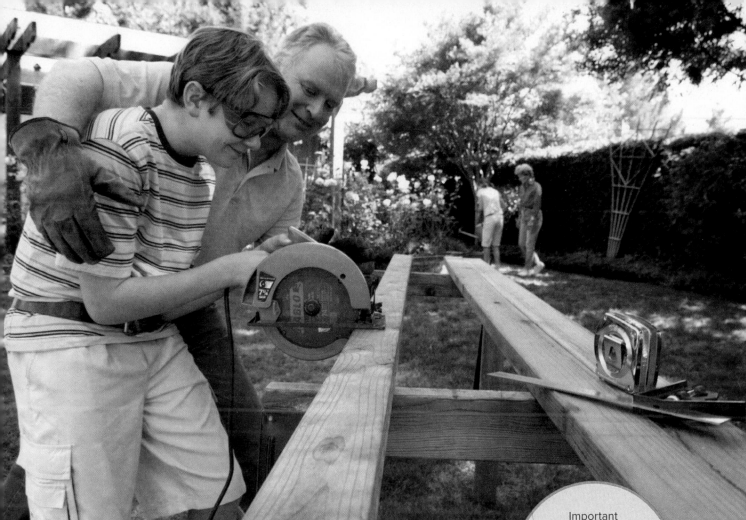

Paul Simcock/UpperCut Images/Getty Images

Improving Your Self-Esteem

MAIN IDEA You can improve your self-esteem and your overall mental and emotional health.

You can control many factors that affect your self-esteem. One important step is to avoid criticizing yourself or spending time with others who criticize you. Set realistic expectations, and don't expect perfection. If you try to be perfect, then you may be unable to enjoy your successes because you will always be thinking that you could have done even better. Here are some additional strategies to improve your self-esteem:

- Choose friends who respect and value you.

- Focus on your positive qualities.

- Replace negative self-talk with supportive self-talk.

- Try new activities to discover your talents.

- See your mistakes as learning opportunities.

- Write down your goals and the steps you will take to achieve them.

- Exercise regularly to feel more energized.

- Volunteer your time to help others.

- Accept the things you can't change and focus your energy on changing the things you can.

Important people in your life play a role in shaping your self-esteem. **How has someone important to you affected your self-esteem?**

Developing Self-Awareness

MAIN IDEA Understanding your needs and meeting them in healthy ways will help you reach your highest potential.

Self-awareness is the ability to understand your thoughts, emotions, and values and how they can influence your behavior. For example, if you are feeling angry about doing poorly on a test, you might snap at a friend even though they had nothing to do with the test or your results. Developing self-awareness includes knowing your strengths and weaknesses and building confidence.

The psychologist Abraham Maslow created a theory that explains human development and motivation. His concept is known as the **hierarchy of needs**.

Reading Check

Explain Why is joining a gang an unhealthy way to meet the need to be valued?

Maslow's model helps us understand our needs. Meeting these needs in healthy ways strengthens our mental/emotional health.

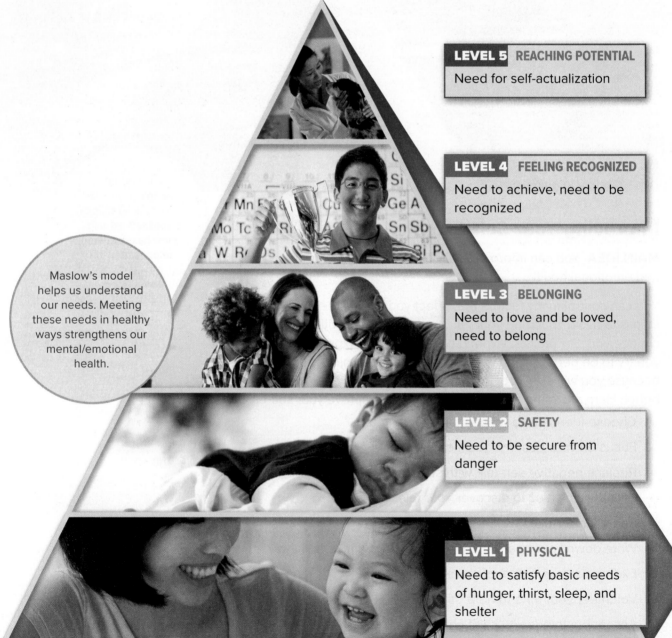

LEVEL 5 REACHING POTENTIAL
Need for self-actualization

LEVEL 4 FEELING RECOGNIZED
Need to achieve, need to be recognized

LEVEL 3 BELONGING
Need to love and be loved, need to belong

LEVEL 2 SAFETY
Need to be secure from danger

LEVEL 1 PHYSICAL
Need to satisfy basic needs of hunger, thirst, sleep, and shelter

(t)Comstock Images/Alamy Stock Photo, (tc)Corbis/SuperStock, (c)Rido/Shutterstock, (bc)Ingram Publishing, (b)Jose Luis Pelaez Inc/Blend Images LLC

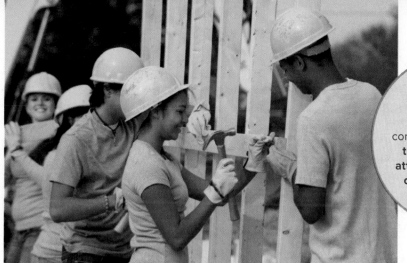

These teens have found a way to contribute to their community. **Why do you think taking time to attend to the needs of others is beneficial to self-esteem?**

Maslow's hierarchy shows that our earliest motivations are to satisfy our physical needs. As infants, we rely on others to meet our basic needs, including food, clothing, and physical safety and comfort. Once these basic needs are met, we become interested in meeting mental and emotional needs. These include the need to belong and to be loved, the need to be valued and recognized, and finally, the need to achieve **self-actualization**. Self-actualization means to strive to be the best you can.

Once you understand your mental and emotional needs, you can learn how to meet them in healthy ways. Trying to fulfill a need in a way that involves a health risk will not promote sound mental/emotional health in the long term. For example, some teens may try to meet their need for belonging by joining gangs. However, joining a gang is a high-risk behavior that can harm all sides of your health triangle. It can lead to involvement with drugs or crime that will hurt you physically, mentally/emotionally, and socially.

Try applying Maslow's model to your personal development. What needs are you most focused on at this point in your life? How are you meeting those needs? By becoming more self-aware, you can begin to take more control of your personal growth. For example, you can reach out to others to form deeper relationships and a stronger support group.

Fitness Zone

My team lost the last game of the season, and I thought about quitting the sport. Then my dad told me that Michael Jordan was cut from the varsity basketball team when he was in tenth grade. Imagine if he had quit! He wouldn't have become one of the greatest basketball players in history. I decided to be like Mike and not give up on exercise or sports.

Lesson 1 Review

Facts and Vocabulary

1. List the characteristics of good mental/emotional health.

2. Define the term *self-esteem*.

3. Identify the five levels of Maslow's hierarchy of needs.

Thinking Critically

4. **Analyze.** Explain how being mentally and emotionally healthy contributes to the quality of your life.

5. **Identify.** What are three ways that you can demonstrate healthy self-esteem and good mental/emotional health?

Applying Health Skills

6. **Practicing Healthful Behaviors.** Keiko just found out that she didn't make the track team. Write a script showing how she can use positive self-talk to deal with this disappointment.

Writing Critically

7. **Descriptive.** Imagine a teen whose suggestions are ignored during a group project. With healthy self-esteem, how might the teen respond?

Developing Personal Identity and Character

BEFORE YOU READ

Create a Cluster Chart. Draw a center circle and label it "Character." Draw circles around it and use these to define and describe this term. As you read, continue filling in the chart with more details.

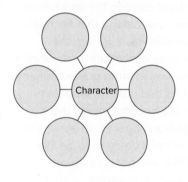

Vocabulary

personal identity
personality
role model
character
integrity
constructive criticism

BIG IDEA Healthy identity is based on being a person of good character.

REAL LIFE ISSUES

Choosing a Path. Casey is in the process of deciding what to do after he graduates high school. He visits the school guidance counselor to discuss his options. The counselor begins by asking, "What are you interested in? What are your talents?" *What are your interests and talents? Write an essay describing how these interests and talents might play a role in your future.*

After completing the lesson, review and analyze your response to the Real Life Issues question.

Your Personal Identity

MAIN IDEA Your personal identity describes who you are.

How do you introduce yourself when you meet someone? At first, you would probably start by giving your name. Later on, you might share more information about yourself, such as "I'm in the tenth grade" or "I like to swim." All these facts about you are part of your **personal identity**, your sense of yourself as a unique individual. Developing your identity is one of the most important tasks you will accomplish during your teen years.

Some parts of your personal identity depend on your age and your situation in life. You share these aspects of yourself with many other people. For example, your identity as a student is one you share with every other student in your school. However, other parts of your identity are unique to you. One aspect of your identity is your **personality**. This is a complex set of characteristics that makes you unique. Your personality sets you apart from other people and determines how you will react in certain situations.

Many factors help form your identity. One major influence is your relationships and experiences with family and friends. As you mature, you'll meet a greater number and variety of people, and some of them may become **role models** for you. This is someone whose success or behavior serves as an example for you.

Other ingredients in your personal identity include:

- your surroundings and cultural background.
- your personal tastes (likes and dislikes).
- your values and beliefs.
- your interests.
- your personal and occupational goals.

The Importance of Good Character

MAIN IDEA Character plays a significant role in your decisions, actions, and behavior.

One important aspect of your identity is your **character**, which is the distinctive qualities that describe how a person thinks, feels, and behaves. Good character is an outward expression of inner values and is a vital part of a healthy identity. A person of good character demonstrates *core ethical values,* such as responsibility, honesty, and respect. Such values tend to be held in high regard across all cultures and age groups.

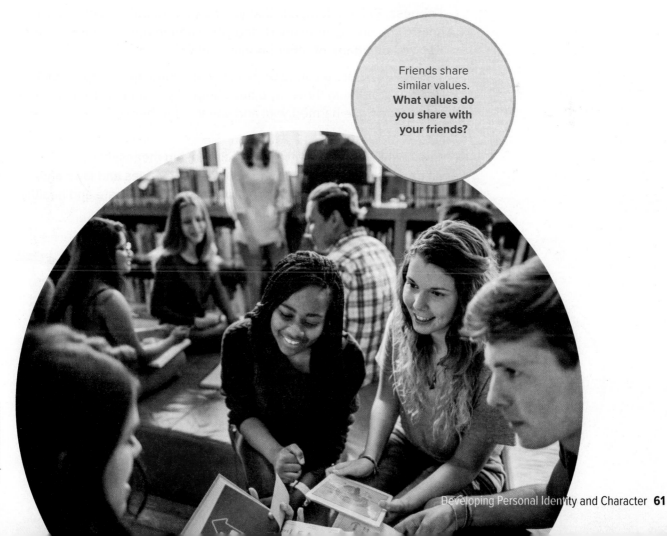

Friends share similar values. **What values do you share with your friends?**

Traits of Good Character

There are six basic traits that are commonly recognized as signs of good character. By demonstrating these traits consistently, you show others that you have **integrity**, or a firm observance of core ethical values.

- **Trustworthiness.** Being trustworthy means that you are honest, loyal, and reliable. If you say you will do something, you do it. For example, if you promise to meet a friend at a certain time, then you will do everything you can to keep that promise. You have the courage to do the right thing, and you don't lie, steal, or cheat.

- **Respect.** You show respect by being considerate of others and accepting of their differences. Even if you disagree with another person's point of view, you will still treat that person with courtesy. You also make decisions that show you care about your health and the health of others.

- **Responsibility.** Being responsible means that you hold yourself accountable for your choices and decisions. Because of this, you practice self-control, thinking before you act and considering the consequences of your actions. You try your best and complete projects you start, even when things don't go as planned. If you don't succeed, you accept responsibility and don't try to blame others for your own actions.

- **Fairness.** Being fair means that you play by the rules, take turns, and share. You are open-minded, and you listen to others. You don't try to take advantage of other people or blame them.

- **Caring.** If you are a caring person, you are kind and compassionate. You are grateful to those who have helped you and forgiving toward those who have harmed you, and you want to help others who are in need.

- **Citizenship.** Demonstrating good citizenship means that you take an interest in the world around you. You obey rules and laws and show respect for authority. You also advocate for a safe and healthy environment at school and in your community.

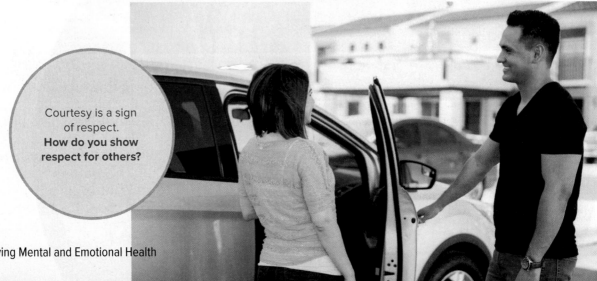

Courtesy is a sign of respect. **How do you show respect for others?**

antoniodiaz/Shutterstock

Working Toward a Positive Identity

MAIN IDEA You can develop a healthy identity.

When you think about who you are right now, it may seem as if your family and your circumstances play the biggest role in forming your identity. There is some truth in this, but remember, *you* control who you *become*. As you mature, you will make more personal choices and decisions, such as choosing a career. Your teen years are a good time to start shaping your identity in positive ways and making yourself into the person you want to be. Here are some tips for promoting a healthy identity:

- **List your skills and strengths.** Include physical, mental/emotional, and social strengths. Read the list when you're feeling down.

- **Surround yourself with positive, supportive people.** Choose friends who support and respect your rights and needs.

- **Find something that you love to do, and do it frequently.** If you're always too busy to do the things you enjoy, you're not taking care of yourself.

- **Stop making life a contest.** Recognize that there will always be people more and less able that you in areas of life. Be content with doing the best you can in all areas that matter to you.

- **Help someone else.** One way to feel good about yourself is to see the positive effects of your own words or actions on someone else's life.

Recognize Your Strengths and Weaknesses

One step in understanding your identity is to analyze your strengths and weaknesses. Be honest and realistic as you do this. If you are a trustworthy friend or a talented singer, you can take pride in these good qualities. At the same time, acknowledge your weaknesses without being too critical, and set realistic goals to improve. For example, if you tend to put things off, such as homework, set a goal to develop new habits. With planning and commitment, you can improve your habits and change weaknesses into strengths.

Demonstrate Positive Values

Practicing good character is not always easy, but it helps you build a positive identity. For instance, suppose that you are an honors student and getting good grades is an important part of your identity. As a result, you might feel pressured to cheat on exams to make sure that you would not lose your identity as a good student. However, giving in to this impulse could damage your identity in other ways. It could harm your reputation and your self-esteem if you get caught, and even if you don't. Instead of thinking of yourself as a good student, you might start thinking of yourself as a liar and a fraud. A truly positive identity will always be built on strong, positive values.

Fitness Zone

I've noticed that there's definitely a connection between having a positive outlook on life and feeling healthy. One day last week, no one could go skateboarding with me. I was bored and started to feel sad. Then I remembered that a family with a girl about my age moved in down the street. I stopped by and introduced myself, and we went for a walk. We got some fresh air and exercise and I had a chance to make a new friend—it felt great!

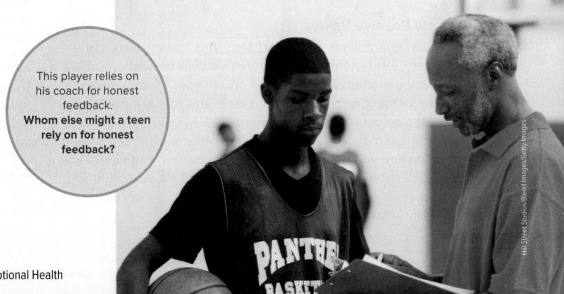

Develop a Purpose in Your Life

A sense of purpose helps you set positive goals and work to achieve them. It also provides you with a framework to build a healthy identity. Some of your goals will be short term, like studying for and passing an exam. Others will be long term, such as planning for higher education and acquiring job skills. Keeping your goals in mind will give direction to your life and help shape the person are becoming.

Take Appropriate Risks and Avoid Harmful Risk Behaviors

Risk taking is a part of life. Playing sports, taking part in artistic or creative activities, public speaking, and making friends all involve some risk. These risks are healthful because they challenge you to develop new skills and to mature in new ways. However, high-risk behaviors, such as reckless driving, joining a gang, or using tobacco, alcohol, or other drugs, are dangerous and harmful.

Form Meaningful Relationships

Meaningful relationships, such as those with your family and friends, are **crucial** to the development of your identity. Relationships provide a support system that can help you build confidence and develop a sense of security and belonging. Within a meaningful relationship, you can also give and receive **constructive criticism**. For example, if a friend doesn't do well in a school debate, you might make helpful suggestions without judging your friend or offering blame.

Contribute to the Community

Your community is your extended support system. It provides services and resources to meet many of your needs. For a community to remain strong, however, all of its members must participate in making it work. Giving back to the community by volunteering is part of being a good citizen. When you volunteer within your community, you improve the quality of people's lives, gain a sense of accomplishment, and raise your self-esteem.

Reading Check

Explain How is developing a purpose for your life helpful?

ACADEMIC VOCABULARY

crucial (adjective): important or essential

This player relies on his coach for honest feedback. **Whom else might a teen rely on for honest feedback?**

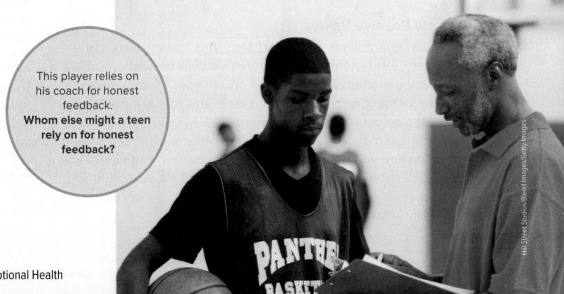

Hill Street Studios/Blend Images/Getty Images

Your Sources of Support

People around you regularly provide support. Some fulfill material needs, others offer comfort and honest opinions, and others provide information. One thing that all of these people have in common is a genuine concern for you. Together they form your support system. Identify your support system. Make a chart with the different types of support: **Material** (providers of money, transportation, physical help), **Emotional** (providers of comfort, sympathy, encouragement), **Information** (providers of knowledge and referrals), and **Appraisal** (providers of feedback, praise, suggestions). Under each category, identify who you count on and why. List those people whose names appear often. These individuals make up your core support group.

Activity: Technology

Pick one person from your core support group.

1. Create a streaming video to express your appreciation for his or her support and encouragement.
2. Identify ways that the person has supported you and helped build your identity.
3. Describe to the person how his or her support has influenced you to support others throughout your life.
4. Tell that person how his or her support has shaped your goals for the future.

Lesson 2 Review

Facts and Vocabulary

1. Define the term *personal identity*.
2. Identify the six traits of good character.
3. Explain the benefit of constructive criticism.

Thinking Critically

4. **Analyze**. Describe how role models help in forming identity.
5. **Describe**. Explain how healthful risk taking can help you mature in new ways.

Applying Health Skills

6. **Communication Skills**. With a classmate, role-play situations where constructive criticism is given.

Writing Critically

7. **Expository**. If you were to choose a role model, who would it be? Write a short essay explaining your choice.

Expressing Emotions in Healthful Ways

. . . .

BEFORE YOU READ

Create a K-W-L Chart.
Make a three-column chart. In the first column, list what you know about emotions and ways to express them. In the second column, list what you want to know about this topic. As you read, use the third column to summarize what you learned about the topic.

K	W	L

Vocabulary

emotions
hormones
empathy
defense mechanisms
hostility

. . . .

BIG IDEA Managing your emotions allows you to express them in healthful ways.

REAL LIFE ISSUES

Expressing feelings. Learning how to manage strong emotions, like anger and sadness, can reduce the risk of violence and improve health. According to the CDC's Youth Risk Behavior Survey (YRBS) of 2015, 485,610 teens were involved in a physical fight that required treatment in an emergency room. In addition, 31 percent of teens reported that they stopped doing some of their usual activities because they felt sad or hopeless. *Write a paragraph describing ways to manage strong emotions and reduce the risk of violence.*

After completing the lesson, review and analyze your response to the Real Life Issues question.

Understanding Your Emotions

MAIN IDEA Recognizing and acknowledging your emotions is a sign of good mental and emotional health.

Have you ever watched a movie that made you feel happy, sad, or scared? These feelings are all examples of **emotions**. Emotions are signals that tell your mind and body how to react. Often, the most intense emotions you feel will be related to events in your life. How you respond to your emotions can affect not only your mental/emotional health but your physical and social health as well. Learning to recognize your emotions and to understand their effects on you will help you learn to manage them in healthful ways. Common emotions include:

- **Happiness.** You may experience happiness as a feeling of being satisfied or positive about life. When you are happy, you usually feel energetic, creative, and sociable.

- **Sadness.** Feeling sad is a normal, healthy reaction to difficult life events. Feelings of sadness may be mild, like the disappointment you might feel if you don't do well on a test, or they can be deep and long lasting, such as the grief you feel when a family member or pet dies.

- **Love.** Strong affection, deep concern, and respect are all aspects of love. Loving someone means that you support that person's needs and growth and respect that person's feelings and values.

- **Fear.** You may feel fear when you are startled or alarmed by someone or something. Fear can be a useful emotion. Feelings of fear can increase your alertness and help you escape from possibly harmful situations. However, some people let fear of imagined threats prevent them from taking healthful risks.

- **Guilt.** Guilt is the feeling of shame and regret that occurs when you act against your values. Although guilt is often appropriate, sometimes people feel guilt over situations that are not under their control. For instance, some children and teens may blame themselves if their parents divorce.

- **Anger.** Anger is a normal reaction to being physically or emotionally harmed. However, anger that is not handled in a constructive way can lead to violence. Anger is often a complicated emotion because it can hide another emotion, such as hurt or guilt.

During adolescence, it's common to feel as if your emotions are swinging from one extreme to another. These emotional changes are triggered by **hormones**. Hormones are chemicals produced by your glands that regulate the activities of different body cells. Feeling overcome by your emotions at this time of your life is normal and is not a cause for concern.

Reading Check

Explain How do hormones affect emotions?

Actors portray strong emotions by using body language and changing their tone of voice. **How might an actor use body language to convey each of the emotions described above?**

U.S. Air Force photo by Master Sgt. Val Gempis

Managing Your Emotions

MAIN IDEA Knowing how to recognize your emotions can help you manage them in healthful ways.

Emotions are neither good nor bad. The way you express your emotions, however, can have good or bad consequences. Learning to express emotions in a healthful way not only helps you cope with emotional upsets, but also helps those around you to better handle their own emotions.

Dealing with Emotions in Positive Ways

As a young child, you learned about how to express your emotions from parents, teachers, and friends. Some emotions, such as happiness and love, are shown through facial expressions like smiles and glances, and through behaviors like laughing and hugging. **Empathy**, or the ability to imagine and understand how someone else feels, is expressed by supporting a friend who is going through a difficult time.

You may know some people who are uncomfortable expressing their feelings. They may prefer to keep all emotions private. You may also know people who sometimes deal with their feelings in harmful ways. They may exaggerate their emotions, pretend they have no feelings, or even express emotions like anger and fear by deliberately hurting others.

Healthful expression of feelings lets you enjoy life more. **What are some positive ways to express emotions?**

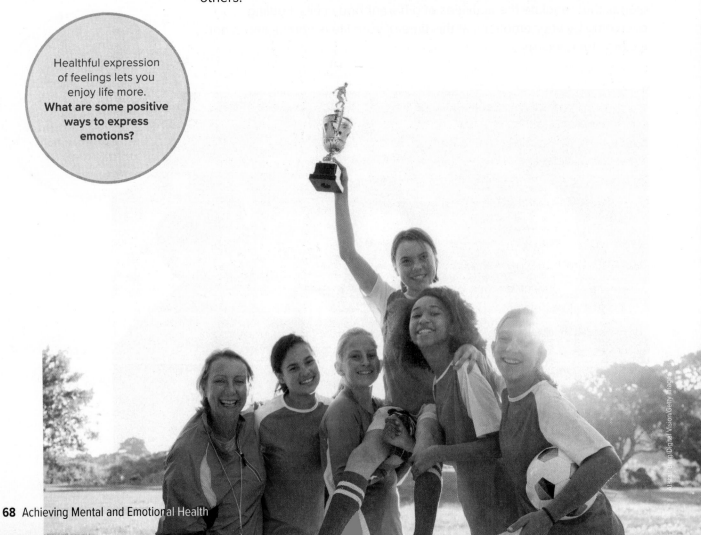

To avoid problems like these, it helps to recognize your emotions and think about positive ways to express them. Try asking yourself these questions:

- Why do I feel the way I do?
- Will this event matter later on in my life?
- Should I wait before responding?
- What can I do to feel better?
- Who can help me deal with my negative feelings?

Responding to Difficult Emotions

It's normal to feel emotions such as fear and sadness in response to problems in your life. These feelings, however, can be managed so they don't become overwhelming. Some techniques to reduce the intensity of your emotions include

- taking several deep breaths.
- relaxing your muscles.
- getting away from the situation until you calm down.
- analyzing your emotions by writing about them in a private journal.
- talking to someone you trust about the way you feel.

Some people choose to manage difficult emotions by avoiding situations that make them uncomfortable. **Defense mechanisms** are mental processes that protect individuals from strong or stressful emotions and situations. Using a defense mechanism, however, will only work for a short time. Eventually, the problem causing the person to use a defense mechanism will need to be worked through in order to solve the problem. Some emotions, such as fear, guilt, and anger, have the potential to cause a lot of damage. People may respond to these emotions without thinking about the consequences. However, by analyzing the causes of these feelings, you can learn to manage them better. Some common mechanisms include:

- **Repression.** Involuntarily pushing unpleasant feelings out of one's mind.
- **Regression**. Returning to behaviors characteristic of a younger age, rather than dealing with problems in a mature manner.
- **Denial**. Unconscious lack of recognition of something that is obvious to others.
- **Projection**. Attributing your own feelings or faults to another person or group.
- **Suppression**. Consciously and intentionally pushing unpleasant feelings out of one's mind.
- **Rationalization**. Making excuses to explain a situation or behavior, rather than taking responsibility for it.
- **Compensation**. Making up for weaknesses and mistakes through gift giving, hard work, or extreme efforts.

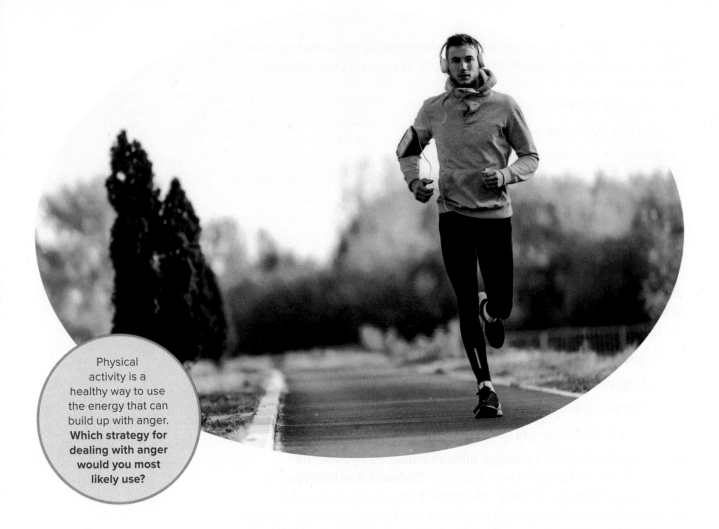

Physical activity is a healthy way to use the energy that can build up with anger. **Which strategy for dealing with anger would you most likely use?**

ACADEMIC VOCABULARY

resource *(noun)*: a source of supply or support

Reading Check

Explain How do people use defense mechanisms?

Handling Fear. Nearly everyone is afraid of something. You can overcome some fears just by recognizing that you're afraid and figuring out what is causing the fear. For example, you may be nervous about giving a presentation in front of a group because you're afraid you will do a bad job and look foolish. You might deal with this fear by getting a friend or a trusted adult to help you prepare for the presentation.

Other fears, such as the fear of going to college or learning to drive a car, may require you to get help from **resources** within your community. If you experience fear that you're unable to control, consider seeking the help of a mental health professional.

Dealing with Guilt. Guilt can also be a very destructive emotion. If it is not managed, it can harm your self-esteem. If you feel guilty about something, think about the cause. Have you hurt someone? In this case, admitting your mistake, apologizing, and promising to be more thoughtful in the future may help relieve your feelings of guilt. However, in other cases, you may discover that your feelings of guilt are misplaced. For instance, if your parents are divorcing, it may upset you, but it's not your fault. Look at the circumstances realistically and honestly, and acknowledge that some situations are out of your control.

Managing Anger. Anger is one of the most difficult emotions to handle. Uncontrolled anger can turn into **hostility**, which can result in harm to the hostile person and to others. As with guilt, it is best to figure out what is causing your anger and then address the problem in a healthy way. When you first feel anger building up inside you, take time to calm down. You might try deep breathing or slowly repeating a calming word or phrase. If this doesn't work, physically remove yourself from the situation. Then try one of these strategies:

- **Do something to relax.** Listen to soothing music, read a book, or picture yourself sitting on a beach or walking through the woods.

- **Channel your energy in a different direction.** Use the energy generated by your anger to do something positive. Take a walk, go for a bike ride, play a musical instrument, or write your feelings down in a private journal.

- **Talk with someone you trust.** Sharing your thoughts and feelings with a trusted friend or family member may help you see the situation from a different point of view. Not only will you feel better, but the listener may also be able to give you some helpful advice on how to handle the situation.

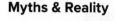

Myths & Reality

We've all heard that it's never good to express emotions such as anger. It's better to use a defense mechanism than to show any emotion.

Myth: Using defense mechanisms is always an unhealthful way to manage emotions.

Reality: Using defense mechanisms is not healthful when they are used as long-term solutions to problems. However, using a defense mechanism can be helpful in coping with difficult emotions, such as anger, on a short-term basis.

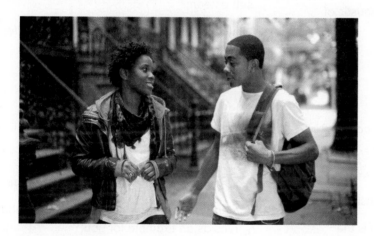

Lesson 3 Review

Facts and Vocabulary

1. What are emotions? How can emotions affect your behavior?

2. What are five common defense mechanisms?

3. List three strategies for handling anger in a healthful way.

Thinking Critically

4. **Analyze.** What role do hormones play in affecting a teen's emotions?

5. **Explain.** Describe what can happen when you take time to think before you respond to a strong emotion. How can this help you stay healthy?

Applying Health Skills

6. **Communication Skills.** Write a one-page script describing how a teen helps a friend manage an emotion such as fear or excitement.

Writing Critically

7. **Descriptive.** Write a poem describing a situation that was emotional for you. Tell how you managed your emotions in a healthful way.

Vocabulary Review

Use the correct vocabulary term to complete the following statements.

1. Having enough skills to do something is called _____.

2. Valuing, respecting, and feeling confident about yourself describes _____.

3. Having the ability to adapt successfully and recover from disappointment, difficulty, or crisis is called being _____.

Understanding Key Concepts

After reading the question or statement, select the correct answer.

4. Which of the following is *not* a characteristic of good mental and emotional health?
   a. Sense of purpose
   b. Pessimistic outlook
   c. Autonomy
   d. Healthy self-esteem

5. Which statement about self-esteem is *not* true?
   a. Self-esteem is always the same.
   b. Self-esteem develops over time.
   c. Self-talk affects self-esteem.
   d. Feedback from others affects self-esteem.

6. Which need within Maslow's hierarchy is the highest-level need?
   a. A safety need
   b. An esteem need
   c. A physical need
   d. The need to reach your potential

Thinking Critically

After reading the question or statement, write a short answer using complete sentences.

7. **Explain.** Why do you think one person can be considered mentally healthier than another when neither has a serious mental problem?

8. **Describe.** How can poor mental health affect your physical health?

9. **Synthesize.** Select one of the suggestions for improving self-esteem. Explain a practical way to make the action or behavior part of your life.

10. **Compare and Contrast.** How might a person with healthy self-esteem respond to a difficult challenge differently than a person with poor self-esteem?

11. **Explain.** Describe how self-esteem can affect your ability to reach your potential.

Vocabulary Review

Correct the sentences below by replacing the italicized term with the correct vocabulary term.

12. A *friend* is someone whose success or behavior serves as an example for you.

13. *Trustworthiness* is a firm observance of core ethical values.

14. *Judgment* involves positive comments that point out problems and encourage improvement.

15. Your *personal identity* is the complex set of characteristics that make you unique.

Understanding Key Concepts

After reading the question or statement, select the correct answer.

16. A person's unique characteristics and group affiliations are known as
    a. features of character.
    b. strengths and weaknesses.
    c. features of identity.
    d. examples of core ethical values.

17. Which quality of good character reflects the importance of community concerns, such as obeying laws and voting?
    a. Responsibility
    b. Trustworthiness
    c. Caring
    d. Citizenship

18. Choosing not to cheat is an example of
    a. recognizing your strengths and weaknesses.
    b. demonstrating positive values.
    c. developing a purpose in your life.
    d. forming meaningful relationships.

19. The groups you belong to help you define
    a. characteristics that you share with other people.
    b. ways to get along with other people.
    c. how people are different.
    d. none of the above.

Thinking Critically

After reading the question or statement, write a short answer using complete sentences.

20. **Discuss.** Name some values that parents likely pass on to their children.

21. **Synthesize.** Why do you think responsibility, honesty, and respect are values that exist across cultures?

22. **Explain.** How might unhealthful risk behaviors affect your health and identity?

23. **Identify.** What are some examples of healthful risk behaviors?

24. **Describe.** What are some ways that good character is related to healthy identity?

LESSON 3

Vocabulary Review

Use the correct vocabulary term to complete the following statements.

25. A chemical produced by your glands that regulates the activities of different body cells is a(n) _____.

26. The intentional use of unfriendly or offensive behavior is called _____.

27. The ability to imagine and understand how someone else feels is called _____.

28. Mental processes that you use to protect yourself from strong or stressful emotions or situations are called _____.

Understanding Key Concepts

After reading the question or statement, select the correct answer.

29. Which of the following is *not* true about anger?
    a. It can result in violence.
    b. Often another emotion is involved.
    c. You become angry as you think about a situation.
    d. It causes little emotional harm.

30. A cause of guilt is
  a. acting against your values.
  b. doing a good deed.
  c. repressing an unpleasant feeling.
  d. recognizing you are not the cause of a negative situation.

31. Which is *not* a positive way to express an emotion?
  a. Hugging
  b. Smiling
  c. Yelling
  d. Laughing

32. Which of the following defense mechanisms uses excuse-making to explain a situation?
  a. Repression
  b. Rationalization
  c. Denial
  d. Compensation

Thinking Critically

After reading the question or statement, write a short answer using complete sentences.

33. **Analyze.** How do peers, family, and friends influence the way you express and manage emotions?

34. **Evaluate.** What might the effects of changing hormone levels during the teen years have on emotions?

35. **Explain.** Why are emotions neither good nor bad?

36. **Identify.** Name one positive characteristic that can be developed when you learn to recognize and express emotions in healthful ways. Discuss how acquiring this characteristic might affect your relationships.

37. **Evaluate.** What are possible consequences to everyone involved when a person responds violently to anger?

┌─ PROJECT-BASED ASSESSMENT ─

Watching for Signs of Mental Illness

BACKGROUND

Good mental health is important to the well-being of everyone. The signs of mental illness, however, are sometimes easy to miss. Recognizing the early signs can help address and treat these problems.

TASK

Conduct an online search and create a podcast describing the early warning signs of one or two mental illnesses.

AUDIENCE

Students at your school

PURPOSE

Help students recognize the warning signs of mental illness. Encourage them to seek help for themselves and others.

PROCEDURE

1. Work in groups to review the information in Module 3 regarding mental health. Assign tasks and responsibilities to each group member.

2. Visit various websites that discuss the early warning signs of the mental illnesses the group has chosen.

3. Create a podcast which includes clear examples of the warning signs.

4. Be sure to explain how mental illness affects teens, and give resources for help.

5. Present your podcast to the students in your class.

6. Ask your teacher for help to create a unified podcast that represents the entire class, to be presented to the principal and possibly added to the school's website.

Math Practice

Interpret Graphs. A survey of 500 U.S. teens ages 14 to 17 shows that participating in after-school activities can improve grades. Use the graph to answer Questions 1–3.

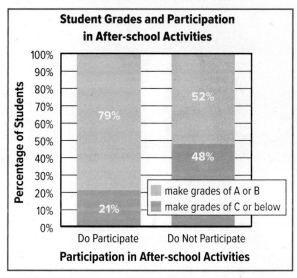

Student Grades and Participation in After-school Activities

Percentage of Students

- 79% — Do Participate (make grades of A or B)
- 21% — Do Participate (make grades of C or below)
- 52% — Do Not Participate (make grades of A or B)
- 48% — Do Not Participate (make grades of C or below)

make grades of A or B
make grades of C or below

Participation in After-school Activities

Adapted from "The YMCA's Teen Action Agenda" by Nels Ericson, *Office of Juvenile Justice and Delinquency Prevention Fact Sheet,* May 2001.

1. Among 1,000 teens who do not participate in after-school activities, how many receive grades of A or B?
   a. 210
   b. 480
   c. 520
   d. 790

2. Choose the fraction of teens who participate in after-school activities and receive grades of A or B.
   a. 1/8
   b. 1/7
   c. 1/4
   d. 4/5

3. Using the information in the chart, what could you conclude about teens between the ages of 14 and 17?
   a. Most make grades of A or B.
   b. Most make grades of C or below.
   c. Most are in after-school activities.
   d. Most are not in after-school activities.

Reading/Writing Practice

Understand and Apply. Read the passage below, and then answer the questions.

Rob had a social studies project due on Monday. "I've got plenty of time," he decided on Thursday. On Friday, he waited for a brilliant idea before giving up. Saturday he went to a baseball game. Rob finally sat down Sunday and worked late into the night. His grade reflected the lack of time and planning he spent on the project.

Rob experienced two common reasons why people procrastinate, or put things off: waiting for inspiration to strike and lack of planning. There are several ways to overcome procrastination. Break large tasks into smaller, more manageable parts. Make a list of everything that needs to be done. Work on each item separately. Tell friends and family your deadlines to help reduce distractions.

1. Which statement best sums up the main point? Procrastination
   a. can be overcome by approaching a task in a variety of ways.
   b. prevents you from starting projects.
   c. creates negative consequences.
   d. causes delays starting for fear of not doing a good enough job.

2. Which of the following does not summarize a suggestion for overcoming procrastination?
   a. Break down the task into smaller, more manageable parts.
   b. Make a list of everything you need to do.
   c. Just sit down and do the work.
   d. Set a deadline for completing.

3. Write a brief essay describing three ways you can avoid Rob's dilemma.

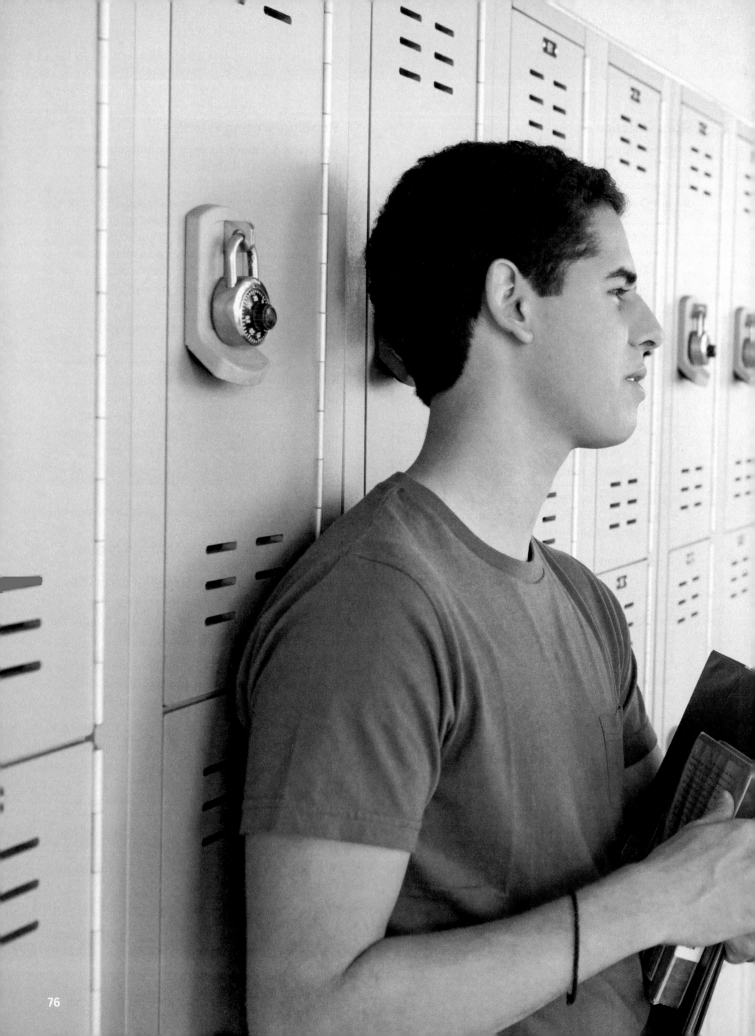

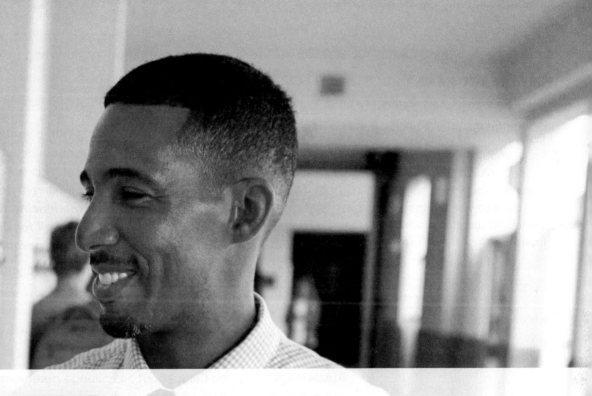

MODULE 4

Managing Stress and Coping with Loss

LESSONS

1 Understanding Stress

2 Managing Stress

3 Coping with Loss and Grief

Understanding Stress

. . . .

BEFORE YOU READ

Create a K-W-L Chart. Make a three-column chart. In the first column, list what you know about stress. In the second column, list what you want to know about this topic. As you read, use the third column to summarize what you learned.

K	W	L

Vocabulary

perception
distress
stressor
psychosomatic response

. . . .

BIG IDEA Stress can affect you in both positive and negative ways.

REAL LIFE ISSUES

Stage Fright. Cari woke up this morning with a vague sense of dread. Now, sitting at her desk in school, she has butterflies in her stomach and her palms are sweaty. Today is oral report day, and Cari is next. She is nervous about speaking in front of her classmates. *Why do you think Cari is experiencing these symptoms? How might she try to calm herself for the presentation? Explain your thoughts in a paragraph.*

After completing the lesson, review and analyze your response to the Real Life Issues question.

What is Stress?

MAIN IDEA How you think about a challenge determines whether you will experience positive or negative stress.

Have you ever described yourself as being "stressed out"? Stress is the way your body and mind react to everyday challenges and demands. Sometimes, stress comes on quickly, like when you are late and running to catch the bus. In other cases, stress can build slowly for days, like when you feel the pressure to perform well in a sports event or on a final exam.

Stress is a natural part of life. In many cases, the situations that cause it are unavoidable. How much a stressful event affects you, however, depends partly on your **perception** of it. Perception is the act of becoming aware through the senses. For example, you might believe that a disagreement with a friend has ruined your friendship. Your friend, on the other hand, might believe that you'll be able to work out the problem in the end. Because of the way you perceive the argument, you will probably feel more stress over it than your friend does.

Your reaction to stressful events depends partly on your previous experiences. For instance, if you enjoy playing in a band, you might not feel nervous about having a solo performance. However, if you've made a mistake during a band performance, you might worry about how well you'll play during your solo.

Reacting to Stress

Stress is not always a bad thing. Sometimes stress can have a positive effect. Feeling stress can be a motivator. Actions that you take to reduce stress are called coping strategies. These are the actions that you take to manage stress. For example, a student who wants to focus on a career as an engineer may feel stress when a big math exam is coming up. The stress a student feels can motivate him or her to study harder for the test in order to get a good grade.

Stress, however, can also have a negative effect. This is called **distress** and it can impair your ability to function. Distress is negative stress that prevents you from doing what you need to do, or stress that causes discomfort. Distress can make a person feel distracted, overwhelmed, impatient, frustrated, or angry.

Causes of Stress

MAIN IDEA Stressors vary among individuals and groups.

Think back to the last time you felt stress in your life. Can you remember what caused it? A **stressor** is anything that causes stress. Stressors can be real or imagined, **anticipated** or unexpected. People, objects, places, events, and situations can all be sources of stress.

The way stressors affect you personally can depend on your experiences and perceptions. What causes stress for you may not cause stress for someone else. For example, public speaking can be terrifying for some people, while others barely feel any nervousness about it at all. However, there are some stressors, like sirens, that affect most people in the same way—by causing heightened alertness.

Reading Check

Explain How can your perception of an event affect the amount of stress you feel?

ACADEMIC VOCABULARY

anticipate (*verb*): to expect

Meeting the demands of an active schedule can be stressful. **How do you deal with the stresses of a regular school day?**

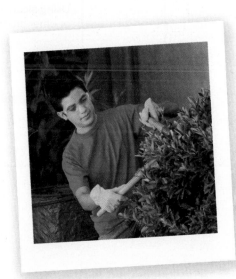
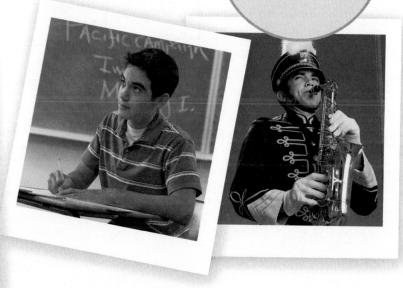

(l to r)Tim Fuller Photography

Your Body's Response to Stressors

MAIN IDEA Stressors activate the nervous system and specific hormones.

Reading Check

List What are the three stages of the body's stress response?

When you perceive something to be dangerous, difficult, or painful, your body automatically begins a stress response. For example, if you are walking by your neighbors' house and their dog suddenly starts barking, you might feel startled and your heart might start racing. The sudden, loud noise is a stressor that affects you automatically, without any thought.

The body's response to stress is largely involuntary, or automatic. It involves both your nervous system and your endocrine, or hormonal, system. The physical stress response is the same regardless of the type of stressor. It involves three stages:

- **Alarm.** Your mind and body go on high alert. This reaction is sometimes called the "fight-or-flight response" because it prepares your body either to defend itself or to flee from a threat.

- **Resistance.** If your exposure to the stressor continues, your body adapts and reacts to the stressor. You may perform at a higher level and with more endurance for a short period.

- **Fatigue.** If exposure to stress is prolonged, your body loses its ability to adapt. You begin to tire and lose the ability to manage other stressors effectively.

STRESSORS FOR TEENS				
Life Situations	**Environmental**	**Biological**	**Cognitive (Thinking)**	**Personal Behavior**
• School demands • Problems with friends, bullying • Peer pressure • Family problems, abuse • Moving or changing schools • Breaking up with a girlfriend or boyfriend	• Unsafe neighborhood • Media (TV, magazines, newspapers, Internet) • Natural disasters • Threat of terrorist attacks • War • Global warming	• Changes in body • Illness • Injury • Disability	• Poor self-esteem • Personal appearance • Not fitting in	• Taking on a busy schedule • Relationship issues • Smoking • Using alcohol or other drugs

Stress and Your Health

MAIN IDEA Ongoing stress affects all aspects of your health.

The physical changes that take place during the stress response can take a toll on your body. Prolonged stress can lead to a **psychosomatic response**, or a physical reaction that results from stress rather than from an injury or illness. Physical effects of stress can include:

- headache.
- a weakened immune system.
- high blood pressure.
- bruxism (clenching the jaw or grinding the teeth).
- digestive disorders.

Mental/emotional and social effects of stress include mood swings, irritability, and difficulty concentrating. Some people attempt to counter the effects of stress by using alcohol or drugs. However, this only creates more problems, especially if the person begins abusing these substances.

The Alarm Response

Alarm begins when the hypothalamus, a small area at the base of the brain, receives danger signals from other parts of the brain. The hypothalamus releases a hormone that acts on the pituitary gland. The pituitary gland secretes a hormone that stimulates the adrenal glands. The adrenal glands secrete adrenaline. Adrenaline is the "emergency hormone" that prepares the body to respond to a stressor.

The physical symptoms of the alarm response include:

- Dilated pupils.
- Increase in perspiration.
- Faster heart rate and pulse.
- Rise in blood pressure.
- Faster respiration rate.
- Narrowing of arteries to internal organs and skin.
- Increased blood flow to muscles and brain.
- Increase in muscle tension.
- Release of blood sugar, fats, and cholesterol.

Character Check

Responsibility Although you cannot control external events, you *can* control how you respond to them. For example, you can choose to adapt to and learn from each situation and challenge you face. Think about a recent disappointment or difficulty you have experienced. How did you bounce back from the situation? How can you apply what you learned about yourself and how you handle stress to similar events in the future?

How Stressed Out Are You?

School is a cause of stress for many teens. In a study that examined what worried teens most about going back to school, nearly a third named schoolwork. Almost as many teens reported that they were worried about social concerns and physical appearance issues. The results of the study found that:

• 32 percent reported schoolwork issues.

• 30 percent reported social issues.

• 25 percent reported physical appearance issues.

• 3 percent reported extracurricular issues.

• 10 percent reported no worries about returning to school.

Identifying the causes of stress in your life is the first step to handling it. If you know the cause, you can figure out how to prevent it or at least reduce its effects on you.

Activity: Mathematics

The study received completed surveys from 600 teens.

1. How many teens felt that issues other than schoolwork caused them stress?
2. How many teens experienced no worries about returning to school?
3. What worries you about returning to school? How do you cope with the stress of new classes?

CONCEPT Ratios and Proportional Relationships: Percents

A percent is a ratio comparing a number to 100. It can also be represented as a fraction with 100 as the denominator. To find the percent of a number, change the percent to a fraction or decimal, then multiply by the number.

Lesson 1 Review

Facts and Vocabulary

1. Define the word *perception*.
2. What are three cognitive stressors for teens?
3. Identify the two body systems involved in the stress response.

Thinking Critically

4. **Synthesize.** Identify one way that stress has had a positive effect on your performance.
5. **Analyze.** Explain how a person in an extremely high-stress situation is able to accomplish an incredible feat of strength, such as lifting a car to free a person trapped underneath.

Applying Health Skills

6. **Analyzing Influences.** Describe ways that peer influence might increase the amount of stress that teens experience.

Writing Critically

7. **Expository.** Write a paragraph describing the positive and negative effects that stress has on your emotions.

Managing Stress

BIG IDEA You can manage stress by learning skills to reduce the amount and impact of stress in your life.

REAL LIFE ISSUES

Ways to Handle Stress. Learning how to manage stress will help you feel more comfortable and confident. When you feel stressed, what types of activities help you relax? The American Psychological Association asked people to report the most common ways they manage stress. Those responses included listening to music, exercising, and spending time with family and friends. *Write a paragraph describing how you manage stress.*

After completing the lesson, review and analyze your response to the Real Life Issues question.

When Stress Becomes a Problem

MAIN IDEA Identifying what is stressful is the first step in learning how to manage stress.

Sometimes, the cause of stress is obvious. It can happen because you're late for an appointment, your computer crashes while you're doing homework, or you realize that you've left an important assignment at home. When you know the cause of stress, you can find ways to resolve the problem. Unfortunately, people often don't recognize the stressors in their lives. In many cases, they realize that they're feeling stressed only after the stress has begun to affect their health.

The effects of stress are *additive,* meaning that they build up over time. Unless you find ways of managing stress, it will take a physical and mental toll on you. In today's demanding world, increasing numbers of teens are experiencing **chronic stress**, which is stress associated with long-term problems that are beyond a person's control. For these teens, stress has become a constant burden that can last for months.

Fortunately, there are some positive steps you can take to deal with stress. Although you can't eliminate all stress from your life, you can learn to manage it. The trick is to use strategies to keep stress from building up and to deal with individual stressors effectively.

BEFORE YOU READ

Create a Cluster Chart.
Draw a circle and label it "Stress-Management Skills." Use surrounding circles to define and describe this term. As you read, continue filling in the chart with more details

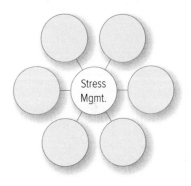

Stress Mgmt.

Vocabulary
chronic stress
relaxation response

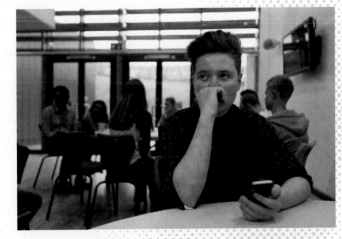

Stress-Management Techniques

MAIN IDEA You can develop strategies to both avoid and reduce your stress.

Stress-management skills help you deal with stressors in a healthful, effective way. Some of these skills involve using coping strategies to prevent stress. Others focus on coping with the impact of stress on your body and mind.

Avoiding and Limiting Stress

One of the easiest ways to reduce the effects of stress in your life is to avoid the situations that cause it. While you can't avoid stressors entirely, you can try to restrict or limit the amount of stress you're exposed to. Here are a few effective strategies you can try:

- **Use refusal skills.** Determine whether you have time for a new activity before deciding to take it on. If the new activity will raise your stress level too much, then use refusal skills to say no.

- **Plan ahead.** Manage your time wisely by planning tasks in advance. For example, think about how stressed you feel before a test. You can reduce this stress by planning for tests well in advance and studying a little each night. You may find that it helps to outline class material, highlighting and numbering the most important points to learn them quickly.

- **Think positively.** We are not able to control the events in our lives, but we *can* control how we respond to them. A positive outlook can limit stress by shifting your perception of stressors and the way you react to them. For example, try viewing a typical stressor, like an upcoming exam, as a learning opportunity. You can also try using positive self-talk, such as "I can do this!" or "Way to go!"

- **Avoid tobacco, alcohol, and other drugs.** Using tobacco, alcohol, and other drugs in an attempt to relieve stress will actually harm the body, leading to more stress.

OVERCOMING TEST ANXIETY
Plan for tests well in advance, studying a little each night.
Learn to outline material, highlighting and numbering important points to learn them quickly.
During a test, do some deep breathing. Get comfortable in your chair. Use positive self-talk such as "I can do this!" or "Way to go!"
Answer all the questions you are sure of, then go back and answer the ones that are more difficult.
After getting your corrected test back, examine your mistakes. If you don't understand the correction, ask your teacher.

Handling Stress

Some stressors in life are unavoidable. Some days you may find yourself running late for school because traffic is bad, or the bus had a flat tire. If you have a part-time job, you may find that your workday becomes more stressful when your boss is also feeling stressed. If you cannot avoid a stressor, try to find ways to reduce its negative effects that will enable you to achieve a **relaxation response**. To lower the impact of stress on your health, try these tips:

- **Practice relaxation techniques.** Deep breathing, thinking pleasant thoughts, stretching, taking a warm bath, getting a massage, and even laughing can relax your body and relieve your stress. For instance, during a test, you can try to do some deep breathing **techniques** and make sure you are sitting comfortably in your chair.

- **Redirect your energy.** When stress causes tension to build up in your body and mind, the best thing to do is use that extra energy in a constructive way. You can put nervous energy to good use through physical activity: going for a walk or a swim, jogging, riding your bike, or playing a game of pickup basketball. Working on a creative project can also be a good way to channel your stress into something positive.

- **Seek support.** Sometimes just talking about a problem can make you feel better. When you feel stressed, try confiding in someone you trust, such as a parent, guardian, sibling, teacher, or close friend. People who care about you may be able to give you a new perspective and possibly some useful advice.

Reading Check

Explain How can refusal skills help you avoid stress?

ACADEMIC VOCABULARY

technique *(noun)*: a method of accomplishing a desired aim

Planning ahead can help you avoid or limit stress. **What other actions can you take to manage stress?**

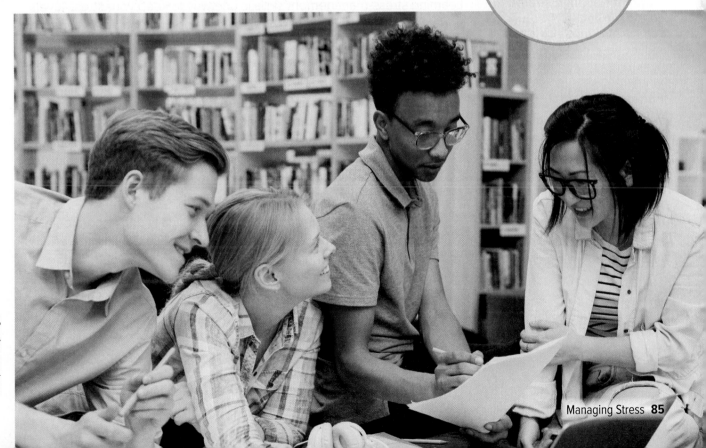

mediaphotos/Getty Images

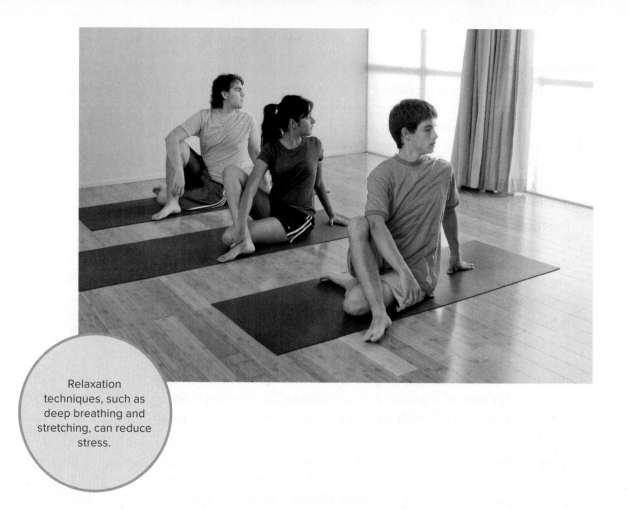

Relaxation techniques, such as deep breathing and stretching, can reduce stress.

Staying Healthy and Building Resiliency

MAIN IDEA Taking care of your health is essential to stress management.

Learning stress-management skills is one way to keep your stress levels under control. However, it also helps to develop good habits that maintain your general health. These habits are a form of self-maintenance. They can help you prevent or reduce stress, deal with stress in positive ways, and recover mentally and physically from stress.

- **Get Adequate Rest.** Too little sleep can affect your ability to concentrate. This, in turn, can affect your schoolwork, athletics, and even relationships. By contrast, getting plenty of sleep can help you face the challenges and demands of the new day. Practicing good time management will allow you to get the eight to nine hours of sleep that most teens need each night.

- **Get Regular Physical Activity.** Being physically active on a daily basis benefits your overall health. And if you are feeling the effects of stress, participating in physical activity can help you manage them. Physical activity can release pent-up energy and clear your mind. Regular exercise also improves your energy level and endurance and helps you sleep better.

Reading Check

Identify What three self-maintenance habits can reduce your level of stress?

Fitness Zone

With school, work, and everything else, my friends and I can get really stressed out. I found that working out is the best stress reliever. When I'm feeling really stressed, I go for a run, swim, or just shoot some baskets on my own. Afterward, I always feel less stressed out.

Tim Fuller Photography

- **Eat Healthful Foods.** Eating a variety of healthful foods and drinking plenty of water helps your body function properly every day. Proper nutrition can reduce the effects of stress, while poor eating habits can cause weakness, fatigue, and inability to concentrate. These can add to your overall stress level. Overeating and undereating can also put your body under stress. Beverages high in sugar and caffeine, such as coffee drinks or energy drinks, can increase the effects of stress.

- **Become Resilient.** Making self-maintenance and stress-management strategies a part of your daily routine can help you become more resilient. You'll be able to adapt more effectively to new situations. Resiliency also lets you recover from disappointments, difficulties, or crises. For example, you would probably feel disappointed if you tried out for a part in a school play and didn't get it. However, if you are resilient, you will bounce back from this disappointment and resolve to work harder for the next audition. Resiliency helps you handle difficulties and challenges in healthful ways and achieve long-term success in spite of problems.

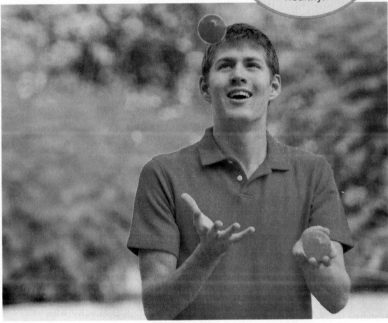

Sometimes you may feel like you are juggling lots of things at once. Developing good habits to reduce and manage daily stressors will help you stay healthy.

Lesson 2 Review

Facts and Vocabulary

1. Define *chronic stress*.

2. Identify four strategies to avoid or limit stress.

3. Identify three relaxation techniques.

Thinking Critically

4. **Synthesize.** It's Wednesday, and Ariana's biology test is on Friday. As she sits down to study, her friend Conner calls and asks her to go out. How might Ariana balance her activities and manage her stress?

5. **Describe.** Explain the role of positive thinking as a stress-management strategy.

Applying Health Skills

6. **Practicing Healthful Behaviors.** Some of the habits that you practice to maintain overall health can also help manage stress. Design a poster illustrating the habits that can help you manage stress.

Writing Critically

7. **Personal.** Evaluate your own wellness in regard to stress. Write a paragraph to explain your assessment.

Coping with Loss and Grief

BEFORE YOU READ

Create Vocabulary Cards.
Write each new vocabulary term on a separate note card. For each term, write a definition based on your current knowledge. As you read, fill in additional information related to each term.

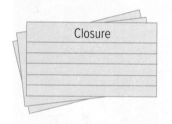

Closure

Vocabulary
stages of grief
closure
coping
mourning
traumatic event

. . . .

BIG IDEA Understanding the grieving process helps you cope with loss and manage your feelings in healthy ways.

┌─ **REAL LIFE ISSUES** ───────────────────

Losing a Close Relative. Kelly has always been close to her grandfather. Every weekend they would spend time together, taking walks, watching movies, playing chess, or just talking. Last week, he died quietly in his sleep at the age of 92. Kelly misses him terribly and feels as if there is a big hole in her life. *If you were Kelly's friend, how might you comfort her as she tries to cope with the loss of her grandfather? Write a dialogue between you and Kelly in which you offer support and sympathy.*

After completing the lesson, review and analyze your response to the Real Life Issues question.

└──

Acknowledging Loss

MAIN IDEA Acknowledging a loss is one way to help begin the healing process.

At least once in your life, you have probably experienced a loss that left you feeling sad. Perhaps your best friend moved to another state, or your girlfriend or boyfriend broke up with you. You may have had to change schools and leave behind some good friends. You may even have had to deal with the death of someone you love—perhaps a friend, family member, or pet. Loss, and the sorrow that it brings, is an unavoidable part of life.

Grieving is a common and natural reaction to any loss that brings on strong emotions. Loss feels hurtful, but it does not have to be harmful. Immediately after a loss, you may feel that you will never recover and that your life will never be the same. Again, these feelings are natural. Acknowledging and understanding your grief is the first step in the healing process. Over time, you will learn to cope with the loss and manage your feelings related to it.

Expressing Grief

MAIN IDEA The grieving process can help people accept the loss and start to heal.

Feelings of loss are very personal. In addition to sadness, some people feel guilt or even anger. Some feel the need to talk about their loss, while others want to be alone. Sometimes people experience different, conflicting reactions at different times.

The Grieving Process

While all people have their own ways of grieving, there are some parts of the grieving process that many people go through. Swiss-American psychiatrist Elisabeth Kübler-Ross identified five **stages of grief**, a variety of reactions that may surface as an individual makes sense of how a loss affects him or her. These are common parts of the grieving process. Not everyone goes through each stage, and the order may be different for each person. However, most people will experience many of these stages:

- **Denial or Numbness**. At this stage, it seems difficult to believe that the loss has really happened.

- **Anger**. The person may feel powerless and unfairly deprived. These feelings are often experienced as anger.

- **Bargaining**. As the reality of the loss sets in, the person may try to make promises to change in the hope of bringing back what has been lost.

- **Depression**. The person may become preoccupied with thoughts about how the loss could have been prevented.

- **Acceptance**. The person faces the reality of the loss and experiences **closure**, or the acceptance of a loss.

Letting yourself experience and accept these feelings as you grieve is necessary for healing These feelings are part of **coping**, or dealing successfully with difficult changes in your life.

Reading Check

Identify List the five stages of grief.

Grieving is a process that you need not experience alone. **How might receiving comfort and support help you through a loss?**

Antonio Guillem/Shutterstock

Coping with Death

MAIN IDEA Coping with death involves receiving and showing support.

Death is one of the most painful losses anyone can experience. Even if a person dies after a long illness, it's normal for the survivors to grieve. If a death was sudden, painful, or violent, the survivors may experience shock as well.

Most people respond to death by **mourning**. Mourning is the act of showing sorrow or grief. Acts of mourning may include talking about the person, experiencing the pain of the loss, and searching for meaning. For some people, it may take a long time to move out of the mourning process. While the grieving process can't be rushed, dwelling on things that can't be changed will only add to the pain. Thinking about happy memories of the person and your relationship, by contrast, may help ease the pain of a death.

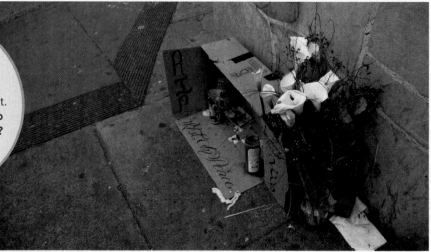

Memorial services and sites help people grieve and show respect. **What are other ways to remember a loved one?**

Showing Empathy

The grieving process is more difficult when you feel that you have to go through it alone. The friendship and support of other mourners may make the process easier. If you don't feel that you can talk to your family and other loved ones about the loss, try confiding in a supportive friend. Likewise, if you know someone who is grieving, there are ways you can show support. Showing empathy for a friend who is grieving is one way to help a person through their grief.

- Help the person to recall happy, positive memories.

- Be a sympathetic listener. This includes allowing silence where appropriate. Sometimes, just nodding your head, rather than trying to respond, is the best way to show that you understand what the person is saying.

- Don't rush the grieving process or try to **resolve** the person's grief in a single day. Remember, no one can lead another person through this process or make it go faster.

ACADEMIC VOCABULARY

resolve *(verb)*: to deal with successfully

Community Support

A person's cultural background can also influence his or her ways of grieving. Common mourning rituals, such as memorial services, wakes, and funerals, are events that celebrate the life of the person who has died and bring comfort to the mourners. Telling stories or describing why the person was special can help you move through the grieving process. Clergy members and mental health professionals who specialize in grief can also provide support.

Coping with Traumatic Events

MAIN IDEA Support from family, friends, and community resources can help individuals recover from a traumatic event.

Traumatic events, such as accidents, violent assaults, suicides, and natural disasters, are sudden and shocking. After a traumatic event, you may feel unsafe and insecure about the future. Support from family members, friends, and community groups or agencies can help you manage your shock and grief. Remember that others in your community are likely to be grieving as well. By sharing your feelings, you can provide mutual support to each other and help each other learn to cope. Trying to resume your normal activities, or at least some of them, can also be a part of the healing process.

Myths & Reality

Grieving is a natural reaction to any loss that brings on strong emotions. However, one myth says that the grief response refers only to a loss through death.

Myth: We grieve only death.

Reality: All losses cause grief. Losing a friend who is moving away can be just as painful. The friend will not be part of your life in the same way, and that creates a sense of loss.

Lesson 3 Review

Facts and Vocabulary

1. Identify the stages of grief.

2. Define the term *coping*.

3. List three examples of a traumatic event.

Thinking Critically

4. **Analyze.** How might coping with a death resulting from a long-term illness differ from coping with a sudden death caused by an accident?

5. **Apply.** Recall a story of personal loss that you read about in a book or saw in a movie. Write a paragraph that describes the process of grieving that the main character went through.

Applying Health Skills

6. **Communication Skills.** Write a letter expressing caring and empathy to a friend who is grieving for a loved one.

Writing Critically

7. **Expository.** Write a paragraph describing ways that people in the community and community support groups can help someone who is coping with a loss.

Vocabulary Review

Use the correct vocabulary terms to complete the following statements.

1. _____ is the reaction of the body and mind to everyday challenges and demands.

2. Anything that causes stress is called a(n) _____.

3. A physical reaction that results from stress rather than from an injury or illness is called a(n) _____.

Understanding Key Concepts

After reading the question or statement, select the correct answer.

4. The amount of stress that you experience mostly relates to
   a. the type of friends that you have.
   b. where you go to school.
   c. your perception of stressors.
   d. how your parents respond to stress.

5. During which stage of the body's stress response are hormones released?
   a. Resistance
   b. Alarm
   c. Fatigue
   d. Recovery

6. Which of the following is *not* a physical symptom of the alarm response?
   a. Faster heart rate and pulse
   b. Decreased blood flow to muscles and brain
   c. Increase in perspiration
   d. Increase in blood pressure

Thinking Critically

After reading the question or statement, write a short answer using complete sentences.

7. **Identify.** What are the five categories of stressors?

8. **Infer.** How would trying an activity for the first time affect your stress level?

9. **Synthesize.** Suppose you've been assigned to work on a project with three students you don't know. How might this affect your perception of doing the project?

10. **Analyze.** Describe how mental fatigue that results from stress can affect your ability to study.

11. **Describe.** List three physical symptoms of stress.

12. **Infer**. You've spent three months feeling stressed while studying for an important exam. What impact could this stress have on your health?

Vocabulary Review

Correct the sentences below by replacing the italicized term with the correct vocabulary term.

13. Using refusal skills, planning ahead, and practicing relaxation techniques are examples of *chronic stress.*

14. You are *relaxed* if you are able to adapt effectively and recover from disappointment, difficulty, or crisis.

15. Practicing stress-management techniques can help you achieve a state of calm, or a *chronic stress,* when stressed.

16. Stress associated with long-term problems beyond one's control is known as *resilient.*

Understanding Key Concepts

After reading the question or statement, select the correct answer.

17. Which is *not* a relaxation technique?
- **a.** Taking a warm bath
- **b.** Laughing
- **c.** Eating a comfort food
- **d.** Deep breathing

18. One way to prevent taking on an activity that will add to your level of stress is to
- **a.** procrastinate.
- **b.** use refusal skills.
- **c.** think positively.
- **d.** redirect your energy.

19. Which of the following is *not* a way to redirect energy that may build up as a result of stress?
- **a.** Going for a walk
- **b.** Watching TV
- **c.** Riding your bike
- **d.** Working on a creative project

20. Which is *not* an effect of physical activity on stress?
- **a.** Clears your head
- **b.** Increases energy level
- **c.** Helps you sleep better
- **d.** Helps you avoid stress

Thinking Critically

After reading the question or statement, write a short answer using complete sentences.

21. Explain. How does identifying personal stressors help in the development of a stress-management plan?

22. Analyze. Why are the effects of stress additive? How can additive stressors affect your health?

23. Synthesize. What might be some important considerations when planning ahead for a research project that is due in three weeks?

24. Analyze. Why shouldn't people smoke cigarettes as a way to relieve stress?

25. Analyze. Explain how having resiliency can help you manage your stress.

LESSON 3

Vocabulary Review

Choose the correct term in the sentences below.

26. *Closure/Coping* is acceptance of a loss.

27. *Coping/Mourning* is the act of showing sorrow or grief.

28. A stressful event that overwhelms your coping strategies is called a *traumatic event/stage of grief.*

Understanding Key Concepts

After reading the question or statement, select the correct answer.

29. Which is *not* a stage of grief?
- **a.** Remorse
- **b.** Empathy
- **c.** Acceptance
- **d.** Denial

30. The needed outcome of grieving is
- **a.** anger.
- **b.** sympathy.
- **c.** remorse.
- **d.** closure.

31. You can show support to someone who is grieving by
- **a.** helping the person recall happy memories.
- **b.** being a sympathetic listener.
- **c.** not rushing the grieving process.
- **d.** all of the above.

32. During which stage of grief do people make a promise to change if what was lost can be returned?
  a. Denial
  b. Depression
  c. Bargaining
  d. Hope

33. Which of the following strategies can help someone cope with a traumatic event?
  a. Spending time alone
  b. Delaying getting back to a daily routine
  c. Putting off grieving
  d. Seeking support from the community

Thinking Critically

After reading the question or statement, write a short answer using complete sentences.

34. **Describe.** What are four examples of loss that could cause someone to experience the grieving process?

35. **Evaluate.** How do you think the ability or inability to remain open to relationships could affect the way a person responds to loss?

36. **Analyze.** What is necessary in order for healing to occur after a loss?

37. **Explain.** At which stage of the grieving process might a person become unable to move on? What should people do if they have difficulty moving through the stages of grief?

38. **Explain.** How do mourning rituals following a death help individuals during the grieving process?

39. **Identify.** Who is available in a community to respond to the needs of survivors of a traumatic event?

PROJECT-BASED ASSESSMENT

The Stages of Grief

BACKGROUND
We all have to cope with a significant loss some time in our lives. A best friend may move to another city, or a close family member may pass away. The grieving process occurs in stages, and understanding those stages will help you cope with loss.

TASK
Conduct an online search about the grieving process. Create a podcast describing the grieving process.

AUDIENCE
Students in your class

PURPOSE
Help other students learn about the grieving process and how they can help someone who is grieving.

PROCEDURE

1. Form small groups. Divide the tasks. Some members may want to conduct the Internet search or write the script for the podcast. Others may want to perform in the podcast.

2. Using the information in Module 4, as well as additional Internet resources, research the stages of grief.

3. Write the script for a podcast about a student who has suffered a significant loss. The podcast should describe the student moving through all the stages of grief.

4. Record the podcast to be played in class.

Math Practice

Interpret Tables. Angelika conducted a survey of 296 students at her school to determine what caused them the most stress. The results of her survey are shown in the table below. Use the table to answer Questions 1–3.

STUDENT STRESSORS AT WASHINGTON HIGH	
Greatest Stressor	**Number of Students**
Grades	93
Peer conflict	81
Family issues	64
Work responsibilities	24
After-school activities	8
Personal health	8
Other	18

1. What percentage of students did not feel that work responsibilities were a stressor?
   a. 88%
   b. 76%
   c. 19%
   d. 92%

2. What number of students reported that family issues caused them the most stress?
   a. 64
   b. 78
   c. 192
   d. 53

3. What could you conclude from the information given in the table?
   a. Most students are stressed about work responsibilities.
   b. After-school activities are stressors for many teens.
   c. Peer conflict ranked second as the greatest stressor for students surveyed.
   d. Personal health issues are stressful for students.

Reading/Writing Practice

Understand and Apply. Read the letter below, and then answer the questions.

Dear Maya,

Things have changed since you moved away. The factory closed and more than 3,000 people are unemployed. I'm sure more people will be leaving town like your family did. Manuel and his family moved, too. Now both of my best friends have left. My parents don't want to tell me, but I can tell that things are not good. I overhear them talking, but they clam up whenever I ask anything. Dad has a new job, but he is making less money. Please write back and let me know how things are going for you. Do your parents have jobs? Have you made new friends? I miss you!

Love,
Isabel

1. Which word *best* describes the tone of this letter?
   a. Angry
   b. Worried
   c. Bitter
   d. Resigned

2. What does this letter reveal most about Isabel?
   a. It's hard for her to make new friends.
   b. She understands life outside her town.
   c. The factory closing led to lost jobs and wages.
   d. She feels stress due to all the changes.

3. Pretend you are Maya and write a reply to Isabel's letter. As Maya, explain what life is like now for you and your family, and how you are dealing with the stress of moving.

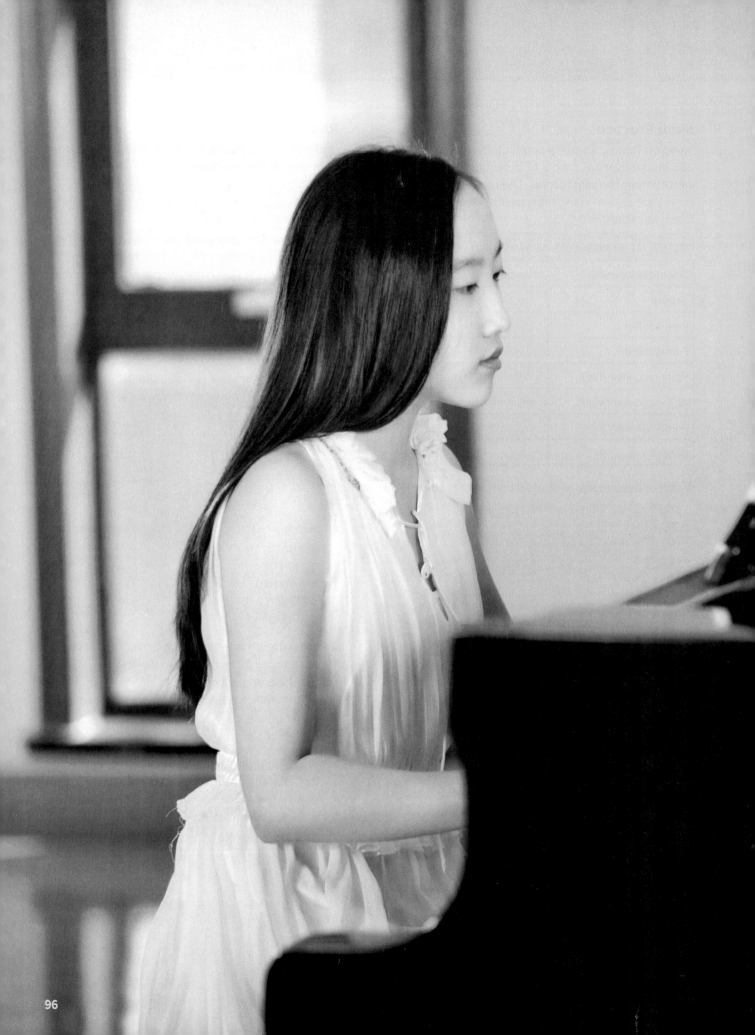

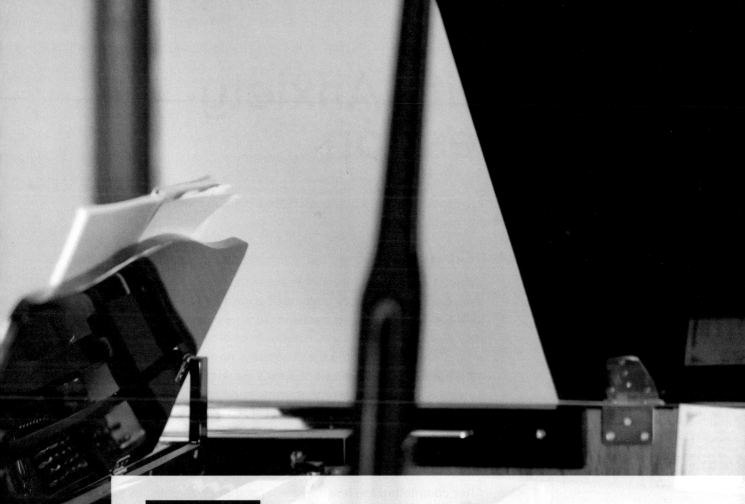

Mental and Emotional Problems

LESSONS

1 Dealing with Anxiety and Depression

2 Mental Disorders

3 Suicide Prevention

4 Getting Help

Dealing with Anxiety and Depression

BEFORE YOU READ

Create an Outline. Look through the lesson to find the headings and subheadings. Write down the headings to make an outline. As you read, fill in details beneath each heading or subheading.

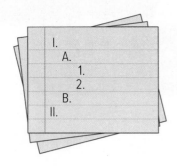

Vocabulary

anxiety
depression
apathy

BIG IDEA Anxiety and depression are treatable mental health problems.

> ### REAL LIFE ISSUES
>
> **Difficult Times.** Tony's parents are separating. He's not really surprised, because they have been arguing a lot lately, but he still feels sad about their decision. Tony worries about how the family will get by financially without both of his parents living at home. The constant feelings of sadness and uncertainty are starting to affect every part of Tony's life. He feels tired all the time, has withdrawn from his friends, and has lost his appetite. All he wants to do is stay home and sleep. *Write a dialogue between you and Tony, as if you were Tony's friend. In your conversation, show him empathy and support during this difficult time. What advice might you give him?*
>
> After completing the lesson, review and analyze your response to the Real Life Issues question.

Understanding Anxiety

MAIN IDEA Occasional anxiety is a normal, manageable reaction to short-term, stressful situations.

Can you remember the last time you felt angry, or scared, or upset? Chances are, it wasn't that long ago since events can happen every day that anger, scare, or upset us. Managing difficult emotions is a normal part of life. They can occur for a variety of reasons, including hormonal changes, relationship issues, grief, or stress.

One common feeling that can be difficult to manage is **anxiety**. Anxiety is the condition of feeling uneasy or worried about what may happen. You may, for example, feel anxious when you have to make an important presentation in front of your class. Occasional anxiety is a natural response to life events. Feelings of worry, insecurity, fear, self-consciousness, or even panic can be common responses to stress. Usually, once the stressful situation is over, the anxiety it caused goes away too.

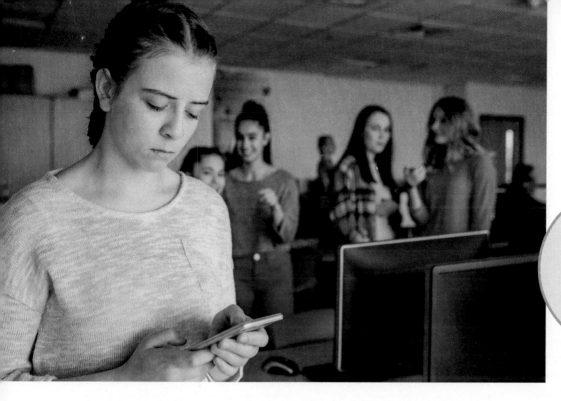

Depression can cause a person to withdraw and suffer alone. **Why might this symptom be dangerous?**

Knowing that anxiety is common, however, doesn't make it easy to handle. To do that, you have to use stress-management techniques. Stress management techniques are tools that you can use to become more resilient. If you feel anxious about an upcoming math test, try using time management techniques to spend a few minutes more each day studying the concepts you need to know for the test. Similarly, if talking in front of a crowd makes you anxious, practice your talk in front of your family or a group of friends.

Some people try to escape from anxiety by using alcohol or drugs. These substances produce a temporary, false sense of relaxation. In the long term, however, they lead to new problems—physical, mental/emotional, social, and legal.

Understanding Depression

MAIN IDEA Depression can linger or be severe enough to disrupt daily activities.

Like anxiety, sadness is a feeling that affects everyone from time to time. **Depression**, however, usually lasts longer and may produce additional symptoms, like prolonged feeling of helplessness, hopelessness, and sadness, that do not go away over time. Depression is a serious condition that **requires** medical help.

About 11 percent of all teens display some signs of depression at one time or another. It's one of the most common mental health concerns among teens. The teen years are a time when most teens experience many changes. Some are good changes. Teens become more independent from family. They think about their adult life and the types of things they want to achieve in the future.

Reading Check

Analyze How can stress management techniques help a teen who suffers from anxiety.

ACADEMIC VOCABULARY

require *(verb)*: to demand as necessary

SolStock/Getty Images

Other changes might be difficult. For example, one teen may become sad or depressed if a friend moves away. The two friends won't be able to spend time together in the future. Another teen may wish to avoid alcohol and drug, and ends a friendship with another teen who uses these substances. Although the teen is protecting his or her future, the person may become sad thinking about the good aspects of the friendship that have also been lost. Resiliency skills can help the teen focus on the positive aspects of growing older and becoming more independent. Using stress management techniques, such as thinking positively and avoiding alcohol and other drugs, can build resiliency and help teens cope with life changes.

In some cases, a bout of depression may pass after a few days. Other times, feelings of depression may last longer. If feelings of sadness do not pass after a few weeks, it may be necessary to seek help from a mental health professional. A person suffering from depression may feel ashamed and unwilling to ask for help. In reality, sometimes a depression will not pass without help from a mental health professional. In some cases, if a depression is not treated, a chemical imbalance may occur in the brain that makes the depression worse. People who suffer from depression should never be made to feel ashamed of asking for help. Depression is a medical condition and may require the help of a medical expert to treat.

When a mental health expert treats a person for depression, the first step is to determine the severity of depression. The severity may depend on the type of depression a person experiences. Sometimes, depression can occur after a difficult life event, such as the death of a loved one. Mental health experts have identified three forms of depression. Forms of depression include:

- Major depression, which is intense and can last for weeks or months.

- Mild or chronic depression, also known as also known as *dysthymia*, which has less severe symptoms, but can persist for years.

- Adjustment disorder is a reaction to a specific life event such as the death of a loved one. Adjustment disorder can also take the form of anxiety that lasts much longer than normal anxiety.

The National Institutes of Health provides valid information on depression and other mental health disorders. To read more, go to http://www.nlm.nih.gov/ and search for the term "depression."

Five or more of these symptoms must persist for two or more weeks before a diagnosis of major depression is indicated.

WARNING SIGNS OF DEPRESSION	
Persistent sad or irritable mood	Loss of energy
Loss of interest in activities once enjoyed	Feelings of worthlessness or inappropriate guilt
Change in appetite or body weight	Difficulty concentrating or making decisions
Difficulty sleeping or oversleeping	Recurrent thoughts of death or suicide
Restlessness or irritability	Feeling hopeless

Causes and Effects of Depression

Depression can have a physical, psychological, or social cause. Sometimes it is a symptom of a medical condition. It may be caused by illness. It may also appear during or after traumatic life events. Social or environmental factors may also play a role. Living in poverty or in a physically or emotionally harmful environment can cause depression. People who are depressed may experience symptoms such as:

- **Changes in thinking.** People who suffer from depression may have trouble concentrating and making decisions. They may also have self-destructive thoughts.

- **Changes in feelings.** People who are depressed may feel sad or irritable and angry. They may also experience a general **apathy** toward life, or a lack of strong feeling, interest, or concern. They may not feel pleasure in things they once enjoyed. They may be sad, or irritable and angry.

- **Changes in behavior.** People with depression may become more or less emotional in their behavior. They may begin eating too little or too much. Often, they have trouble sleeping and seem tired. On the other hand, they may sleep much more than usual. The person may also begin to neglect basic hygiene and withdraw from social situations.

Reading Check

Analyze How might changes during the teen years build resiliency skills.

Getting Help for Depression

MAIN IDEA Depression is a treatable illness.

Depression is serious, but it is treatable. Treatments can include taking medication, making changes in the home or school environment, or counseling. Treating depression takes time, persistence, and patience. If you recognize signs of depression in yourself or a friend, discuss your concerns with a trusted adult. If a friend asks you not to tell anyone that he or she is depressed, it's okay to break that promise. It could literally save your friend's life.

Reading Check

Identify Whom can a depressed teen ask for help?

Lesson 1 Review

Facts and Vocabulary

1. Define the term *anxiety*.

2. What are the causes of depression?

3. Describe changes in thinking that might be effects of depression.

Thinking Critically

4. **Explain.** What is the difference between "feeling down or depressed" and "having depression." Provide examples to show the difference.

5. **Synthesize.** If you believe a friend might be depressed, what can you do to help?

Applying Health Skills

6. **Analyzing Influences.** Divide a sheet of paper into three columns. Label the columns "Family," "Friends," and "School." Use this chart to describe how depression can affect each aspect of your life.

Writing Critically

7. **Expository.** Write a paragraph discussing why it is important for someone with depression to get professional help.

Mental Disorders

BEFORE YOU READ

Create Vocabulary Cards. Write each new vocabulary term on a separate note card. For each term, write a definition based on your current knowledge. As you read, fill in additional information related to each item.

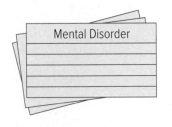

Mental Disorder

Vocabulary

mental disorder
stigma
anxiety disorder
mood disorders
conduct disorder

. . . .

BIG IDEA Gaining an understanding of mental health disorders builds insight and empathy.

REAL LIFE ISSUES

Cutting. Bree has been having a difficult time at school. Some girls that she was friends with in elementary school have begun to bully her. She recently began cutting herself in an effort to release emotional pain. She wears long-sleeved shirts to hide her scars because she doesn't want anyone to lecture her about it. Bree's friends, Kris and Emily, have been discussing the marks ever since they noticed them. They're afraid other students will start whispering about Bree, too, and they don't want to embarrass her or subject her to more bullying. They want to help their friend, but they're not sure how to help or where to turn. *Pretend that you are Bree's friend. You are scared by the cuts on her arms. Write a letter to Bree telling her you care for her and want her to get help.*

After completing the lesson, review and analyze your response to the Real Life Issues question.

Understanding Mental Disorders

MAIN IDEA Mental disorders are medical conditions that require diagnosis and treatment.

Each year, approximately 57.7 million people in the United States are affected by some form of **mental disorder**—an illness of the mind that can affect the thoughts, feelings, and behaviors of a person, preventing him or her from leading a happy, healthful, and productive life. That's about one in every four Americans. Many of these people do not seek treatment because they feel embarrassed or ashamed of their condition. Others fear the **stigma** associated with mental disorders. A stigma is a mark of shame or disapproval that results in an individual being shunned or rejected by others. This is unfortunate, because many mental and emotional problems cannot be solved without professional help.

Mental disorders are illnesses. These medical conditions require diagnosis and treatment, just like a physical illness and injury. Acceptance and understanding encourages people to seek medical help early.

Types of Mental Disorders

MAIN IDEA Mental disorders can be identified by their symptoms.

Mental disorders are medical conditions that can begin as early as childhood. In many cases, they require treatment from health professionals. Types of mental illness include anxiety disorders, impulse control disorders, eating disorders, conduct disorders, personality disorders, and schizophrenia.

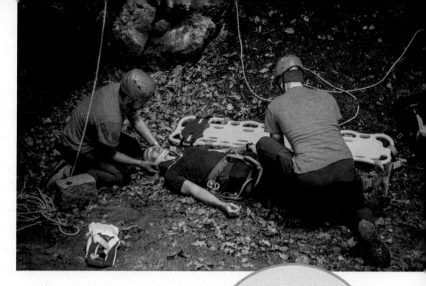

Anxiety Disorders

Anxiety disorders are one of the most common mental health problems among children and teens. An anxiety disorder is a condition in which real or imagined fears are difficult to control. Reports have shown that as many as 25 **percent** of children under the age of 18 experience general anxiety disorders. Types of anxiety disorders include:

- **Phobias.** A phobia is a strong, irrational fear of something specific, such as heights or social situations.

- **Obsessive-compulsive disorder.** This disorder involves persistent thoughts, fears, or urges (obsessions), which lead to uncontrollable repetitive behaviors (compulsions). One common example is an obsessive fear of germs that leads to constant hand washing.

- **Panic disorder.** People with this disorder experience attacks of sudden, unexplained feelings of terror. These "panic attacks" are accompanied by physical symptoms such as trembling, increased heart rate, shortness of breath, or dizziness.

- **Post-traumatic stress disorder.** This condition may develop after exposure to a traumatic event, such as a car accident or a violent attack. Symptoms include flashbacks (reliving the event mentally), nightmares, emotional numbness, guilt, sleeplessness, and trouble concentrating.

- **Generalized anxiety disorder (GAD).** People with GAD feel excessively worried and tense for no reason. They startle easily and have difficulty concentrating, relaxing, and sleeping.

People with anxiety disorders often try to cope with the problem by avoiding the situations that make them feel nervous or fearful. This can make it hard for them to lead normal lives.

Impulse Control Disorders

People with impulse control disorders cannot resist the urge to engage in hurtful behaviors. These actions may be physically or socially harmful. Impulse control disorders may begin in childhood or the teen years, and can continue into adulthood.

Post-traumatic stress disorder may occur in the aftermath of a crisis. **What can community members do to support one another during a crisis?**

ACADEMIC VOCABULARY

percent *(noun)*: one part in a hundred

astarot/Shutterstock

Some examples include:

- **Kleptomania,** the uncontrollable urge to steal.

- **Self-harm.** People deliberately injure themselves. Examples of self-harming behaviors including cutting or burning the skin or pulling out hair.

- **Pyromania,** deliberately setting fires to feel pleasure or release tension.

- **Excessive (or compulsive) gambling.** People continue gambling despite heavy losses, even if they feel the desire to stop.

- **Compulsive shopping.** People uncontrollably spend money on items that they can't afford and don't need.

People with impulse control disorders may physically hurt themselves and others. They may also cause financial harm through behaviors such as gambling or overspending. Often, their behavior damages or destroys their relationships with friends or family members.

Eating Disorders

Eating disorders may surface during the teen years. As teens reach puberty, their bodies go through changes that they may find unsettling. It is not uncommon for some teens to feel that they are overweight while other teens who are experiencing puberty may feel that they are underweight. As they contrast their growing bodies with images of "perfect" bodies that they see in the media, they may feel pressure to change the way they look. This can lead them to develop harmful eating behaviors. The best-known eating disorder is anorexia nervosa, which causes people to starve themselves to become as thin as possible. Other eating disorders include bulimia nervosa and binge eating disorder. Eating disorders are most common among girls, but they affect boys as well. Eating disorders can lead to unhealthful weight loss or weight gain and even cause death.

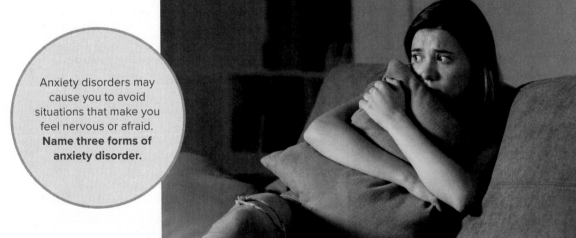

Anxiety disorders may cause you to avoid situations that make you feel nervous or afraid. **Name three forms of anxiety disorder.**

Mood Disorders

People with **mood disorders** experience extremes of emotion much more severe than the normal highs and lows of daily life. Depression is one type of mood disorder. Another example is *bipolar disorder,* also known as manic-depressive disorder. People with this condition go through extreme changes in their mood, energy level, and behavior.

Conduct Disorder

Children and teens with **conduct disorder** engage in destructive behaviors such as stealing, cruelty, lying, aggression, violence, truancy (skipping school), arson (setting fires), and vandalism. Treatment includes learning to adapt to the demands of everyday life.

Personality Disorders

Teens with personality disorders are unable to regulate their emotions. They may feel distressed in social situations or behave in ways that are distressing to others. The cause of personality disorders is unknown, yet some in the medical community believe that genetics and environmental factors play a role in the development of personality disorders.

Schizophrenia

Schizophrenia (pronounced skit-suh-FREE-nee-uh) is a mental disorder in which a person loses touch with reality. Schizophrenia affects about one percent of the population. Both men and women can suffer from this disease. Its symptoms include delusions (believing things that are untrue and unreasonable), hallucinations (seeing or hearing things that are not there), and thought disorders. People with this disorder often behave unpredictably. Professional help and medication are needed to overcome this illness.

Reading Check

List What are examples of conduct disorder?

Character Check

People who suffer from mental disorders are sometimes seen as different. Although some people think it is fun to tease someone who is "different," such teasing is cruel and hurtful. When you show your disapproval of such behavior, you demonstrate consideration and caring for the person being teased. What are some other ways of showing caring and respect for someone who is seen as "different"?

Reading Check

Explain Explain one way of showing caring and respect for someone who is seen as "different."

Lesson 2 Review

Facts and Vocabulary

1. Define the term *stigma*. How can a stigma affect your health?

2. Identify the five types of anxiety disorders.

3. Identify: Which mental disorder can cause a person to have hallucinations?

Thinking Critically

4. **Evaluate.** Explain why mental disorders should be viewed like any other physical illness. Why is it important not to stigmatize someone with a mental disorder?

5. **Analyze.** Why are eating disorders both a mental health problem and a physical health problem?

Applying Health Skills

6. **Advocacy.** Teens suffering from mental disorders often feel confused, isolated, scared, or ashamed. Create a poster promoting awareness of and empathy toward mental illnesses. Focus on specific ways to be supportive, patient, and understanding.

Writing Critically

7. **Expository.** Choose one of the mental disorders you read about in this lesson. Explain why you chose this particular disorder, and how you would learn more about it.

Suicide Prevention

BEFORE YOU READ

Create a K-W-L Chart. Make a three-column chart. In the first column, list what you know about the prevention of suicide. In the second column, list what you want to know about the topic. As you read, use the third column to summarize what you learned.

K	W	L

Vocabulary

alienation
suicide
cluster suicides

Myths & Reality

There are many common misconceptions about suicide. What do you think about this statement about suicide?

Myth: People who talk about suicide won't really attempt it.

Reality: People who talk about suicide are usually considering it and should be taken seriously.

BIG IDEA Professional intervention and support from friends and family can often help prevent suicide.

REAL LIFE ISSUES

Helping a Friend. Nick's friend Ryan has been feeling down lately. Even though Ryan is a good student, he has failed several important tests. As a result, he was suspended from the basketball team. To make matters worse, his girlfriend broke up with him. To Nick, Ryan seems depressed all the time and doesn't care about anything anymore. When Nick tries to talk with him, Ryan just says he wants to get away from it all. *Write a brief paragraph describing how you might respond to Ryan if you were in Nick's position.*

After completing the lesson, review and analyze your response to the Real Life Issues question.

Knowing the Facts About Suicide

MAIN IDEA Certain risk factors increase thoughts of suicide and suicide attempts.

As you have learned, stress is a part of everyone's life. Most people are able to manage stress—at least most of the time—in a healthful way. For some people, however, stress can cause **alienation**, which is feeling isolated and separated from everyone else. These people do not know how to cope with difficult life experiences. They may lack the support that other people receive from family, friends, and community resources. Unable to deal with their emotional pain, some of them seek to escape by ending their lives.

Suicide is the act of intentionally taking one's own life. Suicide is the third leading cause of death among teens aged 15 to 19. Each year, about 4,000 teens commit suicide. Many times, someone who is considering suicide may indicate their intentions to someone close. If you feel that a friend is considering suicide, tell a trusted adult. People who commit suicide may feel hopeless about the future. However, help is available to solve problems.

Suicide Risk Factors

Two risk factors are common among people who commit suicide. More than 90 percent of them either suffer from depression or another mental disorder, or have a history of abusing alcohol or other drugs—or both. Some people abuse alcohol or other drugs to relieve their depression. However, the effects of alcohol and many drugs can actually make depression worse. These substances can also lower a person's inhibitions, making self-destructive behavior more likely.

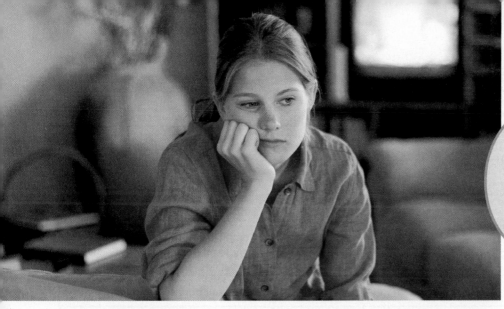

The Centers for Disease Control and Prevention has asked the media to report fewer details about suicide attempts. **How might this effort help reduce the number of suicides?**

Although these are the most common risk factors for suicide, they are not the only ones. Some other risk factors include:

- experiencing a stressful situation or loss.
- having a family history of mental disorders, substance abuse, or suicide.
- making previous suicide attempts.
- having access to firearms.

Finally, some teens who hear about a teen committing suicide may decide to commit suicide themselves. Exposure to other teens who have died by suicide can also be a risk factor. In some cases, it can lead to **cluster suicides**. These are a series of suicides occurring within a short period of time and involving several people in the same school or community. Cluster suicides account for about 5 percent of all teen suicides. Some cluster suicides result from pacts made among groups of peers. In other cases, the teens involved may not know each other, but they all share a common stressor in their environment, such as a tragic event in their school or community. When the news media carries reports of teen suicides, it may encourage other teens who are experiencing stress and depression to try suicide too. Teens may also learn of the suicides of other teens through the news media.

Strategies to Prevent Suicide

MAIN IDEA Recognizing the signs of suicide may help prevent it.

Most suicidal thoughts, behaviors, and actions are expressions of extreme distress. A person **displaying** only a few of these signs may not actually be thinking about suicide. However, any time a person talks about committing suicide—whether it's done in a serious, casual, or even humorous way—*take it seriously.* Any discussion or suggestion about suicide calls for immediate action. Never agree to keep it a secret if a friend tells you he or she is considering suicide. Tell an adult without delay.

ACADEMIC VOCABULARY

display *(verb)*: to make evident

Reading Check

Describe What are some behaviors that might indicate a person is thinking about suicide?

Suicide Prevention **107**

RECOGNIZING THE WARNING SIGNS OF SUICIDE	
• Direct statements such as "I wish I were dead."	• A sense of guilt, shame, or rejection; negative self-evaluation.
• Indirect statements such as "I can't take it anymore."	• Deterioration in schoolwork or recreational performance.
• Writing poems, song lyrics, or diary entries that deal with death.	• Giving away personal belongings.
• Direct or indirect suicide threats.	• Substance abuse.
• An unusual obsession with death.	• Complaints about physical symptoms, such as stomachaches, headaches, and fatigue.
• Withdrawal from friends.	• Persistent boredom and indifference.
• Dramatic changes in personality, hygiene, or appearance.	• Violent actions, rebellious behavior, or running away.
• Impulsive, irrational, or unusual behavior.	• Intolerance for praise or rewards.

Reading Check

Describe What steps can you take to help someone who may be considering suicide?

How You Can Help

If someone you know may be considering suicide, that person needs help. Here are some strategies you can try:

- **Start a meaningful conversation.** Show interest, compassion, patience, and understanding. Don't trivialize the problem by saying things like "You don't really want to do that," or "Everyone feels sad sometimes."

- **Show empathy.** People who are considering suicide often feel that their death will not matter to anyone. Let the other person know that you care and are concerned.

- **Offer support and ask questions.** Remind the person that all problems have solutions, and that suicide is not the answer. Tell the person that most survivors of suicide attempts later express gratitude that they did not die.

Suicide survivor support groups are available in most communities. **How might such support groups prevent suicides?**

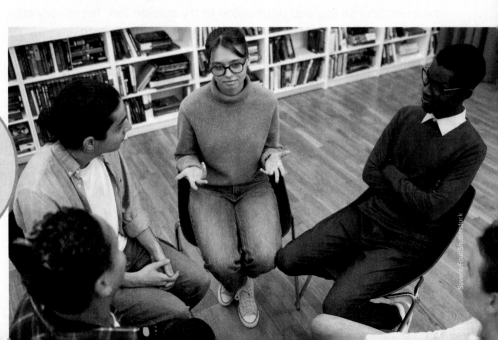

- **Try to persuade the person to seek help.** Encourage the person to talk to a parent, counselor, or other trusted adult. Offer to go with him or her to get help.

Regardless of the outcome of your conversation, tell an adult about the problem. If the adult doesn't seem to believe the threat is serious, then talk to other adults until someone agrees to take action. You can also contact community resources, such as a crisis center or suicide hotline.

REAL WORLD CONNECTION

Depression and Suicide

Untreated depression is the leading cause of suicide. People who consider suicide feel that they don't matter to others. People who appear to have a mental health problem and may be considering suicide need to be encouraged to seek help.

What can you, as a friend, do to help prevent suicide? Should you tell someone that a friend has mentioned suicide, even if that friend asked you to keep the information private? What can people in the community do to help prevent suicides? In small groups, conduct an online search for reliable information about seeking help for depression.

Activity: Writing

Once you have gathered your information as a group, complete the following activity:

1. Write a script for a skit that urges teens to seek help if they are depressed and considering suicide.

2. Record a video of the skit and include a statement encouraging teens to get help.

3. Remind the audience that all problems can be solved and that depression is treatable.

4. Encourage teens who may be depressed to talk to a parent, teacher, or other trusted adult.

5. Provide contact information for local crisis centers and suicide hotlines.

Lesson 3 Review

Facts and Vocabulary

1. Define the term *alienation*.

2. Name the two risk factors that have the strongest association with suicide.

3. Name five warning signs of suicide.

Thinking Critically

4. **Synthesize.** Make a list of three direct statements and three indirect statements that could indicate a teen is considering suicide.

5. **Explain.** Define the term *cluster suicide* and explain what factors sometimes lead to cluster suicides.

Applying Health Skills

6. **Decision Making.** Imagine that you have a friend who shares negative comments about herself. Use the six steps of decision making to determine what actions to take.

Writing Critically

7. **Descriptive.** Write a note to a teen who has exhibited some suicidal warning behaviors. Use the suggestions listed in the lesson to help the teen rethink his or her situation.

Getting Help

BEFORE YOU READ

Create a Cluster Chart. Draw a circle and label it "Getting Help." Use surrounding circles to identify professionals in the community who can help individuals with mental health problems. As you read, continue filling in the chart with more details.

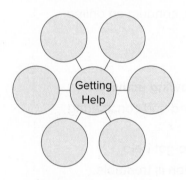

Vocabulary

psychotherapy
behavior therapy
cognitive therapy
family therapy
group therapy
drug therapy

• • • • • • • • • • • •

BIG IDEA Mental health professionals and related agencies provide treatment and support for people with mental health problems.

REAL LIFE ISSUES

No One to Turn To. Angie is desperate. She feels as though her life is spiraling out of control. She's confused, but tries to hide her fears and frustrations. Angie knows she needs help, but wonders who she should talk to for help. She's afraid of what a friend or teacher will think of her if she lets someone know she's feeling confused. ***Write a letter to Angie encouraging her to talk to a trusted adult and ask for help. Make sure the tone of your letter is understanding and considerate.***

After completing the lesson, review and analyze your response to the Real Life Issues question.

When Help is Needed

MAIN IDEA The first step to getting help for a mental health problem is recognizing that help is needed.

Many teens with mental health problems do not seek help. Either they do not recognize how serious their condition is, or they do not understand that help is available. In fact, most mental health disorders in adults have their roots in untreated problems from childhood and adolescence. More than half of all suicidal youths had symptoms of a mental illness for more than a year prior to their deaths.

It can help to remember that mental problems are illnesses, just like physical illnesses. If you had a serious physical problem, such as a broken arm, you probably would not hesitate to see a doctor about it. In the same way, no one should ever feel embarrassed to talk with someone about mental or emotional problems. Teens should seek help if they experience any of the following:

- Feeling trapped or worrying all the time.
- Feelings that affect sleep, eating habits, schoolwork, job performance, or relationships.
- Becoming involved with alcohol or other drugs.
- Becoming increasingly violent, aggressive, or reckless.

Often, friends and family members are the first to realize that a problem is affecting a teen's life and relationships. Their concern may encourage the teen to seek help.

Overcoming the Stumbling Blocks

MAIN IDEA The benefits of treatment encourage people to overcome a reluctance to get help.

Seeking help for a mental health problem can be difficult. However, it is often a crucial step toward getting the problem under control. Talking about problems may make a person feel more vulnerable, at least at first. It may help to remember these facts:

- Admitting a problem does not mean that you are weak or helpless. In fact, asking for help shows that you have the inner strength to take responsibility for your own wellness.

- Serious disorders, compulsions, and addictions are complex problems. They usually cannot be resolved without professional care.

- Sharing your thoughts and feelings with an objective, helpful individual can be a great relief.

- Financial help may be available to help with the costs of care.

Reading Check

Explain What does asking for help from a mental health professional show?

Where to Go for Help

MAIN IDEA People in your community are available to help.

It takes courage to confront a problem and try to solve it. Talking with a trusted adult, such as a parent, guardian, or teacher, is a good first step. Many teens receive help for mental health problems at school. A counselor or the school nurse can identify and contact support services. Other sources of help in the community include clergy members and crisis hotlines. Crisis hotlines allow people to talk anonymously. The workers are trained to deal with difficult mental and emotional situations.

The treatment for mental health problems is unique to each individual. Sometimes, the first treatment plan you try may not work. If that happens, talk to someone else. It may be necessary to try several different treatments. People with mental health problems should continue to seek help from different sources until they find the solutions they need.

Mental Health Professionals

Many types of mental health professionals can be found in your community. They work in schools, clinics, hospitals, and family agencies. These specialists are trained to help people with a wide variety of mental and emotional problems. Types of mental health professionals include:

- **Counselors.** These professionals handle both medical and educational matters. They may or may not have medical training.

Adults working at a crisis hotline are usually volunteers motivated by the desire to help people who are suffering. **How might a person who is caring and yet objective be helpful during an emotional crisis?**

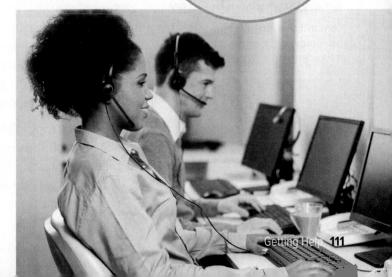

leaf/123RF

• • • • • • • • • •

Reading Check

List Name some people who can help teens with mental and emotional health problems.

• • • • • • • • • • •

• **School psychologists.** These professionals specialize in treating the problems of schoolchildren, including learning, emotional, and behavioral problems.

• **Psychiatrists.** These are medical doctors who can diagnose and treat medical disorders and prescribe medications.

• **Neurologists.** These physicians specialize in physical disorders of the brain and nervous system.

• **Clinical psychologists.** These professionals diagnose and treat emotional and behavioral disorders through counseling. Although they are not medical doctors, some can still prescribe medicine.

• **Psychiatric social workers.** These professionals provide guidance and treatment for emotional problems in hospitals, mental health clinics, and family service agencies.

Treatment Methods

MAIN IDEA Several methods can be helpful in treating a mental health problem.

Mental health professionals may use different treatments depending on their area of expertise and on the needs of the patient. The following are the most commonly used therapy methods.

• • • • • • • • • • •

Reading Check

Explain What types of treatment methods can help those with a mental disorder?

• • • • • • • • • • •

• **Psychotherapy.** This is an ongoing dialogue between a patient and a mental health professional. The dialogue between patient and doctor is designed to root out the cause of a mental problem in order to devise a solution.

• **Behavior therapy.** This is a treatment process that focuses on changing unwanted behaviors through rewards and reinforcements. Rewards and reinforcements help patients successfully learn more healthful behaviors.

• **Cognitive therapy.** This is a treatment method designed to identify and correct distorted thinking patterns that can lead to feelings and behaviors that may be troublesome, self-defeating, or self-destructive. The doctor or therapist and the patient work together to change harmful thinking patterns.

• • • • • • • • • • •

ACADEMIC VOCABULARY

constructive *(adjective):* promoting improvement or development

• • • • • • • • • • •

• **Family therapy.** This treatment focuses on helping the family function in more positive and **constructive** ways by exploring patterns in communication and providing support and education. This treatment method is most successful when every member of the family attends the sessions. The goal is to help family members deal with problems in a constructive way.

• **Group therapy.** This involves treating a group of people who have similar problems and who meet regularly with a trained counselor. In this type of treatment, group members agree that whatever is said in the group is private. They agree not to reveal any information heard during their group sessions to outsiders.

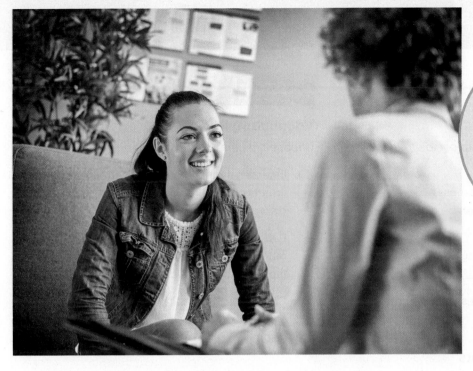

A mental health specialist respects a patient's concern for confidentiality. **What are other benefits of seeking help from a mental health specialist?**

· · · · · · · · · · ·

Character Check

Lately I feel so overwhelmed by all my responsibilities. My dad's away from home in the army and my mom works part time. I watch my brother and sister after school, and I start dinner. I started feeling stressed and missed some homework assignments. When my grades came in, my mom asked some of the other army wives to help me out. She also talked to me about how it's important that I tell her when I'm overwhelmed. It's the responsible thing to do for myself.

· · · · · · · · · · ·

- **Drug therapy.** This therapy is the use of certain medications to treat or reduce the symptoms of a mental disorder. Medications may be used on their own or combined with other treatment methods, such as those listed above.

In some cases, a mental health problem may be serious enough to require hospitalization. In a hospital, a patient can receive intensive care and treatment from doctors, nurses, and a variety of mental health specialists. These specialists are available 24 hours a day to help the patient.

Lesson 4 Review

Facts and Vocabulary

1. Define *behavior therapy.*

2. Identify which mental health professional treats physical disorders of the brain.

3. Name a person a teen might reach out to at school about a mental health problem.

Thinking Critically

4. **Analyze.** What protective factors do you have or can you develop to help you deal with stress in your life?

5. **Synthesize.** How does developing a positive outlook strengthen your resiliency?

Applying Health Skills

6. **Accessing Information.** Compile a list of local resources for mental health problems. Include mental health professionals, school counselors, hospital emergency rooms, and hotlines.

Writing Critically

7. **Persuasive.** Write an editorial about the importance of seeking help for mental health problems. Include strategies for getting help.

LESSON 1

Vocabulary Review

Use the correct vocabulary terms to complete the following statements.

1. Prolonged feelings of helplessness, hopelessness and sadness can be a sign that you are suffering from _____.

2. Feelings of unease or worrying about what may happen are signs of _____.

3. A lack of strong feeling, interest, or concern is called _____.

Understanding Key Concepts

After reading the question or statement, select the correct answer.

4. Which of the following is *not* a change in behavior one might expect with depression?
   a. Trouble sleeping
   b. Eating too much
   c. Eating too little
   d. Running alone

5. Which of the following is *not* a warning sign of depression?
   a. Boredom
   b. Increased interest in life
   c. Poor concentration
   d. Increased irritability

Thinking Critically

After reading the question or statement, write a short answer using complete sentences.

6. **Identify.** What are three feelings you may experience when you are depressed?

7. **Explain.** How might depression affect your sleep?

8. **Analyze.** How might community violence cause someone to become depressed?

9. **Discuss.** While being treated for depression, what else can you do to help the healing process?

LESSON 2

Vocabulary Review

Choose the correct term in the sentences below.

10. Illnesses that involve mood extremes that interfere with everyday living are called *mood disorders/ stigma*.

11. Patterns of behavior in which the rights of others or basic social rules are violated are typical of a *mental disorder/conduct disorder*.

12. Conditions in which real or imagined fears are difficult to control are called *stigma/anxiety disorder*.

Understanding Key Concepts

After reading the question or statement, select the correct answer.

13. Which is *not* an anxiety disorder?
    a. Phobia
    b. Pyromania
    c. Panic disorder
    d. Post-traumatic stress disorder

14. Kleptomania is
    a. an anxiety disorder.
    b. a mood disorder.
    c. an impulse control disorder.
    d. a conduct disorder.

15. Bipolar disorder is
    a. a conduct disorder.
    b. a personality disorder.
    c. an anxiety disorder.
    d. a mood disorder.

Thinking Critically

After reading the question or statement, write a short answer using complete sentences.

16. **Explain.** Describe how misconceptions of mental illness can be overcome.

17. **Analyze.** Explain why some people with a mental disorder may not seek help for their problem.

18. **Describe.** Identify several examples of anxiety triggers for teens.

19. **Infer.** Consider the types of problems that people with impulse control disorders have. Explain what problems people with this disorder may face before getting treatment.

LESSON 3

Vocabulary Review

Correct the sentences below by replacing the italicized term with the correct vocabulary term.

20. The act of intentionally taking one's own life is called *alienation*.

21. A series of suicides occurring within a short period of time and involving several people in the same school or community is referred to as *suicide*.

Understanding Key Concepts

After reading the question or statement, select the correct answer.

22. Suicide is the _____ leading cause of teen deaths.
    a. first
    b. second
    c. third
    d. fourth

23. Of the following risk factors for teen suicide, which should probably be of most concern?
    a. A stressful situation or loss
    b. Substance abuse
    c. Family history of mental disorders
    d. Exposure to other teens who have died by suicide

24. Which is *not* a warning sign of suicide?
    a. Withdrawal from friends
    b. An overwhelming sense of guilt
    c. Persistent indifference
    d. Preoccupation with buying new things

Thinking Critically

After reading the question or statement, write a short answer using complete sentences.

25. **Analyze.** Explain why drinking alcohol is not an effective way to try to relieve depression.

26. **Describe.** What are five warning signs of suicide?

27. **Explain.** Why might cluster suicides occur in a community where the individuals may not even know one another?

28. **Evaluate.** Explain why it is important never to keep secret a person's threat to commit suicide.

LESSON 4

Vocabulary Review

Use the correct vocabulary term to complete the following statements.

29. A treatment method designed to identify and correct distorted thinking patterns is known as _____.

30. The use of certain medications to treat symptoms of a mental disorder is called _____.

Understanding Key Concepts

After reading the question or statement, select the correct answer.

31. A mental health professional who handles personal and educational matters is a
    a. counselor.
    b. school psychologist.
    c. psychiatrist.
    d. neurologist.

32. A treatment method that uses ongoing dialogue between a patient and a mental health professional is
   a. family therapy.
   b. cognitive therapy.
   c. psychotherapy.
   d. group therapy.

33. Which is *not* true regarding crisis-hotline workers?
   a. They are trained to deal with difficult mental/emotional situations.
   b. They are usually volunteers.
   c. They know about your personal situation.
   d. They allow you to remain anonymous.

Thinking Critically

After reading the question or statement, write a short answer using complete sentences.

34. **Describe.** Identify the behaviors that help you recognize that a friend needs help.

35. **Analyze.** What are the possible consequences of not getting help for an adolescent mental disorder?

36. **Synthesize.** What criteria would be important to you when choosing someone to talk with about a mental health problem?

PROJECT-BASED ASSESSMENT

Phobias

BACKGROUND

A phobia is a strong fear of something specific. For example, arachnophobia is a fear of spiders. Other phobias include agoraphobia, the fear of being in an open space, or claustrophobia, the fear of being in a closed space.

TASK

Conduct an Internet search to learn about different types of phobias. Create a web page describing types of phobias and how they are treated.

AUDIENCE

Students at your class

PURPOSE

Develop awareness of one kind of mental illness that affects many children, teens, and adults.

PROCEDURE

1. Conduct research on the Internet to learn more about phobias.

2. Select three to four phobias that you will describe on your web page.

3. Identify the kinds of professional help and solutions available for treating specific phobias.

4. Research online about what might occur if a person's activities should put him or her near the object or situation that is the source of the phobia.

5. Create sections on your web page for each type of phobia, giving as much information as possible.

6. Present your web page to your class.

Math Practice

Understand and Apply. Read the paragraph below, and then answer the questions.

Nearly everyone is mildly depressed at some time, but 16 percent of the U.S. population will suffer from major depression in their lifetime. A study was conducted on more than 9,000 people ages 18 and older. Fifty-seven percent of those who had major depression sought help. This rate is almost 40 percent higher than the rate reported 20 years before the study. Even though the number of patients treated is increasing, it is estimated that only 21 percent are receiving adequate care.

1. If the size of the general population is 200 million people, how many people will experience major depression at some time during their lives?
   a. 14 million
   b. 42 million
   c. 75 million
   d. 92.8 million

2. What function can be used to find the number of people who are seeking help for depression if you know the size of the population with depression? (Hint: The variable N is the number of people seeking help, and P is the size of the population.)
   a. $N = P$
   b. $N = (0.57)(0.07)P$
   c. $N = 0.57P$
   d. $P = 0.07N$

3. Examine the percentages reflecting how many people have major depression, how many of these people seek help, and how many who seek help receive adequate care. Of 20,000 people, how many people would you expect to be receiving adequate care for major depression? Justify your answer.

Reading/Writing Practice

Analyze and Infer. Read the passage below, and then answer the questions.

John F. Nash Jr. is known for his work as a creative mathematician. He is also an example of how one person can succeed in his chosen field even if he is battling a difficult mental health challenge: paranoid schizophrenia. While working at Princeton University in the 1950s, Nash made great strides in a field of mathematics called game theory. This research later earned him a share in the 1994 Nobel Prize in Economics. However, soon after completing this work, he began to suffer what was later diagnosed as paranoid schizophrenia. After taking a break for nearly 30 years, Nash returned to mathematics and continued to do research and write at Princeton.

1. What information supports the claim that Nash is successful?
   a. Nash was born in West Virginia.
   b. Nash has paranoid schizophrenia.
   c. Nash stopped his research for 30 years.
   d. Nash won a Nobel Prize in Economics.

2. Why did the author write this passage?
   a. To cite examples of famous people with various mental disorders
   b. To describe how a mathematician came up with his prize-winning research
   c. To explain how schizophrenia affects mental and physical health
   d. To show how a person can be successful in spite of a mental disorder

3. Write a paragraph describing the effects of schizophrenia on a person's mental and emotional health.

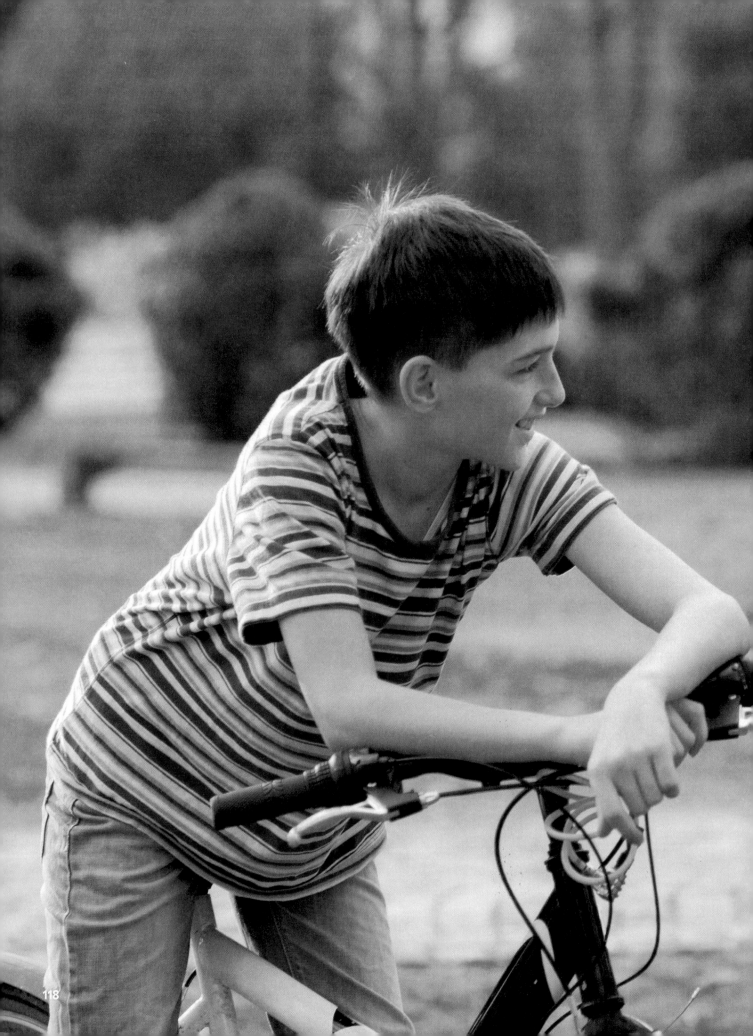

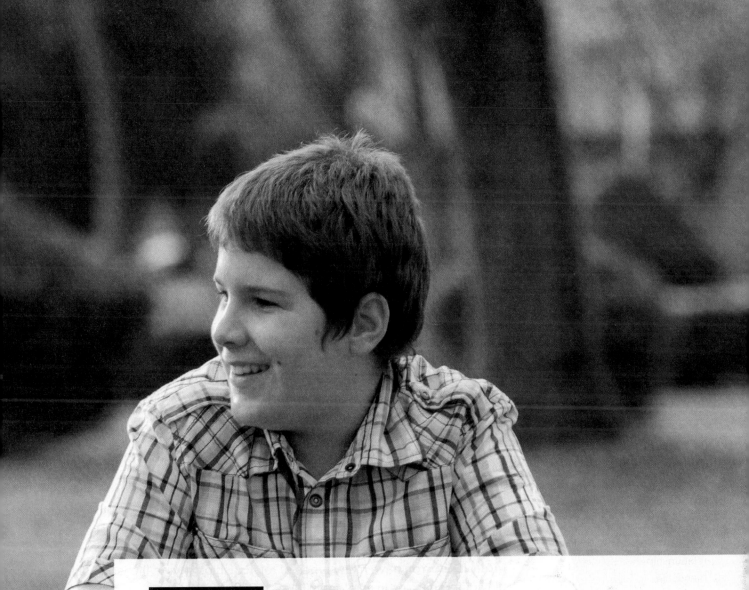

MODULE 6

Skills for Healthy Relationships

LESSONS

1 Foundations of a Healthy Relationship

2 Respecting Yourself and Others

3 Communicating Effectively

Foundations of a Healthy Relationship

BEFORE YOU READ

Create a K-W-L Chart. Make a three-column chart. In the first column, list what you know about relationships. In the second column, list what you want to know about this topic. As you read, use the third column to summarize what you learned.

K	W	L

Vocabulary

relationship
friendship
citizenship
role
cooperation
compromise

BIG IDEA Building strong relationships is important to your overall health.

REAL LIFE ISSUES

Important Relationships. Andrew's classmate has an extra ticket to a sold-out concert on New Year's Eve. Andrew really wants to go, but he already promised his best friend that he would attend his New Year's Eve party. Andrew doesn't want to let his best friend down, but he may not have another chance to see this band in concert. *If you were Andrew, how would you respond? How can you reassure the people in your life of their importance to you? Write a paragraph explaining your choice and how it might impact your friendship.*

After completing the lesson, review and analyze your response to the Real Life Issues question.

Relationships in Your Life

MAIN IDEA You have many types of relationships in your life, and you play different roles in all of them.

One of the most basic human needs is the need to belong and to feel loved. Building and maintaining healthy **relationships** can help you meet this need. A relationship is a bond or connection you have with other people. Although some people use the word relationship to refer to a romantic involvement, there are actually all kinds of relationships that can be important in your life. For instance, you have relationships with family members, friends, teachers, classmates, and people in your community. All of these relationships can affect your health in positive or negative ways.

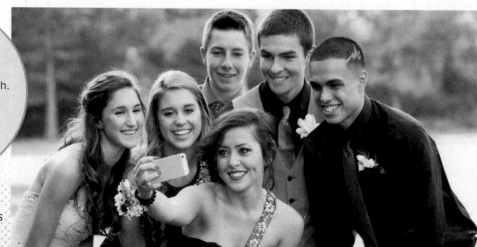

Strong friendships have a positive influence on your health. **What friendships are most important in your life?**

Relationships with Family

Think for a minute about the most important relationships in your life. Chances are, some of the people who came to your mind are the family members who share your home, such as parents or guardians, brothers, and sisters. You may also have thought about other relatives, such as grandparents, aunts, uncles, and cousins. One thing that makes family relationships special is that they last your entire life. The friends you have in high school may not be your friends ten years from now, but your family is your family for life.

Healthy family relationships strengthen every side of your health triangle. Parents or guardians take care of your physical needs for food, clothing, and shelter. The love, care, and encouragement they provide are important to your mental and emotional health. They also help build your social health by teaching you the values and social skills that will guide you in all your other relationships.

Relationships with Friends

Who are your closest friends? How do you know them, and what do you have in common? Although you probably have many friends your own age, **friendships** can form between people of any age. A friendship is a significant relationship between two people that is based on trust, caring, and consideration. You may choose your friends because you have similar interests, because they share your values, or maybe just because they live nearby. Whatever the reason, good friends can benefit your health in many ways. They can boost your self-esteem and help you resist harmful behaviors.

Relationships with Dating Partners

Dating relationships are a new type of relationship for many teens. Dating during the teen years should be fun. It should not add more stress to your life. Healthy dating relationships are built on respect. A partner who is controlling or violent does not respect the other partner. Abuse in a dating relationship can include physical, emotional, or psychological abuse. A dating relationship that becomes abusive or violent should be reported to a parent, guardian, or other trusted adult.

Relationships in Your Community

Your community includes all the people and places that are a part of your daily life. Being part of a strong community has a positive impact on every aspect of your health. Community groups and activities, such as sports programs, can promote healthful behaviors. Your community can also provide resources to help you when you're in trouble. For instance, your local library may offer tutoring programs to help you with schoolwork. A neighborhood watch program may help prevent and report crimes in your community.

Reading Check

Explain How can friends benefit your health?

You reinforce your ties to the community through good **citizenship**—the way you conduct yourself as a member of the community. Good citizens work to strengthen their communities by obeying laws, being friendly to and respecting their neighbors, and taking part in efforts to improve the places where they live.

Roles in Relationships

There is one person who is involved in all of your relationships: you. But even though you are just one person, you fill many different **roles** in your relationships. A role is a part you play in your relationships. In the course of a single day, you may play many roles with different people. You might be a son or daughter at home, a student at school, a friend when you're hanging out with your buddies, a teammate during gym class, and an employee at an after-school job.

Sometimes you can even play more than one role with the same person. For instance, when you babysit a younger brother or sister, you temporarily take on the role of caregiver in that relationship. Your role in a relationship may also change over time. For example, someone you work with might become a friend.

Balancing all the different roles in your life can be tricky. You may feel at times as if you can't handle all the demands that different people are making on you. Trying to manage several conflicting roles can cause personal stress and interfere with your relationships. In situations like this, the decision-making process can help you to figure out the best course of action. You might decide, for example, that even if you care about two people equally, you need to focus more on one relationship right now.

This diagram illustrates the many overlapping roles that one teen, Felicia, plays in her relationships at home, at school, and in her community. **What different roles do you play in your life?**

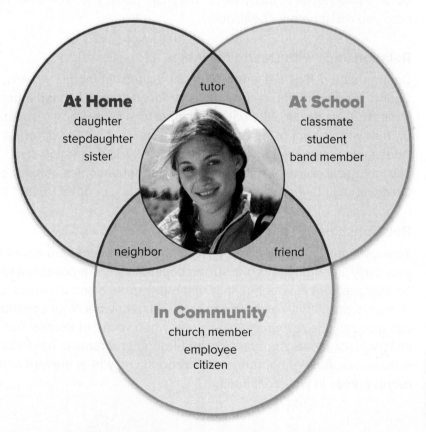

At Home
daughter
stepdaughter
sister

tutor

At School
classmate
student
band member

neighbor

friend

In Community
church member
employee
citizen

Traits of Healthy Relationships

MAIN IDEA In a healthy relationship, people respect and support each other.

Healthy relationships nurture you. They bring out the best in you and encourage you to make healthful choices in your life. There are several qualities that healthy relationships share.

- **Mutual respect.** You treat the people in your life with respect, and they respect you in turn. You accept each other's opinions, tastes, and traditions, even if they are different. At times, you may agree to disagree instead of trying to force your opinions on each other.

- **Caring.** You treat each other with kindness and consideration. During difficult times, you show empathy and support. You're also willing to help each other out in difficult times.

- **Honesty.** You are honest and open with each other. You do not conceal your thoughts, feelings, or actions.

- **Commitment.** You both contribute to the relationship and work to keep it strong, even if it means making some sacrifices. You face your problems in a positive way and work together to overcome them.

Reading Check

Identify What are the characteristics of a healthy relationship?

Skills for Building Healthy Relationships

It takes work to maintain a healthy relationship. The people involved need to make an effort to understand each other and get along in different situations. Three skills that can help are communication, **cooperation**, and **compromise**—sometimes known as the three Cs of healthy relationships.

Communication. Good communication is an important part of any relationship. As you have learned, interpersonal communication is the exchange of thoughts, feelings, and beliefs between two or more people. Effective communication skills help you express your thoughts, feelings, and expectations to others, and to understand theirs in return. For example, suppose you have a friend who always shows up late whenever you make plans together. Good communication means you can tell your friend how you feel and work together to resolve the problem.

Cooperation. Have you ever had to move a heavy desk or other large piece of furniture? Tasks like this are nearly impossible without cooperation. Cooperation is working together for the good of all. Cooperating with others to reach a common goal can strengthen your relationships. For example, when Jonah and his mom worked together to build a set of shelves for his room, they learned to interact better together and they were able to share a sense of accomplishment in the project.

Communication is more than just talking. It's getting your message across to others and hearing their response. **Describe three different ways you might communicate with someone.**

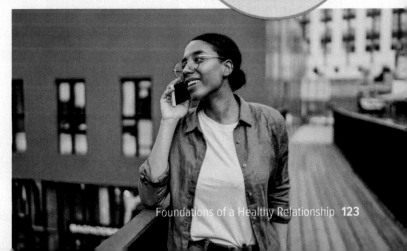

GaudiLab/Shutterstock

Compromise. Suppose you and a friend are discussing how to spend the afternoon. One of you wants to take a bike ride and the other wants to go to the movies. To settle the question, you and your friend might decide on a compromise, such as going for a short ride and then watching a video. Compromise is a problem-solving method in which each participant gives up something to reach a solution that satisfies everyone.

The give and take of effective compromise strengthens relationships. It allows you to resolve disagreements in a way that everyone can accept. Remember, though, that compromise only works when all the people involved are happy with the solution. You should not compromise on things that really matter to you, like your values and beliefs. The art of getting along with others involves knowing when it's appropriate to compromise and when you need to stand your ground

Character and Relationships

Do you remember the six traits of good character? Each of these traits contributes in its own way to healthy relationships. Here are some examples of how each one can strengthen a relationship.

- **Trustworthiness.** Maribel has promised to go to the movies with her friend Noriko on Friday night. On Friday afternoon, a guy Maribel likes asks her if she wants to go out that evening. She'd like to say yes, but she doesn't want to break her promise to Noriko. By keeping her promise, Maribel shows that Noriko can count on her.

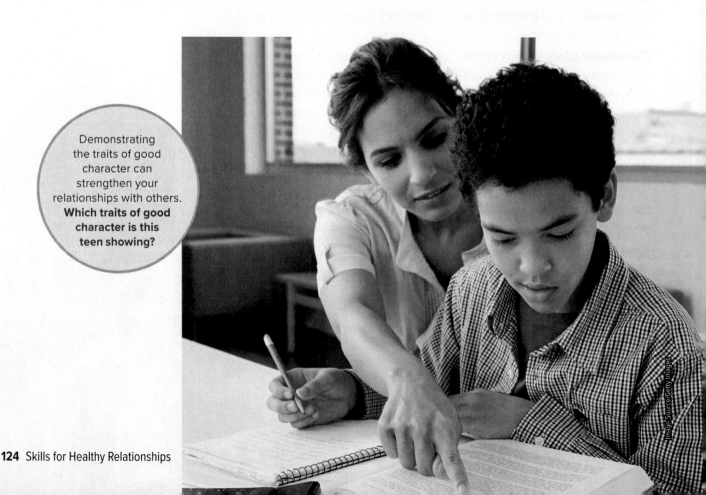

Demonstrating the traits of good character can strengthen your relationships with others. **Which traits of good character is this teen showing?**

Image Source/Getty Images

- **Respect**. Kyle's parents have taught him always to listen when someone else is talking and to avoid interrupting. By extending this courtesy to each other whenever they talk, Kyle and his parents improve their communication as a family.

- **Responsibility**. While she's at a party, Tara accidentally knocks over a glass and breaks it. She immediately apologizes to the host, helps clean up the broken glass, and offers to pay to replace it. Her responsible action improves her host's opinion of her.

- **Fairness**. Enrique and his brother take turns using their computer at home to do schoolwork, send email, and play games. Sharing the **computer** fairly keeps Enrique and his brother from fighting over it.

- **Caring**. When her friend Carl is having trouble with math, Alison offers to help him study for the upcoming test. Carl considers her a good friend for caring about him and helping him out.

- **Citizenship**. Ruby's family bought a snow blower to help her keep their sidewalk and driveway clear. Now, in addition to clearing her own driveway, Ruby offers to do her neighbor's as well. Her actions improve her relationship with her neighbor and her reputation in the community.

ACADEMIC VOCABULARY

computer *(noun)*: a device that can store, retrieve, and process data

Fitness Zone

I always work out with a friend for a couple of reasons. A friend helps keep me motivated when I'm struggling to complete a workout. The other reason is that it's safer to work out with someone else.

Lesson 1 Review

Facts and Vocabulary

1. Identify three kinds of relationships you have in your life.

2. Define *citizenship* and give an example of good citizenship.

3. What are the three Cs of healthy relationships?

Thinking Critically

4. **Analyze.** Explain how relationships with family members are important to all three sides of your health triangle.

5. **Synthesize.** Think about your interactions with other people over the course of a day. Analyze these interactions to identify what roles you played in your relationships that day. Summarize your findings.

Applying Health Skills

6. **Advocacy.** Brainstorm a list of ways that students can demonstrate good citizenship at school. Based on these ideas, create a flyer encouraging students to be good citizens of the school community.

Writing Critically

7. **Narrative.** Write a conversation between two characters who share a relationship. In your narrative, show how the communication between these characters affects their relationship in a positive or negative way.

Respecting Yourself and Others

● ● ● ● ● ● ● ● ● ● ●

BEFORE YOU READ

Create a T-Chart. Draw a two-column chart. Label the left column "Self-Respect" and the right column "Respect for Others." As you read, fill in the columns with information about how each type of respect can improve your relationships.

Self-Respect	Respect for Others

Vocabulary

prejudice
stereotype
tolerance
bullying
hazing
zero tolerance policy

● ● ● ● ● ● ● ● ● ● ●

Reading Check

Explain Why might being unsure about values complicate your relationships?

● ● ● ● ● ● ● ● ● ●

BIG IDEA Family members support and care for one another, especially during difficult times.

REAL LIFE ISSUES

Bullying. Many teens have experienced bullying in schools. According to a 2020 report from the National Center for Education Statistics, 20 percent of teens said that they had been bullied at school during the school year. 15 percent of teens reported being cyberbullied anywhere during the school year. And 4 percent of students reported they were afraid of attack or harm at school. *Write a journal entry describing how being bullied can make someone feel.*

After completing the lesson, review and analyze your response to the Real Life Issues question.

Respect for Yourself

MAIN IDEA Self-respect will strengthen your relationships.

As you have learned, having self-respect is an important part of your mental and emotional health. It can also help you develop healthy relationships with others. When you respect yourself, you're more likely to seek out relationships with other people who also treat you with respect. You're also less likely to let other people talk you into taking risks that could harm your health.

The Need for Strong Values

During your teen years, you may be searching for your personal identity—your sense of who you are and where you belong in the world. Part of this search includes developing your personal value system. Values, as you have learned, are the beliefs, ideas, and attitudes about what is important that help guide the way you live.

Being unsure of your values can really tangle up your relationships. If you aren't clear about your values, it's much harder to communicate them to others. If the people around you don't know what is important to you, you may be more likely to face pressure to take part in unhealthful behaviors. In contrast, being clear about your values can strengthen your relationships. Other people will know what you believe in and understand what's important to you. Upholding your values shows that you respect yourself, and communicating those values to others can help them respect you, too.

Respect for Others

MAIN IDEA It's important to treat people with respect.

Think for a minute about how you would like other people to treat you. Chances are, you'd like respect from everyone you deal with—from strangers on the street to your best friends. You can strengthen your relationships with all the people in your life by treating them with the same respect you'd like them to show you. With strangers and casual acquaintances, you can show respect through common courtesy. For instance, you might hold a door open for someone or say "Thank you" to the checker at the grocery store. With closer friends and family members, you can show respect in more significant ways:

- Listen to other people. Be willing to hear and consider their points of view, even if you disagree with them.

- If someone is upset or experiencing a problem, listen to and empathize with them. Offer to help with problem-solving or in another way.

- Be considerate of others' feelings. Before you say or do something, think about how it might make the other person feel.

- Develop mutual trust. Let others know they can trust you by being honest and dependable. Show that you trust them by believing what they say and being willing to confide in them.

- Have realistic expectations. For example, you can't expect friends and family members to always make you their top priority.

Tolerance

Sometimes people treat others with disrespect because of **prejudice**. Prejudice is an unfair opinion or judgment of a particular group of people. For example, a teen might decide he dislikes all cheerleaders because a cheerleader once turned him down for a date. Some forms of prejudice involve **stereotypes**. A stereotype is an exaggerated or over-simplified belief about people who belong to a certain group. Assuming that all boys like sports, for instance, is an example of a gender stereotype.

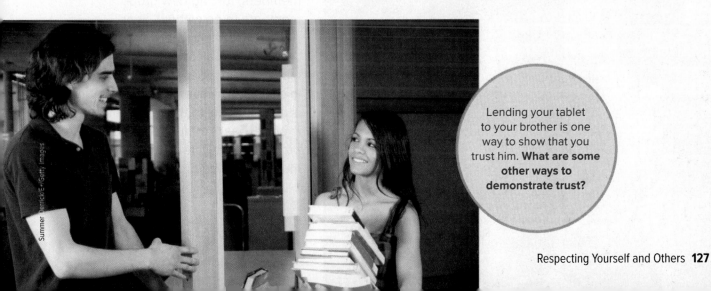

Lending your tablet to your brother is one way to show that you trust him. **What are some other ways to demonstrate trust?**

Prejudice is a barrier to healthy relationships. It can keep people from getting to know others as individuals. Demonstrating **tolerance**, by contrast, can help you build healthy relationships. Tolerance is the ability to accept others' differences. People who are tolerant value diversity. They can appreciate the differences in other people's cultures, interests, beliefs, and perspectives.

Disrespectful Behaviors

Has a fellow student ever picked on you for no reason? Perhaps this person called you names or even threatened you with physical violence. This disrespectful behavior is an example of **bullying**. Bullying is deliberately harming or threatening other people who cannot easily defend themselves. Bullies may tease their victims, spread nasty rumors about them, or try to keep them out of a group. They may even attack others physically, pushing, shoving, or hitting them. Some bullies use technology to target others. Using the Internet, email, or other online tools to harass people, threaten them, or spread rumors is called cyberbullying. This type of bullying allows one person to bully another without ever seeing him or her in person. Because of this lack of face-to-face contact, the bully may not even realize how much his or her actions hurt the other person.

Some bullies push other people around because it makes them feel superior. They may also do it as a way to be part of a group or to keep from being bullied themselves. Kids and teens who are bullied at school may stay home out of fear. They may even try to harm themselves because the bullying has done so much damage to their self-esteem. Bullying behavior is also harmful to the bullies themselves. They are more likely to drop out of school and to have problems with alcohol or violence.

A related problem is **hazing**. Hazing means making others perform certain tasks in order to join the group. Hazing activities can be physically or emotionally harmful. Hazing typically occurs when a group or club includes new members. The new members may be asked to "prove" their value to the other club members. Examples of hazing can include yelling or swearing at new members, forcing new group members to go without sleep, physically beating them, or forcing them to drink alcohol. Severe hazing incidents have been known to result in deaths. However, even mild hazing is disrespectful to the new members. It is often meant to humiliate them or prove that they are inferior to existing members of the group.

Bullies may intimidate others through verbal attacks, malicious rumors, or even physical force. **How would you feel if you were facing the bully in this picture?**

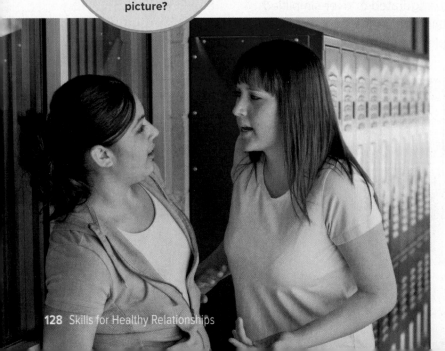

Tim Fuller Photography

Why Teens Become Bullies

Bullies target other teens in order to meet an unmet need. Some are angry because of problems in their lives, and hurting others makes them feel as if they have control over their lives. Other reasons teens become bullies include the need to fit into a group or to feel superior, to avoid being bullied by others, a lack of tolerance for those who are different, or because they lack parental supervision.

Many bullies have been bullied by other teens. They may bully as a way to be part of a group or to keep from being bullied themselves. When one teen bullies others so that he or she won't be bullied, that teen has created a negative cycle of bullying. This negative cycle will continue unless it is broken. To break the negative cycle of bullying, refuse to bully others.

Reading Check

Explain How can a teen break the negative cycle of bullying?

Why Teens Are Bullied

Our differences are what make us unique. One teen may prefer playing video games, while another prefers to play sports. Each choice is based on individual likes and dislikes, and each is acceptable. The teen years, however, are a time when people desire to fit into a group. In order to fit into a group, most teens feel that they must share the same likes and dislikes as other teens. They may be uncomfortable with differences. A teen who is uncomfortable with differences might become a bully and target teens who are different. Reasons that teens are targeted by bullies include:

- being different, such as being overweight or underweight, not sharing interests in activities and sports, needing glasses to see clearly, wearing unusual clothing, being new to a school, or not having popular items.

- being weak and unable to defend oneself.

- being depressed, anxious, or insecure with low self-esteem.

- having few friends or not being part of a clique

Reading Check

Describe How can the desire to fit into a group lead a teen to become a bully?

The Effects of Bullying

MAIN IDEA Bullying has a negative effect on everyone.

When a teen is bullied, he or she is not the only person affected. Everyone involved with bullying is affected, including the bully, the person bullied, and those who watch the bullying. Each of these – the bullied person, the bully, and those who watch – will experience negative effects related to the bullying.

A bully might be trying to gain some control over his or her life. The bully may have been bullied by others. He or she may suffer from low self-esteem and anger. A bully is at higher risk of dropping out of school, becoming violent and using illegal substances.

Teens who are bullied may experience the following effects:

- feeling fearful, helpless, depressed, and lonely.
- have low self-esteem.
- miss school, or drop out of school.
- health problems, such as stomach problems and depression.
- a change in sleep patterns.
- commit self-harm.

Even a teen who witnesses bullying may be affected by it. Watching someone else be bullied may remind that teen of a time when he or she was bullied. It could also create worry that they may be the next target of the bully. Even if that teen does not participate in the bullying, he or she may experience:

- increased use of tobacco, alcohol, or other drugs.
- increased mental health problems, including depression and anxiety.
- missing or skipping school.

Reading Check

Explain Why might a bully also suffer the effects of bullying?

Stop a Bully

MAIN IDEA Several strategies can stop bullying from occurring.

Teens can prevent bullying from happening. They can also help to stop it when it does occur. Strategies to stop bullying include those that are used on-the-spot. Other strategies can be used to stop bullying in the future. However, if the threat of violence exists, a teen should walk away from the bullying and find an adult. On-the-Spot strategies to stop bullying include:

- Tell the bully to stop. Look at the person and speak in a firm, positive voice with your head up. Say that if it continues, you will report the bullying.

- Try humor. This works best if joking is easy for you. Respond to the bully by agreeing with him or her in a humorous way. It could catch the bully off guard.

- Walk away and stay away. Do this if speaking up seems too difficult or unsafe.

- Avoid physical violence. Try to walk away and get help if you feel physically threatened. If violence does occur, protect yourself but do not escalate the violence.

- Find an adult. If the bullying is taking place at school, tell a teacher or a school official immediately.

Teens who are being targeted by a bully can use these future strategies to avoid the bully. These include:

- Talk to an adult you trust. A family member, teacher, or other adult can help. Telling someone can help you feel less alone. They can also help you make a plan to stop the bullying.

- Avoid places where you know bullies may wait to target other students. Stairwells, hallways, courtyards without supervision, and playground areas can be risky locations.

- Stay with a group or find a safe place to go. Bullies are less likely to target a student who is not alone.

Recognize Bullying Behavior

Some teens may not understand how their behavior might be considered to be bullying. If you like to joke with your friends, you can avoid becoming a bully by watching how your friend responds to your jokes. If your friend seems hurt, stop the behavior. A friend who jokes with others may not intend to hurt the feelings of another person. These teens may need help to recognize bullying behavior. If you have already been called a bully or you think you might have bullied another person, try following these steps:

- Stop and think before you say or do something that could hurt someone.

- If you feel like being mean to someone, think about why you want to be mean to that person.

- Talk to an adult you trust. Describe what upsets you about the other person.

- Remember that everyone is different, and that our differences make us interesting and unique.

- If you think you have bullied someone in the past, apologize to that person.

Reading Check

Explain Why is using humor a good strategy for stopping bullying?

Reading Check

Describe Why is it important to pay attention to a friend's response to your jokes?

Reading Check

List What are three ways you can help someone who is being bullied?

Character Check

Fairness is an important quality in any relationship. Whether you are facing an opponent in a student council election or competing with a friend on the tennis court, fairness is a principle that respects the abilities, needs, and contributions of all parties.

Stand Up to a Bully

If you see someone else being bullied you can try to take action to stop it. Even if the person being bullied is not a friend, stopping bullying shows good character. Of course, if you feel that the bully might become violent, it is best to find an adult to intervene to stop the bullying. Some ways that you can stop bullying include:

- Help the person escape the situation by saying that a teacher, parent, or other adult is looking for him or her.

- Tell the bully, "He's okay. Leave him alone," if it feels safe to do so.

- Distract the bully or offer an escape to the person being bullied by saying something like, "Mr. Smith needs to see you right now," or "Come on, we need you for our game," if it feels safe to do so.

- Avoid using violence or insults. It takes a lot of courage for someone to step up on behalf of a bullied person. However, using threats and insults is the same as the bully.

- Encourage the person being bullied to tell an adult.

- Report the bullying to school authorities, a parent, or other adult.

Finally, students can work together to stop bullying at their school. Ask if your school has a zero tolerance policy to bullying. In some schools, a **zero tolerance policy** may extend to bullying and cyberbullying that takes place off of the school property. This is a policy that makes no exceptions for anybody for any reason. This type of policy offers students who feel helpless and isolated a way to stop the bullying.

Lesson 2 Review

Facts and Vocabulary

1. Identify four ways to show respect in your relationships.

2. Define stereotypes.

3. List three reasons some teens bully others.

Thinking Critically

4. **Synthesize.** Give an example of how demonstrating strong values can strengthen your relationships with others.

5. **Analyze.** How is bullying different from hazing?

Applying Health Skills

6. **Decision Making.** Ahmed has just made the swim team, but he's concerned about reports that the varsity swimmers haze the new members. Use the decision-making process to analyze how Ahmed might deal with this problem.

Writing Critically

7. **Persuasive.** Write an editorial about the problem of bullying in schools. Your article should encourage students to help create a positive climate in which bullying is not tolerated.

Communicating Effectively

BIG IDEA Effective communication is a key to building healthy relationships.

REAL LIFE ISSUES

A Pushy Friend. Erin's friend Louise is the kind of person who always wants to have her own way. When they go out together, Louise always decides where they'll go and what they'll do. If Erin ever offers a suggestion, Louise dismisses it. Erin wants to stay friends with Louise, but she's getting tired of being pushed around. She wishes she knew how to stand up for herself without being rude. *Write a letter from Erin to Louise. In it, Erin should discuss how Louise's behavior makes her feel and explain that she'd like to have a say in what they do.*

After completing the lesson, review and analyze your response to the Real Life Issues question.

BEFORE YOU READ

Create a Word Web. Write the phrase "Effective Communication" in the center of a piece of paper. Jot down characteristics of effective communication. As you read, add more notes to your word web.

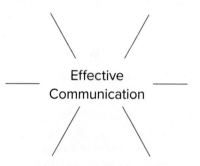

Effective Communication

Vocabulary

aggressive
passive
assertive
"I" messages
active listening
body language

Reading Check

Identify What are the three styles of communication?

Communication Styles

MAIN IDEA There are three types of communication.

Do you know someone who's like Louise, always insisting on doing things her or his own way? How about someone who's like Erin, always going along with what other people suggest? These two characters reflect two of the three major styles of communication. The three major styles are **aggressive**, **passive**, and **assertive** communications:

- Aggressive communication may involve bullying or intimidation. People with an aggressive communication style may not pay attention to other people's thoughts, feelings, or needs.

- Passive communicators put other people's needs ahead of their own. People may adopt a passive communication style because they dislike conflict and will go out of their way to avoid an argument.

- Assertive communication involves standing up for your own rights and beliefs while also respecting those of others. Dealing with a disagreement in an assertive way can involve negotiating with others to find the best solution to the problem.

Using an assertive communication style will improve your relationships with others. It will help ensure that your own needs are met, along with those of other people. In order to communicate assertively, you have to express your own views clearly and also hear and understand what other people have to say.

Ways to Communicate

MAIN IDEA To communicate effectively, you need to learn speaking skills, listening skills, and nonverbal communication.

Communication is a two-way street. It's not enough just to get your own messages through to the other person. You also need to receive the messages being sent to you. This means that while speaking is important to good communication, listening plays an equally important role. It's also necessary to understand nonverbal communication—the messages people send without using words. Knowing how to send and interpret these nonverbal messages will help you communicate better with others.

Speaking Skills

The key to good communication is to say what you mean. It's not reasonable to expect other people to read your mind or be able to pick up on subtle hints. If something is on your mind, you need to say what it is. For example, if a friend has hurt your feelings, you need to let that person know—as clearly and directly as you can.

Of course, being clear and direct doesn't mean being disrespectful of others. In fact, speaking in a way that seems disrespectful can actually make it harder to get your message across. When people feel that they are being attacked, they may be less willing to listen. One way to make sure you don't sound disrespectful when talking about a touchy subject is to use **"I" messages**. An "I" message is a statement that focuses on your feelings rather than on someone else's behavior. Using "I" messages helps you communicate your feelings in a positive way without placing blame on someone else.

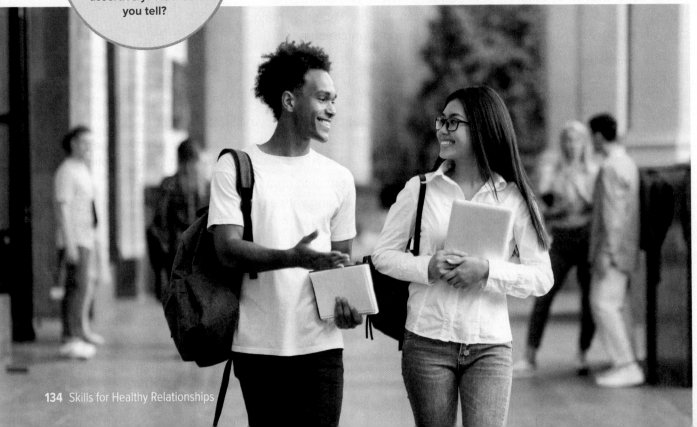

Communicating assertively makes your relationships run more smoothly. **Which teen in this photo would you say is communicating assertively? How can you tell?**

Prostock-Studio/Getty Images

"YOU" MESSAGES AND "I" MESSAGES	
"You" Messages	"I" Messages
"Why can't you ever show up on time?"	"I really don't like to be left waiting—it makes me feel like you don't think I'm important."
"You never listen to anything I say."	"I feel like my suggestions aren't being taken seriously."
"I said I'd take out the trash, and I will! You don't have to nag me about it every five minutes!"	"I'm feeling stressed because I have a big project due tomorrow. I'll take out the trash as soon as I finish working on this."
"You're always taking my things without asking."	"It bothers me when I get home and find my belongings in your room."
"You always ignore me when your other friends are around."	"I feel hurt when I'm left out of a conversation."

Compare the messages in these two columns. **How might a listener react to each message?**

Listening Skills

To communicate effectively, listening is just as important as speaking. You can make sure other people's messages get through to you by practicing **active listening**. This means paying close attention to what someone is saying and communicating. Active listening is a cooperative social skill because it shows that you are actively trying to understand what someone else is saying. Here are some ways to practice active listening:

- **Don't interrupt.** Give your full attention to what the speaker is saying.

- **Show interest.** Face the speaker and make eye contact to show that you are paying attention. You can also encourage the speaker by nodding or making comments such as "I see," "Go on," or "I understand" at appropriate times.

- **Restate what you hear.** Rephrase or summarize the speaker's words to make sure that you understand what you're hearing. For instance, you might say, "It sounds like you're not really sure whether you want to be part of the team anymore."

- **Ask questions**. Asking questions, such as "How do you feel about that?" Asking questions can help you understand what the speaker is saying. It can also help the speaker get a clearer idea of his or her own thoughts and feelings.

- **Show empathy.** Let the other person know that you can relate to his or her feelings. One way to do this is by describing a similar experience you may have had. However, don't steer the conversation away from the speaker's problem to your own problem. Also, avoid comparing the speaker's behavior with your own. Try not to pass judgment on the speaker's attitudes and actions.

Reading Check

Describe What does active listening involve?

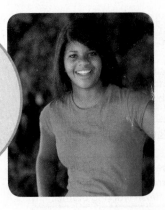
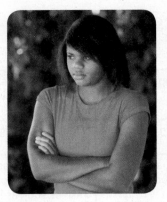
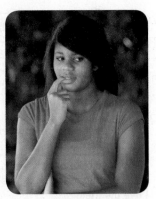

Body language is an important part of nonverbal communication.

Nonverbal Communication

Sometimes, what you say isn't as important as how you say it. A comment such as "Nice outfit" can actually sound like an insult if it's delivered in a sarcastic tone. Your tone of voice is an example of nonverbal communication.

Your **body language** can also affect the meaning of the messages you send to people. Body language is nonverbal communication through gestures, facial expressions, behaviors, and posture. Body language includes everything from nodding your head, which shows that you agree, to turning away, shows that you have stopped listening.

Sometimes you send messages through body language without even realizing it. For example, if you're feeling embarrassed, you may look at the ground instead of at the person you're talking to. In some cases, your body language may even **contradict** what you're saying in words. For instance, saying "I'm fine" in an angry growl with your arms folded will probably make people think you're anything but fine. Being aware of your body language can help you avoid sending mixed messages that may confuse your listeners.

ACADEMIC VOCABULARY

contradict *(verb)*: to imply the opposite of

Encouraging your friends to pursue their interests is one way to show your appreciation for them. **What are other ways to let people in your life know you value them?**

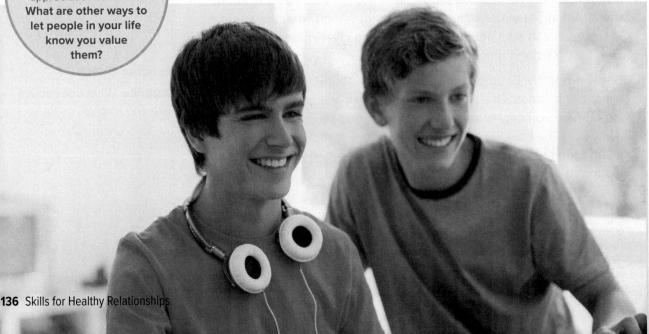

(l, c, r)Tim Fuller Photography, (b)Paul Bradbury/age footstock

Offering Useful Feedback

MAIN IDEA Offering constructive feedback can improve your relationships with others.

Even in a strong relationship, every now and then people say or do things that bother each other. For example, you might have a friend who's lots of fun to be around, except that he drives you crazy by interrupting you whenever you're talking. If you want your friend to change his behavior, you have to let him know how you feel—but in a way that doesn't come across as a personal attack. In other words, you need to offer constructive criticism, nonhostile comments that point out problems and encourage improvement.

The goal of constructive criticism is to bring about positive changes. Thus, it's counterproductive to give it in an aggressive way. Attacking someone isn't going to encourage him or her to change. Instead, use "I" messages that focus on the problem, not the person. To offer constructive criticism, point out a specific problem, explain why it bothers you, and suggest a specific solution. For example, you might say, "I feel that sometimes my ideas don't get heard. I'd really appreciate it if you could let me finish talking. Then I'll be happy to hear what's on your mind."

Letting people know how their actions make you feel isn't something you should do only when there's a problem. It's also important to let people know you appreciate what they do for you. If a friend goes out of her way to help you and doesn't get so much as a "thank you," she might feel that her actions went unnoticed or unappreciated. Let the people in your life know you value them. Tell your dad how much you enjoyed a meal that he prepared, or compliment a friend on her terrific skill as an artist. A little appreciation can go a long way to strengthen a relationship.

Reading Check

Explain What is the goal of constructive criticism?

Myths & Reality

Think you know all there is to know about effective communication? This fact might change your mind.

Myth: I need to use a "You" message to get someone to change his or her behavior or actions.

Reality: "I" messages are a more effective way to communicate because they do not place blame. "You" messages seem disrespectful and often this language makes it harder to get your message across.

Lesson 3 Review

Facts and Vocabulary

1. List the three main styles of communication.

2. List three ways to show interest in what another person is saying.

3. Define the term body language and give an example.

Thinking Critically

4. **Evaluate.** Leah is an aggressive communicator. When somebody says something she disagrees with, she always says, "You're wrong!" How could Leah's communication style affect her relationships with others?

5. **Synthesize.** In a paragraph, discuss how having strong communication in your relationships can contribute to your personal health and safety.

Applying Health Skills

6. **Analyzing Influences.** Think about different factors that can influence how you communicate with others. Factors may include family, peers, culture, or personality. In a paragraph, discuss how one of these factors affects your personal communication style.

Writing Critically

7. **Narrative.** Write a dialogue in which one character offers constructive criticism to another. Follow the guidelines for giving constructive criticism.

LESSON 1

Vocabulary Review

Choose the correct word in the sentences below.

1. A bond or connection you have with other people is called a *relationship/friendship*.

2. *Communication/Citizenship* lets you express your thoughts, feelings, and expectations to others.

3. In *cooperation/compromise,* each participant gives up something to reach a solution that satisfies everyone.

Understanding Key Concepts

After reading the question or statement, select the correct answer.

4. Which of the following is an example of good citizenship?
   a. Looking after a younger brother or sister
   b. Helping a friend study for a test
   c. Taking part in an effort to clean up a local river
   d. Getting good grades in school

5. Jeanne and her father have very different political views. However, they accept their differences and do not try to change each other's opinions. Which quality of strong relationships does this action show?
   a. Mutual respect
   b. Caring
   c. Honesty
   d. Commitment

Thinking Critically

After reading the question or statement, write a short answer using complete sentences.

6. **Describe.** Identify and describe three roles you play in your relationships with others.

7. **Explain.** How does cooperation strengthen your relationships?

8. **Evaluate.** Give an example of a situation in which you should *not* be willing to compromise.

9. **Synthesize.** Identify one trait of good character, and give an example of how it can strengthen a relationship.

LESSON 2

Vocabulary Review

Use the correct vocabulary terms to complete the following statements.

10. _____ is an unfair opinion or judgment of a particular group of people.

11. People display _____ when they recognize and appreciate the differences among people.

12. Deliberately harming or threatening other people who cannot easily defend themselves is known as _____.

Understanding Key Concepts

After reading the question or statement, select the correct answer.

13. Teens who respect themselves probably will choose friends who
    a. are the smartest students in the class.
    b. participate in a wide variety of school activities.
    c. share all of their beliefs, tastes, and values.
    d. treat them with respect.

14. Which of the following statements is *not* an example of prejudice?
    a. I get nervous when I'm in large groups of strangers.
    b. I think kids from private schools are stuck-up.
    c. I don't want girls on our baseball team because they can't throw.
    d. I want to be friends only with Asian American kids because they're such good students.

15. Which of the following is *not* an example of bullying?
    a. Repeatedly making fun of the way a classmate talks
    b. Threatening to beat up a student if he doesn't hand over his lunch money
    c. Accepting someone into your group regardless of the clothing brand she wears
    d. Shoving a younger kid on the school bus

16. If you are being bullied at school, you should
- **a.** just ignore the bully until she goes away.
- **b.** stay home from school to avoid the bully.
- **c.** get a group of friends to gang up on the bully and attack him.
- **d.** tell a trusted adult about the problem and ask for help.

Thinking Critically

After reading the question or statement, write a short answer using complete sentences.

17. Discuss. How might you demonstrate respect in your relationship with a teacher?

18. Explain. In what ways can prejudice harm relationships?

19. Analyze. Explain how bullying can be harmful both to victims and to bullies themselves.

20. Evaluate. At Corinne's school, students who are new to the drama club usually get assigned to sing in the chorus or paint the sets. In contrast, more experienced students get the lead roles in the plays. Is this an example of hazing? Explain why or why not.

LESSON 3

Vocabulary Review

Correct the sentences below by replacing the italicized term with the correct vocabulary term.

21. Trying to get your own way through bullying or intimidation is an example of *passive* communication.

22. Someone using *assertive* communication is unwilling or unable to express his thoughts and feelings.

23. When you use *body language,* you focus on your own feelings rather than on someone else's behavior.

Understanding Key Concepts

After reading the question or statement, select the correct answer.

24. Some of the friends in your group want to go out for Thai food, but you don't like Thai food. Which of the following would be an assertive way to respond?
- **a.** Tell them Thai food is not your favorite and politely suggest an alternative.
- **b.** Go with them for Thai food, but don't eat anything.
- **c.** Just go along with whatever the group wants.
- **d.** Insist on going for Mexican food instead.

25. Which of the following skills is *not* a part of active listening?
- **a.** Listening without interrupting
- **b.** Making eye contact with the speaker
- **c.** Asking questions for clarification
- **d.** Using "I" messages

26. If you stand with your hands on your hips and your lips in a frown while someone is talking, what message might you be sending with your body language?
- **a.** "I'm really interested in everything you're saying."
- **b.** "I'm feeling angry."
- **c.** "I'm embarrassed about something."
- **d.** "I am respectfully considering your opinion."

27. Which of the following is an example of constructive criticism?
- **a.** "Do you always have to leave all your junk out in the hall?"
- **b.** "I can't stand the way you interrupt me all the time."
- **c.** "Haven't you ever heard of knocking? You're always barging into my room!"
- **d.** "Next time, would you mind calling first to let me know you're coming over?"

Thinking Critically

After reading the question or statement, write a short answer using complete sentences.

28. **Evaluate.** Which communication style will most enhance your relationships? Explain how.

29. **Analyze.** Describe the roles that speaking, listening, and body language play in communication.

30. **Synthesize.** A friend calls to tell you that she just broke up with her boyfriend. Explain how you might use active listening in this situation.

31. **Explain.** Why are "I" messages an important part of constructive criticism?

PROJECT-BASED ASSESSMENT

Effective Communication Skills

BACKGROUND

As you've learned, effective communication involves strong speaking and listening skills. The use of technology can play a major role in communication.

TASK

Show two scenarios of people communicating to one another through e-mail. The first scenario should show how someone with weak communication skills may end up sending confusing messages. The second scenario should demonstrate how using effective communication skills can prevent the problems shown in the first example.

AUDIENCE

Other students in your class.

PURPOSE

Demonstrate and practice communication skills.

PROCEDURE

1. Create an example of communication between two people through e-mail. The topic can involve going to the movies, going on a date, or something similar.

2. The first example of communication should show how a teen can experience problems in communication, such as sending an unclear message.

3. Create the second communication example in which the teen avoids communication problems by using effective strategies.

4. Present your communication examples to the class.

Math Practice

Calculate Percentages. Bullying occurs more frequently among middle school students, but it also happens in high school. This diagram shows the estimated number of students affected by bullying.

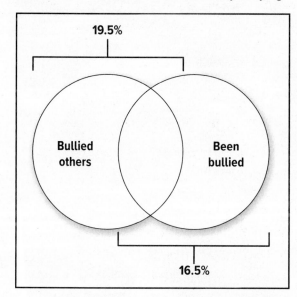

1. About 6% of all students have both bullied other students and have been the victim of a bully. From this information and the diagram, what percentage of students have either been bullied or have bullied another student, but not both?
   a. 3.5% c. 30%
   b. 6% d. 36%

2. Suppose there are 842 students in your school. Using the percentages shown in the diagram, estimate the number of students in your school who have bullied another student.
   a. 25 c. 139
   b. 51 d. 164

3. Using the percentages given above, explain how you would determine the number of students in your school who have neither bullied another student nor been bullied.

Reading/Writing Practice

Understand and Apply. Read the passage below, and then answer the questions.

1. Will: Hey, Jim, are you busy on Sunday? We could catch the afternoon showing of that new action movie. 2. Jim: Actually, I saw that last week with my brother. 3. Will: Well, that's the only movie I want to see. 4. Jim: Oh, it's okay. I don't mind seeing it again. 5. Will: Good. Meet me there at one. 6. Jim: Um, I have church that day, so that will be cutting it close . . . but don't worry about it. 7. Will: Who's worried?

1. What does line 3 reveal about Will's personality?
   a. He does not like movies.
   b. He treats his friends with respect.
   c. He is used to getting his own way.
   d. He is unwilling to express his thoughts and feelings.

2. Jim could best be described as
   a. enthusiastic.
   b. passive.
   c. inconsiderate.
   d. uncommunicative.

3. Rewrite this dialogue with Jim using a more assertive communication style. Your new dialogue should show how being assertive results in an outcome that is more acceptable for both teens.

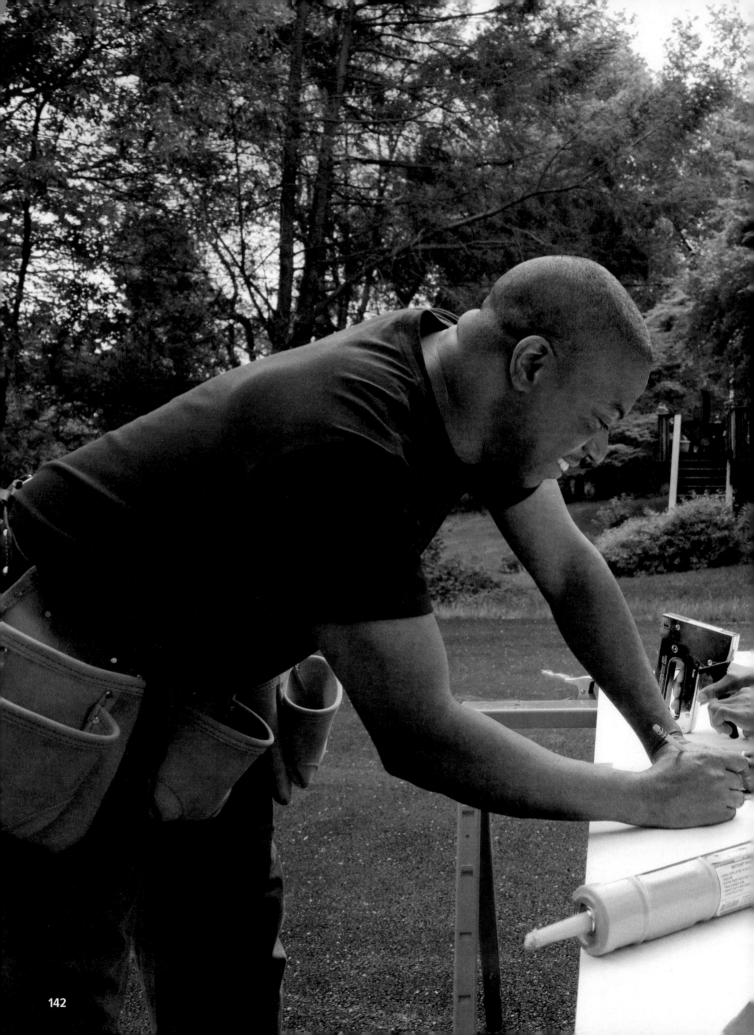

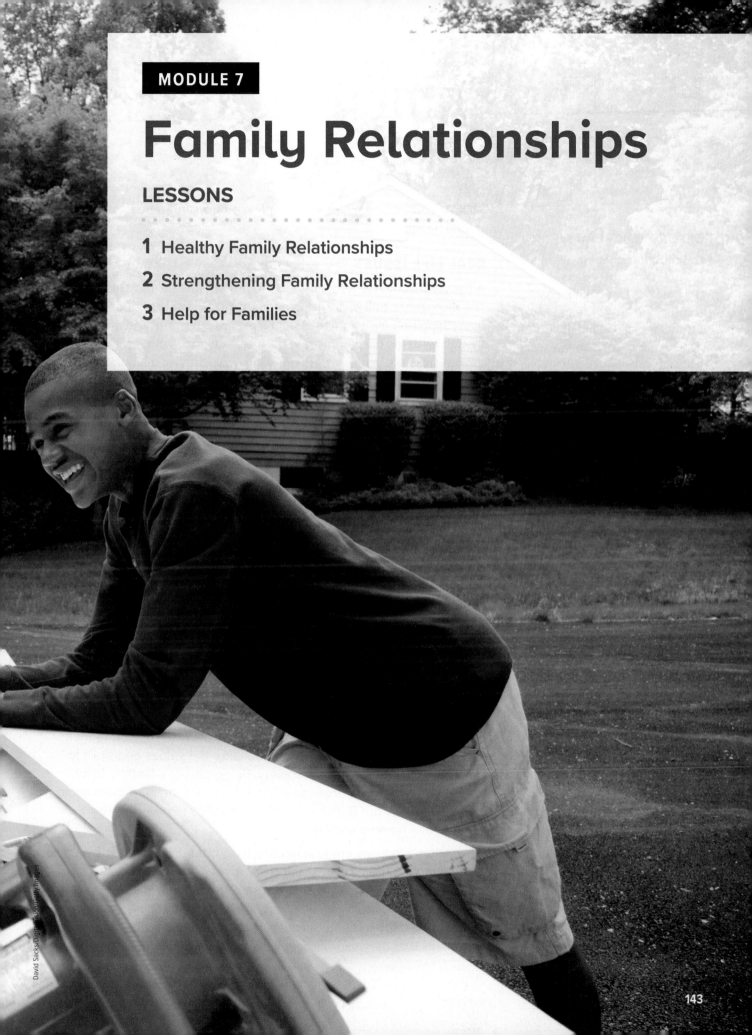

Family Relationships

LESSONS

1 Healthy Family Relationships

2 Strengthening Family Relationships

3 Help for Families

David Sacks/Digital Vision/Getty Images

Healthy Family Relationships

• • • • • • • • • • • •

BEFORE YOU READ

Organize Information. Draw a triangle. Label the sides "Physical," "Mental/Emotional," and "Social." As you read, record information about how families affect each area of health.

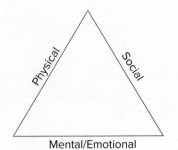

Vocabulary

siblings
nuclear family
single-parent family
blended family
extended family
adoptive family
foster family
affirmation

• • • • • • • • • • • •

BIG IDEA Your relationships with family members influence your total health.

REAL LIFE ISSUES

A Family Discovery. Recently, Jack found out that he's adopted. The discovery came as a shock, and now he's starting to question everything he's ever known about himself and his family. Even though he loves his parents and brother and knows they love him too, he still feels confused. He doesn't know whether to think of them as his "real" family anymore, and he also wonders about his biological parents. *Write a journal entry from Jack's point of view. In it, Jack should express his feelings about being adopted and reflect on how this discovery could affect his life.*

After completing the lesson, review and analyze your response to the Real Life Issues question.

The Family Unit

MAIN IDEA There are many kinds of families, but all family members have certain responsibilities toward each other.

What is a family? This question is not as simple as it sounds. There are many different types of families. Family members may be related to each other by birth, marriage, or adoption. People in the same family may live together or separately.

No matter who is in your family, your relationships with them are some of the most important in your life. Family relationships have a strong influence on your total health. Healthy families provide support to their members and help children and teens develop the values and skills to become successful members of society. Being part of a healthy family can also be an important protective factor for teens, helping them avoid behaviors that may put their health at risk. Healthy families are the foundation of a healthy society.

However, some families are less healthy than others, which may create a disadvantage in the type of support some teens receive. But this does not mean that they cannot set and accomplish goals. Teens who are part of unhealthy families can ultimately develop into healthy, happy adults. Finding a trusted adult to talk to can help these teens manage the problems that they experience.

Types of Families

When you think about families, you may picture your own parents or **siblings**, which are your brothers and sisters. You may also think of other families you know, which may be different from your own. To some people, the word family suggests a **nuclear family**— two parents and one or more children living in the same place. Although this is a common family structure in America, increasing numbers of children and teens live in other types of families, such as the **single-parent family**, **blended family**, **extended family**, **adoptive family**, or if a child or teen is in foster care, a **foster family**:

- **Single-parent families.** These are families with only one parent caring for one or more children. For example, children and teens may live with one parent after a divorce or the other parent's death.

- **Blended families.** These families form when a single parent remarries. The new couple may decide to add to their blended family by having more children.

- **Extended families.** Some people live with members of their extended family, such as grandparents, aunts, uncles, or cousins. Other people have such relatives but see them only on visits. Some people live in intergenerational families, which have three or more generations living together.

- **Adoptive families.** These families consist of a parent or parents and one or more adopted children. Some families have both biological children and adopted children.

- **Foster families.** Children or teens may be placed in foster care because they have lost their parents or because of problems in their original families, such as abuse. Some foster children will eventually return to live with their natural parents. Others may go to live with relatives or be adopted. In some cases, foster parents may decide to adopt a child or teen who has been living with them.

Reading Check

Compare and Contrast How do adoptive families differ from foster families?

Families may include members who are related by birth, by adoption, or both. **What do you think makes someone part of a family?**

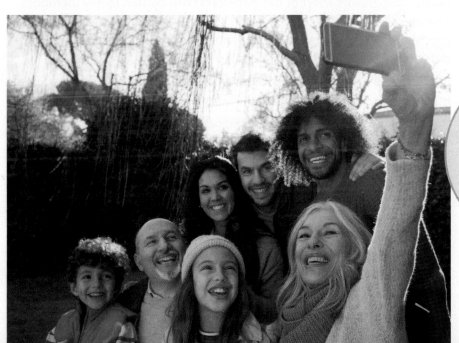

Tim Macpherson/Cultura/Getty Images

America's Families

The structure of American families has shifted over the past several decades. The table below shows how the living arrangements of American children under 18 have changed since 1960. Review the statistics and use the table to answer the questions.

Activity: Mathematics

1. In the year 1960, what percentage of all children lived in each type of household?

2. In the year 2019, what percentage of all children lived in each type of household?

3. What factors do you think contributed to the shift in family structure during this 53-year period?

LIVING ARRANGEMENTS OF AMERICAN CHILDREN UNDER 18						
Year	Total children under 18	Two parents	Mother only	Father only	Other relatives	Nonrelatives
1960	63,727	55,877	5,105	724	1,601	420
1970	69,162	58,939	7,452	748	1,546	477
1980	63,427	48,624	11,406	1,060	1,949	388
1990	64,137	46,503	13,874	1,993	1,421	346
2000	72,012	49,795	16,162	3,058	2,160	837
2010	74,718	51,823	17,283	2,572	2,380	662
2019	75,525	51,561	15,764	3,234	2,319	647

Source: https://www.census.gov/data/tables/time-series/demo/families/children.html

CONCEPT Number and Operations: Percents

A percent is a ratio comparing a number to 100. To calculate percentage, divide the given amount by the total amount. Then multiply the answer by 100 and add a percent sign (%).

Family Interactions

Think for a minute about the roles that different people play in your family. Who makes most of the decisions? Are certain family members responsible for particular jobs, such as sweeping floors or buying groceries? Do you personally have more responsibilities now than you did when you were younger?

In a family, each member plays certain roles and has certain responsibilities. In general, parents or guardians are in charge of meeting the family's basic needs, such as food and shelter. Parents also serve as teachers in the family, establishing rules and setting limits to protect their children's health and safety. They teach their children about the reasons for these rules, as well as teaching the values and skills that will guide them once they are grown.

Children and teens, meanwhile, have roles and responsibilities of their own. When they are young, their main job is to respect the **authority** of parents or guardians. As they get older, they may take on more responsibilities, such as doing chores or caring for younger siblings. By taking on such jobs, teens can help the family run more smoothly and boost their own self-esteem.

ACADEMIC VOCABULARY

authority *(noun)*: the right to make decisions and give commands

Other relatives play a role in the family as well. For example, grandparents may help care for children and teach them about the family's history. Aunts and uncles may serve as mentors and role models. Cousins who are close in age may be friends and playmates to children in the family.

Your Family and Your Health

MAIN IDEA Your family members contribute to your health.

People live together in families for a simple reason: it helps them live longer, better lives. Being part of a family helps you meet your basic needs. Beyond that, being part of a healthy family can strengthen all three aspects of your health.

Promoting Physical Health

The most obvious way your family promotes your physical health is by providing for your basic physical needs. Your parents and guardians make sure that you receive food, clothing, and shelter. They also promote your physical health in a variety of other ways.

- **Providing medical care**. Your parents or guardians take you to the doctor when you are sick. It is their responsibility to make sure you get medical and dental checkups and necessary immunizations. As you get older, you will become more responsible for your own medical care.

- **Setting limits on behavior.** Do your parents set rules about things like how much TV you are allowed to watch or how late you can stay out at night? Although it may not always be obvious, the purpose of these rules is to promote your safety and health. For instance, setting a curfew can protect you from risky situations and also help make sure you get enough sleep.

- **Teaching health skills.** When you were young, your parents helped teach you the skills you'd need to control your own behavior as you got older. For example, they may have taught you basic safety skills, such as wearing a helmet when you ride a bike. They may also have encouraged you to develop healthy habits, like eating nutritious foods and being physically active.

Fitness Zone

It feels good to do something nice for someone, and it can be good for your health too. That's why I like to take my little brother and sister to the park to play catch or basketball. I want to be a good role model and teach them just how important exercise is. Besides, the smiles on their faces make it all worthwhile.

By encouraging healthful behaviors such as physical activity, parents and other family members can promote physical health. **What are other ways your family influences your physical health?**

Promoting Mental and Emotional Health

As you get older, you may rely less on your family to meet your physical needs. However, it is likely that your family still plays an important role in meeting your mental and emotional needs. For example, your family can provide a safe environment for you to express and deal with your emotions. Family members can also give you love and support, helping to meet your basic need to feel that you belong. This sense of belonging, in turn, can help boost your self-esteem.

Your family can also help meet your need to feel valued and recognized. Family members may provide **affirmation** in a variety of ways. Affirmation is positive feedback that helps others feel appreciated and supported. For instance, they can celebrate your achievements with you or show appreciation for the things you do to help out at home.

Promoting Social Health

Your family also plays an important role in your social development. In the first few years of your life, family members helped you learn how to communicate and get along with others. As you grew, your family may have helped you learn other important social skills, such as how to cooperate with others and how to resolve conflicts. The social skills you learned from your family will help you to make your own way in the world as an independent adult.

Family members can provide affirmation by celebrating each other's achievements. **What are other ways family members can support each other mentally and emotionally?**

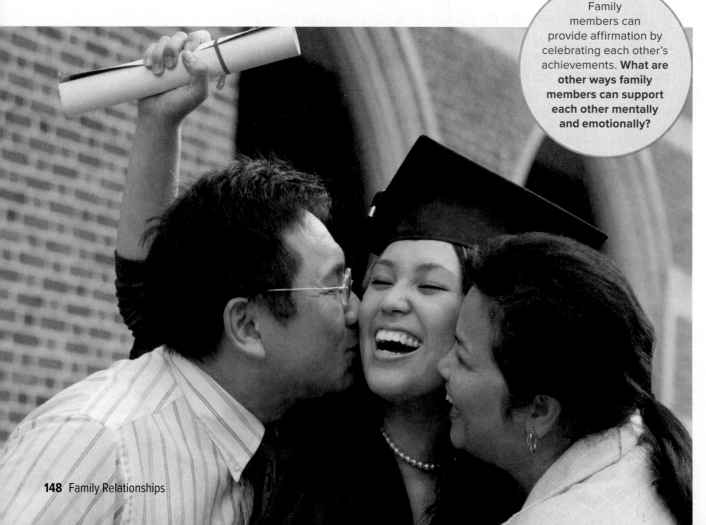

Ariel Skelley/Getty Images

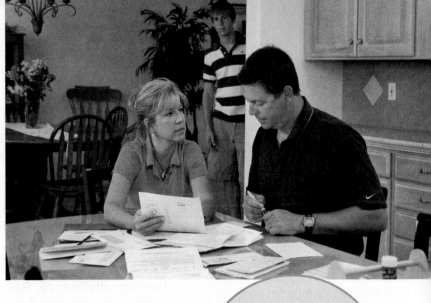

Values. One of the most important ways families promote social health is by instilling values. Parents play an important role in helping children develop core ethical values, such as responsibility, honesty, and respect. Learning these values is a key to developing strong character.

Families can teach values in different ways. One way is simply to explain them. For instance, if two siblings are fighting over a toy, a parent might sit down with them and explain why it's important to share. Teaching by example can be an even more powerful way to promote good values. Let's say a parent is shopping with a child and receives too much change back for his or her purchase. By immediately returning the extra money, the parent teaches the child about honesty and fairness. Likewise, parents who demonstrate kindness and respect in their daily behaviors reinforce these same values in their children. By being positive role models, parents and other family members help children develop strong values.

Cultural Heritage. Families also promote social health by sharing their culture and traditions. For instance, families may light candles together for Kwanzaa or enjoy a barbecue and fireworks on the Fourth of July. Sharing their culture in this way enriches the lives of family members and helps them develop a sense of cultural identity. This awareness of being part of a larger culture can create important social bonds that extend beyond the family.

Parents play a significant role in the development of children's ethical values and sense of responsibility. **How might sharing family financial matters with teens help them develop strong values?**

Lesson 1 Review

Facts and Vocabulary

1. What is a sibling?

2. Name three kinds of families.

3. Identify four ways in which families promote the physical health of children and teens.

Thinking Critically

4. **Synthesize.** Explain how the role you play within your family has changed over time.

5. **Analyze.** How does providing affirmation within the family promote mental and emotional health?

Applying Health Skills

6. **Communication Skills.** Work with a classmate to write and perform a scene that shows family members supporting each other mentally and emotionally. The scene should include "I" messages, active listening, and appropriate body language.

Writing Critically

7. **Personal.** Write a personal essay about your family. Describe how you interact, and discuss how family members contribute to each other's total health.

Strengthening Family Relationships

BEFORE YOU READ

Create a T-Chart. Make a two-column table. Label the columns "Change in Family Structure" and "Change in Circumstances." As you read, fill in each column with examples of changes that can affect families, and strategies strong families can use to deal with these changes.

Change in Structure	Change in Circumstances

Vocabulary

separation
divorce
custody

BIG IDEA Family members support and care for one another, especially during difficult times.

REAL LIFE ISSUES

Dealing with Divorce. Beth has just learned that her parents are getting a divorce. Her father will be moving across town, and she knows that she's going to be asked where she wants to live. Beth is close to both her parents, and she doesn't want to have to choose between them. She'd like to tell her parents how she feels, but she doesn't want to add to their problems. *Write a dialogue in which Beth discusses her feelings with one or both of her parents. Each character should demonstrate good communication skills.*

After completing the lesson, review and analyze your response to the Real Life Issues question.

Characteristics of Strong Families

MAIN IDEA Strong families support their members in a variety of ways.

Different families interact together in different ways. For example, Joyce's family tends to be reserved around each other. They tend to discuss ideas calmly and rationally. When Joyce goes to her friend Ted's house, she's always amazed at how freely his family expresses emotions. Ted and his family laugh and cry easily together. They tease each other and even get into arguments, but they always make up.

This doesn't mean that Ted's family is healthier than Joyce's, or vice versa. They just interact in different ways. The important thing is that both Ted and Joyce feel secure and loved. Both of their families demonstrate traits of strong families, like the ones listed below.

- **Good communication.** Healthy families can share their thoughts and feelings honestly with each other. They listen to each other and demonstrate empathy.

- **Caring and support.** Family members show that they love each other through their words and actions. They express appreciation for each other and help each other through difficult times.

- **Respect.** Family members accept each other as they are. They respect each other's opinions, tastes, and abilities. They show consideration by sharing, being courteous, respecting each individual's privacy, and helping out with household tasks.

- **Commitment.** Healthy families make time for each other. They work together to solve problems, and they're willing to make sacrifices for the good of the family.

- **Trust.** In a healthy family, parents earn their children's trust by being honest and keeping their promises. Children show that they are worthy of trust by being honest, loyal, and reliable.

Reading Check

Identify How can family members show respect for each other?

Coping with Change

MAIN IDEA Family members can help each other cope with changes in the family's structure or circumstances.

Real-life families aren't always like the ones you see in movies and television shows. Families in sitcoms, for instance, may never seem to have any problems that they can't solve by the end of a half-hour episode. In real life, family relationships can be much more complicated.

Families can face a variety of problems, major and minor. Many of these problems have to do with changes in the family's structure or circumstances. A parent losing a job, for example, or the serious illness of a family member, can lead to long-term stress for the whole family. Even positive events, such as a move or the marriage of a relative, can create stress. Since change is a normal part of life, healthy families must be prepared to deal with changes and help each other cope.

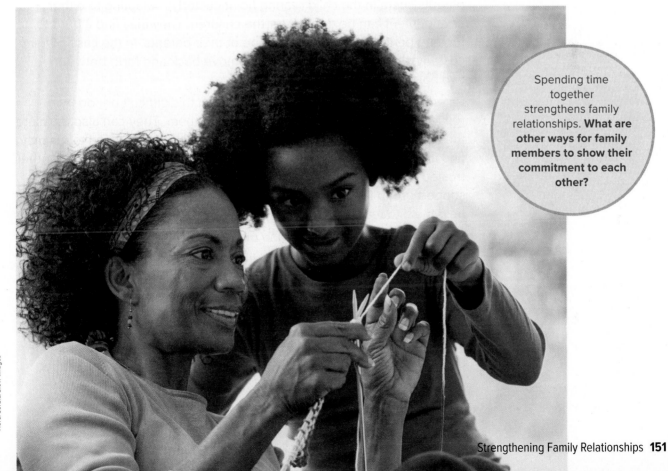

Spending time together strengthens family relationships. **What are other ways for family members to show their commitment to each other?**

Hero/Corbis/Glow Images

• • • • • • • • • • • •

Reading Check

Compare and Contrast What is the difference between separation and divorce?

• • • • • • • • • • • •

Changes in Family Structure

The structure of a family changes when someone new joins the family or when a family member moves out of the home. Both kinds of changes can be stressful for family members. Examples of changes in family structure include births, adoption, separation, divorce, remarriage, and the death of a family member.

Birth and Adoption. Welcoming a new baby or an adopted child into the family is a joyful event. However, adjusting to the new situation isn't always easy. Making room for the new child means that everyone else has to make do with less space. Also, as parents devote time and emotional energy to the new child, they may have less time for the other children—and for each other. All these changes can create stress for everyone. Family members can help each other through this time by sharing the responsibility for taking care of the new child. They can also make an effort to find time for each other.

Separation and Divorce. Separation and divorce are difficult, especially since they result in a family member leaving the home environment. **Separation** is a decision by two married people to live apart from each other. Couples who separate may hope to eventually work out their differences and live together again. **Divorce**, by contrast, is a legal end to a marriage contract.

When parents divorce, they need to come to an agreement about where the children will live. **Custody** is the legal right to make decisions affecting children and the responsibility for their care. Custody may be granted to only one parent (sole custody) or divided so that both parents share in the child rearing (joint custody). Adapting to either arrangement can be difficult for the children. They may find it hard to go for long periods without seeing one of their parents. In the case of joint custody, they may find it stressful to move back and forth between two homes.

Parents can help their children get through this difficult period by reminding them that both parents still love them. They can also reassure the children that the divorce was not their fault. Children and teens may find it easier to cope if they discuss their feelings with parents and other trusted adults. In some cases, they may want to consider joining a support group for children of divorce. Being part of such a group may help them to realize that they are not alone.

Remarriage. After a divorce, one or both parents may decide to marry again. A parent may also remarry after the death of a spouse. When a parent remarries, the children must adjust to dealing with, or even living with, a stepparent. Children may be reluctant to open up to a new stepparent because it feels like they are being disloyal to their parent or their parent's memory. If the stepparent has children from a previous marriage, all members of the blended family will need time to adjust to their new relationships. Good communication and mutual respect will make this process easier.

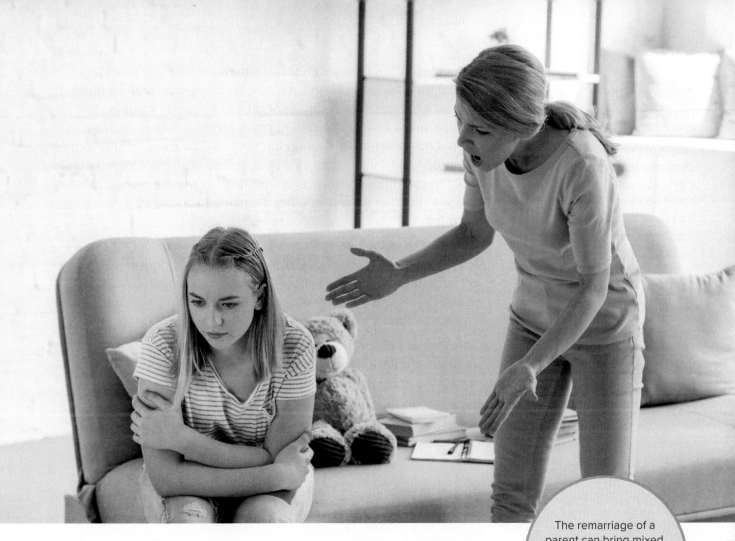

Death of a Family Member. Perhaps the most difficult change a family can go through is the death of a family member, with all the feelings of grief that it brings. Family members can help each other through this difficult time by sharing their feelings and memories about the person they've lost. It's also important for family members to respect each other's feelings. They should remember that the process of grieving is different for everyone. Joining a support group or seeking help from a counselor may also help people who have lost a loved one to recover from their pain.

Changes in Family Circumstances

Changes in a family's **circumstances** can also be a source of stress. Family members can help each other deal with these changes by communicating honestly and showing as much support as possible. Examples of changes in family circumstances include:

- **Moving to a new home.** When a family moves, especially over a long distance, family members may miss their old friends and familiar surroundings. Teens may be anxious about making new friends and adjusting to a new school. When a move results from the breakup of a marriage, it can add to the stress already caused by the divorce.

> The remarriage of a parent can bring mixed feelings. **How can teens show support for a parent's decision to remarry?**

ACADEMIC VOCABULARY

circumstance *(noun)*: an event that influences another event

Character Check

When you seek help for a problem that affects the health of the family, you are demonstrating caring. Make a list of people you think you could approach for assistance if a family member has a substance abuse problem.

- **Changes in the family's financial situation.** Financial problems can result from the loss of a job, a medical emergency, or the inability to follow a budget. Not having enough money to pay the bills can cause stress for all family members. It can also lead to arguments about how the family's limited funds should be used. Interestingly, a sudden financial gain can also be a source of stress. Unaccustomed wealth can trigger anxiety and confusion as people wonder what to do with the money and whether it's going to change the way people see them.

- **Illness and disability.** A serious illness or disability can disrupt a family's normal routine. One or more family members may need to change their schedules to care for the sick or disabled person. Coping with this situation may be easier if all family members play a role in caring for the sick or disabled person.

- **Alcohol or other drug abuse.** Substance abuse is one of the most serious problems that a family can face. Family members must seek outside help to deal with the situation. Teens may wish to consult teachers, other trusted adults, or organizations such as Alateen.

Talking with a parent or other trusted adult can help you deal with the stress of family changes. **To whom do you turn when you need to talk?**

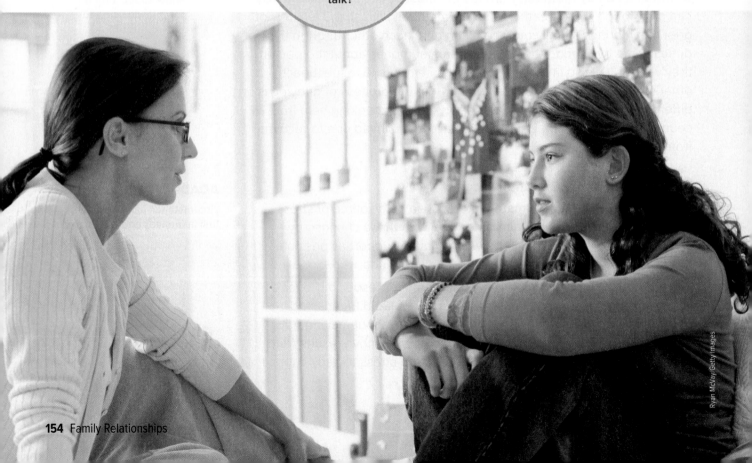

Ryan McVay/Getty Images

Coping With Changes

One of the most important strategies for coping with changes in the family is to talk honestly and openly with other family members. Just talking about your feelings can help reduce the stress. Letting family members know about your needs and wants can also make it easier for them to help you.

You, in turn, can make an effort to support your family members during a difficult period. For example, if your parents are also dealing with stress, you can offer to lighten their load by taking on more chores and responsibilities at home. You can also make a point of being there for family members if they want to talk and showing empathy for their feelings.

If sharing their problems with each other is not enough, family members may find it helpful to talk to someone outside the family. This person could be a counselor, teacher, or member of the clergy. Family members can also try to learn more about the situation they're dealing with, either by reading books or by talking to people who have been through similar experiences. Finally, families should be willing to seek professional help if they need it.

Lesson 2 Review

Facts and Vocabulary

1. How can family members demonstrate good communication?

2. Name the two main types of changes that cause stress in families?

3. Identify three situations that can lead to a change in family structure.

Thinking Critically

4. **Analyze.** Compare and contrast the difficulties sole custody and joint custody can pose for teens whose parents are divorced.

5. **Synthesize.** Give an example of a positive or negative event that could cause stress within a family. Explain what strategies the family might use to deal with this stress.

Applying Health Skills

6. **Stress Management.** Think of a stressful family situation. Then list five stress-management techniques that can help you handle this stress.

Writing Critically

7. **Narrative.** Children sometimes go through stages of grief (denial, anger, bargaining, depression, and acceptance) in response to their parents' divorce. Write a story about a teen who goes through several of these stages. Describe how the teen expresses his or her feelings at each stage.

Help for Families

. . . .

BEFORE YOU READ

Create a Word Web. In the center of a sheet of paper, write the phrase "Sources of Support." As you read, add information about sources of help for families in trouble.

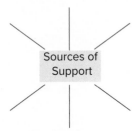

Sources of Support

Vocabulary

abuse
domestic violence
coercion
spousal abuse
child abuse
neglect
elder abuse
cycle of violence
crisis center

. . . .

BIG IDEA Families may require outside assistance to deal with serious problems.

REAL LIFE ISSUES

Worried About a Friend. Mark is worried about his friend Sofia. Sofia says her parents argue a lot, and she thinks that her dad hits her mom. One evening, Mark called Sofia to ask her a question about a homework assignment and heard her parents arguing in the background. Another time, Mark thought he saw Sofia crying at school. *Write a dialogue in which Mark encourages Sofi a to confide in him and seek help. Make sure Mark uses good communication techniques.*

After completing the lesson, review and analyze your response to the Real Life Issues question

---

Violence in Families

MAIN IDEA Violence in families can cause lasting harm.

All families have problems from time to time, and that is normal. In most cases, families can work through their problems with the help of good communication and mutual support. However, some problems are too serious for family members to handle on their own. One of the most dangerous problems a family can face is **abuse**. Abuse is the physical, mental, emotional, or sexual mistreatment of one person by another. Forms of abuse in families include **domestic violence**, which is abuse involving family members, as well as emotional and sexual abuse. Another form of domestic violence is **coercion**. Coercion is using force or threats to persuade another person to do something. One person may use coercion to have another person do something that they don't want to do, such as become sexually active or commit a crime.

Spousal Abuse

Spousal abuse can occur in all kinds of families, regardless of income, ethnicity, or education level. Spousal abuse is domestic violence or any other form of abuse directed at a spouse. It can involve physical or sexual violence as well as emotional abuse. Abusers may threaten or intimidate their victims and try to keep them away from family or friends.

Spousal abuse is a criminal act that can be prosecuted by law. However, this crime often goes unreported. Victims may blame themselves for their partners' abusive behavior, thinking that they somehow deserve the mistreatment. They may also be unwilling to break the family apart by leaving an abusive spouse. Many victims fear they will be unable to financially support themselves or their families if they leave. Some victims simply have nowhere else to go. In some cases, the abuser may threaten to hurt or even kill the victim—or their children—if the spouse attempts to leave.

Child Abuse

Child abuse, which is domestic abuse directed at a child, includes any action that harms or threatens a child's health and development. Like spousal abuse, child abuse can be physical, emotional, or sexual. It may also involve **neglect**. Neglect is failure to provide for a child's basic needs. Neglected children may lack adequate food, clothing, shelter, or medical support. Leaving children alone and unsupervised for long periods of time is also a form of neglect.

Parents who abuse their children don't always want to hurt them. Some parents do not have the knowledge to take care of children. Abusive parents may have been abused themselves as children and don't know any other way for a family to function. Alcohol and drug abuse also increase the risk of violence in the home. Whatever the reasons behind it, abusing a child is always unacceptable and dangerous.

Abuse can harm children emotionally as well as physically. **What forms can child abuse take?**

polya_olya/Shutterstock

Stopping Sexual Abuse

Sexual abuse is a serious crime. In 2012 Erin's Law was introduced to raise awareness of sexual abuse and to stop it from happening. Erin's Law provides tools to help adults recognize the signs of child sexual abuse. The law requires that states provide students with information telling them what they can do if they are being abused or know someone who is being abused. As of 2019, Erin's Law was the law in 37 U.S. states. Supporters of the law hope to have it passed in all 50 U.S. states soon.

Elder Abuse

Elder abuse, which is the abuse or neglect of older family members, is a problem that often goes unnoticed. Elder abuse can occur both within the family and in institutional settings, such as nursing homes. Like children, older family members may suffer physical, emotional, and sexual abuse, as well as neglect. Elder abuse can also be financial. For instance, caregivers may take advantage of elders by taking control of an elder's money and other assets.

Effects of Abuse

Victims of **domestic** abuse may suffer physical injuries, such as bruises, burns, or broken bones. In the worst cases, physical abuse can lead to permanent injury or death. For many victims, however, the emotional scars left by abuse last even longer than the physical injuries. Victims often experience feelings of shame and worthlessness. Abused children may be anxious or depressed and have difficulty in school. Without treatment, abused children often grow up to become abusers themselves—a pattern known as the **cycle of violence**.

Children who live in abusive homes may try to escape the abuse by running away. Others may be forced to leave the family home by an abusive parent or guardian. Many runaways and "thrownaways" end up living on the street or in the company of predatory adults. They are at risk for drug problems, crime, and continuing physical or sexual abuse.

To avoid these risks, children suffering abuse at home need to seek help from an adult they can trust, such as a relative, teacher, medical professional, or religious advisor. The police can also connect these teens with social services that can help them. Short-term shelters can provide a safe place to stay on a temporary basis. "Drop-in" services can provide food, clothing, medical attention, and crisis counseling.

Stopping Domestic Abuse

Stopping domestic violence depends on the three Rs: *recognize, resist,* and *report*. The first step is to *recognize* the problem. Victims and others need to be aware that abuse is a crime and *resist* the urge to excuse or explain away the abuser's behavior. Any claim of abuse should be taken seriously, even if it sounds unbelievable.

ACADEMIC VOCABULARY

domestic *(adjective)*: of or relating to the household or the family

Reading Check

Define What is the *cycle of violence?*

Victims of domestic abuse can also *resist* their abusers. If someone tries to harm you physically or sexually, you can try to escape or to prevent the attack. Once you escape, seek help from a trusted adult. However, resistance may not always be possible. That's why *reporting* the abuse is the third step in putting a stop to it. If you or someone you know is being abused, report the problem to someone who can help you. You can try talking to a trusted adult, such as a family member or a school nurse. You can also contact an abuse hotline or a crisis center. Finally, you can go directly to the police. The victim may also require counseling and medical care. If the abuser is a member of the family, reporting the abusive behavior to authorities will make sure that the family gets help, including the abuser. Abusers may be required to take classes to learn how to deal with stress and other issues in a healthy way, rather than abusing family members or others.

Victims of domestic violence need help. Their abusers need help too. Through counseling and other strategies, they can learn to manage their feelings and break the cycle of violence.

Sources of Support

MAIN IDEA Communities offer many forms of support to families in crisis.

Communities offer resources to help families deal with a variety of problems, including abuse. What type of help they need depends on the seriousness of the problem. Some problems, such as domestic violence, may require notifying the police. Others, such as substance abuse, may require medical help. Some sources of help for troubled families include:

- family counseling services.
- support groups.
- shelters.
- community services.
- law enforcement officials.
- hospitals or clinics.
- faith communities.
- counseling.

Family counseling is therapy to restore healthy relationships in a family. Families come in as a group to meet with a counselor, discuss their problems, and seek solutions. Counseling can help some families to deal with changes such as separation or divorce. It can also help in cases when one family member has a problem that affects the entire family. Such problems may include anger, depression, or substance abuse. Sometimes individual counseling is also helpful.

Myths & Reality

Many myths exist regarding domestic violence. What do you think about this one?

Myth: Children who misbehave may be to blame if they are abused.

Reality: Children are never to blame for abuse. All children misbehave at some time. A child could be tired or hungry and express those feelings through bad behavior.

SUPPORT GROUPS	
Organization	**Provides Support For**
Alcoholics Anonymous	Alcoholics
Al-Anon & Alateen	Family members and friends of alcoholics
Narcotics Anonymous	Drug abusers
Overeaters Anonymous	Compulsive overeaters
Eating Disorders Anonymous	People with anorexia, bulimia, or binge eating disorder
SAFE (Stop Abuse For Everyone)	Victims of domestic violence and abuse
Bereaved Parents of the USA	Parents who have lost a child

These are just a few of the many support groups in the country.

In family counseling, the family meets with the counselor as a group to learn ways to resolve their problems. **Give an example of a problem that a family might seek to solve through family counseling.**

Support Groups

A support group is a gathering of people who are all coping with the same problem. The group meets regularly to discuss their problems and get advice from each other. Support groups can help many people just by reassuring them that they are not alone.

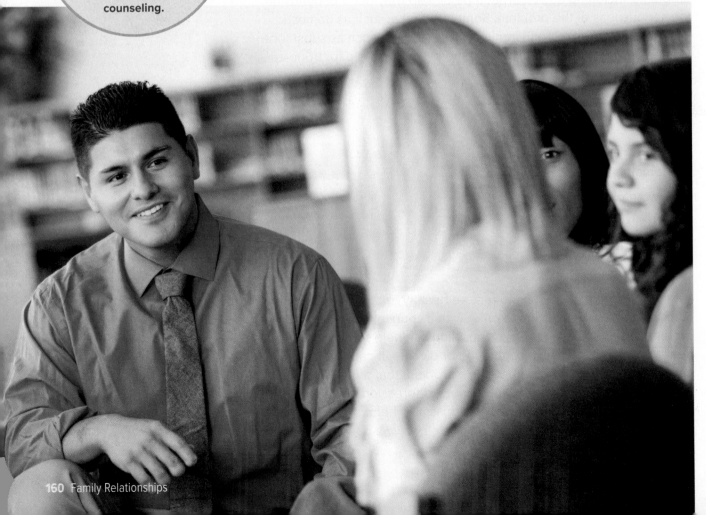

asiseeit/Getty Images

Community Services

Families seeking help may also turn to resources in their community. Troubled family members may seek help from a **crisis center**, a facility that offers advice and support to people dealing with personal emergencies. People might turn to a crisis center to help them get through problems such as substance abuse or domestic violence. Some communities also have crisis hotlines. These are special telephone numbers people can call to receive help 24 hours a day. Hotlines may deal with a variety of personal problems, ranging from stress to thoughts of suicide.

Communities also provide a variety of other services to families in need. For instance, public or private agencies may offer classes on parenting and conflict resolution. Social services can help provide food, clothing, shelter, and medical care. Public agencies can also help adults find a job or receive job training.

Finally, community services offer help for victims of domestic abuse. Social agencies can remove children from abusive homes and place them in foster care. Victims can also seek help by contacting an organization that deals with domestic violence. Many communities provide shelters where spouses and children can go to escape an abusive home. They may also help victims obtain counseling and legal services.

Reading Check

Identify Name three places that can provide help for families in crisis.

Lesson 3 Review

Facts and Vocabulary

1. Identify four different forms of child abuse.

2. Describe the physical and emotional effects of abuse.

3. What is family counseling?

Thinking Critically

4. **Analyze.** Explain how neglect might affect each part of a child's health triangle.

5. **Evaluate.** Hector's dad recently moved out of the house. Hector feels lonely and guilty about his parents' separation. He believes no one understands how he feels. What source of support do you think would be most helpful for Hector, and why?

Applying Health Skills

6. **Accessing Information.** Consult phone directories, bulletin boards, and websites to find resources in your community that help families in crisis. Based on your findings, create a brochure that describes sources of support and how to contact them.

Writing Critically

7. **Expository.** Write an article discussing the problem of domestic abuse. Describe the effects of abuse and identify ways victims can seek help.

Vocabulary Review

Correct the sentences below by replacing the italicized term with the correct vocabulary term.

1. A(n) *single-parent family* consists of a married couple and their children from previous marriages.

2. Two parents and one or more children living in the same place form a(n) *extended family*.

3. *Adoption* is the temporary placement of children in the homes of adults who are not related to them.

Understanding Key Concepts

After reading the question or statement, select the correct answer.

4. Relatives such as aunts, uncles, and grandparents are part of a person's
   a. nuclear family.
   b. blended family.
   c. extended family.
   d. foster family.

5. In a family, children are often responsible for
   a. meeting the family's basic needs, such as food and shelter.
   b. setting limits on family members' behaviors.
   c. teaching values and skills.
   d. performing household chores.

6. Parents promote their children's mental and emotional health by
   a. providing for basic needs, such as food, clothing, and shelter.
   b. providing medical care.
   c. providing affirmation.
   d. sharing cultural traditions.

Thinking Critically

After reading the question or statement, write a short answer using complete sentences.

7. **Describe.** What is one purpose of foster care?

8. **Explain.** How can setting limits on children's behavior promote physical health?

9. **Give Examples.** Name two healthful behaviors children may learn from their parents.

10. **Evaluate.** Why might teaching values by example be more powerful in some cases than teaching by explanation?

Vocabulary Review

Use the correct vocabulary term to complete the following statements.

11. During a(n) _____, a couple may attempt to work out their problems so that they can live together again.

12. A(n) _____ is a legal end to a marriage contract.

13. After a divorce, sole or joint _____ of the children may be granted to one or both parents.

Understanding Key Concepts

After reading the question or statement, select the correct answer.

14. Helping a younger sibling with a difficult school assignment is an example of
    a. good communication.
    b. support.
    c. respect.
    d. trust.

15. Which of the following is an example of a change in family structure?
    a. The birth of a new baby
    b. The loss of a parent's job
    c. A family member's serious illness
    d. Moving to a new home

16. Joint custody is an arrangement in which
    a. the children live with their mother.
    b. the children live with their father.
    c. both parents share responsibility for the children.
    d. the children are placed in foster care.

17. Which of the following is *not* a helpful way to cope with changes in the family?
    a. Talking openly with other family members
    b. Making more of an effort to help out with chores and other responsibilities
    c. Keeping feelings to yourself to avoid worrying family members
    d. Showing empathy for family members' feelings

Thinking Critically

After reading the question or statement, write a short answer using complete sentences.

18. **Describe.** What are five traits of a healthy family?

19. **Compare and Contrast.** Explain how families in movies and TV shows may differ from real families.

20. **Infer.** Why might a divorced parent's remarriage cause mixed feelings for a teen?

21. **Evaluate.** Why can financial gains, as well as losses, be a source of stress for families?

LESSON 3

Vocabulary Review

Choose the correct term in the sentences below.

22. *Cycle of violence/Abuse* is the physical, mental, emotional, or sexual mistreatment of one person by another.

23. Any act of violence involving family members is known as *domestic violence/spousal abuse*.

24. Child *violence/neglect* is the failure to provide for a child's basic needs.

Understanding Key Concepts

After reading the question or statement, select the correct answer.

25. Yelling at or threatening a child is an example of
    a. physical abuse.
    b. emotional abuse.
    c. sexual abuse.
    d. neglect.

26. Older family members are much more likely than young children to suffer
    a. physical abuse.
    b. sexual abuse.
    c. emotional abuse.
    d. financial abuse.

27. If a friend confides that he is being abused, you should
    a. assume the person is just exaggerating.
    b. confront the abuser face-to-face.
    c. keep quiet for fear of putting the victim at further risk.
    d. seek help from a trusted adult.

28. Which type of organization can provide families in need with food, shelter, and medical care?
    a. Counseling services
    b. Support groups
    c. Crisis hotlines
    d. Social services

Thinking Critically

After reading the question or statement, write a short answer using complete sentences.

29. **Analyze.** Explain why some victims of spousal abuse are unwilling to leave their abusers.

30. **Explain.** Why are people who were abused as children more likely to become abusive parents?

31. **Evaluate.** James lives with an abusive, alcoholic parent. He has considered running away from home. What are the possible consequences he might face if he does so?

32. **Compare and Contrast.** What is the main difference between counseling and support groups as a way to deal with family problems?

33. **Explain.** How can community services offer help and support for victims of domestic abuse? Give specific examples.

PROJECT-BASED ASSESSMENT

Coping During Times of Stress

BACKGROUND

A family is a team. For a family to work as a single unit, everyone needs to communicate clearly and carry out their responsibilities. Successful families care for, support, and help each other.

TASK

Create a blog about a fictional family. This family just survived a natural disaster, such as a hurricane or tornado. Some family members live in other areas that were not affected by the disaster. The family members are working together and supporting each other through this difficult time.

AUDIENCE

Students in your class

PURPOSE

Help students learn how family support is especially important in times of stress.

PROCEDURE

1. Organize into small groups. Review the information in Module 7 about family relationships.

2. Conduct an online search on families that have survived natural disasters. How does each family member function independently and as part of a group? Obtain examples of how they support each other.

3. Identify four or five key points to make in the blog.

4. Work together to create a blog about a fictional family supporting each other after a natural disaster. Have each member of your group play the role of a family member. Make sure key points are clearly explained and supported.

Math Practice

Interpret Statistics. The chart below provides marriage and divorce statistics for the U.S. population in 2017 and 2018. Use the statistics to answer Questions 1–3.

Number of marriages in 2017:	2,236,496
Number of marriages in 2018:	2,132,853
Marriage rate in 2017:	6.9 per 1,000 people
Marriage rate in 2018:	6.5 per 1,000 people
Divorce rate in 2017:	2.9 per 1,000 people
Divorce rate in 2018:	2.9 per 1,000 people

National Center for Health Statistics
[source, marriage: https://www.cdc.gov/nchs/data/hestat/marriage_rate_2018/marriage_rate_2018.pdf]

1. By how much did the number of marriages decrease from 2017 to 2018?
   a. 13,643
   b. 10,643
   c. 103,643
   d. 1,030,643

2. What proportion could be used to estimate the total U.S. population in 2018?
   a. $1,000 - 6.5 = x - 2,132,853$
   b. $1,000 - 6.5 = 2,132,853 - x$
   c. $6.5/1,000 = x/2,132,853$
   d. $6.5/1,000 = 2,132,853/x$

3. According to the marriage statistics, which figure best estimates the total U.S. population in 2018?
   a. 328,131
   b. 223,000,000
   c. 297,300,000
   d. 328,131,231

Reading/Writing Practice

Understand and Apply. Read the passage below, and then answer the questions.

There are four people in my family: me, my mom, and my two older sisters. My mom adopted all three of us when I was very young. I don't remember my birth parents, so this is the only family I've ever known. Like any other family, we get into arguments sometimes. But we also take care of each other. My sisters help me with homework, and my mom is always there for us. My mom thinks it's important for my sisters and me to be in touch with our Korean heritage. Even though she's not Korean, she learned to make Korean foods for us. Every year we go to the local heritage festival to celebrate our traditions as a family. It makes me feel valued to know that Mom respects our heritage and doesn't want us to change.

1. In the first sentence, the part after the colon should be changed to read:
   a. me and my mom and my two sisters.
   b. my two older sisters and I and my mom.
   c. my mom, my two older sisters, and me.
   d. I, my mom, and my two older sisters.

2. The author mentions arguments to show that
   a. his family is not healthy.
   b. he gets along with his mother but not with his sisters.
   c. his family is supportive and caring.
   d. his family is much like any other.

3. Think about a cultural tradition that you and your family share. Write a short essay describing this tradition and how it helps bring you together as a family.

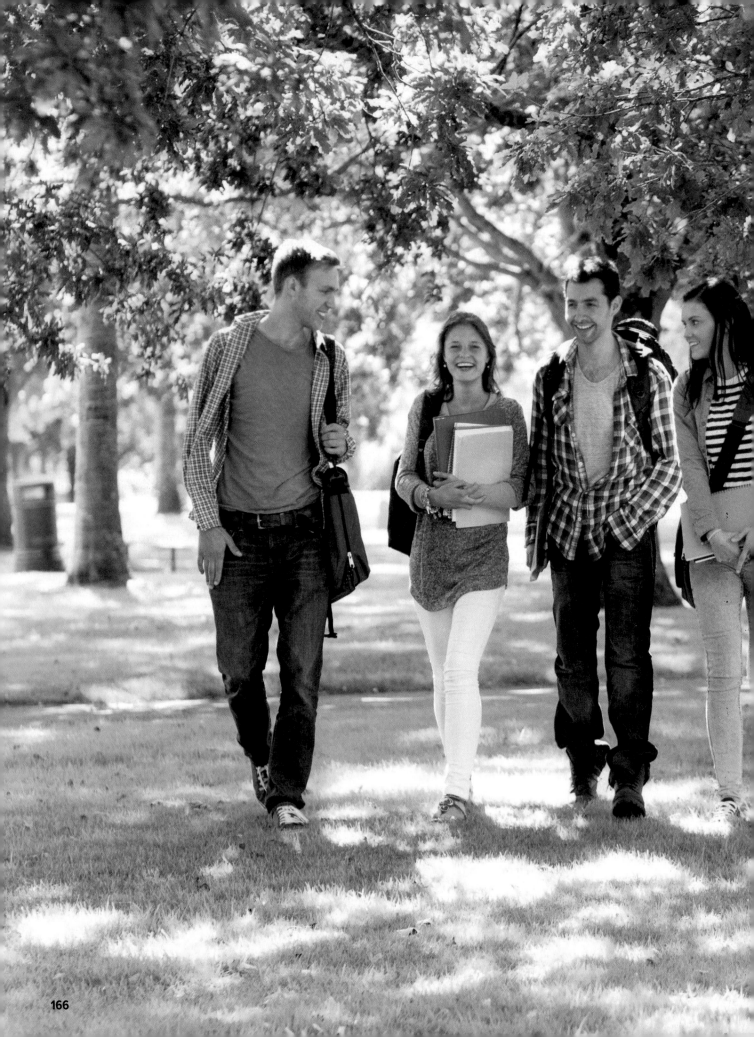

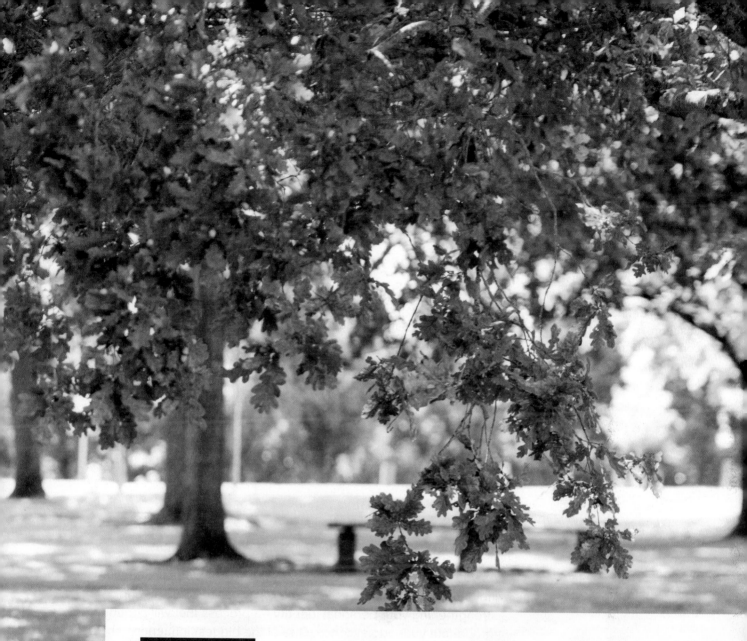

Peer Relationships

LESSONS

1 Safe and Healthy Friendships

2 Peer Pressure and Refusal Skills

3 Practicing Abstinence

Safe and Healthy Friendships

BEFORE YOU READ

Create a Cluster Chart.
Draw a circle and label it "Friendship." Use surrounding circles to define and describe this term. As you read, continue filling in the chart with more details.

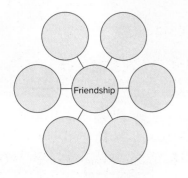

Friendship

Vocabulary

platonic friendship
clique

BIG IDEA Mutual respect and honesty are important characteristics of healthy friendships.

REAL LIFE ISSUES

Maintaining Friendships. Tom and Jarod have been friends since the sixth grade. They promised to join the same clubs and sports teams in high school to stay close friends. Now that they're sophomores, Tom is meeting new friends, and his interests have changed. He wants to try new things but wants to remain friends with Jarod, too. *If you were Tom, how might you express your concerns? Write a brief letter to Jarod explaining your thoughts and feelings.*

After completing the lesson, review and analyze your response to the Real Life Issues question.

Peer Relationships

MAIN IDEA We will all have many types of friends.

As you've probably figured out by now, a lot of things change in your life during your teen years. As a teen, you are developing and strengthening your personal identity—a process that will continue throughout your adolescence. One of the biggest influences on your developing identity is your peers. Peers are people of similar age who share similar interests. Peer relationships can play an important role in your health and well-being. For example, your friends and peers may influence you to try new activities, such as joining the debate club or learning to play tennis. These activities, in turn, can promote all aspects of your health.

You will also have friends who encourage you to take part in unhealthy activities, such as using tobacco, alcohol, and drugs. This type of friend may use intimidation by saying that if you want to be part of his or her group, you must participate in the activity. In these situations, you will need to think about your goals in life and whether the activity is something that is healthy for you.

As you get older, your social groups expand. You may also get a part-time job where you'll meet new people. Over time, you may have opportunities to meet people from different age groups, cultures, races, and religions. Some of the people you meet during your high school years may become lifelong friends.

Friendships

You will form many kinds of friendships throughout your life. Your friendships with others will probably be some of the most significant relationships in your life. Friends not only enjoy spending time together, they also care for, respect, and trust for each other. They may also share interests, hobbies, and other friends. Common **attributes** of friendship include:

- Similar values, interests, beliefs, and attitudes
- Open and honest communication
- Sharing of joys, disappointments, dreams, and concerns
- Mutual respect, caring, and support
- Concern about each other's safety and well-being

You probably have several types of friendships, including casual, close, and platonic friends. With the widespread use of the Internet today, many teens are also forming online friendships.

• • • • • • • • • • • •

ACADEMIC VOCABULARY

attribute *(noun)*: a quality or characteristic

• • • • • • • • • • • •

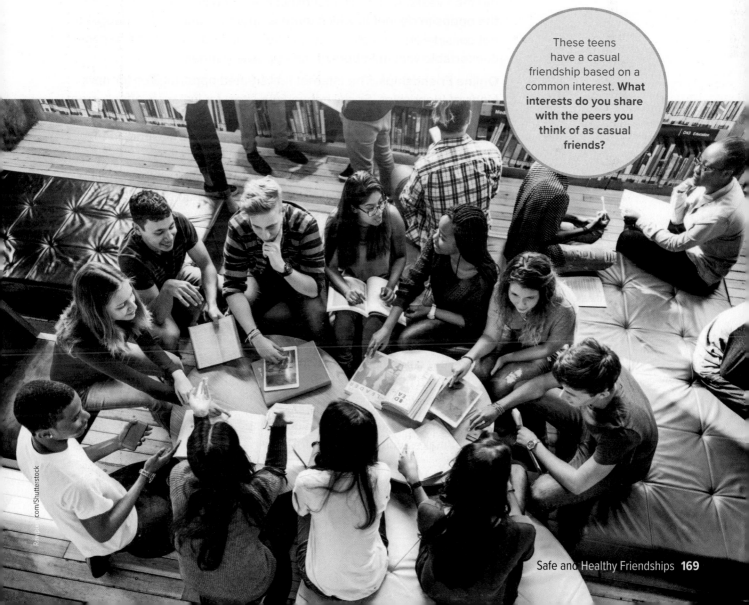

These teens have a casual friendship based on a common interest. **What interests do you share with the peers you think of as casual friends?**

Reu.../com/Shutterstock

Casual and Close Friendships. Think about the people you call your friends. Some of them may be people you only get together with to play sports or pursue hobbies. You enjoy spending time with them, but you wouldn't feel comfortable talking to them about something really personal. These are casual friends—people with whom you share interests but not deep emotional bonds. However, as you get to know a casual friend better, your relationship may develop into a close friendship.

Other friends may be people you feel very close to and would trust with your deepest secrets. These are your close friends, people who have strong emotional ties to you. Close friends share their thoughts, feelings, and experiences with each other. When something is bothering you, a close friend will listen to your concerns without passing judgment and will offer support and encouragement. Close friends also feel comfortable talking about problems that may arise in the friendship.

Platonic Friendships. Your friends can include both males and females. Some people may assume that any relationship between a male and female of dating age must be a romantic relationship, but this is not true. **Platonic friendships** are actually quite common and normal during the teen years. A platonic friendship is a friendship with a member of the opposite gender in which there is affection, but the two people are not considered a couple. They can help you understand and become comfortable with members of the opposite gender.

Online Friendships. The Internet has created opportunities for new kinds of friendships. Social networking sites, for instance, offer a great way to interact with others. Online friendships can be rewarding because you can get to know people from all over the world. In this way, you can learn about other cultures and traditions.

However, online friendships can also be dangerous. People you meet online may not always be telling the truth about themselves. For instance, people who claim to be teens may really be adults. Some of them may even be sexual predators looking for young people to exploit. To protect yourself, keep these guidelines in mind when you communicate with online friends:

- Avoid sharing personal information or photos of yourself with anyone you've only met online.

- Avoid giving out your phone number or street address.

- Be very cautious about taking online friendships offline. If you ever decide to meet an online friend in person, arrange to meet in a public place and have a parent or other trusted adult present.

- Always tell a trusted adult if an online friend asks you to do anything that makes you feel uncomfortable.

Reading Check

Describe Identify and describe three types of friendships.

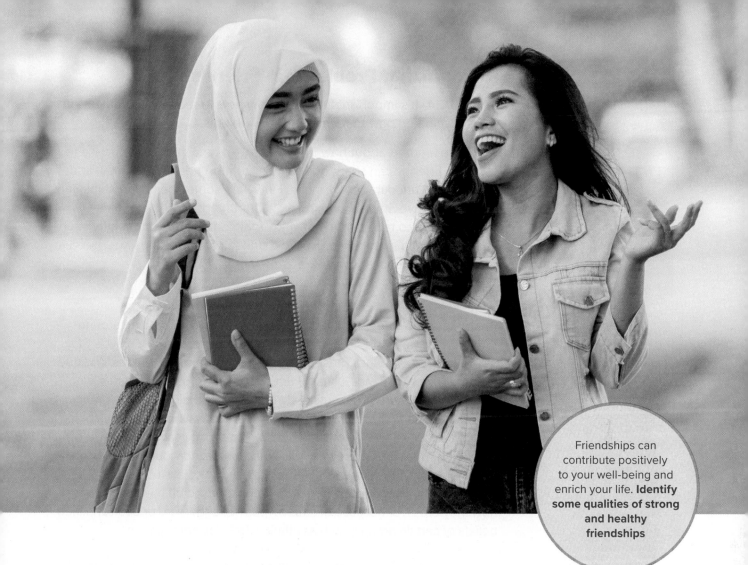

Friendships can contribute positively to your well-being and enrich your life. **Identify some qualities of strong and healthy friendships**

Building Strong Friendships

MAIN IDEA Good friends offer loyalty, support, and motivation.

Over time, you may find some of your friendships changing. You may grow closer to some friends as you share more serious thoughts and feelings. You may also find that some friendships become more complex as they grow closer. It's natural for friendships to grow and change, but always remember that strong friendships are based on mutual respect, caring, honesty, and commitment. Here are some additional features you should expect to see in a healthy friendship:

- **Empathy.** Does your friend consider your needs and feelings? Does he or she demonstrate understanding?

- **Fairness.** Does your friend treat you fairly?

- **Shared interests.** Do you enjoy the same things?

- **Shared values.** Does your friend reinforce your values and motivate you?

- **Acceptance.** Do you and your friend accept and appreciate each other's differences?

- **Support.** Does your friend support you during difficult times?

- **Loyalty.** Does your friend keep your confidences? Does she or he stay true to your friendship?

Recognizing Problems in Friendships

MAIN IDEA It's important that you know how to recognize problems in a friendship and how to resolve those problems.

You have learned about how friendships can be a positive influence in your life. Friends can share good times, comfort you in bad times, and support and encourage you in life. However, sometimes friendships can have a negative effect. For example, your friends may sometimes influence you to take part in activities that could harm your health, such as using alcohol or tobacco. To avoid unhealthy friendships, you need to recognize and resolve problems as they arise.

Cliques

Are there some students at your school who always seem to go around together? Perhaps they're all members of the soccer team, or maybe they all like a particular band. These groups of teens are called **cliques**. A clique is a small circle of friends, usually with similar backgrounds or tastes, who **exclude** people viewed as outsiders. Members of a clique often share interests, dress similarly, and behave in the same way. In some ways being part of a clique can be helpful for teens because it gives them a sense of belonging. However, cliques may also discourage individual members from thinking and acting for themselves. Cliques may also exclude people because of prejudice. They may judge people based on how they look or how they dress, or because of stereotypes—exaggerated or oversimplified beliefs of certain groups, such as ethnic or religious groups.

Managing Feelings of Envy or Jealousy

Another problem that can arise in friendships is envy or jealousy. For example, one friend might feel envious of another who is a better student, a better athlete, or more popular with the opposite gender. Feelings like these can damage a friendship. However, the friendship can survive as long as both people remain focused on the reasons they are friends. If you ever feel jealous of a friend, try asking yourself the following questions:

- What is making me feel jealous?
- Is my friend deliberately trying to make me feel this way?
- What can I do to manage or relieve these feelings?
- How can I feel better about myself? What are my own unique talents and the positive aspects of my life?
- Are these feelings of jealousy more important than our friendship?
- What positive qualities make this person a good friend?

When Friendships Change

Think about the people you considered your closest friends when you were a young child—say, four or five years old. Are they still your friends now? Are you closer to them than you are to any other friends? It's not surprising if the answer is no.

. . . .

Reading Check

Explain What is one way of dealing with feelings of jealousy in a friendship?

. . . .

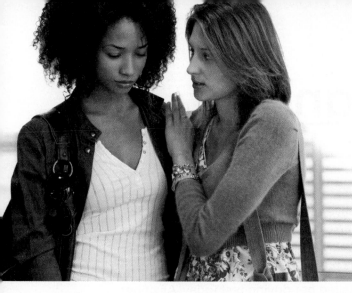

Talking with a trusted friend can help you deal with difficulties in other peer relationships. **What are some other strategies for handling problems in friendships?**

As you grow older, you and a close friend might spend less time together and develop new interests. When close friends grow apart, the friendship may become more casual.

In other cases, you might make a conscious choice to end a friendship because it is becoming harmful. Here are some reasons for choosing to end a friendship:

- A friend pressures you to do something that is unsafe or goes against your values.
- A friend says or does things that are hurtful and insulting to you.
- A friend pressures you to change your beliefs or behaviors.

If you decide to end a friendship, communicate your feelings to that friend in a clear and respectful way. Use "I" messages to explain your feelings and your reasons for ending the friendship. Give your friend a chance to respond with his or her point of view. Although it may be difficult, sometimes ending a friendship is the best decision for both individuals. Remember, you can always talk to another friend or to a trusted adult for advice about dealing with this kind of situation.

Fitness Zone

My friends and I aren't "sports nuts," but we want to be more active. We asked our PE teacher to suggest some activities. He said we should try noncompetitive activities like walking in the park, playing a round of miniature or disc golf, or just hitting tennis balls (but not keeping score).

Lesson 1 Review

Facts and Vocabulary

1. Define the word peers.

2. Define friendship. Identify four traits of healthy friendships.

3. List two problems that may affect friendships.

Thinking Critically

4. **Evaluate.** What actions can you take to promote safe and healthy friendships?

5. **Describe.** Name two possible outcomes of lying to a friend. How might this affect the friendship?

Applying Health Skills

6. **Communication Skills.** With a classmate, role-play a scenario in which close friends communicate needs, wants, and emotions in healthful ways.

Writing Critically

7. **Expository.** Write a dialogue in which peers express disagreement about an issue while still showing respect for their self and others.

Peer Pressure and Refusal Skills

BEFORE YOU READ

Create Vocabulary Cards. Write each new vocabulary term on a separate note card. For each term, write a definition based on your current knowledge. As you read, fill in additional information related to each term.

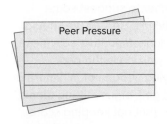

Peer Pressure

Vocabulary

peer pressure
harassment
manipulation

• • • • • • • • • • •

BIG IDEA Learning effective refusal skills will help you deal with negative peer pressure.

REAL LIFE ISSUES

Peer Pressure. Kelly failed her driving test today. All of her friends have their driver's licenses. Now she doesn't want to go back to school and tell her friends what happened. Kelly worries that some of her friends will make fun of her. She's embarrassed that her mom still drops her off at school every morning while all of her friends have their own cars. *Kelly is experiencing unspoken peer pressure. Write a paragraph about a time when you experienced either spoken or unspoken peer pressure. How did you handle the situation?*

After completing the lesson, review and analyze your response to the Real Life Issues question.

Peer Pressure

MAIN IDEA Peers can influence how you think, feel, and act.

Picture this: You are hanging out with friends on a Friday night when someone suggests going to a movie. Everyone else agrees, but you aren't sure because the movie ends late. If you stay until the end, you'll miss your curfew. When you hesitate, your friends say, "Come on! It's the weekend!"

This situation is an example of **peer pressure**, something that most people experience during their teen years. Peer pressure is the influence that people your age may have on you. Peer pressure can have a positive or negative impact on your actions and behaviors. To protect your health and safety, you need to learn how to evaluate forms of peer pressure and respond to it appropriately.

Positive Peer Pressure

Peers can influence you in many positive ways. For example, your peers might inspire you to try a new activity, like an art class, or to try ethnic foods that you've never tasted before. They may also encourage you to take part in community projects, such as a cleanup campaign. Working on a project like this with your peers benefits your social health because it gives you a chance to team up with others to achieve a positive goal. It also benefits your community by providing a cleaner environment. Other volunteer projects you might engage in with peers include serving food at a homeless shelter or working at a Special Olympics event.

Sometimes, positive peer pressure encourages you *not* to participate in certain behaviors or activities. For instance, having friends who do not use tobacco, alcohol, or other drugs may positively influence you to avoid these harmful substances. You can also use positive peer pressure yourself to influence others in healthful ways. For instance, you might encourage a peer to try out for a sports or dance team or to study hard for an important test.

Negative Peer Pressure

In other cases, peer pressure is harmful. Peers sometimes influence each other to take part in risky behaviors or accept harmful beliefs. The members of a clique, for example, may be disrespectful toward people they do not consider acceptable to their group. They may engage in **harassment**, which is persistently annoying behavior, such as name-calling, teasing, or bullying. Negative peer pressure may also lead some teens to behave in ways that go against their values. For example, a peer might pressure a classmate to help him or her cheat on a test.

Positive peer pressure can motivate you to try new activities that can benefit all sides of your health triangle. **What are some examples of positive peer pressure that you have experienced?**

Paul Burns/Getty Images

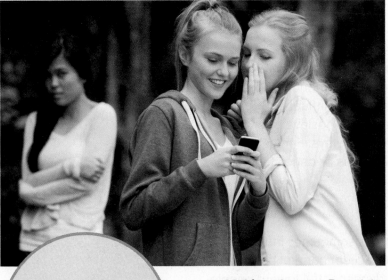

Peer pressure can have both positive and negative effects on your health.

Reading Check

List What are the differences between positive and negative peer pressure?

One way that some people exert negative peer pressure is through **manipulation**. This is an indirect, dishonest way to control or influence other people. Examples of ways in which peers can manipulate one another include mocking, teasing, and making threats. If you witness this kind of hurtful behavior, do what you can to discourage it. Encourage the victim to report the problem to a trusted adult. Some common methods of manipulation include:

- **Making threats.** Promising violence or some other negative consequence if the person does not do what is asked.

- **Blackmail.** Threatening to reveal some embarrassing or damaging information if the person does not do what is asked.

- **Mocking or teasing.** Making fun of another person in mean or hurtful ways.

- **"Guilt trips."** Making a person feel guilty to get desired results.

- **Bargaining.** Offering to make a deal to get what one wants.

- **Flattery.** Using excessive praises to influence another person.

- **Bribing.** Promising money or favors if the person does what is asked.

Resisting Negative Peer Pressure

MAIN IDEA Practicing refusal skills will help you deal with negative peer pressure.

Peer pressure will not stop at the end of your teen years. Throughout your life, you will face situations in which peers, including friends and co-workers, try to influence you to behave in a particular way. They may even make direct requests or demands of you. In some cases, the way you respond to these situations will directly affect your health. For example, getting into a car with friends who have been drinking could result in serious injury or even death. To protect your health and safety, learn and practice effective strategies for resisting harmful peer pressure.

It is important to understand why people sometimes give in to negative peer pressure. One reason is that when facing pressure from a friend, many teens worry about jeopardizing the relationship. They may agree to actions that go against their values in an attempt to maintain a friendship or to make new friends. Teens may also fear that refusing to go along with a group may make them unpopular. They fear that peers will reject them or make fun of their decision. In situations like these, it's important to put your health and safety first. In the end, you are the one responsible for your decisions and your well-being.

One way to resist negative peer pressure is to develop friendships with people who share your values and interests. Friends who respect your health and well-being will be less likely to pressure you into doing anything that goes against your values. You will also find that it is much easier to resist negative peer pressure from others when you have supportive friends who stand by you and respect your decision.

Another important set of tools for resisting negative peer pressure are refusal skills. Learning how to say no effectively can help you protect your health and stay true to your values. Practicing refusal skills will help you to be assertive when a pressure situation arises.

Assertive Refusal

Assertive communication lets you state your position and stand your ground while also acknowledging the rights of others. This is the most effective approach to take when facing negative peer pressure.

Refusal Skills. One important **aspect** of being assertive is being able to use refusal skills when appropriate. Refusal skills are communication strategies that can help you say no to behaviors that are unsafe, unhealthy, or contrary to your values. Effective refusal skills involve three steps:

- **Step 1: State Your Position.** The first step in resisting negative peer pressure is simply to say no. You need to do this clearly and firmly, in a way that shows you really mean it. Combining your words with nonverbal messages will make your statement more effective. You can also reinforce your message by giving an honest reason for it, such as, "It's against my values."

- **Step 2: Suggest Alternatives.** When a peer asks you to do something that makes you uncomfortable, try suggesting another activity. For example, if a friend wants to go to a party where there is no adult supervision, you might say, "No, let's go to a movie instead." By offering an alternative, you create an opportunity to spend time with your friend in a way that's comfortable for both of you. Keep in mind that alternatives are most effective if they take you away from the dangerous or unpleasant situation.

ACADEMIC VOCABULARY

aspect *(noun)*: a feature or phase of something

COMMON METHODS OF MANIPULATION	
• **Making threats**—promising violence or some other negative consequence if the person does not do what is asked	• **"Guilt trips"**—making a person feel guilty to get desired results
• **Blackmail**—threatening to reveal some embarrassing or damaging information if the person does not do what is asked	• **Bargaining**—offering to make a deal to get what one wants
• **Mocking or teasing**—making fun of another person in mean or hurtful ways	• **Flattery**—using excessive praises to influence another person
	• **Bribing**—promising money or favors if the person does what is asked

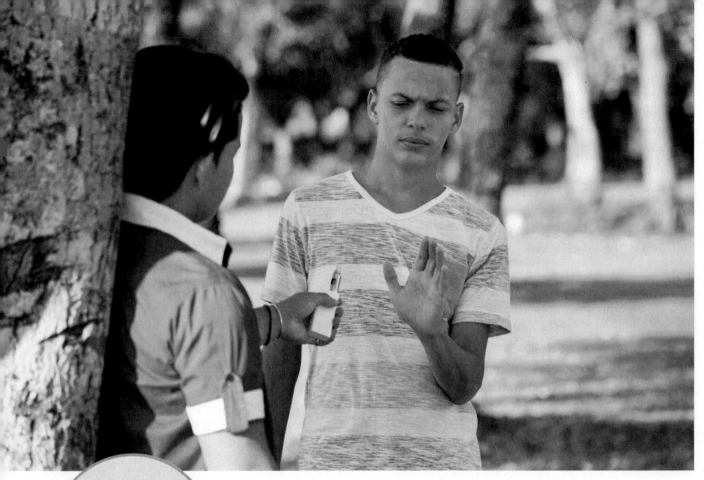

Practicing refusal skills will help you deal with negative peer pressure. **How would you say no if someone pressured you to participate in an unsafe activity?**

- **Step 3: Stand Your Ground.** Even after you've said no, some peers may continue trying to persuade you to join in. Make it clear that you mean what you said. Use strong body language and maintain eye contact, but avoid touching the other person or getting physical in any way. If this doesn't work, remove yourself from the situation. Simply say, "I'm going home," and walk away.

Learning and practicing these three steps can help you avoid unsafe situations. You can feel good knowing that you made the right choice to protect your safety and uphold your values.

Passive and Aggressive Responses

Being assertive may take some practice. To some people, a passive response to negative peer pressure seems easier. Passive communicators are unwilling or unable to express their thoughts and feelings in a direct or firm manner. Teens who respond passively to peer pressure may believe they are making friends by going along with the group. However, being passive all the time may actually cause others to view them as pushovers who aren't worthy of respect.

Other people may respond to peer pressure in an aggressive way. They react by becoming overly forceful, pushy, or hostile. An aggressive response to peer pressure might involve yelling, shoving, or other kinds of verbal or physical force. Aggressive people may get their way, but most people react to aggressive behavior either by fighting back or by avoiding the individual in future. Either reaction can result in emotional or physical harm to both parties.

Learning to use assertive communication, even if it doesn't come naturally, is the most effective way to deal with peer pressure. Being assertive shows that you will stand up for your rights, beliefs, and needs. At the same time, it shows that you respect yourself and those around you.

Reading Check

Explain Why is it important to use assertive refusal skills, rather than using passive or aggressive responses?

Character Check

When parents permit their teens to date, they show that they trust their children to make responsible decisions. A teen who has the self-control and self-discipline to resist peer pressure and avoid high-risk behaviors demonstrates trustworthiness. What are some other ways you can demonstrate trustworthiness?

Lesson 2 Review

Facts and Vocabulary

1. What is *peer pressure*?

2. Identify two examples of manipulation.

3. How might a friend help you resist negative peer pressure?

Thinking Critically

4. **Describe.** Write a paragraph describing how you would respond to someone who says that being aggressive is the only way to get what you want.

5. **Compare and Contrast.** How are harassment and manipulation different? How are they similar?

Applying Health Skills

6. **Refusal Skills.** With a classmate, develop a scenario in which peers try to pressure you to use tobacco or alcohol. Demonstrate refusal strategies for resisting this negative peer pressure.

Writing Critically

7. **Expository.** Write an essay analyzing the positive and negative effects of peer pressure. Explain why it is important to learn how to evaluate and respond to peer pressure.

Practicing Abstinence

BEFORE YOU READ

Create a K-W-L Chart. Make a three-column chart. In the first column, list what you know about dating and abstinence. In the second column, list what you want to know about this topic. As you read, use the third column to summarize what you learned.

K	W	L

Vocabulary

priorities
intimacy
infatuation
self-control
sexually transmitted diseases (STDs)
sexually transmitted infections (STIs)

. . . .

BIG IDEA Setting dating limits and practicing abstinence will benefit all three sides of your health triangle.

REAL LIFE ISSUES

Thinking About Dating. Kayla has a close group of friends. Dan, one of her good friends, recently told her that he wants to date her exclusively. Kayla knows that Dan's been sexually active in the past. She likes Dan and wants to get to know him better, but Kayla does not want to enter into a serious relationship. *Write a dialogue in which Kayla expresses her feelings to Dan. Both individuals should be honest and respectful.*

After completing the lesson, review and analyze your response to the Real Life Issues question.

Dating Decisions

MAIN IDEA Personal values and priorities will influence your dating decisions.

During your teen years, you may start thinking about dating. Dating can be a great way to get to know another person. It also provides opportunities to develop social skills, discover new interests, and reaffirm personal values. Some teens, however, may have personal reasons for choosing not to date. They might not feel ready or they may have other **priorities**, such as focusing on school or spending time with family. Priorities are the goals, tasks, values, and activities that you judge to be more important than others. Talking to a parent or other trusted adult can help you decide whether you're ready to start dating.

If you do decide to date, it's important to establish healthful boundaries. Here are some reasonable expectations to keep in mind:

- Both you and your date deserve to be treated with consideration and respect.

- When you're with someone you are dating, you should be yourself and communicate your thoughts and feelings honestly.

- You should never feel pressured to do anything that goes against your values or your family's guidelines.

Setting Limits

Your parents or guardians may set limits on your dating relationships. For example, they may set a curfew, a time at which you must be home at night. Some parents set limits on whether you can date or where you may go on a date. These limits are not intended to restrict you from trying new things. Limits like these are intended to protect your health and safety.

As you mature, you will begin to start setting your own limits. Talking to a trusted adult can help you with this **process**. For example, it's a good idea to set a limit on the age of the people you date. Dating someone who is much older or younger than you may cause pressure in the relationship. One person may want to do something that the other partner considers an activity for someone younger or older.

You may also need to set limits with your date regarding where you will go, how you will get there, and what you will do when you get there. One important limit you can set is to practice abstinence. When you make a conscious choice to avoid high-risk behaviors, including sexual activity and the use of tobacco, alcohol, and other drugs, you protect your health and safeguard your future. Setting limits and making them clear before a date will protect your safety and help make your dating experience a positive one.

ACADEMIC VOCABULARY

process *(noun)*: a series of actions geared toward an end result

Positive dating relationships are based on mutual respect and caring. **Identify some ways that teens can demonstrate respect for their dates.**

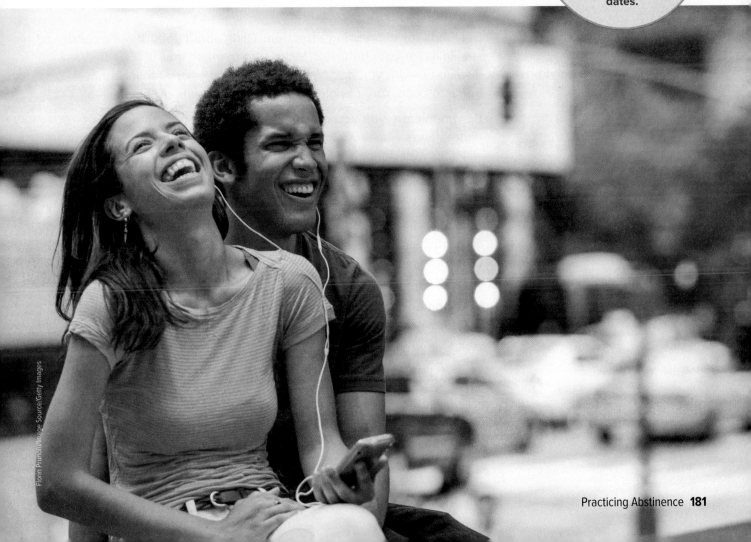

Florin Prunoiu/Image Source/Getty Images

Abstinence

MAIN IDEA There are many strategies that can help you commit to abstinence.

Choosing abstinence in a dating relationship means that you have decided not to become sexually active. When you choose to abstain from sexual activity, you are making the decision to avoid behaviors that could risk your health and your future well-being. Teens who are sexually active are at risk for unintended pregnancy and for sexually transmitted diseases (STDs). Choosing abstinence, however, does not mean doing without **intimacy** or physical contact in a dating relationship. Intimacy is a closeness between two people that develops over time. There are many ways to express affection and develop intimacy without being sexually active. For instance, you can hold hands, hug, kiss, and share your thoughts, feelings, and dreams. Keep in mind, though, that it's important not to confuse genuine affection and intimacy with **infatuation**. Infatuation is an exaggerated feeling of passion.

Practicing abstinence requires planning and **self-control**, which is a person's ability to use responsibility to override emotions. During your teen years, you will notice a surge in sexual or romantic feelings as you move through puberty. It's normal and healthy to have sexual feelings, but you can control these feelings instead of letting them control you. The following tips can help you maintain self-control and stay firm in your decision to practice abstinence.

- **Set limits for expressing affection.** Think about your priorities and set limits for your behavior. Make sure to make this decision *before* you are in a situation where sexual feelings may begin to build. At that point, you may no longer be thinking clearly.

- **Communicate with your partner.** Make sure your dating partner understands what your limits are. Clear and honest communication will help your dating partner understand and respect your limits.

- **Talk with a trusted adult.** Consider asking a trusted adult, such as a parent or guardian, for suggestions on ways to manage your feelings.

- **Seek low-pressure dating situations.** Choose safe dating locations and activities. For example, attend parties only if an adult is present. Consider group dating, which can eliminate the pressure to engage in sexual activity.

- **Date someone who respects and shares your values.** A dating partner who respects you and has similar values will understand your commitment to abstinence.

Sexual Activity and Consent

Sexual activity includes two layers of consent. Each state has a law that defines the age of consent in that state. A teen who is under the age of consent cannot legally agree to become sexually active. If one person is under the age of consent, the other person can be charged with a crime. To find the age of consent for your state, go online to your state's legislature.

Avoiding Risk Situations

Compare the following two dating situations. One is an afternoon picnic in the park with a group of close friends. During the picnic, you and your friends eat, talk, and play catch. The other is a late-night party at the home of a student whose parents are away. Some couples are kissing. In which situation do you think you would be more likely to face pressure to participate in sexual activity or other high-risk behaviors?

As you can see, where you go and what you do on a date can have a big impact on your safety. That's why it's a good idea to take some basic precautions:

- **Before you go on a date, know where you're going and what you will be doing.** Find out who else will be there, and discuss with your parents or guardians what time they expect you home.

- **Avoid places where alcohol and other drugs are present.** The use of alcohol and other drugs can impair a person's judgment. People under the influence of these substances are much more likely to take part in high-risk behaviors. The best way to avoid this risk is not to use alcohol or other drugs and to not associate with people who do use them.

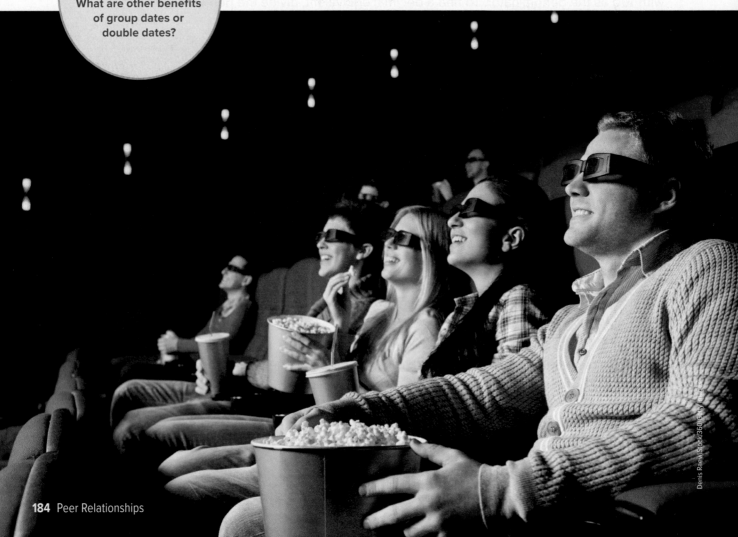

Reading Check

Identify List three behaviors that can help you maintain self-control in a dating situation.

• **Avoid being alone with a date at home or in any isolated place.** You may find it more difficult to maintain self-control when you and your date are alone together. These situations also increase the risk of being forced into a sexual act against your will.

Considering the Consequences

MAIN IDEA Abstinence from sexual activity has a positive effect on all sides of your health triangle.

Sexual activity can result in serious consequences—including, in some cases, legal consequences. It is illegal for an adult to have sexual contact with someone who is under the age of consent (which varies from state to state). In some states, consent laws make it illegal for an unmarried minor to engage in sexual activity at all. For example, if the state's age of consent is 18, two 17-year-olds who engage in sexual activity would be breaking the law. Even when no laws are being broken, sexual activity can still harm a teen's physical, mental/ emotional, and social health.

Going out in a group can reduce some of the pressures of dating. **What are other benefits of group dates or double dates?**

Denis Raev/iStock/360/Getty Images

Effects on Physical Health

Teens also choose to practice abstinence because it is the only guaranteed way to avoid the health risks associated with sexual activity. These risks include unplanned pregnancy and **sexually transmitted diseases (STDs)**, which are infectious diseases spread from person to person through sexual contact. STDs are also known as **sexually transmitted infections (STIs)**.

Unplanned Pregnancy. Every year in the United States, about one million teenage girls become pregnant. Any female teen who has begun to ovulate is physically able to become pregnant. Many rumors exist about pregnancy. A female who is ovulating can become pregnant, even if it's the very first time she has engaged in sexual activity. Teens who become pregnant risk their health and the health of her baby. For example, a teen girl who is pregnant may not get the prenatal care needed to protect her life and that of the growing fetus. The male partners may lack the emotional maturity needed to support them during the pregnancy.

Sexually Transmitted Diseases. Each year, about half of the diagnosed cases of STDs in this country occur among teens and young adults between the ages of 15 and 24. STDs can have serious health effects if they are left untreated. They may cause sterility in males and infertility in females, meaning that their victims will never be able to have a child. Some STDs can even be deadly. Although many STDs can be treated and cured if diagnosed early, some STDs have no cure. These include the herpes virus and HIV, the virus that causes AIDS. This disease is both incurable and life-threatening.

Like pregnancy, many myths exist about STDs. Some teens believe that they cannot catch an STD the first time they engage in sexual activity. Other believe that only some types of sexual activity can result in an STD. Still others believe that if a girl has an STD, she is unable to give it to her partner. All of these myths are untrue. Any type of sexual activity can result in an STD.

Effects on Mental/Emotional Health

Most teens are not prepared for the emotional demands of a sexual relationship. Teens who become sexually active before they are emotionally mature may experience:

- Emotional distress, because the partners are not committed to each other as they would be in a marriage.

- Loss of self-respect, because sexual activity may go against their personal values and those of their families.

- Guilt over concealing their sexual involvement from their parents.

- Regret and anxiety if sexual activity results in an unplanned pregnancy, an STD, or the breakup of the relationship with the partner.

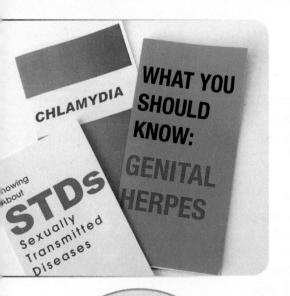

Effects on Social Health

Becoming sexually active can limit the types of relationships a teen may seek in the future. They may tell themselves that the person they are with is "the one" and avoid opportunities to pursue new interests or friendships. A teen who is involved in an exclusive relationship with one other person may not be open to meeting new people. The teen years are a time to meet new people and explore new interests.

In addition, teens who are sexually active run the risk of an unplanned pregnancy. Teen parents face many challenges, such as providing financial and emotional support for their child. Teens who become parents may have to put their own education and career plans on hold. They lose the chance to have a normal adolescence as they have to take on parenthood before they are ready.

Teens may also have unrealistic expectations about the financial resources that are needed to take care of a family. Most teens who have children before finishing high school have no choice but to take low-paying jobs that offer limited opportunity for future growth. Teen parents are unlikely to finish college, making it more likely that their income will stay low. Finally, teen pregnancy and parenthood may also add stress on other family members. Family members of teen parents may not be able to help the teen couple financially, or may resent the burden placed on them to help care for the infant of a teen parent.

Learning the facts about STDs and other negative consequences of sexual activity will help you make informed dating decisions. **How might contracting an STD affect a teen's mental/emotional and social health?**

Committing to Abstinence

MAIN IDEA Honest communication with your dating partner will help you stay committed to abstinence.

Choosing abstinence isn't a decision you can make once and never think about again. It's a choice you will have to recommit to each time you face temptation and pressure from others. To stay committed to abstinence, continue to remind yourself of the reasons you made this choice in the first place. It's also important to talk about your decision with the people you date. Talking about abstinence can be difficult, but the following tips may help the conversation go more smoothly:

- Choose a relaxed and comfortable time and place.

- Begin on a positive note, perhaps by talking about your affection for the other person.

- Be clear about your reasons for choosing abstinence.

- Be firm in setting limits in your physical relationship.

Using Refusal Skills

Committing to abstinence means not letting partners, peers, or the media pressure you to do something you don't want to do. You can use refusal skills to help you stand firm in your decision. Think about some of the reasons why you decided to commit to abstinence and memorize those reasons so that you remember them when you are being pressured.

Reading Check

Identify What are two strategies for staying committed to abstinence?

Ken Karp/McGraw-Hill Education

Recommitting to Abstinence

Teens who have been sexually active in the past may feel that they cannot say no to sexual activity in the future. However, choosing abstinence is *always* an option, regardless of past experiences. In fact, a study by the CDC shows that more than two-thirds of teens who have become sexually active, wish that they had waited. Even if someone has been sexually active in the past, that person can recommit to abstinence.

A teen who has engaged in sexual activity in the past may face pressure from dating partners to continue to be sexually active. A dating partner who knows a teen's history might say that it's not a big deal, or even ask "why that person and not me?" Teens can respond to this pressure by responding that it is a big deal, and that it was a mistake the first time. A partner who knows your history should respect your decisions regarding sexual activity. Teens who recommit to abstinence can feel good about making a positive choice to protect their health and well-being.

USING REFUSAL SKILLS TO SAY NO TO PEER PRESSURE	
Pressure Line	**Your Response**
• "Everybody does it."	• "No. Not everybody is doing it."
• "I thought you were cool."	• "I *am* cool, and the answer's still no."
• "No one will know."	• "I'll know, and I'm the one who matters."
• "If you loved me, you'd do it."	• "If you loved me, you'd respect my decision."

Practicing effective refusal statements will help you resist the pressure to engage in sexual activity.

Lesson 3 Review

Facts and Vocabulary

1. How is *intimacy* different from *infatuation*?

2. What are three negative consequences of teen sexual activity?

3. Identify ways of resisting persuasive tactics regarding sexual involvement.

Thinking Critically

4. **Synthesize.** What are the benefits of practicing abstinence?

5. **Analyze.** How can teen parenthood harm an individual's social development?

Applying Health Skills

6. **Refusal Skills.** Write a scenario in which a teen is being pressured to engage in sexual activity. The teen should demonstrate effective refusal skills to resist the pressure.

Writing Critically

7. **Personal.** Write an essay describing what your life will be like in ten years. Include an explanation of how practicing abstinence will help you achieve your goals.

Vocabulary Review

Correct the sentences below by replacing the italicized term with the correct vocabulary term.

1. When two teens of the opposite gender have affection for each other but are not considered a couple, they are said to have a *romantic friendship*.

2. A *peer* excludes people viewed as outsiders.

3. An exaggerated or oversimplified belief about a group of people is called a *judgment*.

Understanding Key Concepts

After reading the question or statement, select the correct answer.

4. Which of the following attributes is *not* necessary for a friendship to work?
   a. Mutual respect
   b. Concern about each other's safety
   c. Identical beliefs and values
   d. Open, honest communication

5. Which of the following statements is true of online friendships?
   a. They're not *real* friends unless you meet them face-to-face.
   b. It's okay to assume that people are who they say they are.
   c. You should exchange photos and personal information.
   d. They can be a rewarding way to meet people from around the world.

6. If you need to end a friendship, how should you handle the situation?
   a. Give the friend a detailed list of what exactly he or she did wrong.
   b. Give the friend the "silent treatment" until he or she gets the message.
   c. Talk about your own feelings and reasons for ending the friendship.
   d. Have someone else tell the friend that you no longer want to be friends.

Thinking Critically

After reading the question or statement, write a short answer using complete sentences.

7. **Identify.** Name one positive effect and one negative effect of belonging to a clique.

8. **Explain.** How would you tell a friend that your friendship has changed?

9. **Discuss.** Name ways that peers might influence your identity as a teen.

10. **Compare and Contrast.** What qualities do casual friends, close friends, and platonic friends share? How do these social groups differ?

Vocabulary Review

Use the correct vocabulary terms to complete the following statements.

11. Name-calling and bullying are examples of _____.

12. When you stand up for your rights in a firm and positive way, you are being _____.

13. If you are urged to take part in unhealthy behaviors, _____ will help you say no.

Understanding Key Concepts

After reading the question or statement, select the correct answer.

14. Which of the following is an example of positive peer pressure?
    a. Offering friendship in exchange for a favor
    b. Encouraging friends to become volunteers at a homeless shelter
    c. Smoking cigarettes to win approval
    d. Persuading a friend to bully another teen

15. Which of the following behaviors does *not* use manipulation?
    a. Flattering a person to influence her actions
    b. Teasing a person in a hurtful way
    c. Using a "guilt trip" to get desired results
    d. Asking a person to tell you honestly what she thinks

16. Which of the following is *not* part of the three-step process of refusal skills?
    a. Try it once before saying no.
    b. Suggest alternatives.
    c. Stand your ground.
    d. State your position.

17. Shaking your head and raising your hand in a "Stop" signal are examples of:
    a. Peer pressure
    b. Manipulation
    c. Nonverbal assertive refusal
    d. Aggressive behavior

Thinking Critically

After reading the question or statement, write a short answer using complete sentences.

18. **Explain.** What are the risks of responding passively to peer pressure?

19. **Describe.** What behaviors do people use when responding aggressively to peer pressure?

20. **Analyze.** Suppose a group of friends constantly teases a student in your school. How can you show disapproval of this inconsiderate and disrespectful behavior?

21. **Evaluate.** Analyze the similarities and differences between passive, aggressive, and assertive forms of communication.

LESSON 3

Vocabulary Review

Choose the correct term in the sentences below.

22. *Responsibility/Abstinence* is a deliberate decision to avoid high-risk behaviors.

23. The ability to practice responsible behaviors even when you are faced with temptation is called *self-control/priority*.

24. *Infatuation/Intimacy* is the closeness that grows over time between two people who care about each other.

Understanding Key Concepts

After reading the question or statement, select the correct answer.

25. Which of the following statements is true?
    a. STDs can be cured with over-the-counter medications.
    b. Teens under the age of 18 are immune to STDs.
    c. Some STDs have no cure, and some can cause infertility or even death.
    d. The symptoms of all STDs go away after a few months.

26. Which of the following behaviors will help you maintain self-control while dating?
    a. Date someone who respects and shares your values.
    b. Return home from dates before midnight.
    c. Avoid dating someone who goes to your own school.
    d. Limit the number of parties you attend.

27. A person trying to pressure you into sexual activity would probably *not* say:
    a. "Don't worry, no one will ever know."
    b. "If you feel uncomfortable with this, then we shouldn't do it."
    c. "If you love me, then show it."
    d. "Everyone in school is doing it."

28. Approximately how many teenage girls become pregnant every year in the United States?
    a. 1,000
    b. 10,000
    c. 100,000
    d. 1,000,000

Thinking Critically

After reading the question or statement, write a short answer using complete sentences.

29. **Identify.** When might sexual activity result in a loss of self-respect?

30. **Identify.** What are two *risk situations* that could increase your chances of being pressured into sexual activity?

31. **Describe.** How might engaging in sexual activity have a negative effect on your social health?

32. **Describe.** What are some ways that teens and their parents can set limits for dating relationships?

33. **Discuss.** How are teens' attitudes toward sexual activity influenced by the media and popular culture?

34. **Analyze.** Why is abstinence the best choice for teens? Include information on the social, mental/emotional, and physical benefits of abstinence.

PROJECT-BASED ASSESSMENT

Friendship Survey

BACKGROUND

Your peers are important to your development as an individual. During the teen years, you develop a variety of relationships. Some relationships are casual friendships, while others are close friendships. Dating relationships also develop during this time.

TASK

Use an online survey tool to conduct a survey of students in your school to find out what characteristics they consider essential for a close friendship.

AUDIENCE

Students in your class

PURPOSE

Find out what qualities your peers believe differentiate a close friendship from other kinds of relationships.

PROCEDURE

1. Use the information in Module 8 to develop a list of qualities that are essential for a close friendship.

2. Create a ten-question survey using an online survey program. The questions might gauge the importance of each quality as "very important," "important," or "not important."

3. Select 15 or more students for the survey. Use the online survey tool to tally the responses.

4. Examine the results, and make a table showing the responses to each question. Determine the qualities that are considered to be most essential for a close friendship.

5. Discuss the results with your class.

Math Practice

Interpret Graphs. The graph below shows the percentages of young adults who volunteer each year. Use the graph to answer Questions 1–3.

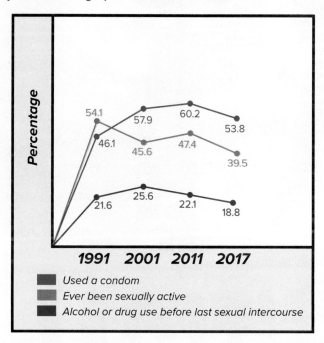

1991   2001   2011   2017

■ Used a condom
■ Ever been sexually active
■ Alcohol or drug use before last sexual intercourse

Adapted from "Volunteering in America: 2007 State Trends and Rankings in Civic Life," Corporation for National and Community Service, April 2007.

1. By what percentage has sexual activity among teens decreased between 1991 and 2017?
   a. 10.2   c. 4.3
   b. 14.6   d. 12.6

2. Which year shows the highest rate of teens reporting alcohol use before engaging in sexual activity?
   a. 2001   c. 1991
   b. 2011   d. 2017

3. Identify the years with the lowest and highest percentage of condom use. What is the difference in percentage between the two years?
   a. 3.2   c. 14.1
   b. 6.0   d. 4.5

Reading/Writing Practice

Understand and Apply. Read the passage below, and then answer the questions.

I have been best friends with Tamara since the first grade. Tamara is nice to me and to other people.

Tamara's kindness shows in many ways. Once she gave her circus tickets to some kids who had never been to the circus. Tamara visits a nearby nursing home at least once a month. She worries about some of the people she has met there because they have no family.

Tamara was a good friend to me when my parents divorced. She listened to me for hours as I talked about how upset I was. She also let me cry and never told me that I was overreacting. I knew that she couldn't do anything to change the situation, but she always made me feel better.

1. How does the author show that Tamara is a good friend?
   a. By comparing Tamara's actions to those of her other friends
   b. By pointing out that Tamara once helped with a canned-food drive
   c. By citing examples of Tamara's kindness
   d. By saying that Tamara does not gossip

2. When Tamara listened to her friend talk about divorce, what characteristics of friendship did she show?
   a. Mutual respect   c. Support
   b. Caring   d. All of the above

3. Describe the qualities that you think make someone a good friend. Give examples and details to support your opinions.

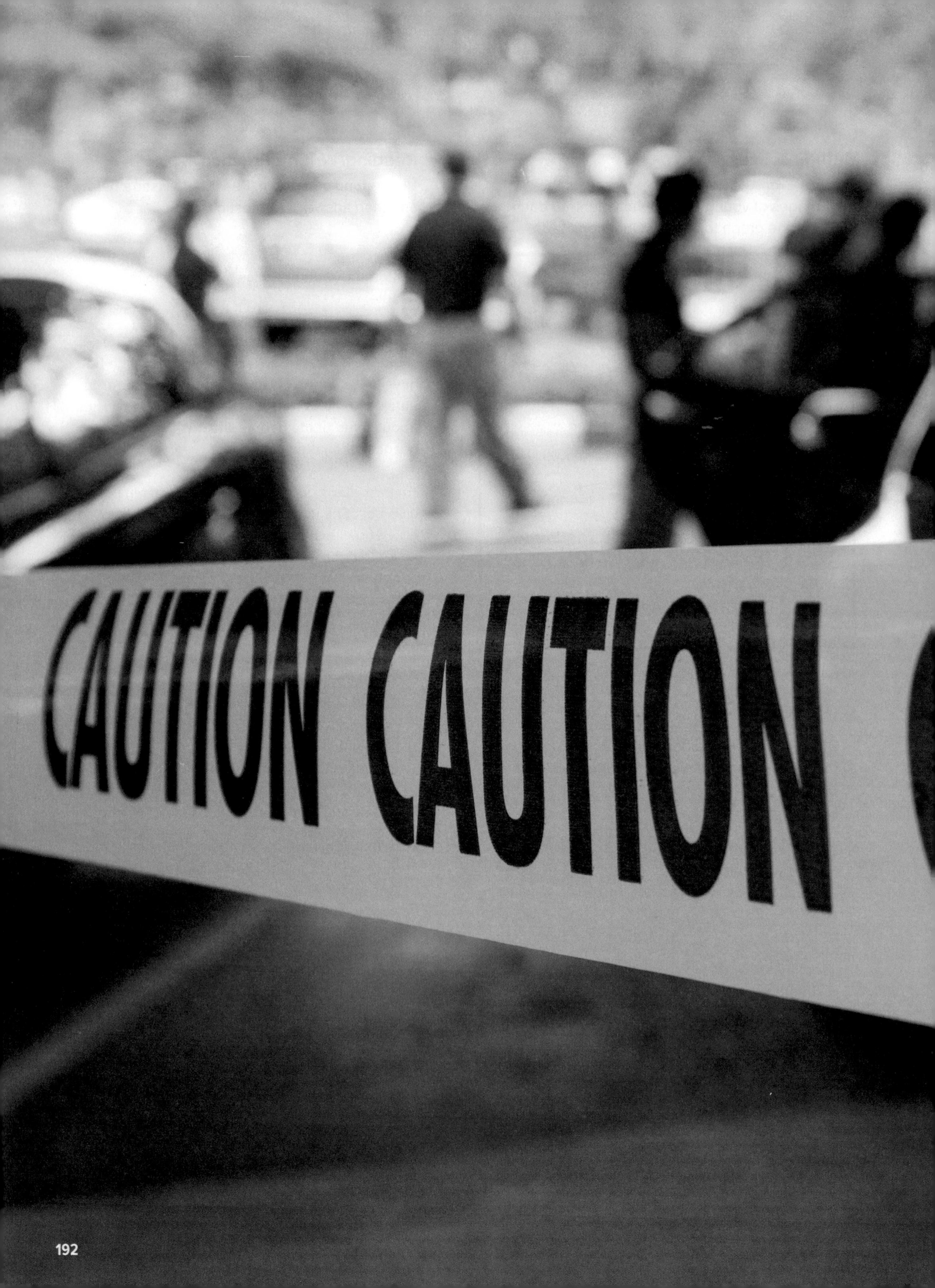
CAUTION CAUTION

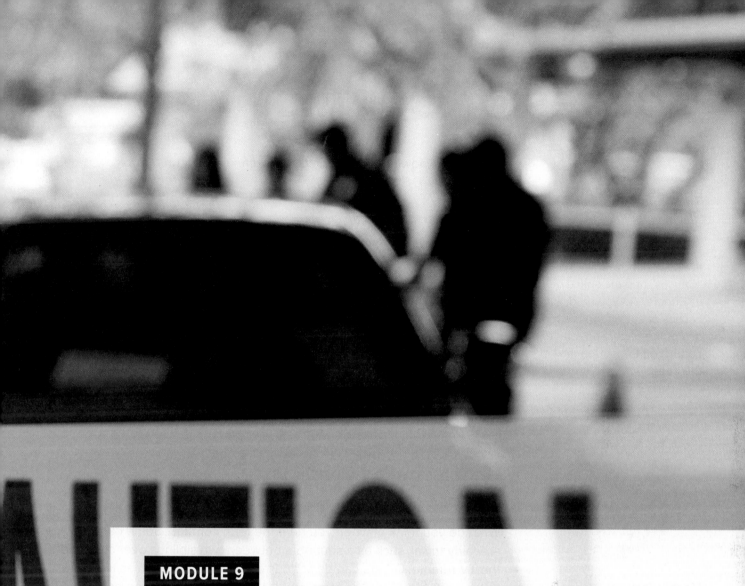

Resolving Conflicts and Preventing Violence

LESSONS

Causes of Conflict

- - - - - - - - - - - -

BEFORE YOU READ

Organize Information. In the center of your paper, write "Conflict" and circle it. Label the space above this circle "Causes" and the space below it "Effects." As you read, list causes of conflict on the top half of the page, and effects of conflict on the bottom half of the page.

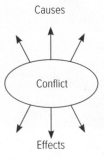

Causes

Conflict

Effects

Vocabulary

conflict
interpersonal conflict
escalate

- - - - - - - - - - - -

Reading Check

Compare and Contrast How are interpersonal conflicts different from internal conflicts?

- - - - - - - - - - - -

BIG IDEA Knowing why conflicts occur can help you prevent them.

REAL LIFE ISSUES

Conflict in Communication. Jessie has been looking for her new coat all evening, and now she is running late for a movie. As she rushes out the door, her sister, Lauren, walks in wearing the coat. Jessie is furious. She yells, "If you can take my clothes without permission, I'll take yours whenever I feel like it!" Jessie walks into Lauren's room, grabs an armful of clothes, and walks out the front door with them. ***Write a paragraph explaining what you think caused this conflict and how it might have been avoided.***

After completing the lesson, review and analyze your response to the Real Life Issues question.

Understanding Conflicts

MAIN IDEA Conflicts can arise for a variety of reasons.

What do you think of when you hear the term **conflict**? Some conflicts are fairly trivial, such as a squabble between two siblings over control of the TV remote. Others can be serious or even deadly, such as turf wars between rival gangs. The term conflict refers to any disagreement, struggle, or fight. There are two major types of conflicts:

- **Interpersonal conflicts.** Interpersonal conflicts are between people or groups of people. They tend to arise when one party's needs, wishes, or beliefs clash with those of another party. Interpersonal conflicts can involve groups of any size, from individual people to entire nations.

- **Internal conflicts.** Internal conflicts take place within an individual. For example, if your best friend's birthday party and your sister's championship soccer game fell on the same day, you might go through an internal conflict over which event to attend.

Common Causes of Conflict

Conflicts between people or groups can arise for a variety of reasons. Some conflicts arise out of misunderstandings. For instance, in the Real Life Issues scenario, Lauren and Jessie got angry at each other over a miscommunication. Sometimes, misunderstandings occur when one person **misinterprets** another person's language, gestures, or sense of humor. This type of conflict might occur between people of different cultures or age groups. In other cases, someone deliberately starts a conflict—for example, by insulting or tripping someone else. Causes of conflict include:

- **Power struggles.** A teen and her parents might have a conflict over how late she is allowed to stay out at night.

- **Personal loyalties.** A teen might be angry with his best friend for taking another person's side in an argument.

- **Jealousy and envy.** A teen might be upset when her friend starts going out with a boy she likes.

- **Property disputes.** A teen might be angry with his brother for borrowing his jacket without permission.

- **Conflicting attitudes and values.** Two friends might have an argument because one wants to hang out only with the "cool" crowd, while the other wants to be friendly to everyone.

- **Lack of respect.** A teen might be rude to an exchange student at school because of a prejudice against that student's ethnic group.

ACADEMIC VOCABULARY

misinterpret *(verb)*: to understand wrongly

Conflicts between people can occur for many different reasons. **Which type of conflict does this picture show?**

Understanding these causes of conflict may help you avoid some conflicts before they start. If it looks like a conflict is developing, you may able to keep it from **escalating**. Escalate means to become more serious. Conflicts can escalate into fights when emotions get out of control. Feelings such as hurt pride, embarrassment, or the desire for revenge can turn a simple conflict into a situation that could be unsafe for everyone involved. In some cases, it's best to simply walk away before the conflict escalates.

Results of Conflict

Conflict is a normal part of life. Because each individual is different, it's inevitable that people will disagree sometimes. Learning to manage conflicts and deal with them before they get out of hand will strengthen all aspects of your health.

Sometimes, conflicts can actually have positive results. Working to resolve a conflict can help people improve their communication and problem-solving skills. It can also improve their social health by teaching them how to get along with people who disagree with them. In addition, dealing with conflicts can strengthen relationships. When two people have a conflict and they make the effort to work through it together, it shows their commitment to each other.

Reminding a friend who often borrows money to get some cash before you go out is one way to prevent a conflict. **What other ways can you think of?**

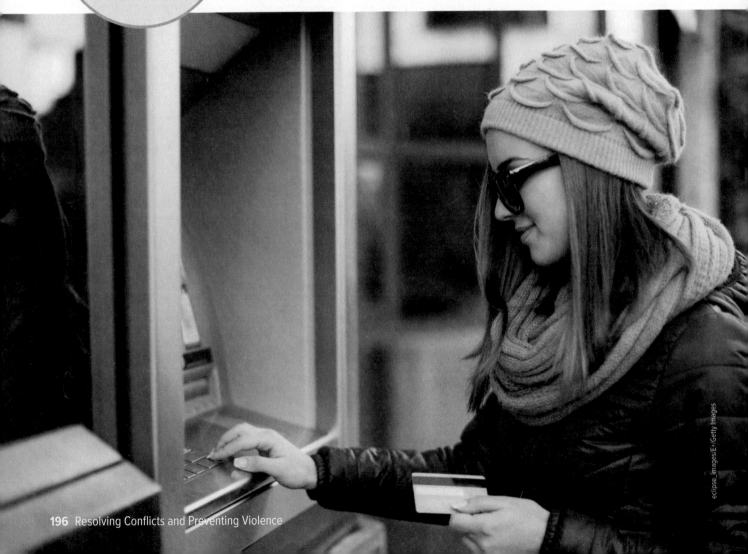

eclipse_images/E+/Getty Images

Unfortunately, conflicts can also have negative effects. They can often be a major source of stress, resulting in physical problems such as headaches and lost sleep. Conflicts can also harm your emotional and social health. They can lead to hurt feelings and cause serious damage to relationships. In addition, conflicts in the workplace sometimes cause people to lose their jobs. In the worst cases, conflicts can escalate to violence, resulting in serious injury or even death.

Preventing Conflicts

It's often easier to prevent a conflict than it is to resolve it. For instance, if you know someone who is always trying to provoke you into an argument, you might decide to avoid that person. If you get involved in a minor disagreement with someone, you can remind yourself that the argument isn't that important in the long run. It's not worth damaging your relationship over something trivial.

Sometimes you can prevent conflicts by adjusting your own behavior. For instance, suppose you have a friend who always forgets to bring money when you go out. Instead of feeling annoyed every time, you might just make a point of reminding this person to stop at the ATM beforehand. Adjusting your attitude can also help. If you tend to interpret any kind of personal remark as an attack, you might try to relax and not be bothered so much by what other people say.

Character Check

I'm working on a group project for one class. One person in the group takes the opposing side every time another group member suggests something we should add to our final project. The person says she's forcing us to look at all sides of the issue. To most of us it seems more like bullying. I asked her to think about what she was doing, and said it feels disrespectful that she constantly argues with others.

Lesson 1 Review

Facts and Vocabulary

1. Identify two common causes of interpersonal conflicts.

2. How can conflicts be positive?

3. Give an example of how conflicts can negatively affect one's health.

Thinking Critically

4. **Analyze.** How might adapting your behavior help prevent conflicts?

5. **Evaluate.** Discuss the benefits and drawbacks of walking away from a developing conflict.

Applying Health Skills

6. **Analyzing Influences.** How might influences such as environment, culture, media, and personal values affect a conflict between two people?

Writing Critically

7. **Expository.** Write an essay about common teen conflicts. Explain how to prevent some of these conflicts.

Resolving Conflicts

BIG IDEA Conflicts can be resolved through negotiation or mediation.

BEFORE YOU READ

Create a Venn Diagram. Draw two overlapping circles and label them "Negotiation" and "Mediation." As you read, fill in the circles with information about these two methods of resolving conflicts. Traits the two methods have in common should go in the overlapping area.

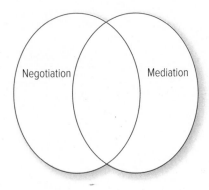

Negotiation   Mediation

Vocabulary
negotiation
mediation
confidentiality
peer mediation

REAL LIFE ISSUES

Two Teens, One Bathroom. Joe bangs furiously on the bathroom door. "Maggie! You've been in there for half an hour! I need to get ready for school too, you know!" His sister, Maggie, flings open the door. "You know it takes me longer to get ready," she says. "I have to wash and blow-dry my hair every morning. Give me a break!" Joe sighs. "Look, we can't go through this every morning. Can't we work out some kind of deal?" *Continue the dialogue between Joe and Maggie. Have them brainstorm a solution to their conflict.*

After completing the lesson, review and analyze your response to the Real Life Issues question.

Responding to Conflict

MAIN IDEA There are various ways to deal with a conflict.

When you have a conflict with someone else, you have two choices: you can walk away or respond to it. If you think the conflict could escalate and become dangerous, getting out is the best approach. This is also true if you are having trouble managing your own anger. Walking away will give you a chance to calm down so that you can approach the conflict rationally.

However, in many cases, walking away from a conflict will not make it go away. You may stop it from escalating, but the same issue is likely to come up again until you find a way to deal with it. Sooner or later, you will need to practice *conflict resolution,* the process of ending a conflict through cooperation and problem solving.

Compromise

You can often resolve minor conflicts with a compromise. If you and your brother disagree about what to watch on TV, you might agree to watch one show and record the other. However, it can be difficult to reach a compromise when both parties have strong opinions about an issue. In addition, it's unwise to compromise when doing so could have harmful consequences or would go against your values.

Effective Negotiation

MAIN IDEA Negotiation involves finding a solution that both sides can accept.

When conflicts are not resolved, they can grow worse, sometimes resulting in violence. It's important to understand that violence does not solve conflicts. One group may be able to force another to do what it wants, but they won't have dealt with the causes of the conflict. As a result, the same conflict is likely to keep coming up again and again. Each time, the violence may escalate, harming more and more people. A better approach to conflicts is **negotiation**. Negotiation is the use of communication and, in many cases, compromise to settle a disagreement.

The Negotiation Process

The negotiation process involves talking, listening, and considering the other party's point of view. The goal is to create a plan to resolve the conflict, which may involve compromise for both parties. Mutual respect is an important ingredient in a successful negotiation. The steps of the negotiation process are:

1. Take time to calm down and think over the situation.

2. Let all parties take turns explaining their side of the conflict without interruption. Remember to use good communication skills, such as active listening and "I" messages.

3. If necessary, ask for clarification to make sure that each party understands the other's position.

4. Brainstorm solutions to the conflict.

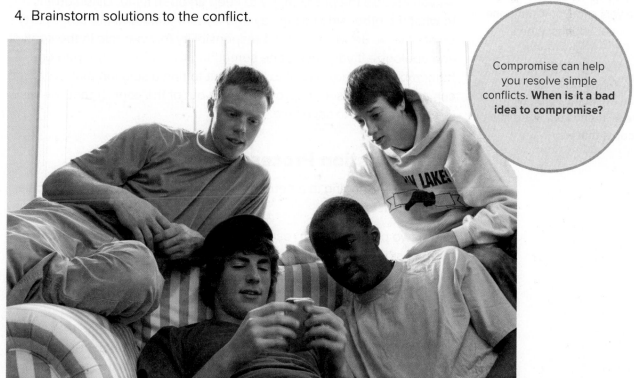

Compromise can help you resolve simple conflicts. **When is it a bad idea to compromise?**

5. Discuss the advantages and disadvantages of each solution.

6. Agree on a solution that is acceptable to both sides. The ideal outcome will be a win-win solution—one that benefits everyone and has no real drawbacks for anyone. If this is not possible, the two parties may need to compromise.

7. Follow up to see whether the solution has worked for each party.

Preparing for Negotiation

Successful negotiations require careful planning. Taking these steps ahead of time will increase the chances that negotiation will work:

- **Choose the time and place carefully.** The negotiation should take place at a time when both parties are calm, not impatient or rushed. Arrange to meet in a quiet place on neutral ground—not at the home of either party or in any other place that "belongs" to one side.

- **Check your facts.** Make sure your understanding of the situation is based on accurate information.

- **Plan what you will say.** Think about how to word your statement respectfully. You may wish to rehearse or write down your statement.

Tips for Successful Negotiation

Staying calm is an important key to successful negotiation. Getting angry or upset could throw off the negotiations. Try to see the other party not as an enemy, but as a partner in the negotiations. Attack the problem, not each other. Avoid blaming and name-calling.

As you discuss the problem, try to keep an open mind. Listen attentively to what the other side has to say and try to understand the other party's point of view. Be willing to take responsibility for your role in the conflict and apologize if you have done something to hurt the other person. Remember, your goal is not to "win," but to find a solution that everyone can accept. Make sure to provide a way out of the conflict that will allow the other person to save face.

The Mediation Process

MAIN IDEA Bringing in a neutral third party to mediate can help solve some conflicts.

When two parties cannot reach a solution through negotiation, they may consider **mediation**. Mediation means bringing in a neutral third party to help others resolve their conflicts peacefully. The word *mediation* literally means "being in the middle." Having a third party "in the middle" helps put some distance between the two opposing parties. The presence of someone who is not on either side can reduce the level of confrontation. Mediation can be especially useful for dealing with conflicts that go on for a long time and threaten to disrupt everyday life.

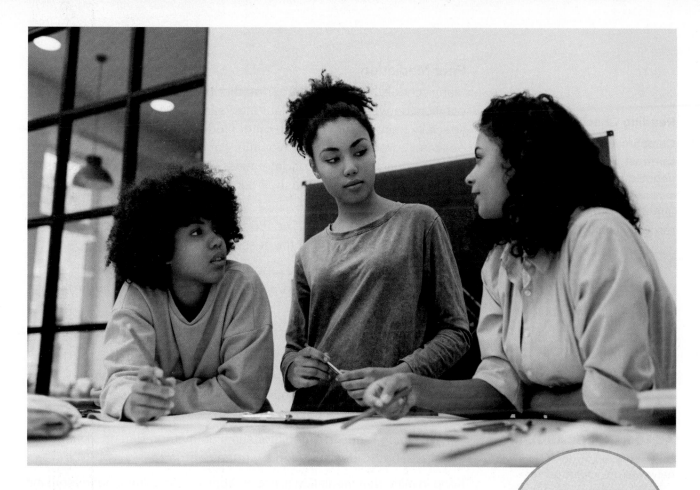

Mediation can help people settle interpersonal conflicts. **What qualities would an effective mediator need?**

Mediation can be formal or informal. Formal mediation involves the help of a mediator who has special training in resolving conflicts. Informal mediation can be as simple as asking a teacher to help settle a dispute with a classmate. Effective mediation depends on the basic principles of neutrality, confidentiality, and well-defined ground rules.

- **Neutrality.** The mediator must always be an outsider who has no stake in the dispute. The mediation session should also take place in a neutral location.

- **Confidentiality. Confidentiality** means respecting the privacy of both parties and keeping details secret. The mediator promises not to reveal to outsiders anything said by either party during the process.

- **Well-defined ground rules.** Both parties must agree to the rules set by the mediator. In some cases, the mediator may ask the two parties to sign an agreement to work out the problem within a given time frame.

In a typical mediation, each party gets a chance to present its side of the argument. The mediator then summarizes the points made by each side and leads a discussion between the two parties. The mediator does not make judgments or impose solutions. Instead, the solutions must come from the two parties. However, the mediator can help them see the advantages and disadvantages of certain ideas.

Reading Check

Compare and Contrast Explain how negotiation and mediation are similar and how they are different as strategies for resolving conflicts.

Peer Mediation

Many schools have started **peer mediation** programs to help resolve conflicts between students. Peer mediation is a process in which specially trained students help other students resolve conflicts peacefully. Peer mediation is voluntary and confidential. Rather than trying to punish students or determine who is right or wrong, it aims to help students move beyond their conflicts. Typically, peer mediation involves:

- **Making introductions.** The mediator explains that he or she will remain neutral and that the session will be confidential.

- **Establishing ground rules.** Both parties must agree to such rules as listening without interrupting, telling the truth, and addressing each other with respect.

- **Hearing each side.** Each student gets to tell his or her story in turn. The mediator may ask questions and take notes.

- **Exploring solutions.** The two sides discuss the situation and propose possible solutions. Each solution is discussed, and both parties try to find a solution they can both accept.

- **Wrapping it up.** The mediator sums up the agreement. In some cases, both sides may sign a written **contract**.

Keep in mind that mediation is not an appropriate solution for every kind of problem in schools. Violence and other crimes, for instance, require action from the school's administration or from legal authorities. However, problems such as teasing and bullying may be solved through peer mediation. Students who have been through the peer mediation process can apply the skills they learn when resolving future conflicts.

Lesson 2 Review

Facts and Vocabulary

1. List three steps you could take to prepare for a negotiation.

2. Determine when it might be necessary to bring in a mediator to settle a conflict.

3. Give two examples of ground rules in a peer mediation process.

Thinking Critically

4. **Evaluate.** Suppose a friend wants to copy answers off your paper during a test. When you refuse, she gets angry. Explain whether this conflict could be resolved through compromise.

5. **Make Inferences.** Why might peer mediation for students work better than bringing in an adult mediator?

Applying Health Skills

6. **Conflict Resolution.** Luke wants to go to a basketball game, but his parents want him to help out with spring cleaning. Write a dialogue in which they use conflict-resolution techniques to settle this problem.

Writing Critically

7. **Narrative.** Write a short story that centers on a conflict between two teens. Show how the characters resolve their conflict through compromise, negotiation, or mediation.

Understanding Violence

BIG IDEA Teens need to know about forms of violence and ways to protect themselves.

REAL LIFE ISSUES

The Costs of Violence. Teens may be involved in various forms of violence both on and off school property. A 2017 survey of youth risk behaviors conducted by the CDC found that 23.6 percent of teens had been involved in physical fights. 8.5 percent of teens had been in a physical fight on school property. ***Write a paragraph explaining how violence in schools can be avoided.***

After completing the lesson, review and analyze your response to the Real Life Issues question.

Causes of Violence

MAIN IDEA Weapons, drugs, and gangs are some factors that can contribute to violence.

Violence in society takes many forms. Violence is the threatened or actual use of physical force or power to harm another person or to damage property. Some acts of violence result from interpersonal conflicts that escalate out of control. However, violence can also be random, affecting people who just happen to be in the wrong place at the wrong time. People may commit violent acts for many reasons, including:

- Uncontrolled anger or frustration.

- A need to control others.

- Hatred or prejudice against a particular group.

- Retaliation, or revenge, for some past harm—whether real or perceived.

Certain risk factors make children and teens more likely to be involved in violence. Children are at a greater risk if their families are poor, have low levels of education, or are involved in illegal activities. For teens, friends and peers play a greater role. Having friends who are involved in violence and crime greatly increases teens' risk of committing violent acts themselves. Fortunately, there are also factors that can help protect teens from becoming involved in violence. Teens who are committed to school and have a negative attitude toward crime are less likely to commit acts of violence, even if they have several risk factors.

BEFORE YOU READ

Create a Word Web. Write "Violence" in the center of a sheet of paper. As you read the lesson, add information about causes of violence and forms that violence can take.

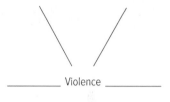

Violence

Vocabulary

violence
assault
random violence
homicide
sexual violence
sexual assault
rape
dating violence

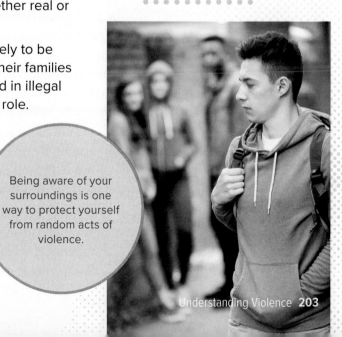

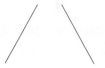

Being aware of your surroundings is one way to protect yourself from random acts of violence.

Alcohol and Drug Use

Many teens who are involved in violence use alcohol or other drugs. Studies have found that alcohol, in particular, plays a role in many violent crimes. There are several possible reasons for this connection:

- Drinking and drug use can lower people's self-control. As a result, they may be less likely to restrain their violent impulses.

- Drinking and drug use can damage people's judgment. They may overreact to something they see as a threat or fail to consider the consequences of their actions.

- Teens may engage in violent crimes as a way to get money to buy drugs.

- People who use drugs and drink alcohol are more likely to engage in other high-risk behaviors, such as fighting, carrying weapons, and engaging in unsafe sexual activity.

Some teens actually become involved with violence before they start to use alcohol or drugs. In other words, for some teens, it isn't using drugs and alcohol that makes them violent. Instead, their violent lifestyle puts them at risk for other problems, including substance abuse.

Mental and Emotional Problems

Low self-esteem is another risk factor for violence among teens. **Insecure** teens may try to use violence to prove themselves. Teens who have had little success in life may use violence as a way of getting back at a system that they think has caused them to fail. Teens with low self-esteem may also be more likely to join gangs as a way to belong. Gang membership puts teens at much higher risk for violence. Stress, depression, and strong emotions such as anger can lead some teens to become violent. Learning to control anger effectively can greatly reduce the risk of violence. Anger-management workshops and counseling can help teens learn to deal with anger and avoid lashing out at others.

Availability of Weapons

A 2017 government survey revealed that more than one in four high school students reported that they had carried a weapon within the past 30 days. Roughly 5 percent of all students said that they had carried a gun. When people are carrying weapons, violence can more easily turn deadly. To protect yourself from the dangers associated with weapons, follow these strategies:

- Do not carry weapons. Some teens carry guns "for protection," but having a gun or other weapon actually makes you less safe, not more. In fact, people who carry guns are twice as likely to become victims of gun violence.

- If you know that another teen is carrying a weapon or that there are weapons in your school, tell a trusted adult, such as a parent or teacher. If you fear that doing this might put you in danger, try to find a way to contact the authorities anonymously.

Reading Check

Describe Name three ways for teens to protect themselves from situations involving weapons.

- If your parents keep a gun at home, encourage them to equip it with a trigger lock and to store it unloaded in a locked cabinet.

Violence in the Media

Every day, children and teens are exposed to violent words and images on television and movies, and in song lyrics, and video games. Recent studies of violence in the media indicate that more than 60 percent of all television shows and more than 85 percent of top-rated video games contain some violence. In addition, scenes that feature violence often fail to show its harmful consequences. The victim's suffering is often unseen. In many cases, the characters who commit violent acts suffer no punishment as a result.

Exposure to violence in the media can influence the way people think about violence. Some young people who view scenes of violence may begin to perceive it as normal or even positive. Studies have found that children and teens act more aggressively right after watching violent scenes. Also, children and teens who are aggressive tend to watch more violent television than their less aggressive peers.

Children and teens are exposed to violence in the media every day. **How might this exposure influence their behavior?**

Gang Violence

Youth gangs are groups of teens or young adults who are involved collectively in violent or illegal activity. Gangs are often involved in drug dealing, robbery, and violent attacks on members of rival gangs. Teens who join gangs may be seeking protection from violence or looking for a way to fit in.

Teens who belong to gangs are much more likely than their peers to commit serious or violent crimes. They are also much more likely to become victims of violence. Being part of a gang reduces a teen's chances of graduating from school and finding a steady job. As a result, teen gang members may become career criminals.

To avoid gang influence, be aware of gang activity in your area, including the colors and symbols used by various gangs. Having this information will enable you to recognize and avoid gang members. It will also help you avoid dressing in a way that could cause you to be mistaken for a gang member. Seek out positive alternatives to gang membership, such as participating in sports or after-school programs. Finally, be prepared to use refusal skills if anyone ever tries to recruit you into a gang.

Hero Images/Getty Images

Violence Among Teens

The National Youth Risk Behavior Survey keeps track of behaviors that put teens' health and safety at risk. The chart below shows how some behaviors related to violence have increased or decreased over time.

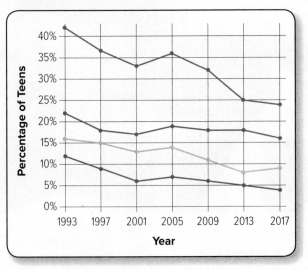

Source: Centers for Disease Control and Prevention, National Youth Risk Behavior Survey, 1991–2017

Key:
- Being in a physical fight (at least once in the past year)
- Carrying a weapon (at least once in the past month)
- Carrying a weapon on school property
- Being in a physical fight on school property

Activity: Mathematics

Use the graph to answer the following questions:

1. What percent of teens were involved in a physical fight in 2013?

2. What overall trend can you detect for all four risk behaviors over the 24-year period shown?

3. Which of these behaviors do you think poses the greatest danger to teens? Why?

CONCEPT Measurement and Data: Interpreting Graphs
A line graph compares the relationship between two variables. It is an effective tool for showing trends.

Types of Violence

MAIN IDEA Violence may be physical or sexual.

In nearly half of all violent crimes, the victims know their attackers. This rate is even higher for certain types of crimes, such as sexual attacks, in which victims are very likely to know their attackers, while robberies are typically random.

Assault and Homicide

An **assault** is an unlawful physical attack or threat of attack. Assault is a crime that includes everything from minor threats to attacks that cause life-threatening injuries. Each year over 4 million assaults take place in the United States, and more than 1 million of those incidents result in injury. Roughly half of all assaults occur between people who know each other. However, assaults may also be a form of **random violence**—violence committed for no particular reason.

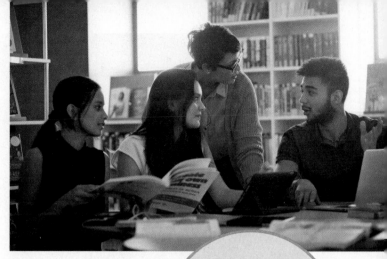

If the victim of an assault dies, the crime becomes a **homicide**. Homicide is the willful killing of one human being by another. Teens can protect themselves from assault and homicide by avoiding the risk factors associated with violence in general. That means avoiding drugs, alcohol, weapons, and gangs. You can also work on developing your protective factors. For instance, strengthening your ties to your family and your school can lower your overall risk of violence.

Sexual Violence

You've probably heard of sexual harassment, or unwelcome sexual conduct. It can include jokes, gestures, or physical contact. In some cases, sexual harassment may escalate to **sexual violence**. This is any form of unwelcome sexual contact directed at an individual. Forms of sexual violence include **sexual assault** and **rape**. Sexual assault means any intentional sexual attack against another person. Rape is any form of sexual intercourse that takes place against a person's will. In 2018, 734,630 rapes or sexual assaults occurred in the U.S. Rape is one of the crimes least likely to be reported to the police. Survivors of rape may be unwilling to go to the police because of shame or fear. In some cases, they may not even see the attack as a crime.

Sexual violence can affect anyone. However, most victims of this crime are female, and most rapists are male. Also, more than half of all female rape victims, and about three-quarters of male victims, are under 18 years old. Of all violent crimes, rape and sexual assault are the ones in which victims are most likely to know their attackers.

Avoiding Sexual Violence. A sexual attack can happen anywhere. To protect yourself, be aware of your surroundings wherever you go. Refuse to go anywhere alone with someone you don't know or trust. Go to parties with friends so that you can all watch out for each other. Avoid alcohol and drugs, which can make you an easier target. Finally, trust your instincts. If a situation feels unsafe, don't hesitate to get out.

Responding to a Sexual Attack. If you are ever sexually attacked, your goal is to survive. In some cases, that may mean resisting the attacker, while in other cases, it may be safer to submit. You may try to stall for time, distract the attacker, or scream to attract attention. Do whatever you need to do to survive the situation.

Reporting a sexual attack to a trusted adult right away gives you the best chance of bringing the attacker to justice. To preserve evidence of the attack, do not bathe or brush your teeth until you have been examined. Seek medical help for any injuries and, if appropriate, get tested for pregnancy and sexually transmitted diseases (STDs).

Survivors of rape and sexual assault need time to heal physically and emotionally. They may suffer feelings of fear, guilt, and shame. Many mistakenly blame themselves for the attack. Counseling can help survivors of a sexual attack recover from the experience.

Teens who are involved in school activities are at less risk of violence, including assault and homicide. **Why do you think involvement with school can lower teens' risk of violence?**

Klaus Vedfelt/DigitalVision/Getty Images

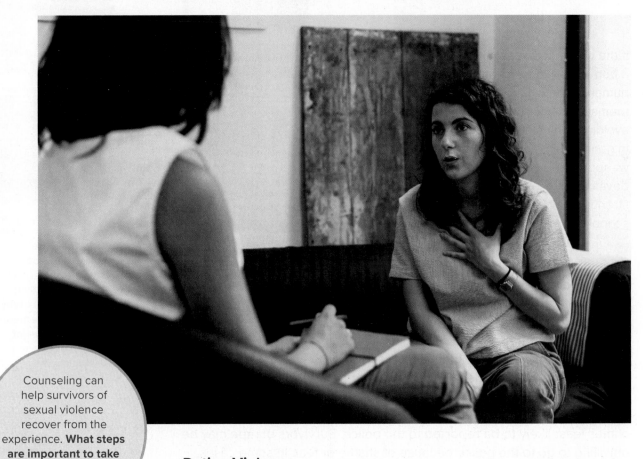

Counseling can help survivors of sexual violence recover from the experience. **What steps are important to take right after a sexual attack?**

Reading Check

Identify What are some ways of responding to a sexual attack?

Dating Violence

Violence of any type is a sign of an unhealthy relationship. When one person behaves violently against another, it shows a lack of respect. **Dating violence** is a form of violence where a person uses violence in a dating relationship to control his or her partner. Any form of violence, including dating violence, is against the law. Dating violence can include physical, emotional, or psychological abuse. Physical abuse includes hitting, kicking, or scratching. Emotional abuse includes name-calling and demeaning a dating partner. Psychological abuse might include preventing a dating partner from spending time with friends that he or she made before the dating relationship began.

If the person who is being abused tries to end the relationship, the abusive partner may apologize for the abusive behavior and promise never to do it again. The abusive partner may try to say that he or she loves the dating partner or that he or she is trying to keep the person safe. These are excuses. They are not true.

It can be difficult to convince someone who is being abused to end the relationship. A person in an abusive dating relationship may need help understanding why the relationship needs to end. Then, that person may need help to end the relationship. Friends can provide emotional support. Ask a parent or other trusted adult for help if you are concerned about breaking off the dating relationship. If you are worried that a friend is in an abusive dating relationship, talk to a trusted adult about this potentially dangerous situation.

Hate Crimes

A hate crime is any crime motivated chiefly by hatred of or prejudice against a particular group. People may be targeted because of their race, religion, culture, sexual orientation, or other difference. Hate crimes can take many forms, such as:

- **Harassment.** This may include racial slurs, stalking, or trying to exclude a targeted group from community life.
- **Vandalism.** Perpetrators may deface buildings with messages or symbols that express hatred of a particular group.
- **Arson.** Criminals may blow up or set fire to buildings associated with a particular group.
- **Assault and homicide.** Criminals may physically attack or even kill members of the targeted group.

Hate crimes don't just harm the individual victims. They affect all members of the targeted group, spreading fear, distrust, and anger throughout the community. They can also provoke the targeted group to strike back with hate crimes of their own.

The best way to stop hate crimes is to change the attitudes behind them. No one is born hating members of a particular group. Those attitudes have to be learned. Practicing and teaching tolerance toward other groups can go a long way toward ending these crimes. When a hate crime occurs, community members can condemn the crime and express support for the targeted group. This may prevent the hate violence from escalating.

Witnesses and bystanders can help prevent violence by reporting dangerous situations. For example, suppose you hear two people at school arguing loudly and the situation is escalating. You should report this to a teacher or other trusted adult. They may be able to defuse the situation before it becomes violent.

Character Check

The past year has been tough on my family. My mom's in the military and stationed overseas. I feel confused, sad, and angry most of the time. I got into a fight at school and the night it happened, my dad talked to me about what I was feeling. He said that it isn't selfish to care for myself by talking about what was bothering me. It's better to care for yourself by talking it out than getting into trouble.

Lesson 3 Review

Facts and Vocabulary

1. Identify two factors that can contribute to violence.

2. What is random violence?

3. Identify two steps you can take to protect yourself from sexual violence.

Thinking Critically

4. **Evaluate.** Why might survivors of rape be reluctant to tell others about the crime?

5. **Analyze.** How can practicing and promoting tolerance help prevent violence?

Applying Health Skills

6. **Refusal Skills.** Write a dialogue between two teens at a party. One teen is trying to persuade the other to go somewhere alone together. The other teen uses refusal skills to avoid the threat of sexual violence.

Writing Critically

7. **Persuasive.** Write an editorial promoting tolerance and condemning hate crimes.

Preventing and Overcoming Abuse

• • • • • • • • • • •

BEFORE YOU READ

Organize Information. Make a chart with three columns. Label the columns "Physical Abuse," "Emotional Abuse," and "Sexual Abuse." As you read, fill in the columns with examples of each type of abuse, possible effects, and ways to prevent or respond to it.

Physical Abuse	Emotional Abuse	Sexual Abuse

Vocabulary

physical abuse
emotional abuse
verbal abuse
sexual abuse
incest
stalking
date rape

• • • • • • • • • • • •

BIG IDEA Abuse can cause physical, mental, and emotional damage.

REAL LIFE ISSUES

A Dangerous Date. Elena smiles at Matt as she hops into his car for their date. On the drive, Matt turns and heads in a different direction. "Where are you going?" Elena asks. "The concert's that way." "Change of plans," Matt says with a sly grin. "There's a party on the other side of town. Some guys figured out how to get into that old abandoned house. I thought it would give us time to be alone." Elena begins to worry. She's afraid that if she and Matt are alone, he might try to take advantage of her sexually. *Write a conclusion to this story that shows how Elena escapes from this potentially dangerous situation.*

After completing the lesson, review and analyze your response to the Real Life Issues question.

Abuse in Relationships

MAIN IDEA All forms of abuse are extremely harmful.

Abuse is the physical, mental, emotional, or sexual mistreatment of one person by another. Abuse can occur in all kinds of relationships, including dating relationships. Both males and females can be affected. A dating relationship may be abusive if one partner:

- Tries to pressure the other into sexual activity.
- Tries to make the relationship serious or exclusive right away.
- Acts jealous or possessive.
- Tries to control the other's behavior.
- Yells, swears, or otherwise emotionally attacks the other.
- Threatens the other with physical violence.

Forms of Abuse

Abuse in relationships can take several forms. The most common forms include physical abuse, emotional abuse, verbal abuse, sexual abuse, and stalking.

- **Physical abuse.** Physical abuse is a pattern of intentionally causing bodily harm or injury to another person. Examples of physical abuse include hitting, kicking, shoving, biting, hair pulling, and throwing objects at another person. Physical abuse can result in serious injuries. It can also leave the victim emotionally scarred. Victims of physical abuse may respond with violence of their own.

- **Emotional abuse.** Emotional abuse is a pattern of attacking another person's emotional development and sense of worth. Emotional abuse can damage self-esteem, leaving the victim feeling worthless or helpless. Victims may even come to feel that they deserve the abuse. Abusers may also humiliate their victims, attempt to control their behavior, threaten them with physical harm, or cut them off from friends and family members.

- **Verbal abuse.** Verbal abuse is the use of words to mistreat or injure another person. Examples of verbal abuse include yelling, swearing, and insults or put-downs.

- **Sexual abuse.** Sexual abuse is a pattern of sexual contact that is forced upon a person against the person's will. Sexual abuse can take many different forms which can include sexual assault, rape, or trying to pressure someone else into sexual activity. Sexual abuse can harm victims physically and emotionally. It may also put them at risk for pregnancy or disease. Another form of abuse that can affect families is **incest.** Incest occurs when a family member commits sexual abuse against another family member. Incest is a crime. It can cause severe emotional damage to the victim.

- **Stalking.** Stalking is repeatedly following, harassing, or threatening an individual. Some stalkers physically follow their victims from place to place. Others harass them by calling or emailing repeatedly and sending letters or gifts. More than 3.3 million people are stalked each year in the United States, and most of them know the stalker. Some people think that being stalked is a form of flattery. Stalkers can be dangerous. If a stalker feels ignored by the victim, he or she might become violent.

Communicating your sexual limits clearly to the people you date can help protect you from being in an abusive relationship. **What are some harmful effects of abuse?**

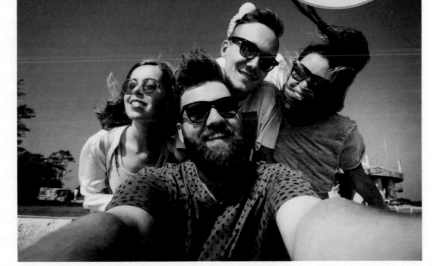

Yulia Mayorova/Shutterstock

Sometimes, teens in abusive relationships don't realize there is a problem. A boyfriend may think that being jealous and possessive of his girlfriend just shows how much he loves her. The girlfriend may accept his efforts to dominate and control her as normal. Teens need to understand that trying to control a **partner** is not a normal or healthy part of a relationship. People in healthy relationships treat each other with respect. They show consideration for each other's feelings and don't hurt or belittle each other.

Protecting Yourself From Abuse

There are several steps you can take to avoid abusive relationships. For starters, you can hang out with others who share your values and treat you with respect. You can also know your own limits with regard to sexual activity and communicate those limits clearly to anyone you date. Avoiding drugs and alcohol is another important step. These substances can limit your ability to make sound decisions.

Know the warning signs of abuse in relationships. If you feel a relationship might be turning dangerous, trust your instincts and get out. If necessary, talk to and seek help from a trusted adult, such as a parent or teacher. If you feel you are in immediate danger, you can contact the police to report the abuse and get help. Finally, remember that no matter what happens, you are not to blame for anyone else's behavior. You can only control your own actions.

Date Rape and Acquaintance Rape

MAIN IDEA Rape that occurs in dating relationships is a form of abuse.

Sometimes, abuse in dating relationships can take the form of sexual violence. **Date rape** is one of the most common forms of rape. More than 40 percent of female rape victims and more than 10 percent of male victims are romantically involved in some way with their attackers. Date rape is related to *acquaintance rape,* in which the attacker is someone the victim knows casually or considers a friend. This is the form of rape that affects male victims most often.

Myths & Reality

It is important to understand the common myths about date rape in order to prevent it. What do you think about this myth?

Myth: Date rape almost always happens between people who have just met each other or don't know each other well.

Reality: It's common for a person to be raped by someone she or he has been dating for a long time.

A dating partner might use intimidation or teasing to coerce a dating partner to become sexually active. A dating partner might also use date rape drugs. Date rape drugs can be added to any drink. Soda, punch, or even milk can be used to deliver date rape drugs. Alcohol can also be used as a date rape drug. Using alcohol makes it harder to think clearly, to make good choices, to say no, or to resist an assault. Dating violence and date rape are crimes. To protect yourself, follow some simple rules:

- Avoid leaving your drink unattended. If your drink has been left unattended, throw the drink out and get a new one.

- Avoid accepting drinks that were obtained from open containers or punch bowls. Drugs may have been added without your knowledge.

- If your drink smells or tastes odd, throw it out.

- If you feel drugged or drunk after drinking a soft drink, get help immediately.

All forms of rape can harm survivors physically, mentally, and emotionally. Minor injuries, such as scratches and bruises, are common. A smaller percentage of survivors suffer major injuries such as broken bones. Long-term effects include chronic pain, headaches, or stomach problems. Survivors are also at risk for pregnancy and STDs. In addition, rape can trigger feelings of shock, anxiety, guilt, and distrust of others. In the long term, survivors may develop mental and emotional problems, such as depression, eating disorders, or post-traumatic stress disorder.

Alcohol, Drugs, and Date Rape

Alcohol often plays a role in date rape. Drinking lowers people's inhibitions and impairs their judgment, making them more likely to take risks they wouldn't normally take. Both females and males are more likely to be sexually attacked when they have been drinking. In addition, males are more likely to commit sexual attacks when under the influence of alcohol.

Some rapists use drugs to subdue their victims. Substances like Rohypnol ("roofies"), GHB, and ketamine are sometimes called "date rape drugs" because they can make someone an easier target. Mixed with food or drink, these drugs are difficult to detect. They work quickly, with effects ranging from drowsiness and dizziness to loss of consciousness. People who have been drugged often cannot remember what happened to them, making it difficult for them to identify their attackers.

Avoiding Date Rape

The tips you learned for avoiding sexual violence also apply to date rape and acquaintance rape. Specific strategies for avoiding date rape include the following:

- Avoid being alone with a dating partner you don't trust or know well, or with anyone who makes you feel uneasy or uncomfortable.

- Avoid alcohol and drugs. Stay sober and aware of what's going on around you.

- Be clear about your sexual limits with dating partners.

- Always get your own beverage at parties, and never leave it uncovered or unattended. Also, don't drink anything that smells or tastes strange.

- Make sure you have a way to get home from any party or social event. Don't depend on your date for a ride. If necessary, carry money for cab fare.

- If you start to feel dizzy, disoriented, or otherwise unwell, it may be a warning sign that you have been drugged. Tell someone you trust and ask for help getting home.

Reading Check

Explain What form of rape most often affects male victims?

Getting your own drink and always keeping an eye on it can help you avoid date rape drugs. **What other strategies can help prevent date rape?**

Overcoming Abuse

MAIN IDEA Counseling can help survivors of abuse recover from its effects.

Victims of abuse or rape may be reluctant to tell others about what has happened to them. Recognizing that they are not to blame can be the first step in recovering from the experience. People need to understand that all forms of abuse, including rape, are illegal. Reporting the incident to a trusted adult or to authorities can help prevent future abuse.

Help for Survivors

People who have survived rape or abuse may feel angry, confused, or ashamed. They may withdraw from friends and family or develop symptoms of depression or anxiety. The experience may lead to a fear of intimacy and an inability to trust others. In the long term, these individuals may be at risk for problems such as alcohol or drug abuse, eating disorders, self-injury, and suicide.

Seeking professional help is the best way to work through these feelings and avoid long-term health consequences. It can be difficult to talk about something as traumatic as rape or abuse, but suppressing the memories will not make them go away.

Taking part in a support group is one way for survivors of abuse to recover from the experience. **What advantages might a support group have over one-on-one therapy?**

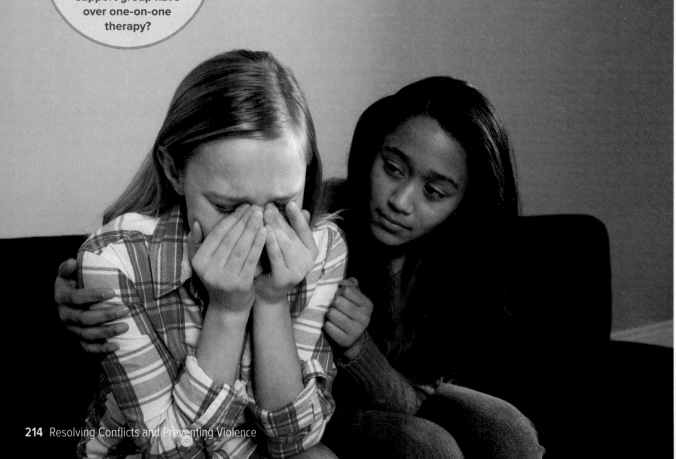

Talking about the experience in a safe, supportive environment is the best way to move toward healing. Survivors can seek support from sources such as:

- Parents, guardians, or other trusted adults.
- Teachers, coaches, or school guidance counselors.
- Members of the clergy.
- Police.
- Private physicians or hospital emergency rooms
- Rape crisis centers or shelters for victims of domestic violence.
- Therapists, counselors, or support groups.

Counseling can take several forms. Some survivors of abuse prefer one-on-one sessions with a trained therapist. Others feel more comfortable with support groups where they can share their experiences with other survivors. Being in a group like this may help them understand that they are not alone.

Reading Check

Evaluate Why is it important to report all forms of abuse to the authorities?

Help for Abusers

In cases of abuse, the victim isn't the only one who needs help. Abuse is a learned behavior, and many abusers were once victims themselves. They need help to break the cycle of violence. Some abusers may see their behavior as normal or justified. They need help to recognize that abusing others is wrong and to learn healthier ways of relating to others. Other abusers understand that their behavior is wrong but feel powerless to stop it. They need to learn that they are responsible for their own behavior and that with help, they can control their violent impulses.

Counseling can help abusers learn to cope with their anger in healthier ways. It can teach them how to communicate better and resolve conflicts peacefully. Abusers should recognize that asking for help is an act of courage. Without it, their violent behavior may increase until it destroys their relationships or causes serious harm to someone they love. By getting the help they need, they may be able to save their relationships and stop the cycle from continuing to the next generation.

Lesson 4 Review

Facts and Vocabulary

1. What is verbal abuse?

2. Identify two warning signs that a dating relationship may be abusive.

3. Identify two strategies for avoiding date rape.

Thinking Critically

4. **Analyze.** Why should you make sure you have a way to get home from a party or social event other than depending on your date for a ride?

5. **Evaluate.** Why is it beneficial for abusers, as well as survivors of abuse, to seek counseling?

Applying Health Skills

6. **Communication Skills.** Suppose a friend has just confided to you about being in an abusive relationship. Write a dialogue between you and your friend in which you show support and encourage your friend to seek help.

Writing Critically

7. **Creative.** Write a poem or song about the problem of abuse in relationships.

Vocabulary Review

Use the correct vocabulary term to complete the following statements.

1. The term _____ refers to any disagreement, struggle, or fight.

2. Disagreements can _____ into fights when emotions get out of control.

3. _____ can arise when one party's needs, wishes, or beliefs clash with those of another party.

Understanding Key Concepts

After reading the question or statement, select the correct answer.

4. Which of the following is *not* an example of an interpersonal conflict?
    a. Two friends disagree over which movie to see.
    b. Two rival gangs fight over control of a neighborhood.
    c. Two political parties clash over tax policy.
    d. A teen feels torn between loyalties to two friends who are not on good terms.

5. Which of the following is a positive result of conflict?
    a. Improved problem-solving skills
    b. Stress
    c. Damaged relationships
    d. Violence

Thinking Critically

After reading the question or statement, write a short answer using complete sentences.

6. **Discuss.** How might cultural differences contribute to interpersonal conflict? What steps could people take to avoid this problem?

7. **Analyze.** Explain how conflicts can both help and harm relationships.

8. **Synthesize.** How could you prevent a friend's frequent forgetfulness from becoming an ongoing source of conflict?

Vocabulary Review

Correct the sentences below by replacing the italicized term with the correct vocabulary term.

9. Solving a disagreement in a way that satisfies everyone involved is called *escalation.*

10. *Discussion* involves bringing in a neutral third party to help resolve conflicts.

11. *Neutrality* means respecting the privacy of both parties and keeping details secret.

Understanding Key Concepts

After reading the question or statement, select the correct answer.

12. Which of the following conflicts most likely could be resolved through compromise?
    a. The school drama club is split over which of two plays to put on.
    b. One group of parents wants the school to adopt a dress code, but the other doesn't.
    c. A teen wants to buy a used car, but his father objects because the car is unsafe.
    d. One friend makes fun of a boy whom the other likes.

13. Which of the following is *not* a good strategy for negotiation?
    a. Choose the time and place carefully.
    b. Refuse to compromise.
    c. Listen attentively to what the other side has to say.
    d. Be willing to take responsibility for your role in the conflict.

14. For a conflict between two teens who are friends, the best peer mediator would be
    a. the parent of one of the teens.
    b. a teen who is friends with one of them.
    c. a teacher.
    d. a student who does not know either teen well.

Thinking Critically

After reading the question or statement, write a short answer using complete sentences.

15. Analyze. Compromise is not always a good way of resolving a conflict. In what type of situation is it unwise to compromise?

16. Evaluate. Is a compromise between two parties the ideal outcome of a negotiation? Why or why not?

17. Explain. Why is it important for mediators in a conflict to be neutral?

LESSON 3

Vocabulary Review

Choose the correct term in the sentences below.

18. *Violence/Assault* is the use of physical force to harm people or damage property.

19. The willful killing of one human being by another is called *homicide/rape.*

20. The term *sexual violence/sexual assault* refers to any form of unwelcome sexual contact directed at an individual.

Understanding Key Concepts

After reading the question or statement, select the correct answer.

21. Teens are *less* likely to be involved in violence if they
   a. have friends or family who are involved in crime.
   b. use alcohol or drugs.
   c. are committed to school.
   d. have an underprivileged background.

22. Which of the following accurately describes the term *youth gang*?
   a. Teens who hang out together
   b. A major drug ring run by young adults
   c. Two teens who have shoplifted
   d. Teens who commit acts of vandalism and assault as a group

23. In most cases of rape, the victim
   a. does not know the rapist.
   b. is female.
   c. is over 18 years old.
   d. reports the crime to the police.

Thinking Critically

After reading the question or statement, write a short answer using complete sentences.

24. Analyze. What are the possible consequences of retaliating for a violent act?

25. Explain. How can media violence influence behavior?

26. Evaluate. What is the advantage of reporting a sexual attack to the police right away, without bathing or showering first?

LESSON 4

Vocabulary Review

Choose the correct term in the sentences below.

27. *Physical abuse/Emotional abuse* is a pattern of intentionally causing bodily harm or injury to another person.

28. Repeatedly following, harassing, or threatening an individual is known as *verbal abuse/stalking.*

29. *Sexual abuse/Date rape* is a pattern of sexual contact that is forced upon a person against the person's will.

Understanding Key Concepts

After reading the question or statement, select the correct answer.

30. Trey insists that his girlfriend ask his permission before she goes out with her friends. He also calls to check up on her whenever she's out. His behavior is an example of
    a. physical abuse.
    b. emotional abuse.
    c. sexual abuse.
    d. stalking.

31. Which of the following behaviors can *reduce* your risk of date rape?
    a. Using alcohol or other drugs
    b. Being alone with a date you don't trust or know well
    c. Relying on your date for a ride home
    d. Going to a party with a group of friends

Thinking Critically

After reading the question or statement, write a short answer using complete sentences.

32. **Explain.** Why is verbal abuse considered a form of emotional abuse?

33. **Analyze.** How does knowing your sexual limits and communicating them clearly to the people you date protect you from abuse?

34. **Evaluate.** Why are some survivors of rape or abuse reluctant to seek counseling? What might convince them that counseling *can help*?

PROJECT-BASED ASSESSMENT

Recognizing the Warning Signs of Violence

BACKGROUND

Recognizing the warning signs of violence can prevent a situation from escalating and becoming violent. Knowing how to prevent a conflict from becoming violent can reduce the risk of injury.

TASK

Create a podcast or a short streaming video public service announcement (PSA) describing the warning signs of violence.

AUDIENCE

Students in grades 6–8

PURPOSE

Help students learn how to stay safe by recognizing the warning signs of violent behavior.

PROCEDURE

1. Conduct an online search for public service announcements on other subjects. Create a list of the characteristics that make these PSAs effective.
2. Review the information in Module 9 on conflicts and violence.
3. Write the script for a PSA podcast or video. Have it reviewed by your teacher or a school counselor.
4. Record or film your PSA.
5. Present your PSA to a middle school class.

Math Practice

Interpret Tables. A study surveyed teachers at schools that implemented a peer-mediation program. The table below lists some of the problems that teachers reported and the percentage decrease in incidents of those problems since the program began. Use the table to answer Questions 1–3.

Problem	Percentage decrease since implementing program
Expulsions	73%
Assaults	90.2%
Discipline referrals	57.7%

Adapted from *Safe and Drug-Free Schools Program Inventory*, 2002.

1. Which problem decreased the most since the peer-mediation program began?
   a. assaults
   b. conflict
   c. discipline referrals
   d. expulsions

2. If the number of assaults reported before the program began was 150 per year, about how many assaults per year occurred after the program began?
   a. 15
   b. 60
   c. 90
   d. 135

3. A student looking at this table concluded that since the peer-mediation program began, problems decreased by 220.9% (the sum of all three percentages). Why would you question his reasoning?
   a. The percentages do not add up to 100%.
   b. 220.9% is not the sum of all three percentages.
   c. The percentage decreases are not likely related to the peer-mediation program.
   d. There might be overlap in the percentages. For example, assault may lead to expulsion.

Reading/Writing Practice

Understand and Apply. Read the passage below and then answer the questions.

If you have a friend in an abusive relationship, you may be tempted to "rescue" her or him. You may try to persuade your friend to leave the relationship by criticizing the abuser. However, criticizing the abuser may simply make the victim less willing to confide in you.

Ask your friend how she or he feels. Express your concerns in a way that focuses on the abusive behavior rather than on the abuser. You might say, "I'm worried that you're getting hurt," rather than "That jerk doesn't deserve you." Let your friend know that she or he can always count on you for sympathy and support. That way, when your friend does feel ready to leave the relationship, she or he will be more likely to turn to you for help.

1. The purpose of this piece is
   a. to describe the consequences of abuse.
   b. to discuss ways to prevent abuse.
   c. to let teens know how to help a friend in an abusive relationship.
   d. to list sources of help for abused teens.

2. Which sentence should be added at the beginning of the second paragraph?
   a. Instead, the best approach is to listen without criticizing.
   b. The victim may deny the abuse.
   c. Abuse can destroy self-worth.
   d. Abuse is never acceptable.

3. Write a letter to a fictitious friend who is involved in an abusive relationship. Use the guidelines provided in this passage to offer sympathy and support.

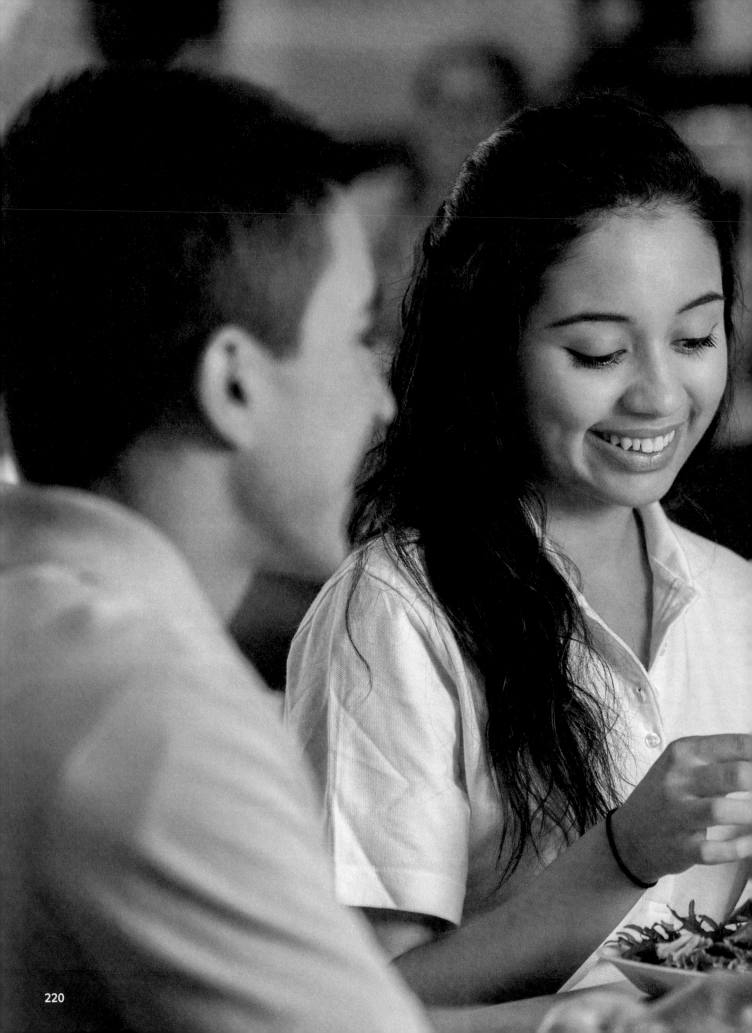

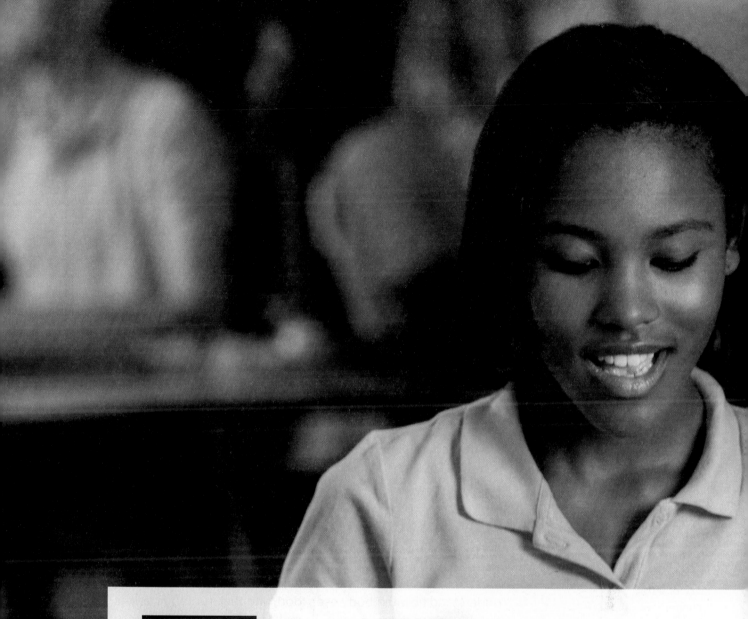

MODULE 10

Nutrition for Health

LESSONS

1 The Importance of Nutrition

2 Nutrients

3 Healthy Food Guidelines

4 Nutrition Labels and Food Safety

The Importance of Nutrition

Create a K-W-L Chart. Make a three-column chart. In the first column, list what you **k**now about nutrition. In the second column, list what you **w**ant to know about this topic. As you read, use the third column to summarize what you **l**earned.

K	W	L

Vocabulary

nutrition
nutrients
calorie
osteoporosis
hunger
appetite

Fitness Zone

I always thought that by skipping meals, I was cutting calories. Well, I was wrong. When you don't eat, your body responds by telling your brain that you might starve. That slows down your metabolism so you don't burn as many calories. It's much healthier to eat smaller and more frequent, healthy meals. That keeps your metabolism high and burns more calories.

BIG IDEA Learning to make healthful food choices will keep you healthy throughout your life.

REAL LIFE ISSUES

Schools can play a major role in the nutrition of teens. What influences students' food choices in your school cafeteria? Take a close look at the cafeteria environment. Are there brightly lit vending machines promoting unhealthful food choices? Are students required to wait in long lines to get their school lunch, leaving them with little time to eat? Environmental factors such as these may have a negative influence on food choices at school. *Write a paragraph describing why it's important for schools to offer students healthful food choices.*

After completing the lesson, review and analyze your response to the Real Life Issues question

Why Nutrition Matters

MAIN IDEA The food you eat affects your health and quality of life.

Most of us know what foods we enjoy eating. However, we may not understand how the body uses food, and that our food choices determine our overall health. To make healthful food choices, you must learn about **nutrition**, the process by which your body takes in and uses food.

Your body relies on food to provide it with **nutrients**, substances in food that your body needs to grow, to repair itself, and to supply you with energy. Energy is measured in **calories**. A calorie is a unit of heat used to measure the energy your body uses and the energy it receives from food. Foods that benefit your health provide fuel for physical activities. They help you stay mentally alert and keep you looking and feeling your best, too. The benefits of good nutrition affect more than your short-term energy and alertness. Good nutrition maintains your health throughout your lifetime. Choosing healthful foods can help you avoid diseases, such as type 2 diabetes, cardiovascular disease, stroke, certain cancers, and **osteoporosis**, which is a condition in which the bones become fragile and break easily.

What Influences Your Food Choices?

MAIN IDEA A variety of factors influence food choices.

Each time you make a food choice, something—perhaps many things—influences you to make that choice. Understanding your influences can help you make healthful choices.

Hunger and Appetite

People eat for two reasons: hunger and appetite. **Hunger** is the way your body signals that it needs fuel. When you are hungry, you may feel tired or weak. Your **appetite**, however, can increase your desire for food through your senses. For example, when you walk past a bakery and smell fresh-baked bread, you may suddenly feel like eating a piece of bread.

Sometimes, choosing foods based on your appetite is called **psychological** eating. Your body may not be hungry for the food. However, if you feel memories of a happy family dinner when that food was eaten, you may feel that eating the food again will bring back those feelings.

Reading Check

Explain In what ways do your eating habits affect your health?

ACADEMIC VOCABULARY

psychological *(adjective):* directed toward the mind

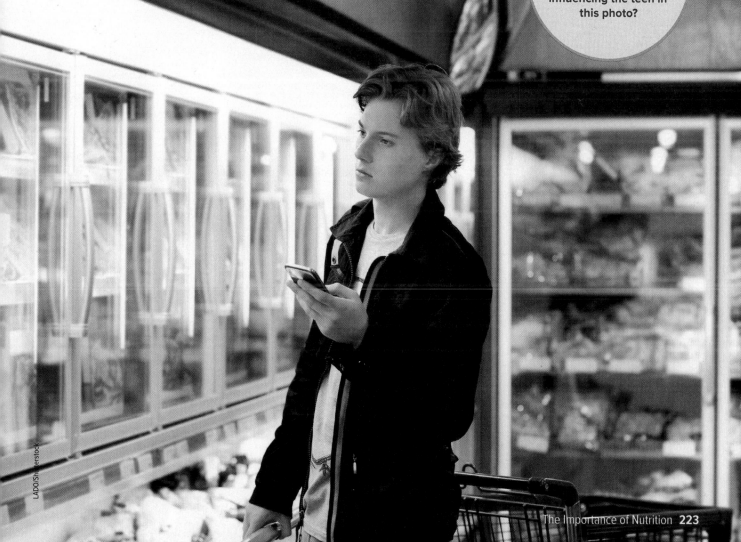

Several factors can influence your food choices.
What might be influencing the teen in this photo?

LADO/Shutterstock

Food and Emotions

At times, some people eat in response to an emotional need. For example, they may choose a particular food or type of food when they feel frustrated, stressed, lonely, or sad—or as a reward when they feel good. Other people may snack continuously while absorbed in another activity, such as watching television or playing games on a computer. This is called *mindless eating.* They may eat even if their body does not need food.

Food and Your Environment

The people and things around you also affect what you choose to eat. These are environmental influences.

- **Family and culture.** If your family eats most meals at home, this will influence where you prefer to eat. Your family's food choices may also influence your own. In many cases, a family's preferences are based on cultural influence.

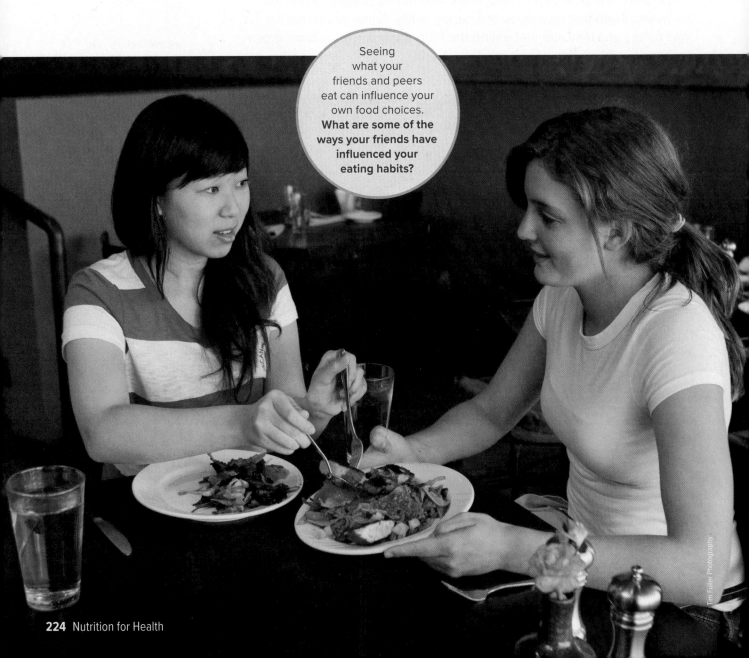

Seeing what your friends and peers eat can influence your own food choices. **What are some of the ways your friends have influenced your eating habits?**

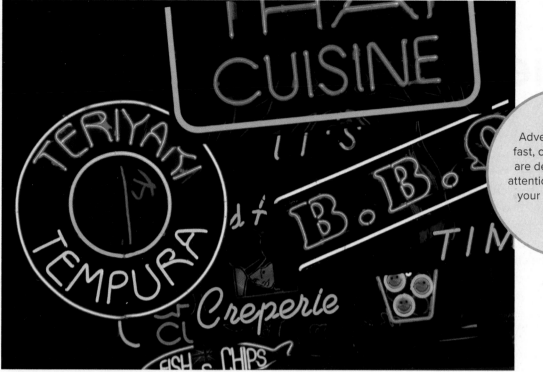

Advertisements for fast, convenient food are designed to grab attention and influence your choice in what you eat.

- **Friends.** If your friends always go out for pizza after school, you're more likely to eat pizza, too. Also, your friends may influence you to try new foods, including those from other cultures.

- **Time and money.** People with busy schedules may choose foods that are quick and easy to prepare, such as convenience foods and microwaveable meals. For other people and families, the cost of food may also be a factor. They may choose to eat expensive foods (such as steak) less frequently.

- **Advertising.** Advertisers try to influence your food choices. They hope that an ad for a juicy hamburger will send you running to visit the nearest fast food restaurant.

Reading Check

Make Inferences Why do advertisers want to influence your food choices?

Lesson 1 Review

Facts and Vocabulary

1. Name three health problems that good nutrition can help you avoid.

2. What is the difference between hunger and appetite?

3. Identify two emotions that influence eating when someone isn't hungry.

Thinking Critically

4. **Analyze.** How can advertising influence your food choices?

5. **Evaluate.** When Emily smells homemade chocolate-chip cookies she cannot resist them. What is influencing her behavior? Describe why you think the influence is healthy or unhealthy.

Applying Health Skills

6. **Stress Management.** Eating when you're not hungry can be a response to stress. List three healthier ways to respond to stress.

Writing Critically

7. **Descriptive.** Write an essay describing two ways in which your family or friends influence your food choices.

Nutrients

BEFORE YOU READ

Create a Cluster Chart. Draw a circle and label it "Nutrients." Draw circles around it and use these to define and describe this term. As you read, continue filling in the chart with more details.

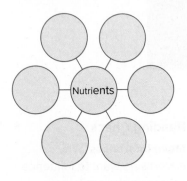

Vocabulary

carbohydrates
fiber
proteins
cholesterol
vitamins
minerals

BIG IDEA Each nutrient in your diet plays a unique and essential role in keeping you healthy.

REAL LIFE ISSUES

Too Much (Nutrition) Information. Lately, Judy has been getting a lot of advice on what to eat—and all of it is different. First her friend Heather told her you need lots of carbohydrates and little fat. Judy's friend, Rob, said eating certain combinations of foods is a good idea. Then Judy read a magazine article stating that eating too many carbohydrates will cause weight gain. Judy is confused by all the information. She's beginning to feel she should just eat whatever she likes. *Write a journal entry from Judy's point of view. Have her describe how she will figure out whether the health information she's getting is valid or not.*

After completing the lesson, review and analyze your response to the Real Life Issues question.

Giving Your Body What It Needs

MAIN IDEA Each of the six nutrients has a specific job or vital function to keep you healthy.

Everything you eat contains nutrients. Nutrients perform specific roles in maintaining your body functions. Your body uses nutrients in many ways:

- As an energy source
- To sustain growth
- To heal, and build and repair tissue
- To help transport oxygen to cells
- To regulate body functions

Six types of nutrients are found in foods. Three types—carbohydrates, proteins, and fats—provide energy. The other three types—vitamins, minerals, and water—perform a variety of other bodily functions. Eating foods that provide your body with a variety of nutrients helps to keep you healthy throughout your life.

Nutrients That Provide Energy

MAIN IDEA Carbohydrates, proteins, and fats provide energy and help maintain your body.

The energy in food comes from three sources: carbohydrates, proteins, and fats. Each gram of carbohydrate or protein provides four calories of energy. Each gram of fat provides nine calories. The body uses these nutrients to build, repair, and fuel itself.

Carbohydrates

Nutrition experts recommend getting from 45 to 65 percent of your daily calories from **carbohydrates**. The three types of carbohydrates are simple, complex, and fiber. Your body uses carbohydrates by breaking them down into their simplest forms. Most of the carbohydrates you consume are turned into a simple sugar called *glucose*.

Simple carbohydrates are sugars; in addition to glucose, these include fructose and lactose. They are the main source of fuel for your body. Fructose occurs naturally in fruits while lactose is found in milk. This type of sugar also occurs naturally in honey and maple syrup. Sugars are added to many processed foods, such as cold cereals, breads, and bakery products.

Complex carbohydrates, or starches, are long chains of sugars that are linked together. Common sources of complex carbohydrates include grains; grain products such as bread; and pasta, beans, and root vegetables.

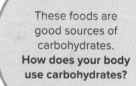

These foods are good sources of carbohydrates. **How does your body use carbohydrates?**

Fiber is the final type of carbohydrate. Fiber moves waste through your digestive system. Eating foods high in fiber can help you feel full, and may reduce the risk of cancer, heart disease, and type 2 diabetes. Although your body cannot digest fiber, it plays an important role by aiding digestion and reducing the risk of disease.

Experts recommend that teen girls ages 14 to 18 eat 26 grams of total fiber daily. Teen boys should eat 38 grams of total fiber. Good sources of fiber include fruits and vegetables, whole grains, and products made from whole grains, nuts, seeds, and legumes.

Proteins

Proteins are made up of chemicals called *amino acids.* Your body produces and uses 20 amino acids that are found in foods. About nine of the amino acids are called *essential amino acids* because the body must get them from food. The rest are known as *nonessential amino acids.*

Types of Proteins Many proteins are from animal sources, such as meat, eggs, and dairy products. These are sometimes called "complete" proteins because they contain all nine essential amino acids. Proteins from plant sources are usually missing one or more of the essential amino acids. People who follow vegetarian diets, however, get all the amino acids needed by eating a variety of plant-based foods that are rich in protein. These include grains, nuts, seeds, and legumes.

The Role of Proteins Protein is the basic building material of all your body cells. Muscles, bones, skin, and internal organs are all constructed of protein. It helps your body grow and will help your body maintain muscles, ligaments, tendons, and all body cells throughout your life.

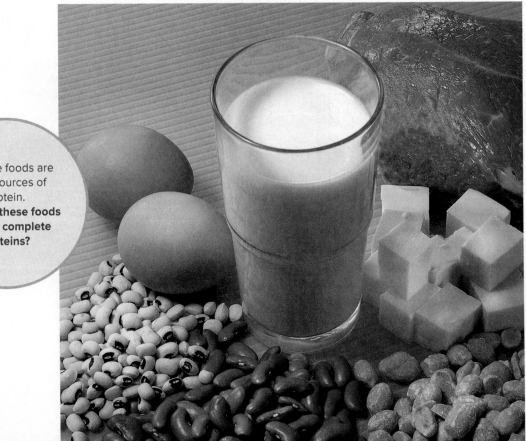

All these foods are good sources of protein. **Which of these foods provide complete proteins?**

Proteins also do a variety of other jobs in the body. For example, the protein hemoglobin in your red blood cells carries oxygen to all your body cells. Proteins may also function as hormones. These are chemicals that regulate the activities of your various body systems. Protein can be used as an energy source, although it does not supply your body with energy as quickly or easily as carbohydrates.

Teen boys between the ages of 14 to 18 should aim to consume about 52 grams of protein per day, and teen girls of the same age need 46 grams per day. Between 10 to 15 percent of your total daily calories should come from protein.

Fats

When you hear about fats in food, what advice comes into your mind? Chances are that you have heard that fats in foods can make you overweight. Does this mean you should avoid eating food with any fat in it? No. Your body needs a certain amount of fat to function properly. You can, however, choose healthier fats.

Types of Fats. Dietary fats are composed of fatty acids. Some of the fats that your body needs but cannot produce on its own are called *essential fatty acids.* All fat in foods is a combination of unsaturated and saturated fats. A third category of fats, trans fats, are formed through a process called *hydrogenation,* which causes vegetable oils to harden.

- **Unsaturated Fats.** When this type of fat is eaten in moderate amounts, it can lower your risk of heart disease. Vegetable oils, nuts, and seeds tend to contain larger amounts of unsaturated fats.

- **Saturated fats.** Consuming too many saturated fats may increase your risk of heart disease. Saturated fat is found mostly in animal-based foods such as meat and many dairy products. A few plant oils (palm, coconut, and palm kernel) also contain high amounts of saturated fat.

- **Trans Fats.** As trans fats harden, they become more saturated. Trans fats are found in stock margarine, snack foods, and packaged baked goods, such as cookies and crackers. Trans fats can raise your total blood cholesterol level, which can increase the risk for heart disease. As a result of the risks posed by trans fats, the USDA now requires that the amount of trans fats be listed on food nutrition labels. Additionally, some cities have passed laws limiting or eliminating the use of trans fats in foods prepared in restaurants.

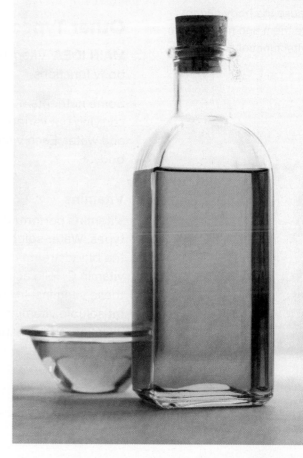

Olive oil is a good source of healthful, unsaturated fat. **Why are unsaturated fats better for your health than saturated fats?**

Reading Check

Cause and Effect What are the benefits of choosing snacks labeled "no trans fat"?

Myths & Reality

Think you know all there is to know about nutrition? This fact might change your mind.

Myth: All fats are bad for your health.

Reality: Saturated fats and trans fats are bad for your health, but unsaturated fats are essential to the diet because the body cannot make them and needs them for vital functions.

Health Issues of Fats

Your body needs a certain amount of fat to carry out its basic functions. Consuming too much fat, however, can be harmful. Because fatty foods are generally high in calories, consuming too much fatty foods can lead to unhealthful weight gain and obesity.

Fats provide a concentrated form of energy. The essential fatty acids are also important to brain development, blood clotting, and controlling inflammation. They also help maintain healthy skin and hair. Fats also absorb and transport fat-soluble vitamins (A, D, E, and K) through the bloodstream. The calories from fats that your body does not use are stored as body fat. Stored fat, known as *adipose tissue,* provides insulation for the body. However, carrying too much body fat increases the risk of health problems, such as type 2 diabetes and cardiovascular disease.

Additionally, consuming saturated fats can increase the levels of **cholesterol** in your blood. Cholesterol is needed to create cell walls, certain hormones, and vitamin D. However, excess cholesterol in your blood can build up inside your arteries. This raises your risk of heart disease. Like saturated fats, trans fats also promote the buildup of cholesterol in your arteries.

Teens should aim to consume less than 25 to 35 percent of their calories from fats. Choose healthful unsaturated fats. Limit your intake of saturated fats, including trans fats, to less than 10 percent of your total calories.

Other Types of Nutrients

MAIN IDEA Vitamins, minerals, and water perform a wide variety of body functions.

Some nutrients do not supply calories. Calories are still necessary for carrying out various body functions. These include vitamins, minerals, and water. Each vitamin and mineral performs a different job in the body.

Vitamins

Vitamins perform different functions in the body, and consist of two types. Water-soluble vitamins dissolve in water and pass easily into the bloodstream during digestion. The water-soluble vitamins include vitamin C, folic acid, and the B vitamins. Your body does not store these vitamins. In contrast, fat-soluble vitamins are stored in fat. The fat-soluble vitamins include A, D, E, and K. Your body stores these vitamins, and consuming large amounts of them can become harmful.

VITAMINS

> This table shows some types of fat-soluble and water-soluble vitamins.

Vitamin/Amount Needed Per Day by Teens Ages 14 to 18	Role in Body	Food Sources
Fat-Soluble Vitamins		
A Teen female: 700 mcg Teen male: 900 mcg	needed for night vision; stimulates production of white blood cells; regulates cell growth and division; helps repair bones and tissues; aids immunity; maintains healthy skin and mucous membranes	carrots, sweet potatoes, tomatoes, fortified cereals, leafy green vegetables, fish, liver, fortified dairy products, egg yolks
D (calciferol) Teen female: 15 mcg Teen male: 15 mcg	helps body use calcium and phosphorus (needed for building bones); aids immune function; helps regulate cell growth	fortified cereals and dairy products, fatty fish such as salmon and tuna Note: Your skin naturally produces vitamin D when exposed to sunlight
E Teen female: 15 mg Teen male: 15 mg	protects cells from damage; aids blood flow; helps repair body tissues	fish, milk, egg yolks, vegetable oils, fruits, nuts, peas, beans, broccoli, spinach, fortified cereals
K Teen female: 75 mcg Teen male: 75 mcg	essential for blood clotting, aids bone formation	green leafy vegetables, vegetable oils, cheese, broccoli, tomatoes
Water-Soluble Vitamins		
B1 (thiamine) Teen female: 1.0 mg Teen male: 1.2 mg	helps the body use carbohydrates for energy; promotes health of nervous system	enriched and whole-grain cereal products, lean pork, liver
B2 (riboflavin) Teen female: 1.0 mg Teen male: 1.3 mg	helps body process proteins and fats; maintains health of skin, nervous system, and digestive system	lean beef, pork, organ meats, legumes, eggs, cheese, milk, nuts, enriched grain products
B3 (niacin) Teen female: 14 mg Teen male: 16 mg	helps body process proteins and fats; maintains health of skin, nervous system, and digestive system	liver, poultry, fish, beef, peanuts, beans, enriched grain products
B6 Teen female: 1.2 mg Teen male: 1.3 mg	helps body use proteins and fats; supports immune and nervous systems; helps blood carry oxygen to body tissues; helps break down copper and iron; prevents one type of anemia; helps maintain normal blood sugar levels	organ meats, pork, beef, poultry, fish, eggs, peanuts, bananas, carrots, fortified cereals, whole grains
B12 (cobalamin) Teen female: 2.4 mcg Teen male: 2.4 mcg	maintains healthy nerve cells and red blood cells; needed for formation of genetic material in cells; prevents one type of anemia	liver, fish, poultry, clams, sardines, flounder, herring, eggs, milk, other dairy foods, fortified cereals
C (ascorbic acid) Teen female: 65 mg Teen male: 75 mg	protects against infection; promotes healthy bones, teeth, gums, and blood vessels; helps form connective tissue; helps heal wounds	citrus fruits and juices, berries, peppers, tomatoes, broccoli, spinach, potatoes
Folic acid (folate) Teen female: 400 mcg Teen male: 400 mcg	helps body form and maintain new cells; reduces risk of birth defects	dark green leafy vegetables, dry beans and peas, oranges, fortified cereals and other grain products

Minerals

Your body cannot produce **minerals**, and must get them from food. One mineral that is especially important to your health is calcium. It promotes bone health. Eating calcium-rich foods helps reduce the risk of developing osteoporosis. While osteoporosis is most common in women over the age of 50, teens can take action now to reduce the risk of osteoporosis later in life. Bone mass builds most rapidly between the ages of 10 and 20, reaching a peak around age 30. Eating calcium-rich foods as a teen can protect your health in the future.

Water

Water is in all of your body cells and is essential for most body functions. These include:

- moving food through the digestive system.
- digesting carbohydrates and protein, and aiding other chemical **reactions** in the body.
- transporting nutrients and removing wastes.
- storing and releasing heat.
- cooling the body through perspiration.
- cushioning the eyes, brain, and spinal cord.
- lubricating the joints.

ACADEMIC VOCABULARY

reaction *(noun)*: a response to a stimulus or influence

Water is essential for just about every function in your body. **When should you make sure to drink extra water?**

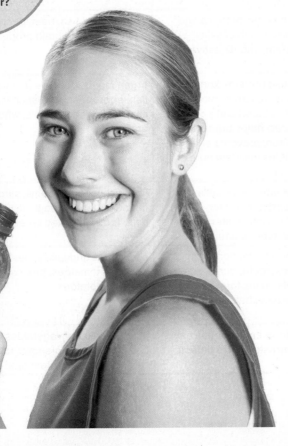

All foods contain water, so about 20 percent of your total daily water intake comes from food. The additional water the body needs can be obtained from drinking with meals and when you feel thirsty. Teen girls need about 9 cups of fluids a day, and teen boys need about 13 cups each day.

Active teens may need to drink more than the recommended amounts of water, because the body loses more water when sweating. Active teens should remember to drink water before, during, and after exercise. Remember to also drink extra fluids when the weather is hot to prevent dehydration. Also, drinks that contain caffeine, such as coffee, tea, and some soft drinks, cause your body to lose fluids. Drinking these fluids can cause your body to become dehydrated.

Paul Bradbury/age footstock

MINERALS

This table shows some types of minerals, their role in the body, and sources.

Mineral/Amount Needed Per Day by Teens Ages 14 to 18	Role in Body	Food Sources
Calcium Teen female: 1,300 mg Teen male: 1,300 mg	forms bones and teeth; aids blood clotting; assists muscle and nerve function; reduces risk of osteoporosis	dairy products, calcium-fortified juice, calcium-fortified soy milk and tofu, corn tortillas, Chinese cabbage, broccoli, kale
Phosphorus Teen female: 1,250 mg Teen male: 1,250 mg	produces energy; maintains healthy bones	dairy products, peas, meat, eggs, some cereals and breads
Magnesium Teen female: 360 mg Teen male: 410 mg	maintains normal muscle and nerve function; sustains regular heartbeat; aids in bone growth and energy production	meat, milk, green leafy vegetables, whole grains, nuts
Iron Teen female: 15 mg Teen male: 11 mg	part of a compound in the red blood cells needed for carrying oxygen; aids in energy use; supports immune system	meat, poultry, beans, fortified grain products

Reading Check

Explain What is the difference between water- and fat-soluble vitamins?

Lesson 2 Review

Facts and Vocabulary

1. Which nutrients can your body use as sources of energy?

2. What are essential amino acids? From what source do you obtain essential amino acids?

3. How does eating calcium-rich foods as a teen protect your lifelong health?

Thinking Critically

4. **Analyze.** How might saturated fats and trans fats cause illnesses later in life, like heart disease?

5. **Synthesize.** What are the health benefits of eating a variety of fruits and vegetables?

Applying Health Skills

6. **Goal Setting.** Examine your school's weekly lunch menu. List the most healthful food choices available each day. Then use the steps for goal setting to create a healthy eating plan.

Writing Critically

7. **Narrative.** Write a story from the point of view of a nutrient. Have the nutrient describe itself, what it does in the body, and why it is important for health.

Healthy Food Guidelines

BEFORE YOU READ

Create an Outline. Preview this lesson by scanning the pages. Organize the headings and subheadings into an outline. As you read, fill in your outline with important details.

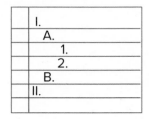

Vocabulary

Dietary Guidelines for Americans
MyPlate
nutrient-dense
food desert

· · · · · · · · · · · · ·

BIG IDEA MyPlate is a tool that can help you choose healthful foods for all your meals and snacks.

REAL LIFE ISSUES

No Time for Breakfast. Ever since she started high school, Tina never seems to have enough time for breakfast. Homework keeps her up late, so when she wakes up the next morning, she barely has time to get dressed and catch the bus. Most mornings in class, she feels weak and sluggish, and by lunchtime she's ravenous. Tina wants to find the time to eat breakfast so she has more energy throughout the day. ***Pretend you are Tina. In a paragraph, write out a plan to fit breakfast into your busy schedule.***

After completing the lesson, review and analyze your response to the Real Life Issues question.

Guidelines for Eating Right and Active Living

MAIN IDEA MyPlate helps you apply what you know about nutrients to choose healthful foods.

The **Dietary Guidelines for Americans** are a set of recommendations about smart eating and physical activity for all Americans. They are published by the U.S. Department of Agriculture (USDA) and the Department of Health and Human Services (HHS). They provide science-based advice for healthful eating. The guidelines also provide information on the importance of active living. This advice can be summed up in three key guidelines:

- Make smart choices from every food group.

- Find your balance between food and activity.

- Get the most nutrition out of your calories.

Making Smart Choices

Choosing a variety of foods from each food group will provide all the nutrients your body needs. The five food groups are: grains, vegetables, fruits, milk, and proteins. Each day, you should aim to eat foods from each of the groups. The quantity of food from each group is determined by your gender, activity level, and age. The USDA offers online tools that can help you learn what quantity of food from each group is right for you. Additionally, the USDA offers another tool called **MyPlate**, an interactive guide to healthful eating and active living. This tool helps you put the Dietary Guidelines into action.

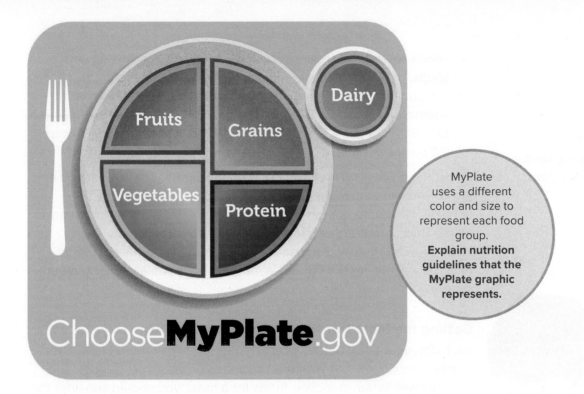

MyPlate uses a different color and size to represent each food group. **Explain nutrition guidelines that the MyPlate graphic represents.**

The MyPlate graphic shows a dinner plate covered with four differently colored triangles. A blue circle to the right side of the plate represents a glass of milk or other dairy product. On the plate, each of the triangles is a different size and is labeled. The size of the triangle represents a proportion. For example, on the plate, you will see that the vegetables portion of the plate is larger than protein. This means that you should eat more vegetables than protein.

The MyPlate website contains tools that provide more information on each of the food groups, as well as other tools. Some of these tools will show you how to develop a personalized eating plan, create a healthy menu, and even to analyze your current diet.

Your Best Choices

Within each food group, some choices are better than others. The Dietary Guidelines offers three tips for choosing the most healthful foods from each food group:

- **Balance Calories.** When choosing foods, think about your total calorie intake for the day. It's important to enjoy your food, but to eat less of those foods that may not be as healthful. One way to do this is to avoid choosing oversized portions. Many times, a couple of bites of a food you enjoy are enough to satisfy your appetite for that food.

- **Foods to Increase.** When planning your meals, aim to fill half of your plate with vegetables and fruit. Eating these foods will help fill you up and reduce the amount of high-fat and high-sodium foods. Also, when choosing grain products, choose whole grains. Whole grains are high in fiber, which helps aid digestion and reduces the risk of disease. Finally, when choosing dairy products, select products that are fat-free or low in fat.

• **Foods to Reduce.** Processed foods, such as frozen meals and soups, tend to be high in sodium. When buying these foods, choose low-sodium items. Choosing water over sugary soft drinks is another good choice. Even low-calorie soft drinks have been linked to health problems. Teens should aim to drink about 2 liters of water (1.8 quarts) per day.

Physical activity is an important part of staying healthy. Even if you eat the correct amount and mix of healthful foods, you might still be unhealthy if you do not get enough physical activity. When planning meals, think about the amount and type of physical activity you will do each day. The Dietary Guidelines recommend that teens should be physically active for 60 minutes almost every day to avoid unhealthful weight gain.

Getting the Most Nutrition Out of Your Calories

Each day, your body needs a certain number of calories as fuel. The number of calories that you need depends on your age, gender, and activity level. When selecting foods for a meal, you should consider the nutrients that foods provide as well as the total calorie count. For example, for lunch you might see a tempting picture outside a restaurant of a person enjoying a fast food meal, and you may decide that you want the same meal. If you do choose that meal, it's likely that you will meet your calorie needs. However, you may not obtain the variety of nutrients that your body needs. To make sure you get enough nutrients from foods, choose **nutrient-dense** foods. These foods have a high ratio of nutrients to calories.

Nutrient-dense foods such as carrots may provide the same number of calories as foods that are not nutrient dense, such as potato chips. By making it a habit to eat more foods such as carrots and fewer potato chips or fast foods, you will get more nutrients out of the same number of calories. At times, eating foods that are high in calories and low in nutrients can be part of a healthy eating plan. Choose to eat a smaller portion of these foods. If your overall diet is nutrient dense, your eating plan can include an occasional treat.

The Dietary Guidelines recommend choosing a variety of fruits and vegetables every day. **What fruits or vegetables would you choose for an afternoon snack?**

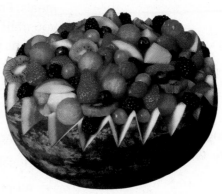
Healthful Eating Patterns

MAIN IDEA Use MyPlate and the Dietary Guidelines to plan all your meals and snacks.

It's Monday morning and you have overslept. You have 20 minutes to get ready before you need to leave for school. Try using MyPlate as a tool to help you plan healthful meals. The plate can help you **visualize** how a healthful meal might look. When you're hurried, it's tempting to skip breakfast. However, you may pay the price later when you feel weak and hungry in the middle of a class. After eight hours of sleep, your body needs to refuel. If you force it to keep going, you will likely run short on energy.

Eating breakfast has many benefits. Children and teens who eat breakfast typically get better grades, are less distracted in school, and are less likely to become overweight. Fitting breakfast into your schedule may take a little planning, but it's worth the time. You can prepare the night before in several ways. For example, you can set the table before you go to bed. When you wake up, all you have to do is fill your cereal bowl or put bread in the toaster. Other ideas for quick and easy breakfasts are making instant oatmeal or grits, hard-cooked eggs (which can be cooked the day before), or toasting a whole-grain muffin.

If you simply don't care for traditional breakfast foods, there are plenty of choices. Try toasting a whole-grain bagel, or have toast with peanut butter or melted cheese. A breakfast burrito (eggs, cheese, and salsa rolled in a tortilla) can also be a quick and healthful alternative. Another healthy choice may be to reheat last night's leftover spaghetti for breakfast.

ACADEMIC VOCABULARY

visualize *(verb)*: to form a mental image of

Reading Check

Analyze List ways that the plate diagram and MyPlate guidelines are consistent.

Burke/Triolo Productions/Brand X Pictures/Getty Images

Sensible Snacks

Healthful snacks can give you energy to keep you going between meals. Enjoying a sensible snack after school, for instance, can keep you from coming to the dinner table so hungry that you eat twice as much as you should. There are plenty of healthful foods that you can easily enjoy when you need a snack:

- Fresh fruit
- Cut-up vegetables, such as celery or carrot sticks
- String cheese
- Unsalted nuts
- Air-popped popcorn
- Fat-free yogurt

Reading Check

Identify What is a *food desert*?

Access to Healthy Foods

In order to eat a healthful diet, families need access to stores that sell healthful foods. This can be difficult in communities with no grocery stores. These areas are referred to as **food deserts**. These are areas where it is difficult to buy affordable or high-quality foods. In food deserts, families shop at convenience stores. In general, prices are higher and the food quality is lower at convenience stores.

A 2012 study reported by the National Institutes of Health shows that low-income communities have fewer grocery stores. These communities have more convenience stores and fast-food restaurants. This lack of access to healthy foods affects the people who live in the area. They must travel farther to purchase healthy foods. They also pay more for foods at convenience stores, and eat more often at fast-food restaurants.

Living in a food desert can cause health issues, such as obesity and diabetes. One objective of Health People 2020 addresses this problem. Meeting the objective will increase access to food retailers offering foods that are encouraged by the Dietary Guidelines for Americans. The Federal Government also works to improve people's health by making healthy foods available through government programs.

Many different foods can be part of a healthful breakfast. **Name three nontraditional breakfast foods that you might like to try.**

Eating Right When Eating Out

While it's tempting to enjoy a treat when eating out, making healthful food choices is just as important when you eat away from home. By reading the menu carefully and asking your server questions, you can find the most healthful, nutrient-dense items available. Here are a few tips to keep in mind:

- Watch portion sizes. Restaurant meals have grown larger over the years. If you think the serving size is more than you need, try splitting the meal with a friend or wrapping up the leftovers to take home.

- Pay attention to how foods are prepared. Fried foods are likely to be high in fat. Grilled, baked, and broiled foods are more healthful choices.

- Add fresh vegetables and fruit. The salad bar can be a health-conscious eater's best friend. If the restaurant doesn't have one, order a salad off the menu or ask the server to provide extra lettuce and tomato for your sandwich.

- Go easy on toppings. High-fat sauces, mayonnaise, butter, and sour cream add fat and calories. Make your meal healthier by asking the server to leave these out or serve them on the side.

- Avoid drinks with high calories. Choose water instead of soft drinks to satisfy your thirst without adding extra calories to your meal.

Character Check

Citizenship means doing what you can to improve your community. For example, there may be people in your community who go to sleep hungry every night. You can help by learning how to organize an effort to collect nonperishable food items for a local food bank or homeless shelter.

Lesson 3 Review

Facts and Vocabulary

1. List the five basic food groups.

2. Identify the kinds of foods that are best to avoid or limit.

3. List two examples of nutrient-dense foods.

Thinking Critically

4. **Analyze.** The Dietary Guidelines recommend regular physical activity. Why is this recommendation made?

5. **Synthesize.** Josh ate a cheeseburger, fries, and a soda for lunch. List the foods he could choose for dinner to balance out his lunch.

Applying Health Skills

6. **Accessing Information.** Search for information from credible sources that provide meal planning based on MyPlate.

Writing Critically

7. **Expository.** Write a description of a meal you had recently. Discuss what foods or cooking methods made this meal healthful or unhealthful.

Nutrition Labels and Food Safety

BEFORE YOU READ

Organize Information. Fold a sheet of paper into quarters. Unfold it and label the four sections "Clean," "Separate," "Cook," and "Chill." As you read, fill in the sections with tips about the four steps in food safety.

Clean	Separate
Cook	Chill

Vocabulary

food additive
foodborne illness
pasteurization
cross-contamination
food allergy
food intolerance

BIG IDEA By reading food labels and handling foods safely, you can avoid many food-related health problems.

REAL LIFE ISSUES

Food Allergies. Alex is allergic to nuts. If he eats anything that contains nuts, his face swells up and he has to be taken to the hospital. He's learned to read food labels carefully to make sure nothing he eats has nuts in it. His friend Lauren has invited him to her house for dinner with her family. He'd like to say yes, but he knows that if anything they serve has nuts in it, he could be in serious trouble. *Write a paragraph explaining how you would handle this situation. How can Alex protect his safety and his friend's feelings at the same time?*

After completing the lesson, review and analyze your response to the Real Life Issues question.

Nutrition Label Basics

MAIN IDEA Food labels provide information about the ingredients and nutritional value of foods.

Each package of food you buy carries a printed label that provides information about the nutritional value of what's inside. The food label also lists all of the ingredients that were used to prepare the food. Among other things, the food label lists:

- the name of the food product.
- the amount of food in the package.
- the name and address of the company that makes, packages, or distributes the product.
- the ingredients in the food.
- the Nutrition Facts panel, which provides information about the nutrients found in the food.

Ingredient List

The ingredients in a food appear on the label in descending order by weight. So, the ingredient that makes up the largest share of the weight listed first, followed by the ingredient that makes up the next largest share, and so on. However, food labels that list several similar ingredients can be misleading. For example, a product that contains three kinds of sweeteners would list each one separately: high-fructose corn syrup, corn syrup, sugar. All three sweeteners will be listed separately and will appear farther down on the list. However, if you add all three together, you might learn that the main ingredient in the food is added sugars.

Food Additives. Some foods contain food additives which are substances added to a food to produce a desired effect. These are used to keep a food safe for a longer period of time, to boost nutrient content, or to improve taste, texture, or appearance. Two food additives that might cause concern are aspartame, a sugar substitute, and olestra, a fat substitute. Many diet soft drinks are sweetened with aspartame. Some potato chips are made with olestra, which passes through the body undigested. Because olestra is not absorbed, some people experience gastrointestinal problems when eating it.

Nutrition Facts

The Nutrition Facts panel provides information about the nutrients found in food. Along with information about specific nutrients, food labels make other types of claims about nutritional value. Federal law provides uniform definitions for the following terms:

- **Free.** The food contains none, or an insignificant amount, of a given component: fat, sugar, saturated fat, trans fat, cholesterol, sodium, or calories. For instance, foods labeled as being *calorie-free* must have fewer than five calories per serving.

- **Low.** You can eat this food regularly without exceeding your daily limits for fat, saturated fat, cholesterol, sodium, or calories. Low-fat foods, for instance, must have 3 grams or less of fat per serving.

- **Light.** A food labeled as *light* must contain one-third fewer calories, one-half the fat, or one-half the sodium of the original version. On some packages, *light* may refer only to the color of the food, such as light brown sugar.

Reading Check

Explain Why are additives used in foods?

- **Reduced.** The food contains 25 percent fewer calories, or 25 percent less of a given nutrient, than the original version. This term may also be worded as *less* or *fewer*. Foods labeled as *reduced* may offer a much healthier option than the original version. However, the reduced version of a high-calorie food may still contain a high number of calories.

- **High.** The food provides at least 20 percent of the daily value for a vitamin, mineral, protein, or fiber. Synonyms for this term include *rich in* and *excellent source of*.

- **Good source of.** The food provides 10 to 19 percent of the daily value for a vitamin, mineral, protein, or fiber. Synonyms for this term include *contains* and *provides*.

- **Healthy.** Foods described as healthy must be low in fat and saturated fat and contain limited amounts of cholesterol and sodium. They must also provide at least 10 percent of the daily value for vitamin A, vitamin C, iron, calcium, protein, or fiber.

The Nutrition Facts panel gives information about the nutrients found in a food. **Why do consumers need this information?**

Dual Columns, Two Forms of the Same Food

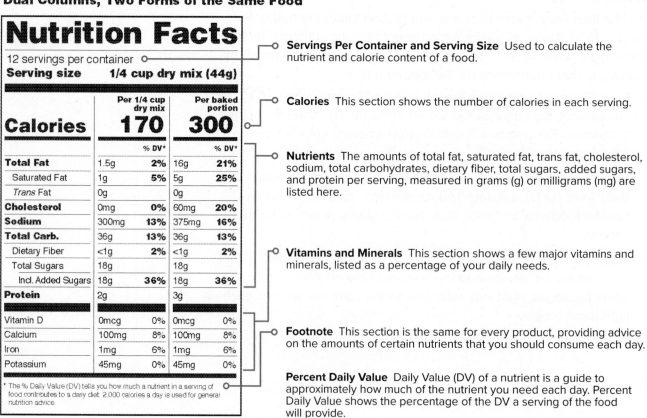

Nutrition Facts

12 servings per container
Serving size   **1/4 cup dry mix (44g)**

	Per 1/4 cup dry mix		Per baked portion	
Calories	**170**		**300**	
		% DV*		% DV*
Total Fat	1.5g	**2%**	16g	**21%**
Saturated Fat	1g	**5%**	5g	**25%**
Trans Fat	0g		0g	
Cholesterol	0mg	**0%**	60mg	**20%**
Sodium	300mg	**13%**	375mg	**16%**
Total Carb.	36g	**13%**	36g	**13%**
Dietary Fiber	<1g	**2%**	<1g	**2%**
Total Sugars	18g		18g	
Incl. Added Sugars	18g	**36%**	18g	**36%**
Protein	2g		3g	
Vitamin D	0mcg	0%	0mcg	0%
Calcium	100mg	8%	100mg	8%
Iron	1mg	6%	1mg	6%
Potassium	45mg	0%	45mg	0%

* The % Daily Value (DV) tells you how much a nutrient in a serving of food contributes to a daily diet. 2,000 calories a day is used for general nutrition advice.

Servings Per Container and Serving Size Used to calculate the nutrient and calorie content of a food.

Calories This section shows the number of calories in each serving.

Nutrients The amounts of total fat, saturated fat, trans fat, cholesterol, sodium, total carbohydrates, dietary fiber, total sugars, added sugars, and protein per serving, measured in grams (g) or milligrams (mg) are listed here.

Vitamins and Minerals This section shows a few major vitamins and minerals, listed as a percentage of your daily needs.

Footnote This section is the same for every product, providing advice on the amounts of certain nutrients that you should consume each day.

Percent Daily Value Daily Value (DV) of a nutrient is a guide to approximately how much of the nutrient you need each day. Percent Daily Value shows the percentage of the DV a serving of the food will provide.

Organic Food Labels

In addition to nutrition claims, another notation on food labels is "USDA Organic." Foods labeled as organic are produced without the use of certain agricultural chemicals, such as synthetic fertilizers or pesticides. These foods also cannot contain genetically modified ingredients or be subjected to certain types of radiation. The USDA Organic label makes no claims, however, that organic foods are safer or more nutritious than conventionally grown foods.

Open Dating

Many food products have *open dates* on their labels. These dates help you determine how long the food will remain fresh. Several types of open dates exist:

- **Sell by date.** This date shows the last day on which a store should sell a product. After this date, the freshness of a food is not guaranteed.

- **Use by or expiration date.** These dates show the last day on which a product's quality can be guaranteed. For a short time, most foods are still safe to eat after this date.

- **Freshness date.** A freshness date appears on **items** that will not last long on the shelves, such as baked goods. The freshness date shows the last date on which a product is considered fresh.

- **Pack date.** A pack date shows the day on which a food was processed or packaged. The pack date does not give the consumer an indication of the product's freshness.

ACADEMIC VOCABULARY

item *(noun):* an object of concern or interest

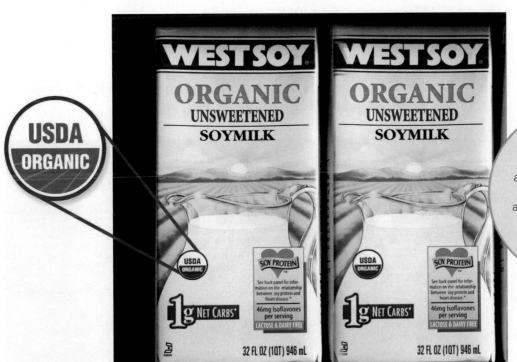

Foods bearing the USDA Organic label are produced without the use of certain agricultural chemicals. **Why might some consumers prefer these foods?**

(l)©USDA, (r)Andrew Resek/McGraw-Hill Education

Food Safety

MAIN IDEA Handling food carefully can help you avoid foodborne illnesses and other hazards.

Have you ever seen a sign in a restaurant restroom reminding employees to wash their hands before returning to work? Requiring restaurant workers, and guests, to wash their hands before leaving the restroom helps prevent the spread of pathogens that can cause illness. It is one strategy for preventing **foodborne illness**, or food poisoning. Each year, about 76 million Americans become ill as a result of foodborne illnesses.

How Foodborne Illness Occurs

Bacteria and viruses cause most cases of foodborne illness. The most common sources are the bacteria *Campylobacter*, *Salmonella*, *E. coli*, and a group of viruses known as the *Norwalk* and *Norwalk-like viruses*.

Some pathogens are naturally present in healthy animals. *Salmonella* bacteria can infect hens and enter their eggs. Shellfish may pick up bacteria that are naturally present in seawater. Fresh fruits and vegetables may become contaminated if they are washed with water that contains traces of human or animal wastes. Finally, infected humans who handle food can spread pathogens from their own skin to the food or from one food to another.

Some common symptoms of foodborne illness are cramps, diarrhea, nausea, vomiting, and fever. In most cases people recover from foodborne illness within a few days. Occasionally, symptoms may be severe and may lead to dehydration. Fluids lost through vomiting and diarrhea can result in dehydration. If the following symptoms are present, consult a doctor:

- A fever higher than 101.5 degrees F

- Prolonged vomiting or diarrhea

- Blood in the stool

- Signs of dehydration, including a decrease in urination, dry mouth and throat, and feeling dizzy when standing.

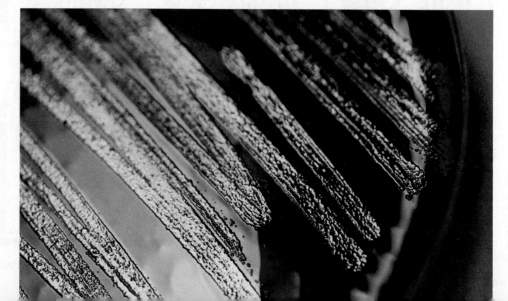

Keeping Food Safe to Eat

Everyone involved in delivering food to people in the United States takes steps to prevent pathogens from entering the food supply. One important process is **pasteurization** of milk and juices. Pasteurization is treating a substance with heat to kill or slow the growth of pathogens. This helps prevent *E. coli* infection. The Dietary Guidelines outline four steps—clean, separate, cook, and chill—to keep foods safe.

Clean. Wash and dry your hands for at least 20 seconds using soap and warm water before handling foods, and frequently while handling foods. Also remember to wash your hands after using the bathroom or touching a pet.

Avoid **cross-contamination**, which is the spreading of pathogens from one food to another, by cleaning utensils and surfaces carefully. Wash cutting boards, dishes, utensils, and countertops with hot, soapy water after you finish preparing each food item. Wash the food itself. Rinse fresh fruits and vegetables under running water, and rub the surfaces of firm-skinned fruits and vegetables.

Separate. The foods most likely to carry pathogens are raw meat, poultry, seafood, and eggs. To avoid cross-contamination, separate these from other foods. Store them separately when shopping and at home. Use separate cutting boards when preparing raw meat, poultry and fish. Transfer cooked food on a clean platter rather than using the same platter that held the raw food.

Cook. Heating food to a high enough temperature will kill the pathogens that cause foodborne illness. To determine whether meat, poultry, and egg dishes are cooked thoroughly, use a food thermometer to measure the internal temperature (the temperature at the center of the food).

Reading Check

Explain Why is it best to always use warm water and soap when washing your hands?

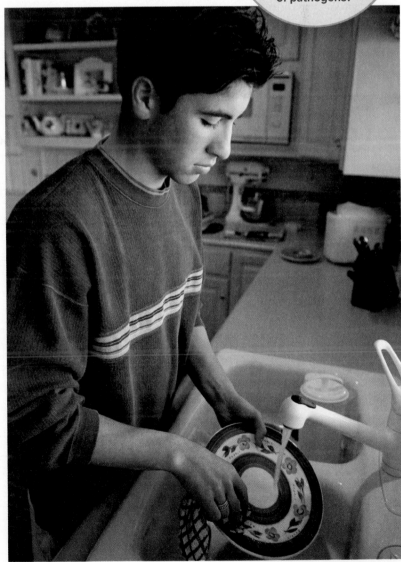

Washing hands, produce, utensils, and surfaces carefully is the first step in preventing foodborne illness.
How does this step prevent the spread of pathogens?

Photodisc/Alamy Stock Photo

Chill. Refrigeration slows the growth of harmful bacteria. Refrigerate or freeze meat, poultry, and other perishable foods as soon as you bring them home from the store. Avoid overpacking the refrigerator. This is important because circulating air will help keep the food cool. Divide large amounts of food into small, shallow containers to help it cool more quickly.

Frozen foods should be thawed safely before cooking. Thaw frozen foods in the refrigerator, in a microwave, or under cold running water. Discard any food that has been sitting out at room temperature for two hours or longer—one hour when the temperature is above 90 degrees F.

The top of this thermometer shows safe temperatures for cooking food, while the bottom shows safe temperatures for storing food. **Why is the area in the middle called the danger zone?**

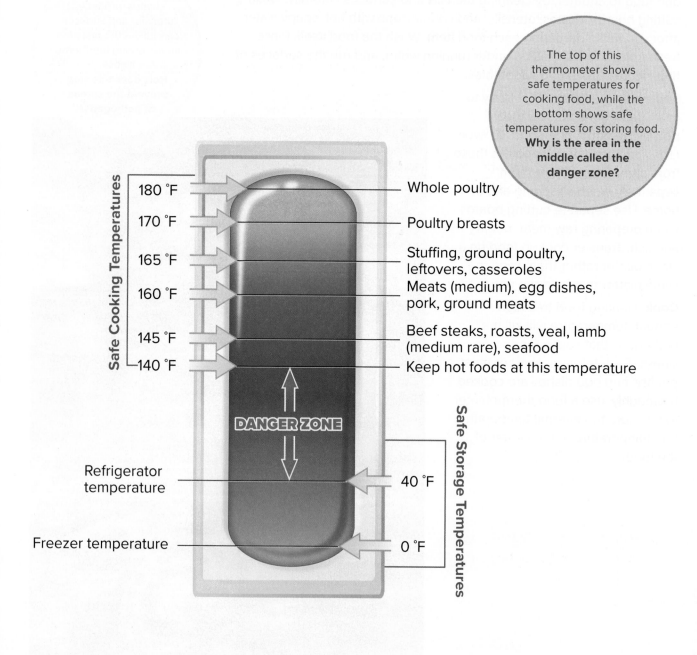

Safe Cooking Temperatures

- 180 °F — Whole poultry
- 170 °F — Poultry breasts
- 165 °F — Stuffing, ground poultry, leftovers, casseroles
- 160 °F — Meats (medium), egg dishes, pork, ground meats
- 145 °F — Beef steaks, roasts, veal, lamb (medium rare), seafood
- 140 °F — Keep hot foods at this temperature

DANGER ZONE

Refrigerator temperature — 40 °F
Freezer temperature — 0 °F

Safe Storage Temperatures

Food Sensitivities

While preventing pathogens from getting into food is important for the health of everyone who eats the food, some foods may only affect certain people. Food sensitivities fall into two groups: **food allergies**, which are a condition in which the body's immune system reacts to substances in some foods, and **food intolerances** which are a negative or dangerous reaction to some foods that doesn't involve the immune system. The most common allergens are found in milk, eggs, peanuts, tree nuts, soybeans, wheat, fish, and shellfish. Food labels are required to tell whether a food product contains any of these ingredients or any protein derived from them.

The symptoms of food allergies vary from mild to life threatening. Some people experience skin irritations, such as rashes, hives, or itching. Others develop gastrointestinal symptoms such as nausea, vomiting, or diarrhea. The most dangerous allergic reaction is anaphylaxis. This is a condition in which the throat swells up and the heart has difficulty pumping. Anaphylaxis can be life threatening and requires immediate medical attention.

A food intolerance is more common than a food allergy. One of the most common is lactose intolerance. This occurs when a person's body does not produce enough of the enzyme needed to digest lactose, a sugar found in milk. People who are lactose intolerant may experience gas, bloating, and abdominal pain.

Reading Check

Compare and Contrast What is the difference between a food allergy and a food intolerance?

Fitness Zone

After we learned to read food labels in health class, I started checking the label on everything I eat. I'm doing it as a part of my overall fitness plan. I was surprised to see that fruit juice is high in calories. It's better to drink water or eat a piece of fruit.

Lesson 4 Review

Facts and Vocabulary

1. Explain what the term light means when used on a food label.

2. Explain the difference between a sell by date and a use by date.

3. Identify another term that refers to foodborne illness.

Thinking Critically

4. **Evaluate.** An instant soup is very low in fat and calories but high in sodium. Can this food be labeled "healthy"? Explain why or why not.

5. **Synthesize.** What are the possible consequences of undercooked eggs?

Applying Health Skills

6. **Practicing Healthful Behaviors.** Summarize the steps for preventing foodborne illnesses. Post the steps in your kitchen as a reminder of food safety.

Writing Critically

7. **Persuasive.** Write an essay that convinces others of the importance of food safety.

Vocabulary Review

Use the correct vocabulary term to complete the following statements.

1. The process by which your body takes in and uses food is called _____.

2. Your body relies on food to provide it with the _____ it needs to grow, to repair itself, and to supply you with energy.

3. A _____ is a unit of heat used to measure the energy your body uses and the energy it receives from food.

Understanding Key Concepts

After reading the question or statement, select the correct answer.

4. Which of the following is not a way that choosing healthful foods affects your total health and wellness?
   a. It gives your body the nutrients it needs for growth and development.
   b. It helps you avoid unhealthful weight gain.
   c. It provides fuel for sports and other activities.
   d. It ensures that you will never get sick.

5. Preferring certain foods because you've grown up eating them is an example of the influence of
   a. family.
   b. friends.
   c. money.
   d. advertising.

Thinking Critically

After reading the question or statement, write a short answer using complete sentences.

6. **Analyze.** Why is emotional eating harmful?

7. **Synthesize.** How might the food choices of a high-powered business executive with a busy schedule differ from those of a part-time worker?

8. **Discuss.** Give an example of a way in which a person's cultural background could influence that person's food choices.

Vocabulary Review

Choose the correct word in the sentences below.

9. Your body's main source of energy is *carbohydrates/proteins*.

10. Consuming saturated fats and trans fats can increase the levels of *fiber/cholesterol* in your blood.

11. *Vitamins/minerals* are elements found in food that are used by the body.

Understanding Key Concepts

After reading the question or statement, select the correct answer.

12. Which of the following is not one of the six basic nutrients?
    a. Carbohydrates
    b. Fiber
    c. Protein
    d. Vitamins

13. Your body uses carbohydrates by breaking them down into
    a. sugars.   c. fatty acids.
    b. amino acids.   d. water.

14. About what percentage of your daily calories should come from fat?
    a. 10 to 15 percent
    b. Less than 25 to 35 percent
    c. At least 30 percent
    d. 50 to 65 percent

Thinking Critically

After reading the question or statement, write a short answer using complete sentences.

15. Describe. How does fiber benefit your body?

16. Explain. Why is it dangerous to consume too much of a fat-soluble vitamin?

17. Explain. Why does your body need more water when you are very active?

LESSON 3

Vocabulary Review

Use the correct vocabulary term to complete the following statements.

18. The _____ contain recommendations about smart eating and physical activity for all healthy Americans.

19. An interactive guide to healthy eating and active living is the _____.

20. Foods that are _____ have a high ratio of nutrients to calories.

Understanding Key Concepts

After reading the question or statement, select the correct answer.

21. Which food group triangle in MyPlate is largest?
   a. Grains
   b. Fruits
   c. Vegetables
   d. Proteins

22. The Dietary Guidelines recommend that teens be physically active for
   a. 20 minutes, three or more times a week.
   b. 30 minutes a day.
   c. 50 minutes, five or more times a week.
   d. 60 minutes a day.

23. Which method of preparation tends to make food high in fat?
   a. Baking
   b. Broiling
   c. Frying
   d. Grilling

Thinking Critically

After reading the question or statement, write a short answer using complete sentences.

24. Explain. How can people who don't eat dairy products get enough calcium every day?

25. Analyze. Why is it important to include nutrient-dense foods in your daily eating?

26. Identify. Give two examples of healthful snacks.

LESSON 4

Vocabulary Review

Correct the sentences below by replacing the italicized term with the correct vocabulary term.

27. *Ingredients* may be used to keep a food fresh longer, to boost its nutrient content, or to improve its taste, texture, or appearance.

28. *Boiling* means treating a substance with heat to kill or slow the growth of pathogens.

29. It is important to clean utensils and surfaces carefully to prevent *foodborne illness,* the spread of pathogens from one food to another.

Understanding Key Concepts

After reading the question or statement, select the correct answer.

30. Which of the following is *not* listed in the Nutrition Facts panel?
   a. The number of servings per container
   b. The number of calories per serving
   c. The vitamin and mineral content of the food
   d. The ingredients found in the food

31. Regular ice cream contains 7.5 grams of fat per serving. Ice cream that contains only 5 grams of fat per serving could be described as
    a. light.
    b. low-fat.
    c. reduced-fat.
    d. fat-free.

32. Which of the following is *not* one of the four basic steps for preventing foodborne illness?
    a. Clean
    b. Chop
    c. Cook
    d. Chill

Thinking Critically

After reading the question or statement, write a short answer using complete sentences.

33. **Compare and Contrast.** What is the difference between a food that is labeled "low-fat" and one that is labeled "reduced-fat"?

34. **Identify.** What are the usual symptoms of foodborne illness?

35. **Identify.** Name two foods that are common sources of allergens.

PROJECT-BASED ASSESSMENT

The Importance of Nutrients

BACKGROUND

Nutrients are the substances in food that your body needs. To have a healthful diet, your body needs six basic nutrients.

TASK

You will work in a small group to create a wiki that a group of friends can use to help each other make healthy food choices.

AUDIENCE

Students in your class

PURPOSE

The purpose of the wiki is to help your peers learn to make healthy food choices based on the six basic nutrients and how the body uses them. The wiki will also show which foods provide the body with each of the nutrients.

PROCEDURE

1. Review the information about the six groups of nutrients discussed in Module 10.

2. Create a wiki with your group that explains and gives examples and tips on how to make healthy food choices based on the six basic nutrients.

3. Be sure the healthy food choices are based on the six nutrients. Make any necessary revisions.

4. Obtain permission from your principal to post the wiki on the school's website.

Math Practice

Interpret Tables. To determine which food intake pattern to use, the following table gives an estimate of individual calorie needs. The calorie range for each age/sex group is based on physical activity level, from sedentary to active. *Sedentary* lifestyles include light physical activity. *Active* lifestyles include the equivalent to walking more than 3 miles per day at 3 to 4 miles per hour and the light physical activity typical of day-to-day life.

CALORIE RANGE		
	Sedentary	Active
Females		
14–18	1,800	2,400
19–30	2,000	2,400
Males		
14–18	2,200	3,200
19–30	2,400	3,000

1. What are the approximate calorie needs of a sedentary 16-year-old male?
   a. 1,800 calories　　c. 2,200 calories
   b. 2,000 calories　　d. 2,400 calories

2. In 2000, the total number of active females age 14–18 in the United States was approximately 4,788,000. This was a 31 percent increase from the total number in 1975. What was the approximate number of active females age 14–18 in 1975?
   a. 274,000　　　c. 2,245,000
   b. 398,000　　　d. 3,655,000

3. About 35 percent of a 16-year-old male's calories should come from carbohydrates. Which most closely matches this number?
   a. 1/4　　　c. 3/5
   b. 1/3　　　d. 5/7

Reading/Writing Practice

Understand and Apply. Read the passage below and then answer the questions.

Last weekend, after a game of basketball at the local community center, we all went to get a snack from the vending machine. Everything in the machine was high in fat, salt, or sugar. I put my money back in my pocket. My friends said, "Why don't you want anything?" Here's why. Last year, my dad found out he has high blood pressure. He's a bit overweight, so his doctor told him to cut out foods high in salt and fat. My parents didn't tell me to stop eating snacks like chips and cookies, but Dad's condition helped me understand that what I eat can affect my health.

1. What was the author's purpose in writing this piece?
   a. To teach friends how to communicate better
   b. To explain that eating better can affect your health
   c. To persuade others to eat cookies rather than chips
   d. To argue that healthy snacks taste better than unhealthy snacks

2. According to this text passage, high blood pressure may be related to
   a. exercising occasionally.
   b. choosing salty foods that are high in fat.
   c. selecting low-fat foods that are salty.
   d. eating foods that are high in fat and salt.

3. Write a paragraph giving your suggestions about how to improve eating habits. Provide details to support your main points.

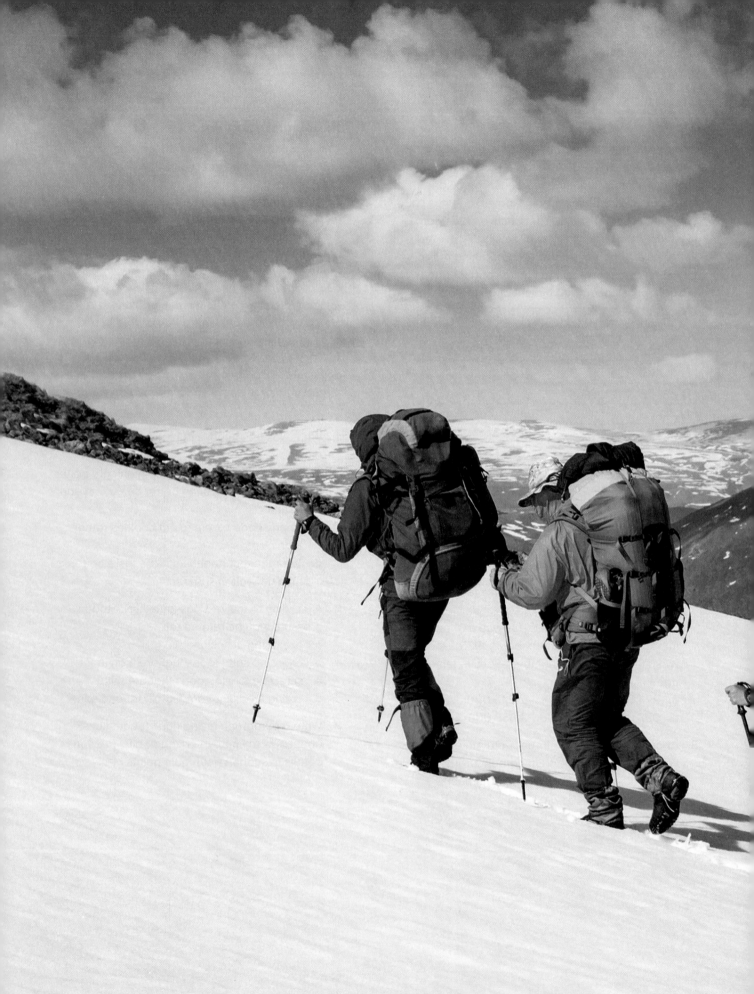

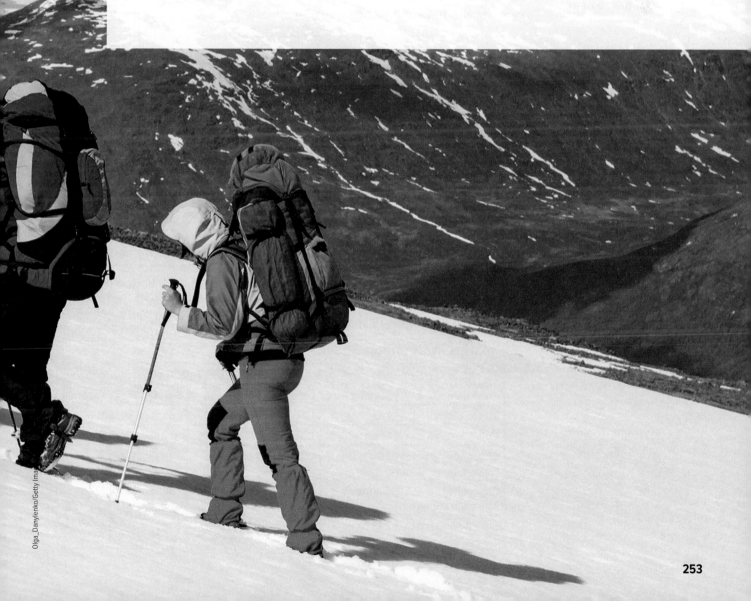

Managing Weight and Eating Behaviors

LESSONS

1 Maintaining a Healthy Weight

2 Body Image and Eating Disorders

3 Lifelong Nutrition

Olga_Danylenko/Getty Ima

Maintaining a Healthy Weight

BEFORE YOU READ

Create a Venn Diagram. Draw two overlapping circles. Label them "Losing Weight" and "Gaining Weight." As you read, fill in the outer area of each circle with useful tips on the corresponding topic. Fill in the overlapping area with advice that is useful to everyone trying to maintain a healthy weight.

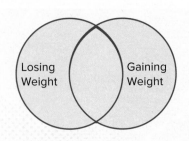

Vocabulary

metabolism
body mass index (BMI)
overweight
underweight
obese
osteoarthritis

BIG IDEA Maintaining a healthy weight helps you protect your health and prevent disease.

REAL LIFE ISSUES

On the Unhealthy Track. In 2017, the CDC conducted a survey called *Youth Risk Behavior Survey* (YRBS). Survey results showed that many teens have unhealthy habits. For example, 15.4 percent of teens do not get 60 minutes of physical activity at least once a week. 43 percent of teens play video games or use the computer for non-school purposes 3 or more hours a day. ***Write a paragraph describing how a person can adopt a healthy habit.***

After completing the lesson, review and analyze your response to the Real Life Issues question.

The Calorie Connection

MAIN IDEA You maintain your weight by taking in as many calories as you use.

Your **metabolism** is the process by which your body breaks down substances and gets energy from food. The energy you get from food is measured in units called *calories*. If you take in more calories than your body needs, you will gain weight. If you use more calories than you take in, you will lose weight.

Your Energy Balance

The balance between the calories you consume and those you burn as fuel is called the *energy balance*. It takes about 3,500 calories to equal 1 pound of body fat. Thus, if you consume 500 fewer calories than you use every day, you will lose 1 pound per week.

Calories in Common Snack Foods

High-Calorie Snack			Lower-Calorie Alternative		
Food Item	Serving Size	Calories	Food Item	Serving Size	Calories
Potato Chips	1 oz.	155	Pretzels	1 oz.	108
Cola	12 oz.	151	Water	16 oz.	0
Chocolate/caramel candy bar	1.6 oz.	208	Apple	1 medium	70
Chocolate sandwich cookies	6 cookies	282	Granola bar, raisin nut	1 oz.	127
Cream-filled snack cakes	2 (3 oz.)	314	Vanilla yogurt (low-fat)	8 oz.	193

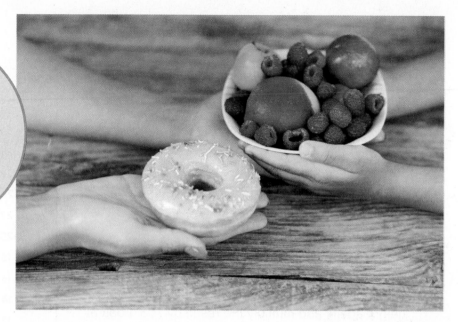

Snacks with lots of sugar, such as this donut, are often high in calories, while fresh produce, like this bowl of fruit, are low in calories. **Which snack should you choose to maintain a healthy weight?**

How Many Calories?

As a rule, foods that are high in fat will also be high in calories. A gram of fat contains nine calories while a gram of protein or carbohydrate contains only four. However, not all high-calorie foods are high in fat. Foods with lots of sugar, for example, are often high in calories. Fresh vegetables and fruits, which contain more water and fiber, are usually low in calories.

The way food is prepared also affects its calorie content. Fried foods, foods with rich sauces, and foods prepared in ways that add extra fats and sugars are likely to be high in calories. To control your weight, eat less of these high-calorie foods, or eat them less often.

Maintaining a Healthy Weight

MAIN IDEA Body mass index and body composition help you judge whether your weight is healthy.

What is a healthy weight for you? The answer depends on several factors, including your age, gender, height, body frame, and stage and rate of growth.

Body Mass Index

One way to learn whether your body weight falls into a healthy **range** is to calculate your **body mass index (BMI)**. BMI is a measure of body weight relative to height. The Real World Connection feature activity in this lesson gives you practice in determining your BMI. The charts that are part of this activity show you whether you're **overweight** (above the standard weight range), **underweight** (below the standards weight range), or at an appropriate weight for your height. However, it's important to understand that every teen grows at his or her own rate. As you move through puberty, your body is undergoing a lot of change. Some teens will gain weight while others may appear to be underweight. Some teen may grow quickly and become tall while others do not. Your goal should be to eat a healthy diet most of the time, get regular physical activity, and to stay within a healthy weight range.

Reading Check

Predict What would probably happen if you increased your activity level without eating more food?

ACADEMIC VOCABULARY

range (noun): the distance between possible extremes

Reading Check

Explain What does body mass index (BMI) measure?

Eviart/Shutterstock

Determining BMI

Here's an example for a 16-year-old male who is 6 feet tall and weighs 182 pounds.

$$182 \div 72 = 2.528$$

$$2.528 \div 72 = .035$$

$$0.035 \times 703 = 24.6$$

$$BMI = 24.6$$

Use this formula to determine your BMI. First, convert your height into inches. Divide your weight in pounds by your height in inches. Divide that result by your height again, and multiply the result by 703. Look at the charts to the right to determine if you're at risk for being overweight or underweight.

Activity: Mathematics

Some problems require more than one step to solve. Think through your approach before choosing an operation to use.

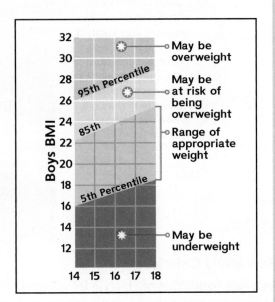

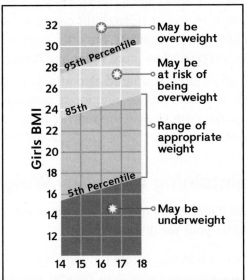

Body Composition

Although BMI is a quick, easy way to evaluate your weight, it doesn't tell the whole story. It's also important to consider your body composition—the ratio of fat to lean tissue in your body. A person who is very muscular, for instance, may have a high BMI but still be healthy.

One common way to check your body composition is a skin-fold test. This involves measuring the thickness of skin folds at different points on the body to figure out how much fat is stored beneath the skin. This test should be performed by a qualified professional.

Your Weight and Your Health

MAIN IDEA Being either overweight or underweight carries health risks.

People whose weight does not fall into a healthy range are at a higher risk for various diseases. This is true whether they are weigh too much or too little. If your BMI suggests that you may be overweight or underweight, ask a health care professional about healthful ways to gain or lose weight.

Weighing Too Much

You've probably heard that more than 15 percent of teens in the United States are overweight. This percentage has tripled since the 1980s. Being overweight or **obese** has serious health risks. Being obese means having an excess of body fat. It can increase your risk for health problems such as heart disease, cancer, asthma, gallbladder disease, or type 2 diabetes. It can also increase risk for **osteoarthritis**, which is a disease of the joints in which cartilage breaks down.

Some people are overweight or obese because of heredity or genetics. A slow metabolism can also lead to weight gain. However, many people who are overweight take in too many calories and get too little physical activity.

Weighing Too Little

Being underweight also carries health risks. Teens who weigh too little may feel weak, tire easily, or have trouble concentrating. Some underweight people may also have trouble fighting off disease.

Some people are naturally thin because of genetics. Others may have a fast metabolism. Teens may also be thin because their bodies are growing very quickly. As their growth slows, their bodies may "fill out." For other teens, however, being too thin can mean that they aren't getting the calories and nutrients their growing bodies need. Teens who exercise a great deal may not be eating enough food to meet their bodies' extra calorie needs.

Managing Your Weight

MAIN IDEA To manage your weight, stay physically active and eat healthful foods.

If your weight seems to be in a healthy range, then you probably don't need to worry too much about the number of calories you consume. If you want to lose or gain weight, however, you'll need to adjust your energy balance. This means changing either the number of calories you take in, the number you burn through physical activity, or both.

Staying active helps you maintain a healthy weight. **What might happen if these teens spent their afternoons playing video games instead of engaging in physical activity?**

Photodisc/Getty Images

Reading Check

Summarize What health problems may underweight teens have?

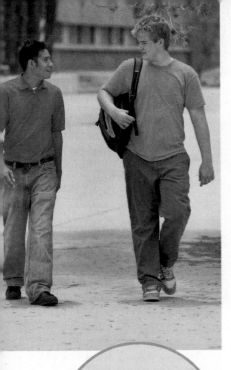

There is a wide range of weights that can be considered healthy. **Why should you avoid comparing your weight to that of your friends?**

The Dietary Guidelines for Americans does not advise teens to diet for weight loss. Instead, teens should try to eat a healthful, well-balanced diet and aim to get at least 60 minutes of physical activity every day to reach a healthy weight. Below are some more healthful strategies for managing your weight.

- **Target a healthy weight.** Use the BMI charts or consult a health care professional to find your ideal weight range.

- **Set realistic goals.** Do not try to gain or lose weight too quickly. Whether you are trying to gain weight or lose weight, a weight change of one to two pounds a week is a healthy recommendation. Aim to eat a healthful diet every day and exercise regularly.

- **Personalize your plan.** Make sure to include foods you enjoy in your daily eating plan. Also, choose physical activities that you will be able to do and that will fit into your schedule.

- **Put it in writing.** Write down your weight goals and your plan to achieve them.

- **Evaluate your progress.** As you track your weight, don't worry too much about daily ups and downs. Instead, focus on the long-term trend: whether your weight is rising or falling from week to week.

Healthful Ways to Lose Weight

If you want to lose weight, MyPlate can be a useful tool. It provides information on food groups, recommended amounts, and the importance of physical activity. Here are some other points to keep in mind for weight loss.

- **Choose nutrient-dense foods.** Fruits, vegetables, and whole grains supply the nutrients your body needs with fewer calories.

- **Watch portion sizes.** Follow MyPlate's advice about the recommended portion size for each major food group.

- **Watch your fats and sugars.** Limit your intake of foods that are high in fats and added sugars. These add calories without many nutrients.

- **Enjoy your favorite foods in moderation.** If you love ice cream, avoid giving it up completely. Instead, try enjoying a small scoop less often.

- **Tone your muscles.** Strength-training exercises can tone your muscles to give you a lean, trim shape. Also, since muscle tissue takes more calories to maintain than fat, increasing your muscle mass means that your body will use more calories even when you're sitting still.

- **Stay hydrated.** Teens need between 9 and 13 cups of water a day to meet their body's needs. Some of this water can come from the foods you eat, but drinking fluids is also important. Fruits and vegetables are the best food sources of water. Have you noticed how juicy watermelon is?

Healthful Ways to Gain Weight

Teens who want to gain weight should aim to increase the amount of healthy muscle on their bodies, rather than adding fat. To gain healthy weight, stick with a regular exercise program while also following the strategies listed below.

- **Select higher-calorie foods from the five major food groups.** High-calorie foods from the five basic food groups are more healthful choices than extra fats, oils, and sweets. For example, choose whole milk instead of fat-free milk. Other higher-calorie, nutrient-rich foods include nuts, dried fruits, cheese, and avocados.

- **Eat nutritious snacks.** Enjoy healthful snacks throughout the day to increase your daily calorie intake.

- **Get regular physical activity.** If you're increasing your calorie intake to gain weight, don't forget to exercise. Physical activity, especially strength training, will help ensure that most of the weight you gain is muscle rather than fat.

Reading Check

Explain How is physical activity important to weight loss?

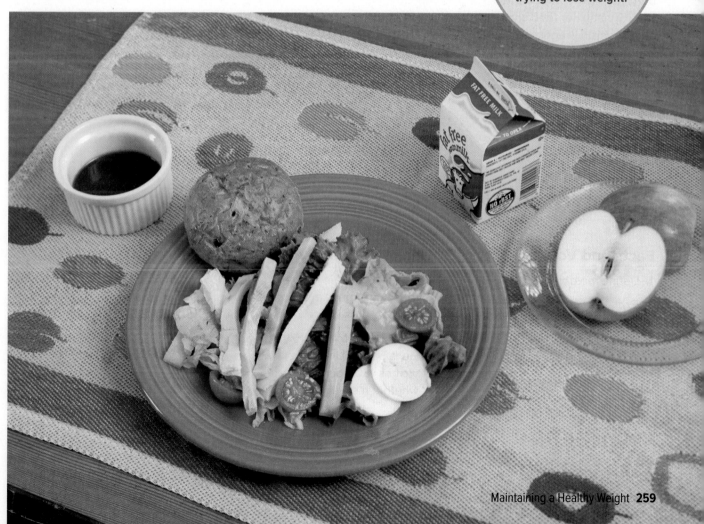

Your food choices can help you either gain or lose weight. **List three nutritional qualities that make this lunch a good choice for someone trying to lose weight.**

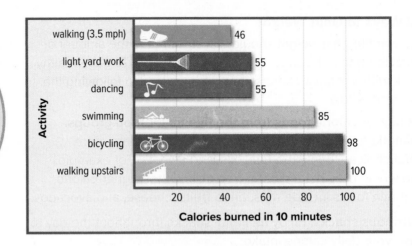

Activity (y-axis)

- walking (3.5 mph): 46
- light yard work: 55
- dancing: 55
- swimming: 85
- bicycling: 98
- walking upstairs: 100

Calories burned in 10 minutes (x-axis: 20, 40, 60, 80, 100)

Fitness Zone

My dad always says, "If you always do what you always did, you'll always get what you always got." I realized he is saying that if you want to change the outcome, you have to change your behavior. I wanted to get into shape, but skipped workouts and ate junk food. When I changed my behavior, I got what I wanted. Making healthier food choices and exercising regularly improved my fitness level, and I felt a lot healthier.

Physical Activity and Weight Management

Physical activity can help you lose or maintain a healthy weight. Some added benefits of regular physical activity:

- It helps relieve stress.
- It promotes a normal appetite response.
- It increases self-esteem, which helps you keep your plan on track.
- It helps you feel more energetic.

Lesson 1 Review

Facts and Vocabulary

1. Define *metabolism*.

2. Explain how to calculate your body mass index.

3. List three health problems associated with being overweight and obese.

Thinking Critically

4. **Analyze.** Explain how exercise that builds muscle can help promote loss of body fat.

5. **Synthesize.** Mike is 15 years old. He is 5 feet 9 inches tall and weighs 180 pounds. Explain whether his weight is in a healthy range.

Applying Health Skills

6. **Practicing Healthful Behaviors.** Write a plan describing strategies you will use to maintain a healthy weight throughout your life.

Writing Critically

7. **Expository.** Write a short article aimed at middle school students describing the causes and effects of the overweight and obesity problem among teens.

Body Image and Eating Disorders

BIG IDEA Poor body image may lead to unhealthful and harmful eating behaviors.

REAL LIFE ISSUES

Warning Signs of an Eating Disorder. People with eating disorders such as anorexia nervosa have an irrational fear of gaining weight. Warning signs of anorexia include: obsession with weight loss, brittle hair and nails, dry and yellowish skin, constant cold body temperature. *Write a dialogue of how you would talk to a friend you suspect may have an eating disorder. What would you say to show caring and concern?*

After completing the lesson, review and analyze your response to the Real Life Issues question.

Your Body Image

MAIN IDEA The media and other influences can affect your body image.

When you look in the mirror, do you like what you see? If your answer is yes, that means that you have a positive **body image**, or the way in which you see your body. Though many teens like the way they look, many others feel insecure about their changing bodies. During your teen years, you will go through many physical changes at a rapid pace. You may feel unhappy with your body type and wish you were taller, shorter, thinner, shapelier, or more muscular.

BEFORE YOU READ

Create a Comparison Chart. Make a chart and label the rows "Anorexia," "Bulimia," and "Binge Eating."

Label the columns "Symptoms" and "Health Risks." As you read, fill in the chart with information about these eating disorders.

	Symptoms	Health Risks
Anorexia		
Bulimia		
Binge Eating		

Vocabulary

body image
fad diet
weight cycling
eating disorders
anorexia nervosa
bulimia nervosa
binge eating disorder

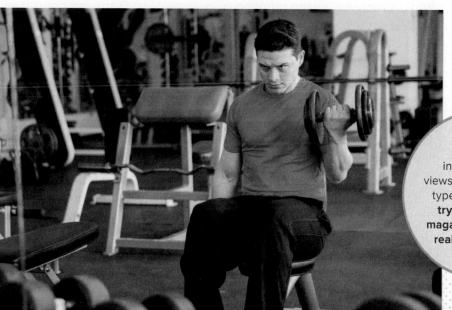

Media images may influence teens' views about ideal body types. **Do you think trying to look like magazine models is a realistic or healthy goal?**

Antoniodiaz/Shutterstock.com

Where does body image come from? There are a variety of answers. Sometimes, teens may compare their bodies to images in the media, such as models, athletes, or actors. However, it's important to remember that these images aren't always realistic. They can be touched up to remove flaws. Peers can also influence a teen's body image. Overweight or underweight teens may face discrimination because of the way they look, and all teens may feel pressure from friends to look a certain way.

Reading Check
Define What is body image?

Accepting Yourself

The rapid pace of physical change you experience during your teen years can affect your body image. Growth spurts may cause some teens to look thin. In other cases, hormonal changes can cause weight gain. Try to accept yourself the way you are. If you feel dissatisfied, talk to a parent or other trusted adult about your feelings. You can't change your basic body type, and you could hurt your health if you try.

Fad Diets

MAIN IDEA Fad diets are neither safe nor reliable ways to lose weight.

Teens who want to lose weight may be tempted to try **fad diets** that promise quick, easy weight loss. People on these diets may lose weight temporarily, but they usually regain it when they go off the diet. As a result, fad diets can lead to **weight cycling**, a repeated pattern of losing and regaining body weight.

Research shows that fad diets are not effective. They often **pose** serious health risks. In fact, most teens should not diet at all. Teens who want to lose weight should talk to a doctor before starting any weight-loss plan. A doctor can refer you to a registered dietitian, an expert in nutrition, who can help you set and reach your nutrition-related goals. In rare cases, teens with a serious weight problem may be advised to follow a low-calorie diet, but only under the supervision of a health care professional. In general, teens who want to maintain a healthy weight should simply follow the nutrition guidelines of MyPlate and get regular physical activity.

ACADEMIC VOCABULARY
pose (verb): to present or set forth

Types of Fad Diets

Some fad diets restrict the types and amounts of food that you eat. Others rely on pills or supplements. Most fad diets fall out of favor when people realize that they're unhealthy and they just don't work. Still, certain types of fad diets keep popping up every few years in a different form. The list below shows several common types of fad diets.

- **Miracle foods.** These plans promise you can "burn fat" by eating lots of a single food or type of food. In reality, there is no single food that can destroy fat. Moreover, eating only certain types of food will not give your body the nutrients it needs.

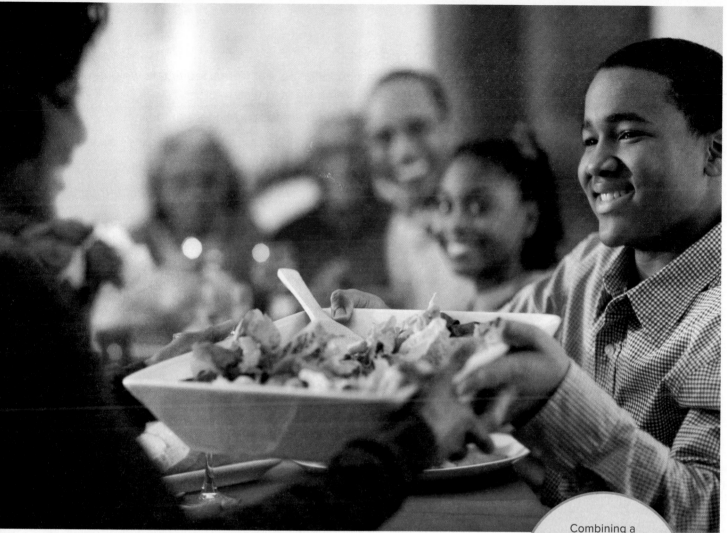

Combining a healthful, lower-calorie eating plan with physical activity is a more reliable way to lose weight than any fad diet. **What are some drawbacks of fad diets?**

- **Magic combinations.** These plans promise that certain foods will trigger weight loss when they're eaten together. The food combinations may be safe to eat as part of an overall healthy diet, but there's no evidence that combining certain foods will lead to weight loss.

- **Liquid diets.** These plans replace solid food with ultra-low-calorie liquid formulas. These diets can lead to dangerous side effects if they are followed incorrectly. However, doctors may recommend them (with medical supervision) for people who are seriously obese.

- **Diet pills.** Some diet pills and supplements claim to suppress your appetite so that you eat less. Others claim to "block" or "flush" fat from the body. Some types of diet pills can be addictive. In addition, they can cause serious side effects, such as drowsiness, anxiety, or a racing heart.

- **Fasting.** *Fasting* means going without food entirely. Some religious and cultural customs require people to fast for short periods, such as specific days of the year or specific times of the day during certain months. This kind of short-term fasting is safe for most people. However, fasting for longer periods is not a safe way to lose weight. It deprives the body of needed nutrients and can result in dehydration.

There are several ways to tell a fad diet from a legitimate weight-loss plan. Here are some warning signs to watch for:

- Food combinations that do not follow MyPlate guidelines
- Promises of ultra-fast weight loss (more than two pounds a week)
- Claims that you can lose weight without physical activity
- Words such as *effortless, guaranteed, miraculous, breakthrough, ancient, or secret*
- Requirements to buy special foods or other products
- Claims that "doctors don't want you to know" about this weight-loss plan

Eating Disorders

MAIN IDEA Eating disorders are extreme and dangerous eating behaviors that require medical attention.

As you have learned, some types of weight-loss diets are unhealthful. Yet some people eat in ways that are even more harmful to their health. These people suffer from **eating disorders**. Eating disorders are classified as mental illnesses. They are often linked to depression, low self-esteem, or troubled personal relationships. Social and cultural forces that emphasize personal appearance can also play a role. Eating disorders often run in families, and research suggests that genetics may play a role in their development.

Reading Check

Explain What are some typical characteristics of fad diets?

People with anorexia can be very thin and still see themselves as overweight. **What are other symptoms associated with anorexia?**

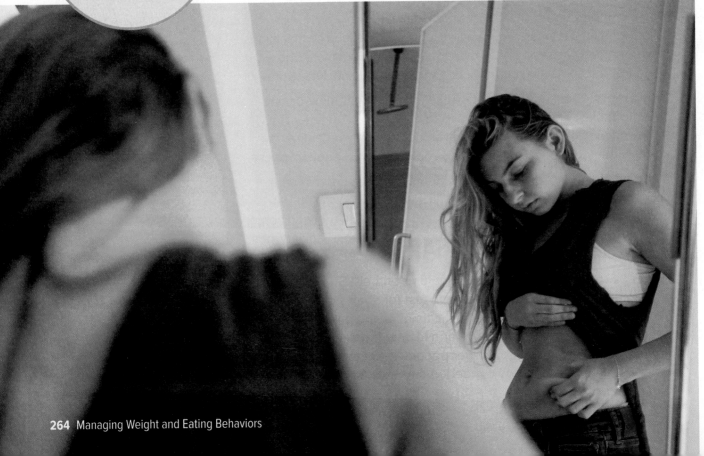

Image Source/PhotoStock-Israel

Anorexia Nervosa

Anorexia nervosa is an eating disorder in which an irrational fear of weight gain leads people to starve themselves. This disorder mainly affects girls and young women, but is not uncommon among males. People with anorexia have an unrealistic self-concept. They may view themselves as overweight even when they are dangerously thin.

Several mental and social factors are linked to anorexia. These include outside pressures, high expectations, a need to be accepted, and a need to achieve. Doctors also say that biological factors, such as genetics, can play a role in the development of this disorder.

People with anorexia often develop obsessive behaviors related to food. These may include:

- Avoiding food and meals.
- Eating only a few kinds of food in very small amounts.
- Weighing or counting the calories in everything they eat.
- Exercising excessively.
- Weighing themselves repeatedly.

Anorexia can cause the same health problems as malnutrition or starvation. Body temperature, heart rate, and blood pressure may drop. The bones may become brittle, and the body's organs may actually shrink. Anorexia nervosa can lead to heart problems and sudden cardiac death.

Bulimia Nervosa

Bulimia nervosa is similar to anorexia in some ways. People with bulimia also fear weight gain and feel dissatisfied with their bodies. However, instead of avoiding food all the time, they regularly go on *binges,* eating a huge amount of food in a single sitting. During a binge, they may feel out of control, often gulping down food too fast to taste it. After the binge, they *purge* to rid their bodies of the excess food. They may force themselves to vomit or take laxatives to flush the food out of their system. Instead of purging, some people with bulimia may fast or exercise frantically after a binge.

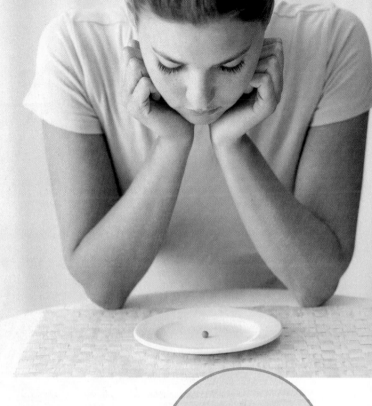

Eating disorders involve an irrational fear of weight gain and an unrealistic self-image. **Give some examples of how eating disorders affect behavior.**

Fitness Zone

Some of my friends skip breakfast to lose weight. Some say they don't have the time to eat it. My dad says that he read a magazine article saying that people who eat breakfast every day are more likely to lose weight and keep it off. Eating breakfast gives you an energy boost. It also increases your metabolism, which means that you burn more calories. I think it's so cool that you can actually eat to maintain a healthy weight or lose weight.

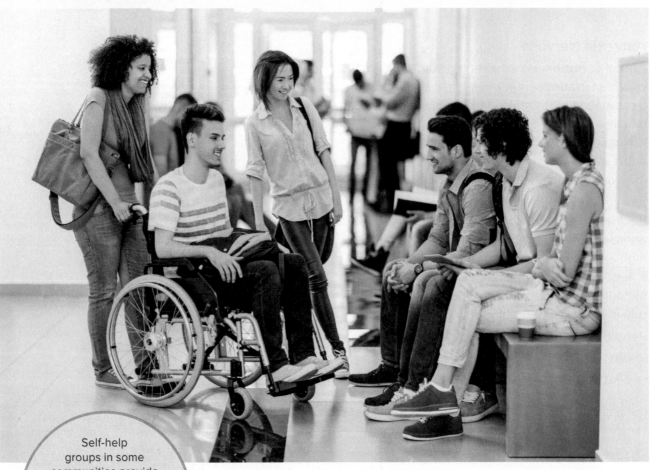

Self-help groups in some communities provide ongoing support for people recovering from eating disorders. **How might being part of such a group be helpful?**

Unlike people with anorexia, bulimia sufferers are usually in the normal weight range for their age and height. However, this disease can cause serious health problems. It can lead to dehydration, sore and inflamed throat, and swollen glands. It can also damage the stomach, intestines, or kidneys. People who purge by vomiting may damage their teeth by exposing them regularly to stomach acid. Purging can also cause chemical imbalances in the body. In severe cases, these imbalances can lead to irregular heart rhythms, heart failure, and death.

Binge Eating Disorder

People with **binge eating disorder** go on eating binges in much the same way people with bulimia do. However, these binges generally do not occur as often. During a binge, people may feel guilty and disgusted about their behavior but powerless to stop it. People with this disorder do not purge after a binge.

Binge eating disorder is more common in males than other eating disorders. Boys and men account for more than a third of all cases. Binge eating disorder can lead to becoming overweight or obese. As a result, it can lead to all the health problems linked to obesity, such as high blood pressure, type 2 diabetes, and cardiovascular disease.

Seeking Help

Eating disorders are serious and dangerous illnesses. People with these disorders need help to overcome them. Medical help may involve counseling, nutritional guidance, and a doctor's care. In extreme cases, a hospital stay may be necessary.

For anorexia nervosa, the goal of treatment is to get the patient's body weight back up to a healthy level. The patient will also receive psychological and family therapy. Family members and friends can also play a key role in treatment. They can create a supportive environment and help the patient learn to eat normally again.

The key to treating bulimia nervosa is to break the cycle of binging and purging. Behavioral therapy can sometimes help with this goal. After that, psychotherapy can address the emotional problems that led to the eating disorder. Similar treatments are used for binge eating disorder.

People with eating disorders often cannot admit that they have a problem. Family members and friends can help them to recognize the problem and seek treatment. Some patients end up needing long-term treatment to recover from an eating disorder. Support groups can help with this process. If you think that you or someone you know may have an eating disorder, your first step might be to talk to a trusted adult, such as a parent, counselor, or school nurse.

Reading Check

Compare and Contrast
How is binge eating disorder different from bulimia nervosa?

Lesson 2 Review

Facts and Vocabulary

1. List two factors that influence body image.

2. Define *fad diets*.

3. List three types of eating disorders.

Thinking Critically

4. **Synthesize.** How might a poor body image result in an eating disorder?

5. **Evaluate.** If you read an ad in a magazine promising you can lose up to 15 pounds in one month while still eating all your favorite foods, would you think this was a fad diet or a legitimate plan? Explain why.

Applying Health Skills

6. **Analyzing Influences.** Write an essay describing how teen magazines portray teens and their bodies. How might the magazine's pictures affect the body image of teens?

Writing Critically

7. **Narrative.** Write a story about a teen who seeks help for an eating disorder. Describe the symptoms and how the disorder affects the teen's life.

Lifelong Nutrition

BEFORE YOU READ

Create a Cluster Chart. Draw a circle and label it "Special Nutritional Needs." Draw surrounding circles and use these to describe nutritional needs for vegetarians, athletes, and those with health conditions. As you read, continue filling in the chart with more details.

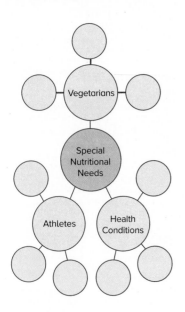

Vocabulary

vegetarian
dietary supplements
autoimmune disease
performance enhancers
herbal supplements
megadoses

BIG IDEA Nutritional needs will change throughout your life.

REAL LIFE ISSUES

A Personal Choice. Miranda is facing a moral dilemma. After spending the summer at a camp where she helped care for farm animals, she's become uncomfortable with eating meat. She thinks of animals as friends, and she doesn't like the idea of eating them. However, food is an important part of her family's traditions. Miranda is afraid her parents won't understand her decision not to eat meat anymore. *Write a dialogue in which Miranda tries to explain to her parents her desire to become a vegetarian.*

After completing the lesson, review and analyze your response to the Real Life Issues question.

Lifelong Nutritional Needs

MAIN IDEA Your age, gender, lifestyle, and health needs can affect your body's food needs.

Everyone has different nutritional needs. An active 16-year-old girl will need more calories and different levels of nutrients than an 80-year-old man. In addition to differing nutrient needs, we all have individual preferences and other considerations when it comes to diet. Some people choose to avoid meat and other animal-based foods. Others must avoid certain foods, such as nuts, due to food allergies. Listed here are factors that can affect your nutritional needs.

- **Age.** When you were a young child, you probably ate a lot less food than you do now. During your teen years, your body's calorie needs have increased to support your growth. As you grow older, your calorie needs will continue to change.

- **Gender.** On average, females need fewer calories than males. However, they have a greater need for specific nutrients such as iron and calcium. This is especially true during pregnancy, when a woman must meet the nutritional needs of her developing baby along with her own. Pregnant women need extra iron, calcium, and folic acid, along with more calories from nourishing foods. Nutrition impacts the reproductive health of both males and females. Malnutrition is associated with an increased risk of infertility which is the inability to become pregnant despite trying for 12 months or more. In females, poor nutrient intake is linked to infertility and miscarriages. In males, consuming lower amounts of nutrients such as folate, vitamin C, and lycopene is associated with infertility. Lycopene is a natural plant pigment that gives foods such as tomatoes and watermelons their red color.

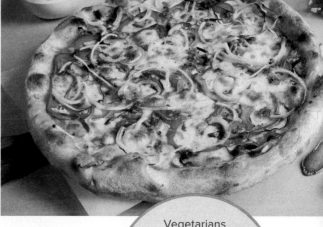

- **Activity level.** The more active you are, the more calories your body needs. Very active people need to take in more calories to maintain their weight. Preferably they should be from nutrient-dense foods.

Vegetarian Diets

A **vegetarian** is a person who eats mostly or only plant-based foods. There are several different types of vegetarian diets. The strictest vegetarians, known as vegans, eat only plant-based foods. Other types of vegetarians include eggs, dairy foods, or both in their diets. Some people choose to follow a modified vegetarian diet, which includes small amounts of certain types of meat, such as fish or chicken.

People may choose a meatless or near-meatless diet for many reasons. Some people do not want to eat animals for moral reasons. Others believe a vegetarian diet is more healthful. Still others are vegetarians for religious, cultural, or economic reasons—or they simply prefer not to eat meat.

The vegetarian-eating style has both advantages and disadvantages to a person's health. Plant-based foods tend to be lower in saturated fat and higher in fiber than most animal-based foods. Additionally, plant-based foods contain no cholesterol, unlike animal-based foods. As a result, a well-planned meatless diet may help reduce the risk of cardiovascular disease and some types of cancer. However, plant-based foods also tend to be lower in certain nutrients, such as protein, iron, calcium, zinc, and some B vitamins. One nutrient, vitamin B12, is found only in animal-based foods. Some vegetarians may need to take **dietary supplements**—products that supply one or more nutrients as a supplement to, not a substitute for, healthful foods—to get all the nutrients they need.

Health Conditions

Sometimes, the foods people eat can **trigger** certain diseases or health conditions. People with these conditions may need to avoid or limit certain foods in order to avoid health problems. Each of the health conditions listed below can affect a person's diet.

- **Diabetes.** People with diabetes have to monitor their eating carefully. They have to make sure their blood sugar stays in a healthy range. Diabetics who use insulin must tailor the amount of insulin they inject to the amount of carbohydrates in the foods they eat. Others may be able to control their diabetes without medication by carefully controlling the carbohydrates in foods and beverages they consume. Those who are overweight may find that losing weight helps control their blood sugar.

- **Food allergies.** Food allergies can range from merely annoying to life-threatening. People with severe food allergies must take great care to avoid the foods and food ingredients they are allergic to. This means checking ingredient lists on packaged foods and questioning waiters at restaurants. This can be troublesome, but not nearly as troublesome as being rushed to the emergency room.

Vegetarians can choose from a wide variety of healthful and tasty foods to meet their protein needs. **Name the foods in each dish that are a source of protein.**

Reading Check

Identify List two kinds of people who might use dietary supplements.

ACADEMIC VOCABULARY

trigger (verb): to initiate or set off

Reading Check

Explain What are some potential health benefits of a vegetarian eating style?

Hans Geel/Shutterstock

- **Lactose intolerance.** People with this intolerance can't easily digest the lactose in milk and some dairy products. Some of them choose to avoid dairy products altogether. Others find they can control the problem by consuming smaller portions of milk or by getting their calcium from cheese and yogurt, which contain less lactose. Some people take lactase (the enzyme needed to digest lactose) in liquid or tablet form when they eat dairy products. Another option is to choose lactose-reduced dairy products, which are available at many supermarkets.

- **Celiac disease.** Also known as *gluten intolerance,* this is an **autoimmune disease**. Autoimmune diseases are a condition in which the immune system mistakenly attacks itself, targeting the cells, tissues, and organs of a person's own body. People with this condition are unable to tolerate a protein called *gluten,* which is found in wheat, rye, and barley. Oats may also be harmful to those with celiac disease. The only treatment is to avoid these grains, and anything made from them, including bread, pasta, and beer. Fortunately, gluten-free alternatives to many of these foods can be found in many food stores these days.

- **High blood pressure.** Consuming salt can raise a person's blood pressure. This effect is stronger in some individuals than in others. People with high blood pressure are often encouraged to keep their salt intake low. Processed and packaged foods are the largest source of sodium in the American diet. Replacing high-sodium foods with foods that are high in potassium, like fresh fruits and vegetables, has been shown to promote healthy blood pressure levels.

- **High cholesterol.** People with high cholesterol levels may need to reduce their intake of saturated fats and trans fats. These fats increase cholesterol production in the body.

Nutrition for Athletes

MAIN IDEA Athletes have special nutritional needs related to their activity level.

Eating right has a strong impact on an athlete's performance. Like everyone else, athletes need a balanced diet that supplies enough nutrients to support health. The most important difference is that when you're very active, you need more calories to keep your body fueled up.

Teen athletes may need anywhere from 2,000 to 5,000 calories per day. The amount of calories depends on the sport and on the intensity, length, and frequency of their training. To get these extra calories, athletes need to choose nutrient-dense foods with plenty of protein and carbohydrates. These foods will help student athletes keep their energy up and maintain a healthy weight for athletic competition.

Fitness Zone

I carry healthy snacks in my backpack every day. When I get hungry, I'm not tempted to buy something that's not healthy. An apple or a small bag of carrots are easy to carry. They're healthier than a candy bar or chips, too.

Making Weight

In some sports, such as wrestling or boxing, your weight is important because you have to compete with others in the same weight class. If your sport requires you to "make weight," then be sure you compete at a weight that's right for you. Your ideal weight will put your BMI in a healthy range and allow you to eat enough to meet your daily nutrient needs.

Some athletes try to compete in a weight class that's too low for them because they think they will have a better chance against smaller opponents. In reality, they are hurting themselves by trying to force their bodies down to a weight that isn't healthy. Extreme measures such as fasting or trying to sweat off extra weight can cause dehydration, harming performance as well as health. If you really do need to lose some weight, stick to a sensible plan that will take off one-half to one pound a week.

Hydration

Everyone needs water to stay healthy. Teen girls need about 9 cups of water a day to stay well-hydrated, and teen boys need about 13 cups. (This water can come from the food that you eat, as well as from beverages.) Student athletes, however, need even more fluids. When you sweat during exercise, your body loses fluids. These fluids must be replaced to avoid dehydration and heatstroke. Dehydration can lead to fatigue, dizziness or lightheadedness, and cramping. It can also cause an imbalance of electrolytes—minerals that help maintain your body's fluid balance. The minerals sodium, chloride, and potassium are all electrolytes. To prevent dehydration, drink water before and after you exercise, and about every 15 minutes or so during a workout.

Eating Before a Competition

Eating before a competition provides your body with the energy it needs to get through the event. Try to eat about three to four hours before a competition so that your stomach is not full during competition. Choose a meal that is high in carbohydrates and low in fat and protein. Fat and protein stay in the digestive tract for a longer period of time. Good choices of foods to eat before a competition include pasta, rice, vegetables, breads, and fruits. Also, remember to drink plenty of water before, during, and after the competition.

Eating After a Workout

During exercise and competition, your muscles use the energy you have supplied it with to fuel activity. It is important to refuel your muscles after hard workouts and competitions so that you can be ready for the next one. Carbohydrates are important after exercise because they supply energy to your muscles. Protein helps repair and rebuild muscles that have been damaged during intense workouts. Good choices of foods to eat after exercise and competition include whole-grain cereal with low-fat milk and fruit, chocolate milk and a banana, or a fruit smoothie made with low-fat yogurt. It is important to replace your sweat losses by drinking plenty of water after a competition.

Drinking plenty of water during a workout helps you avoid dehydration and keep performing at your peak. **What problems can dehydration cause?**

Avoiding Performance Enhancers

Some athletes try to gain an extra edge by using **performance enhancers**. These are substances that boost athletic ability. Many of these substances pose health risks, especially for teens. Many performance enhancers are illegal, and most have been banned under the rules of many sports organizations.

- **Anabolic steroids.** These dangerous drugs, which are illegal without a doctor's prescription, have the same effect as male hormones (known as *androgens*) in the body. Athletes who take them disregard their many health risks in an effort to boost their muscle growth.

- **Androstenedione.** Androstenedione, better known as "andro," is a weaker form of the androgens that the body produces naturally. Although some athletes take it to build muscle, its actual benefits are doubtful. It has many of the same side effects as steroids, and its use is now banned in professional sports.

- **Creatine.** This compound helps release energy. Some athletes take creatine to give them a quick burst of power and reduce muscle fatigue. However, it can actually hurt athletic performance because of its side effects, which include cramps and nausea. Using it at high doses may damage the heart, liver, and kidneys.

- **Energy drinks.** Most energy drinks contain high amounts of caffeine. They provide quick energy in an unhealthful way by increasing your heart rate. Using energy drinks can actually harm you and your athletic performance. Drinking caffeinated beverages may cause your body to lose more fluids, leading to dehydration.

Using any type of performance enhancer, whether it's legal or illegal, is not worth the risk. You can perform at your peak without them by training, eating right, and getting enough rest.

Using Supplements

MAIN IDEA Dietary supplements can help people meet their nutrient needs if they cannot do it with food alone.

Walk down the aisles of any drugstore, and you will see a huge array of dietary supplements. These supplements provide various combinations of vitamins, minerals, protein, and fiber. You may also see **herbal supplements** that claim to promote health in various ways. Herbal supplements are dietary supplements containing plant extracts.

The most important thing to know about supplements is that they are no substitute for eating a variety of healthful foods. Some people, however, may not be able to get all the nutrients they need through food alone. For example, strict vegetarians may use supplements to provide the nutrients they are not getting from animal-based foods. Pregnant or nursing women may use them to make sure they get all the extra nutrients their bodies need. Supplements can also help people who are recovering from illness or taking medications that reduce their bodies' ability to absorb certain nutrients.

Concerns About Dietary Supplements

Most people who follow a nutritious, well-balanced eating plan, such as the one recommended in MyPlate, will not need a multivitamin. However, multivitamin and mineral supplements are generally safe to take, as long as you use them correctly. For starters, do not take supplements that supply more than 100 percent of the Daily Value for any nutrient. Taking **megadoses**, or very large amounts, of any supplement can be dangerous. Some vitamins, including A, D, E, and K, can build up in the body and become toxic.

Many herbal supplements raise additional concerns. Some people take these "natural" products because they believe they are a safe alternative to drugs for treating certain conditions. However, these supplements can actually be dangerous. For instance, using the herb ephedra, or *ma huang,* can lead to a heart attack or stroke. Products containing this herb were banned in 2004. Other herbs, such as kava and comfrey, have been linked to serious liver damage. The National Institutes of Health (NIH) cautions that herbal supplements can have the same dangers as drugs, and should be used with the same care.

Herbal supplements aren't regulated in the same ways as foods or drugs are. However, the U.S. Food and Drug Administration (FDA) can take action to stop the sale of supplements that are unsafe or mislabeled. To be safe, treat supplements with the same caution you would use with any drug. Check with your health care provider before using them, especially if you are already taking other medications.

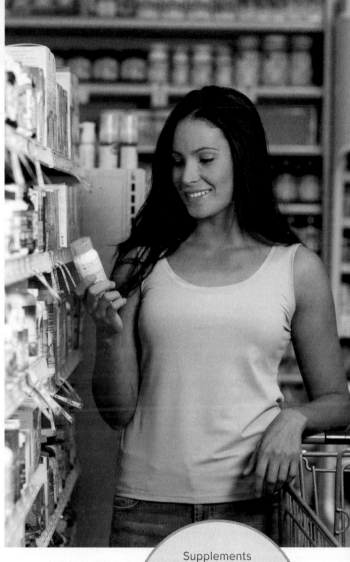

Supplements can help you meet your needs for specific nutrients, but they cannot take the place of healthful foods. **What are some reasons people might use supplements?**

Lesson 3 Review

Facts and Vocabulary

1. Define the term *dietary supplements.*

2. List three factors that can affect your body's nutrient needs.

3. Describe why all athletes should avoid using performance enhancers.

Thinking Critically

4. **Analyze.** How would cutting back on food and water affect the performance of a student athlete?

5. **Evaluate.** Is it safe for a vegan to take a daily supplement that provides the recommended dose of iron, calcium, and B vitamins? Explain why.

Applying Health Skills

6. **Advocacy.** Create a flyer telling teens about the dangers of using dietary supplements. Include warnings about specific types of supplements.

Writing Critically

7. **Expository.** Write an article for the school newspaper. In the article, tell teens the right and wrong ways to improve athletic performance.

LESSON 1

Vocabulary Review

Use the correct vocabulary term to complete the following statements.

1. _____ is a measure of body weight relative to height.

2. Adults who have an excess of body fat may be considered _____.

3. People who are _____ have a BMI that is lower than the healthy range.

Understanding Key Concepts

After reading the question or statement, select the correct answer.

4. Measuring the thickness of skin folds at different points on the body is a way to determine your
   a. body mass index.
   b. body composition.
   c. metabolism.
   d. energy balance.

5. Which of the following is *not* a health risk associated with being overweight?
   a. Hypertension (high blood pressure)
   b. Type 2 diabetes
   c. Osteoarthritis (a joint disease)
   d. Anemia (a condition in which the blood cannot carry needed oxygen to the body)

6. A safe, reasonable rate of weight loss is
   a. 1 pound per day
   b. 5 pounds per week
   c. 1/2 to 1 pound per week
   d. 1 to 2 pounds per year

Thinking Critically

After reading the question or statement, write a short answer using complete sentences.

7. **Explain.** How is your weight related to your energy balance?

8. **Identify.** List three healthful steps you could take if you wanted to gain weight.

9. **Compare and Contrast.** What is the difference between being overweight and obese?

10. **Evaluate.** Why is physical activity important for all teens, regardless of weight?

LESSON 2

Vocabulary Review

Correct the sentences below by replacing the italicized term with the correct vocabulary term.

11. A repeated pattern of losing and regaining body weight is called *binge eating*.

12. *Fad diets* are extreme, harmful eating behaviors that can cause serious illness or even death.

13. *Anorexia nervosa* is an eating disorder in which people overeat compulsively.

Understanding Key Concepts

After reading the question or statement, select the correct answer.

14. Which of the following might cause teens to develop a negative body image?
    a. Focusing on their good qualities
    b. Being picked on at school because of the way they look
    c. Being physically active
    d. Having friends with positive attitudes toward their own bodies

15. Teens who think they need to lose weight should
    a. take diet pills.
    b. follow a liquid diet.
    c. begin a fast.
    d. consult a doctor.

16. Which of the following is *not* a behavior associated with anorexia nervosa?
    a. Avoiding food and meals
    b. Exercising excessively
    c. Eating a large amount of food in a single sitting
    d. Weighing oneself repeatedly

17. The first step in treating bulimia nervosa is to
    a. break the cycle of binging and purging.
    b. get the patient's weight back to a normal level.
    c. address the emotional problems that led to the eating disorder.
    d. provide nutritional guidance.

Thinking Critically

After reading the question or statement, write a short answer using complete sentences.

18. **Explain.** Why are fad diets generally not safe or reliable ways to lose weight?

19. **Explain.** What makes very-low-calorie diets dangerous for teens?

20. **Analyze.** Identify three signs that distinguish a fad diet from a legitimate weight-loss plan.

21. **Explain.** What are three risks associated with using diet pills?

22. **Compare and Contrast.** How are the eating disorders anorexia and bulimia similar? How are they different?

23. **Compare and Contrast.** How are bulimia and binge eating disorder similar? How are they different?

LESSON 3

Vocabulary Review

Use the correct vocabulary term to complete the following statements.

24. People who eat mostly or only plant-based foods are called _____.

25. _____ are dietary supplements containing plant extracts.

26. Taking a _____, or a very large amount, of any supplement can be dangerous.

Understanding Key Concepts

After reading the question or statement, select the correct answer.

27. Which of the following foods would all vegetarians refuse to eat?
    a. Eggs
    b. Milk
    c. Chicken
    d. Bread

28. People with celiac disease must avoid foods that contain
    a. sugar.
    b. lactose.
    c. gluten.
    d. fiber.

29. Which medical condition may require people to limit their salt intake?
    a. Allergies
    b. Diabetes
    c. High cholesterol
    d. High blood pressure

Thinking Critically

After reading the question or statement, write a short answer using complete sentences.

30. **Identify.** List three factors that may influence a person's calorie and nutrient needs.

31. **Analyze.** How can good nutrition enhance your health throughout your life?

32. **Evaluate.** Describe the health advantages and disadvantages of a vegetarian eating style.

33. **Explain.** How are dehydration and electrolyte imbalance related?

34. **Explain.** Why are dietary supplements not a substitute for eating a variety of healthful foods?

35. **Identify Problems and Solutions.** Toby has a milk allergy and is unable to consume dairy products. How might he benefit from dietary supplements?

36. **Describe.** What health problems can result when athletes take performance enhancing drugs or supplements?

PROJECT-BASED ASSESSMENT

Helping a Friend

BACKGROUND

Eating disorders are a serious medical problem that can result in lifelong health problems and even death. Often, people with eating disorders try to hide the disorder from their friends and family.

TASK

With your group of three students, create a streaming video of a short skit that demonstrates how you would talk to a friend who you suspect may have an eating disorder. Encourage your friend to get help. Your video should also demonstrate ways to obtain help for the friend from a trusted adult.

AUDIENCE

Students in your class

PURPOSE

Practice communicating effectively with your peers and with adults

PROCEDURE

1. Conduct an online search on symptoms of eating disorders and review those in your textbook. Choose one eating disorder to focus on in your video.

2. Collaborate as a group to write the script, film, and upload the video with these characters: a student with a suspected eating disorder, the student's friend, and an adult.

3. Be sure your chosen method of communication demonstrates the following: expressing concern and support, telling an adult about the problem, and making sure your friend receives help.

4. When creating the video, remember that a person with an eating disorder may not accept advice.

5. Show your video to the class. Ask permission to upload your group's video to the school's website.

Math Practice

Problem Solving. Some math problems require you to read a text passage. Read the text carefully and answer the questions that follow.

Mohammed's school started a fitness and nutrition program. Mohammed joined the program and developed food and physical activity plans. Exactly two weeks after starting the plan, Mohammed had lost 3 pounds and noticed that he had more energy. Later that week, Mohammed left school feeling restless. He decided to go for a power walk. He burned 37 calories warming up before he went on the walk and 2.3 calories for every minute of walking once he got started. When Mohammed finished his power walk, he spent 10 minutes cooling down.

1. What was Mohammed's average weight loss per day in the first two weeks of his plan?
   a. 0.21 pounds/day   c. 1.50 pounds/day
   b. 0.67 pounds/day   d. 4/67 pounds/day

2. If x represents the number of minutes Mohammed power walked and y represents how many calories he usually burns cooling down, which expression below could be used to figure out how many total calories he burned on the power walk?
   a. $x(2.3 + 37 + y)$
   b. $(2.3 + 37)(x + y)$
   c. $(2.3 \times y) + 37 + x$
   d. $(2.3 \times x) + 37 + y$

3. Mohammed burned 37 calories during his warm-up, 20 calories during his cool down, and power-walked for 43 minutes. How many total calories did he burn?

Reading/Writing Practice

Understand and Apply. Read the passage below and then answer the questions.

About 50 million Americans begin weight-loss diets each year. Very few—perhaps 5 percent—will manage to keep the weight off. Why? Most people approach weight loss the wrong way. They look for "quick fixes" that will let them lose weight with as little effort as possible. They may put their faith in "magic" weight-loss formulas or combinations of food that will "melt away" the pounds. The only sensible approach is to cut your calorie intake by following the MyPlate guidelines, and getting more physical activity. This plan may not be quick—and it may not be easy—but it will produce lasting results, a promise no other diet can live up to.

1. What is the main idea of this article?
   a. Millions of Americans try to lose weight each year.
   b. Weight-loss diets can be harmful.
   c. Nobody really loses weight by dieting.
   d. Only a sensible plan will result in permanent weight loss.

2. Which sentence could be added to introduce the second paragraph?
   a. There are no shortcuts to weight loss.
   b. Fad diets can help some people.
   c. A healthy weight has many benefits.
   d. For many people, losing weight is impossible.

3. Contrast the realities of fad diets with losing weight by following a plan of healthy eating and physical activity.

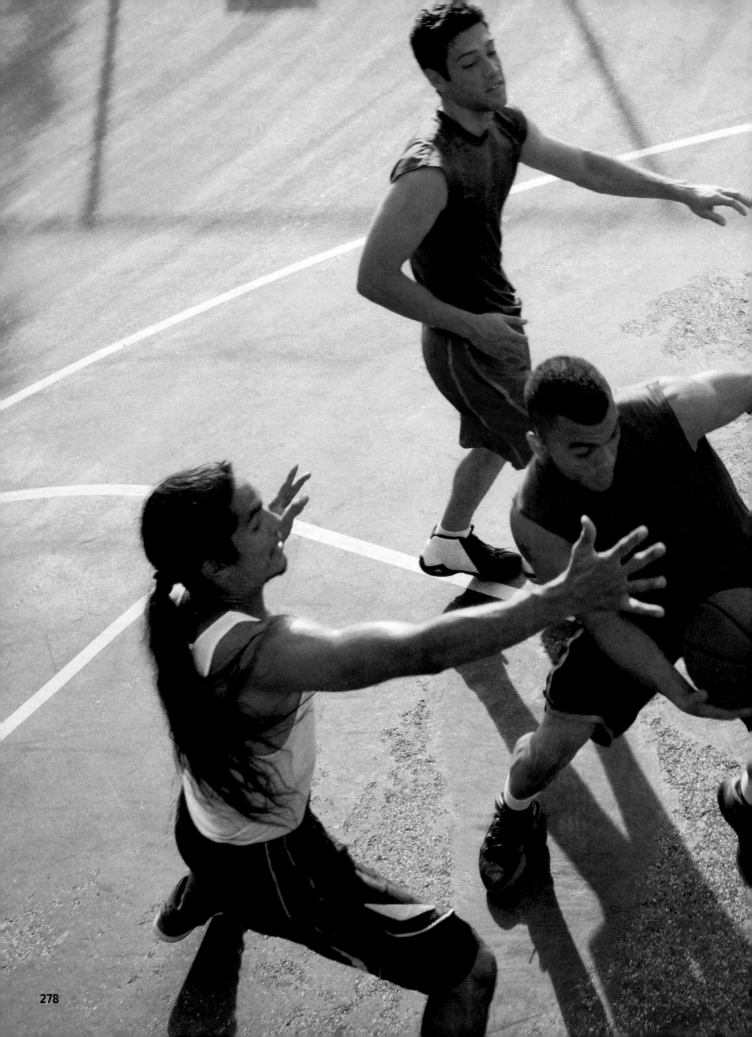

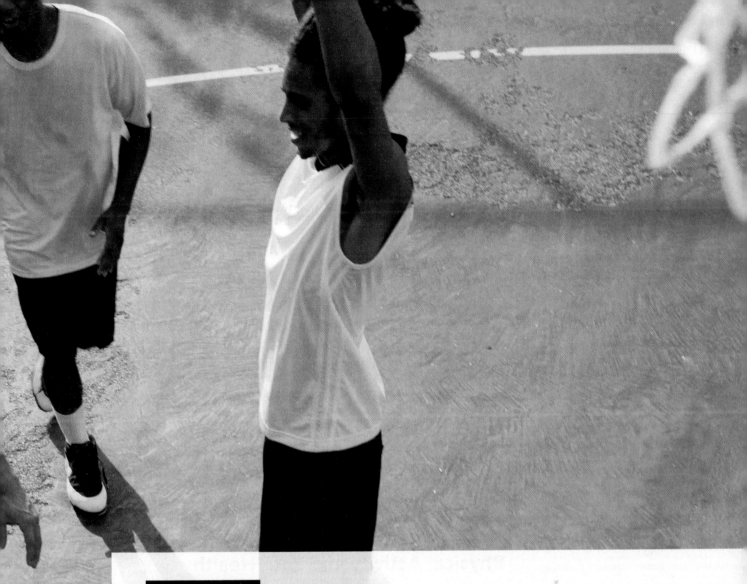

MODULE 12

Physical Activity and Fitness

LESSONS

Benefits of Physical Activity

BEFORE YOU READ

Organize Information. Divide a sheet of paper into three columns. Label them "Physical," "Mental/Emotional," and "Social." As you read the lesson, fill in the chart by listing how physical activity benefits these three aspects of your health.

Physical	Mental/ Emotional	Social

Vocabulary

physical activity
physical fitness
exercise
sedentary

BIG IDEA Being physically active benefits your total health in a variety of ways.

REAL LIFE ISSUES

Trying Something New. Nina and Marianne have been best friends since grade school. When Marianne took up kickboxing last year, Nina was disappointed that her friend had a new activity that she didn't share. Marianne kept talking about how much she enjoyed her new sport and encouraging Nina to try it. In the beginning, Nina was hesitant, but she finally decided to take up the sport as well. Now the two friends have another activity they can enjoy together. *How do your friends affect your choice of sports and other physical activities? Describe an activity that someone you know has influenced you to try.*

After completing the lesson, review and analyze your response to the Real Life Issues question.

Physical Activity and Your Health

MAIN IDEA Physical activity benefits all aspects of your health.

If you could take just one step to improve your health, what would that be? Probably the most important step you could choose would be to lead a more physically active life. **Physical activity** is any form of movement that causes your body to use energy. It benefits just about every system in your body, and it also helps your mental/emotional and social health. Physical activity doesn't just mean "working out." It includes all kinds of activities that you do every day, such as walking to school, cleaning your room, or playing sports. There are lots of different ways to make physical activity a part of your life and enjoy all its health benefits.

Physical Benefits

Getting regular physical activity improves your **physical fitness**, which is the ability to carry out daily tasks easily and have enough reserve energy to respond to unexpected demands. The types of activities you choose can strengthen different parts of your body. For example, some activities can strengthen your muscles and bones, lower blood pressure, or breathe more efficiently.

You can achieve specific fitness goals through **exercise**. This is the purposeful physical activity that is planned, structured, and repetitive, and that improves or maintains physical fitness. However, all kinds of physical activity—not just exercise—will improve your health. Being physically active can help you maintain a healthy weight and reduce your risk of many serious diseases.

Teens should try to be active for at least 60 minutes each day. This may seem like a lot, but you don't have to do it all at once. Dividing the time into smaller segments will help you get in your 60 minutes throughout the day.

This illustration shows just a few of the ways physical activity makes your body stronger. **Which systems in your body benefit from regular physical activity?**

The Active Body

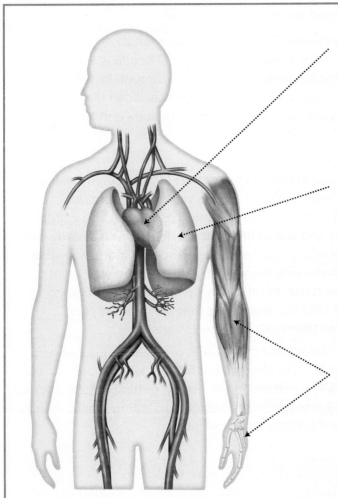

Cardiovascular System
Regular physical activity strengthens the heart muscle so that it pumps blood more efficiently. It reduces blood pressure and lowers the levels of artery-clogging cholesterol.

Respiratory System
As your activity level increases, your lungs begin to work more efficiently, pulling in larger amounts of air and increasing the amount of oxygen delivered to your body. As a result, you can do many activities more easily—for example, running a greater distance without becoming short of breath.

Musculoskeletal System
Physical activity strengthens muscles and bones, reducing your risk of developing fragile bones as you age. Strengthening your bones and muscles can also improve your balance and coordination.

Mental and Emotional Benefits

Being physically active does more than just maintain your physical health. It can also have a positive effect on your mental and emotional health.

- **Stress relief.** Have you ever noticed that you feel better after you exercise? Physical activity stimulates your body to produce chemicals called endorphins. This results in a feeling of well-being, aids relaxation, and relieves physical pain. Some types of physical activity, such as stretching, can also ease tension.

- **Mood enhancement.** If you're ever in a bad mood, try going for a walk. Chances are, you'll be in better spirits when you get home. Physical activity is a natural mood lifter. In addition to endorphins, it promotes the production of other brain chemicals that combat anxiety and depression. For this reason, people with anxiety and depression are advised to get regular physical activity.

- **Better sleep.** Do you get enough rest at night? Research studies have shown that most teens don't get nearly as much sleep as their bodies need. Moderate activity at least three hours before bedtime helps you relax and get to sleep more easily.

- **Improved self-esteem.** Think of the health triangle: If you feel better physically, your mental/emotional and social health will also improve. The physical fitness you develop through increased activity can translate to more self-confidence. It can give you a sense of accomplishment and also help you look and feel your best.

Reading Check

Explain How does physical activity benefit your mental and emotional health?

Social Benefits

Are you a member of a sports team at school? Do you enjoy hiking or exploring trails in nearby parks? If so, you've probably formed friendships through these activities. Physical activity can be a great way to make new friends and spend time with the friends you already have. Being active as part of a group can make exercising more enjoyable. Getting physical activity with friends can also motivate you to get exercise on a regular basis, or on days when you may not want to exercise. It can also help you learn skills that will improve your relationships, such as teamwork and sportsmanship.

The increased self-esteem that comes with physical fitness can help your social life as well. It can give you confidence when meeting new people or dealing with social situations. Finally, getting regular physical activity can help you manage stress, rather than letting it build up until it has a negative impact on your relationships.

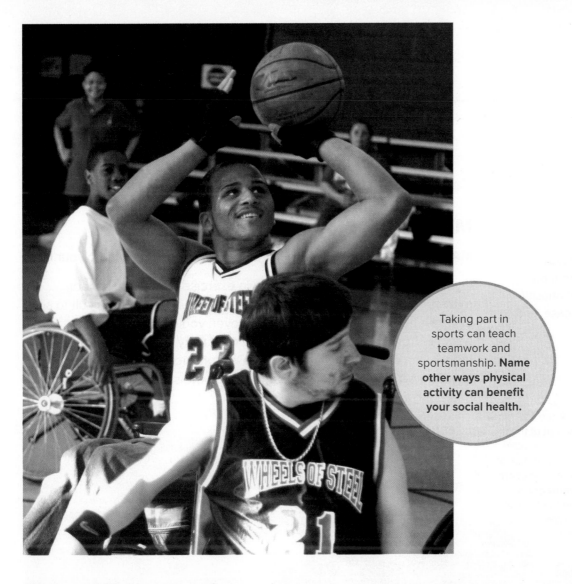

Taking part in sports can teach teamwork and sportsmanship. **Name other ways physical activity can benefit your social health.**

Risks of Being Inactive

MAIN IDEA An inactive lifestyle puts you at risk for a variety of health problems.

Despite the many benefits of physical activity, many teens still lead **sedentary** lives. A sedentary lifestyle involves little physical activity. Sedentary teens may **devote** their free time watching TV, playing video games, or on the Internet. Although everyone should spend some time on these activities, the amount of time should be limited. Being sedentary puts you at risk for a variety of health problems. These include:

- unhealthful weight gain and obesity.
- cardiovascular disease, such as heart attack and stroke.
- type 2 diabetes.
- certain types of cancer.
- asthma and other breathing problems.

Realistic Reflections

- osteoporosis, a condition in which the bones become porous and fragile, making them much more likely to break.

- osteoarthritis, a condition caused by the breakdown of cartilage and bone in the body's joints.

- psychological problems such as stress, anxiety, and depression.

Reading Check

Identify Problems and Solutions How can teens reduce their risk of obesity, cardiovascular disease, and type 2 diabetes?

Making Time for Physical Activity

MAIN IDEA There are several ways to fit physical activity into your life.

If your lifestyle is a busy one, fitting in exercise along with school, extracurricular activities, and other interests may make it difficult to set aside an hour a day for exercise. However, you can get the same benefits from several shorter periods of activity spread out over the course of a day. Try to fit in 10 minutes of physical activity six times a day. Shorter bursts of activity can give you the same benefits as an hour-long workout.

Just by turning off the TV and getting out of the house for a little exercise, you can reduce your risk of health problems. **What are other advantages of participating in physical activities?**

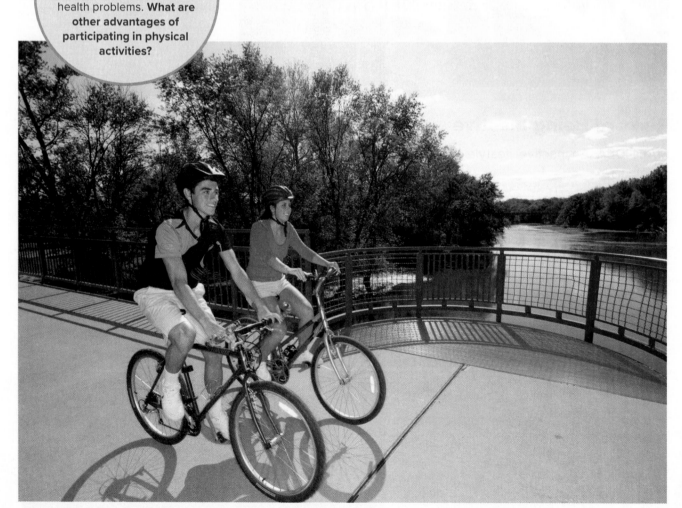

Jason Boyer Photography

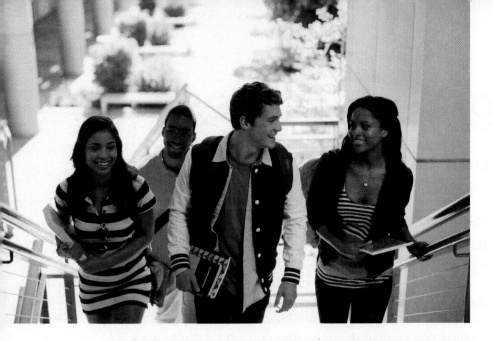

Paul Bradbury/age fotostock

Reading Check

Identify List two ways you can make time for physical activity.

Character Check

By participating in regular physical activity, you take responsibility for your health. By taking care of yourself, you are saying that you are worth investing in. Be positive about the benefits these activities bring you, and don't forget to compliment yourself: "I like how I feel, and I like how I look!"

ACTIVE ALTERNATIVES	
Instead of this . . .	**Try this . . .**
• Taking the elevator	• Taking the stairs
• Using a snowblower	• Shoveling snow
• Getting a ride to school or to a friend's house	• Walking, skating, or riding your bike
• Using a shopping cart	• Carrying your groceries to the car
• Taking the car through a car wash	• Washing the car by hand
• Playing video or computer games	• Playing basketball, soccer, or tennis

Lesson 1 Review

Facts and Vocabulary

1. What is the difference between physical activity and exercise?

2. Name three body systems that benefit from regular physical activity.

3. Identify two types of disease associated with a sedentary lifestyle.

Thinking Critically

4. **Analyze.** Explain how being physically active on a regular basis makes your body better able to respond to physical demands.

5. **Synthesize.** Camilla has a busy schedule and cannot find one hour a day for exercise. What advice would you give her?

Applying Health Skills

6. **Stress Management.** Raul feels stress from taking several honors classes and spending many hours doing homework. How can he incorporate physical activity into his schedule to reduce stress?

Writing Critically

7. **Expository.** Write a one-page essay describing what might influence a teen to choose a sedentary lifestyle. Suggest ways a teen can become physically active.

Improving Your Fitness

BEFORE YOU READ

Create a Comparison Chart. Draw a chart. Label the columns "Define," "Measure," and "Improve." Label the rows "C/E" (cardio endurance), "M/S" (muscular strength), "M/E" (muscular endurance) and "F" (flexibility). As you read, fill in your chart with information from the lesson.

	Define	Measure	Improve
C/E			
M/S			
M/E			
F			

Vocabulary

cardiorespiratory endurance
muscular strength
muscular endurance
flexibility
aerobic exercise
anaerobic exercise

Reading Check

Classify Which elements of fitness would help you run a marathon?

BIG IDEA Different types of exercise can help you evaluate and improve the various elements of fitness.

> ## REAL LIFE ISSUES
>
> **Building Fitness Levels.** Mel is in the process of training for a 12-mile charity run, which will take place in a few months. His goal is to run the whole race, but he has made it through only ten miles during his practice runs. He knows that in order to reach his goal, he will have to improve his cardiorespiratory endurance. *Think of a physically challenging goal that you would like to work toward. Write a short paragraph describing which elements of fitness you would need to focus on in order to meet that goal.*
>
> After completing the lesson, review and analyze your response to the Real Life Issues question.

Elements of Fitness

MAIN IDEA The five elements of fitness can affect your health in different ways.

What does it mean to be physically fit? Are you fit if you can run five miles or do a dozen push-ups in a row? Actually, these are just two of the four elements of fitness. They include endurance, strength, flexibility, and body composition. The endurance element of fitness includes two types, namely heart and lung endurance, and muscle endurance.

- **Cardiorespiratory endurance** is the ability of your heart, lungs, and blood vessels to send fuel and oxygen to your tissues during long periods of moderate to vigorous activity. It allows you to run a mile or go on a long hike without tiring. Good cardiorespiratory health also lowers your risk of cardiovascular disease.

- **Muscular strength** is the amount of force your muscles can exert. It is needed for all kinds of activities that put stress on your muscles, such as lifting, pushing, and jumping.

- **Muscular endurance** is the ability of your muscles to perform physical tasks over a period of time without tiring. It gives you the power to carry out daily tasks without fatigue, such as carrying boxes up and down a flight of stairs.

- **Flexibility** is the ability to move your body parts through their full range of motion. It allows you to touch your toes without bending your legs. Being flexible can improve your performance in many sports and reduce your risk of muscle strain and other injuries.

- Body composition is the ratio of fat to lean tissue in your body. It is also an element of fitness. Having low overall body fat lowers your risk of cardiovascular disease and other health problems.

Evaluating Your Fitness

MAIN IDEA You can use different tests to evaluate each element of your fitness.

So how fit are you? If you're not sure how to answer that, the following tests may help. Each of the tests described below measures a different element of fitness.

Measuring Cardiorespiratory Endurance

You can evaluate your cardiorespiratory endurance with a three-minute step test. You will need a sturdy bench or step about 12 inches high and a watch or clock with a second hand. Follow this procedure:

1. Step up onto the bench with your right foot. Bring up your left foot. Step back down, right foot first, then left foot.

2. Continue stepping up and back down for three minutes. Try to maintain a steady pace of about 24 steps per minute.

3. After three minutes, take your pulse. Place two fingers of one hand on your opposite wrist. (Do not use your thumb, which has its own pulse.) Count the number of heartbeats you feel in 15 seconds. Multiply that number by four to find your pulse rate.

4. View the results below to see how you did on the test.

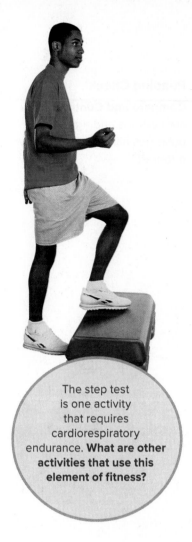

The step test is one activity that requires cardiorespiratory endurance. **What are other activities that use this element of fitness?**

FITNESS TEST SCORING CHART			
Step Test	**Partial Curl-Ups**	**Right-Angle Push-Ups**	**Sit-and-Reach Test**
Male teens: (heartbeats per minute): 85–95: Excellent 95–105: Good 105–126: Fair 126+: Needs improvement	Boys, ages 13–14: 21	Boys, age 14: 12 Boys, age 15: 14 Boys, age 16: 16 Boys, age 17: 18	Boys: 1 inch
Female teens: (heartbeats per minute): 85–95: Excellent 95–106: Good 106–126: Fair 126+: Needs improvement	Girls, ages 13–14: 18	Girls, ages 14–17: 7	Girls: 3 inches

Each of the columns below provides scores for the fitness tests. If you scored at or above the number shown for each of these three tests, you are in good shape. If you scored below the number shown, you need to work on that element of fitness.

Reading Check

Compare and Contrast How are curl-ups and right-angle push-ups alike? How are they different?

Measuring Muscular Strength and Endurance

All of the muscles in your body will benefit from regular exercise. Different muscle groups require different types of exercises. The two exercises below will test the strength and endurance of your abdominal muscles and upper body.

Partial Curl-Ups. Use the following procedure to measure your abdominal strength:

1. Lie on your back with your knees bent and your feet about 12 inches from your backside. Extend your arms forward with your fingers pointing toward your knees.

2. Raise your head and upper body off the floor, sliding your hands forward. Touch your knees with your fingertips. Slowly return to your original position.

3. Continue doing curl-ups at a rate of one every three seconds until you can no longer maintain this pace.

4. View the results below to see how you did on the test.

Good scores are:

Boys, ages 13–14: 21 or more partial curl-ups

Girls, ages 13–14: 18 or more partial curl-ups

If you score below this number, you need to work on abdominal strength and endurance.

Right-Angle Push-Ups. To test your upper body strength and endurance, do right-angle push-ups:

1. Lie facedown in the push-up position. Place your hands under your shoulders, with your legs parallel to each other and resting on your toes.

2. Straighten your arms and push up. Keep your back and arms straight. Bend your arms and lower your body until your elbows form a 90-degree angle, with your upper arms parallel to the floor.

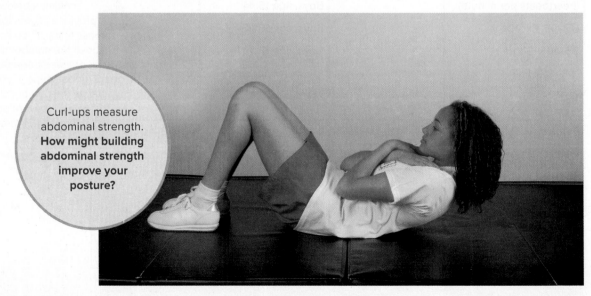

Curl-ups measure abdominal strength. **How might building abdominal strength improve your posture?**

McGraw-Hill Education

3. Continue doing one push-up every three seconds until you can no longer maintain this pace.

4. View the results below to see how you did on the test.

Good scores are:

Boys, age 14: 12 or more push-ups

Boys, age 15: 14 or more push-ups

Boys, age 16: 16 or more push-ups

Boys, age 17: 18 or more push-ups

Girls, ages 14-17: 7 or more push-ups

If you score below this number, you need to work on upper body strength and endurance.

Measuring Flexibility

The sit-and-reach test measures the flexibility of your lower back and hamstring muscles. To set up the test, tape a yardstick to the top of a box with 9 inches protruding over one end. Place the box against a wall, or ask someone to hold the box in place with the yardstick pointing out.

1. Remove your shoes and sit on the floor. Place the sole of one foot flat against the side of the box under the yardstick. Bend the other leg at the knee.

2. Extend your arms over the yardstick, with your hands placed one on top of the other, palms down.

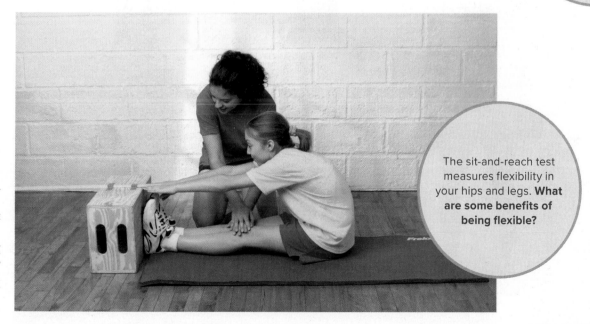

Right-angle push-ups are a way of measuring upper body strength and endurance. **What other activities require upper body strength and endurance?**

The sit-and-reach test measures flexibility in your hips and legs. **What are some benefits of being flexible?**

3. Reach forward in this manner four times. The fourth time, hold the position for at least one second while a partner records how far you can reach.

4. Switch legs and repeat the test.

5. View the results below to see how you did on the test.

Good scores are:

Boys: 1 inch

Girls: 3 inches

If you score below this number, you need to work on your flexibility.

Getting Fit

MAIN IDEA Different forms of exercise will improve various elements of fitness.

Most exercises fall into two basic categories. Jogging, swimming, and riding a bike are examples of **aerobic exercise**. These are rhythmic activities that use large muscle groups for an extended **period** of time. They raise your heart rate and increase your body's use of oxygen. Over time, your heart and lungs adapt to the increased demands. They will begin to work more efficiently. This helps you build cardiorespiratory endurance. Getting regular aerobic exercise will reduce your risk of cardiovascular disease. It also helps you manage your weight. The Real World Connection explains how to find your target heart rate when doing aerobic exercise.

ACADEMIC VOCABULARY

period *(noun)*: the completion of a cycle

Lifting weights is one form of resistance or strength training. **What are the benefits of strength training?**

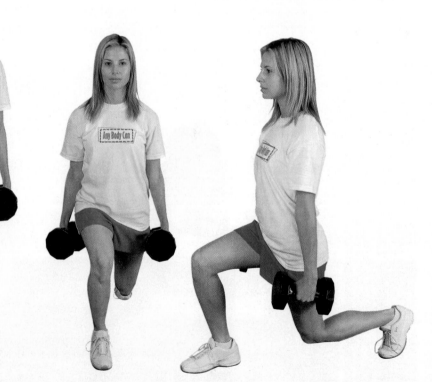

Anaerobic exercise involves intense, short bursts of activity in which the muscles work so hard that they produce energy without using oxygen. Exercises like sprinting or lifting weights can improve your muscular strength and endurance. The more the muscles work, the stronger they will become. Exercises that strengthen the muscles are known as resistance or strength training. The three types of resistance exercises are:

- Isometric exercises that use muscle tension to improve strength with little or no movement of the body part. Pushing against a wall or other immovable object is an example of isometric exercise.

- Isotonic exercises combine movement of the joints with contraction of the muscles. Try lifting free-weights or doing calisthenics, such as pull-ups, push-ups, and sit-ups. These exercises build flexibility as well as strength.

- Isokinetic exercises exert resistance against a muscle as it moves through a range of motion at a steady rate of speed. Various types of weight machines and other exercise equipment provide isokinetic exercise.

Free weights, exercise machines, and your own body weight can all provide resistance that will build muscle. Strength training can also help with weight control because it increases your body's muscle mass. This makes your body use energy faster.

Both aerobic and anaerobic exercise can help strengthen your bones. Any weight-bearing activity, in which your body must work against gravity, can increase bone density and lower your risk of osteoporosis. Strength training, walking, and dancing are all weight-bearing exercises.

One other type of exercise is stretching. It can improve your flexibility, circulation, posture, and coordination, as well as ease stress. It may also lower your risk of injury during other activities. Do stretching exercises slowly, holding each stretch for 10 to 30 seconds without bouncing. If you feel pain, you've pushed too far.

Reading Check

Identify What kind of exercise helps improve bone strength?

Myths & Reality

Do you think you know all there is to know about physical fitness? This fact might prove you wrong.

Myth: Running is the best way to become physically fit.

Reality: There is no best exercise for becoming physically fit. A variety of exercises should be used to address each of the five elements of fitness.

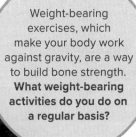

Weight-bearing exercises, which make your body work against gravity, are a way to build bone strength. **What weight-bearing activities do you do on a regular basis?**

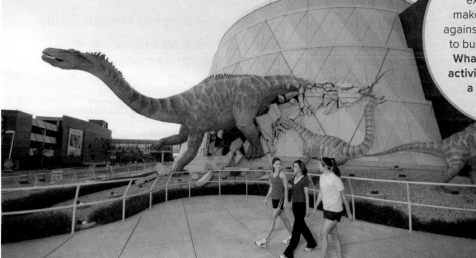

Jason Boyer Photography

Targeting Cardiovascular Fitness

Your target heart range is the ideal range during aerobic activity. To calculate your target heart range:

1. Multiply your age by 0.7.

2. Subtract this number from 208 to get an estimate of your maximum heart rate. If you are 16 years old, your maximum heart rate will be 197 beats per minute.

3. Multiply this number by 50 percent to get your minimum heart rate for moderately intense activity.

4. Multiply the number in step 2 by 70 percent to get your maximum heart rate for moderately intense activity and the minimum for vigorous activity.

5. Multiply the number in step 2 by 85 percent to get your maximum target heart rate for any physical activity. Exercising above this rate is dangerous.

6. To figure out your heart rate during exercise, take your pulse for six seconds and multiply the result by 10.

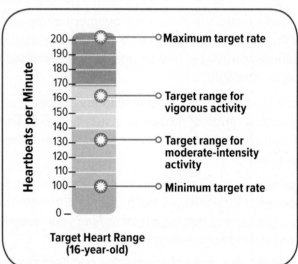

Target Heart Range (16-year-old)

Activity: Mathematics

Calculate your target heart range for moderate activity and for vigorous activity. Explain how you would adjust your activity level to stay within your target range for walking, running, and sprints.

CONCEPT Operations and Algebraic Thinking

To solve this problem, change the percent to a fraction or to a decimal, and then multiply by the number.

Lesson 2 Review

Facts and Vocabulary

1. What are the five elements of fitness?

2. Which element of fitness does the sit-and-reach test measure?

3. What kind of exercise would you do to improve your cardiorespiratory endurance?

Thinking Critically

4. Analyze. How will your target heart range for physical activity change as you grow older? Explain why.

5. Evaluate. Carmen wants to get in shape. She is planning to join a gym and use only the weight machines. Is this a good plan? Why or why not?

Applying Health Skills

6. Goal Setting. Create and perform a plan to improve your cardiorespiratory endurance.

Writing Critically

7. Personal. Create a fitness journal to track your food intake, calories consumed, and energy expended for one week. Analyze your results.

Planning a Personal Activity Program

BIG IDEA Planning your physical activity can help you achieve specific fitness goals.

REAL LIFE ISSUES

Getting Fit. Pete wants to get in better shape. He has decided to create a fitness plan, but he's not sure where to start. He's not even sure he knows how to determine what a good level of fitness is. He doesn't know what exercises to do, how often he should do them, or how long he should do them. *If you were Pete, what steps would you take to create an appropriate fitness plan? In a paragraph, describe the steps you would take.*

After completing the lesson, review and analyze your response to the Real Life Issues question.

Your Fitness Plan

MAIN IDEA When choosing physical activities, think about your fitness goals and activities you enjoy.

If you want to improve your physical fitness, setting a specific fitness goal can help get you motivated. You can develop a plan to reach your goal based on your personal needs, such as your current level of fitness and the resources you have available.

Your Fitness Goals

Measuring your level of fitness can help you set fitness goals. If you learned that you have good cardiorespiratory endurance but not much upper body strength, you could make building upper body strength your goal.

Personal Needs

When planning a personal activity program, try choosing activities that you enjoy and that you can realistically do. Several factors that may affect your activity choices include:

- **Cost.** Some activities require expensive equipment. It may make sense to borrow or rent equipment, rather than buying it, when you try a new sport.

BEFORE YOU READ

Create Vocabulary Cards. Write each new vocabulary term on a separate note card. For each term, write a definition based on your current knowledge. As you read, fill in additional information related to each term.

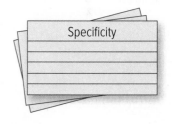
Specificity

Vocabulary
specificity
overload
progression
warm-up
workout
cool-down
resting heart rate

- **Where you live.** Is your local area flat or hilly? What is the climate like? Factors like these will affect the activities that you can do close to home.

- **Your schedule.** If you like to sleep late, planning to jog every morning will probably fail. Choose activities that fit your schedule and habits.

- **Your health and fitness level.** Do you have a health condition that may affect your exercise plan, such as asthma? If so, talk to your doctor before starting a new activity. In any case, start slowly and choose activities that are right for your level of fitness.

- **Personal safety.** When choosing activities, make sure that you have a safe environment to perform them in. For instance, you should not go running on busy streets with no sidewalks.

Types of Activities

Are you someone who enjoys competition? Do you prefer lone activities where your goal is to improve your individual performance? Choosing a variety of activities will help you meet specific fitness goals and keep you from getting bored. An exercise plan can include non-competitive activities such as walking, hiking, or playing a pickup basketball or soccer game with friends, as well as other organized school or community sports.

Reading Check

Determine When might it be important to consult a doctor before trying a new physical activity?

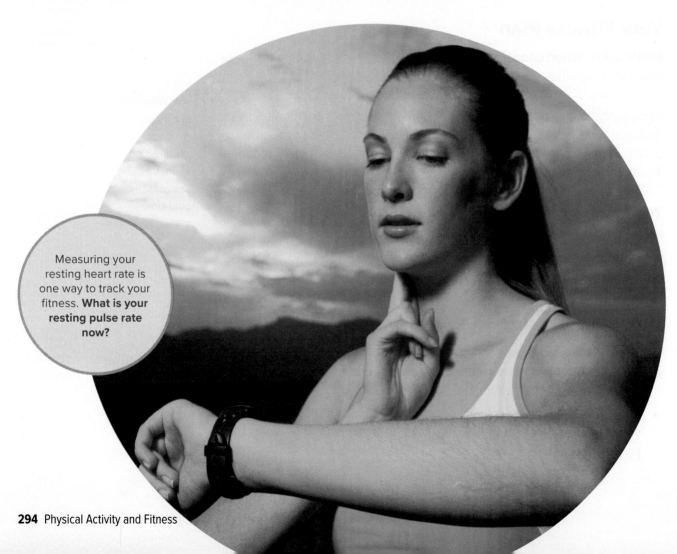

Measuring your resting heart rate is one way to track your fitness. **What is your resting pulse rate now?**

Tetra Images/SuperStock

Sedentary activities, which don't involve much movement, should be limited to a small part of your day. Teens should aim to get at least 60 minutes of physical activity every day, or at least most days. You can include the following types of activity in your fitness plan:

Moderate-Intensity Physical Activities. These count toward your daily dose of physical activity. Examples include walking, climbing stairs, household chores, and yard work.

Aerobic Activities. These activities raise your heat rate. Aim for at least three 20-minute sessions per week of vigorous aerobic activity. Examples include cycling, brisk walking, running, dancing, in-line skating, cross-country skiing, and most team sports.

Strength Training. This develops muscle tone. Aim for at least two or three sessions per week of 20 to 30 minutes each, with at least one day off between sessions. Exercises that tone arm muscles include rowing, cross-country skiing, pull-ups, and push-ups. To tone legs, try cycling, running, or skating. Abdominal muscles can be toned by rowing or cycling and by doing abdominal crunches.

Flexibility Exercises. You can boost your flexibility by stretching for 10 to 12 minutes a day. Other flexibility exercises include gymnastics, martial arts, ballet, Pilates, and yoga.

Principles of Building Fitness

MAIN IDEA Effective fitness programs focus on four principles: specificity, overload, progression, and regularity.

When designing a physical activity program, you will start by considering your needs and interests. However, you should also pay attention to the four key principles of building a fitness plan: specificity, overload, progression, and regularity.

Specificity. This means choosing the right types of activities to improve a given element of fitness. Different types of activities will improve different elements of fitness. For example, aerobic activities such as running or swimming will improve your cardiorespiratory endurance. Strength-training activities such as weight lifting will build muscular strength.

Overload. This means exercising at a level that's beyond your regular daily activities. You must push your body beyond its normal level to increase fitness. As you increase the demands on your body, it will adapt by growing stronger.

Progression. This means gradually increasing the demands on your body. To continue building fitness, you must continue to raise the demands on your body. Try working a little harder or longer during each session or working out more often during the week.

Regularity. This means working out on a regular basis. You need at least three balanced workouts a week to maintain your fitness level. Include different activities to get the recommended hour of physical activity each day.

Reading Check

Make Inferences Why do you need to increase the demands on your body over time to build fitness?

ACADEMIC VOCABULARY

instance *(verb)*: to mention as a case or example

Reading Check

Explain What is the purpose of a warm-up?

Stages of a Workout

MAIN IDEA An exercise session has three stages: warm-up, workout, and cool-down.

Now that you've defined your fitness goals, chosen your activities, and scheduled time to do them, it's time to get moving. To get your body ready for physical activity and to avoid injuries, include three stages in every exercise session: the warm-up, the workout, and the cool-down.

Warm-Up

A **warm-up** is gentle cardiovascular activity that prepares the muscles for work. Warming up before exercise increases blood flow, delivering needed oxygen and fuel to your muscles. It also gradually increases your pulse rate and body temperature. To warm up, choose an activity that will work the same muscles you're going to use during your workout. For **instance**, before a run, warm up by walking or jogging slowly.

Check your resting heart rate. After warming up your muscles, take a few minutes to stretch. Stretching can prepare your muscles for activity and increase your flexibility.

Workout

The **workout** is the part of an exercise session when you are exercising at your highest peak. There are four factors to consider when planning a workout. You can remember them by using the F.I.T.T. formula:

- **F: Frequency of workouts.** Schedule at least three exercise sessions a week, but give your body time to rest between workouts. Include other types of physical activity during the week to get an hour of activity each day.

- **I: Intensity of workouts.** Push yourself hard enough to create overload. For aerobic activities, exercise within your target heart rate range. Check your heart rate during your workout. For strength training, you should feel strain on your muscles, but not pain.

- **T: Type of activity.** Vary your activities throughout the week to build different elements of fitness. If you jog Monday and Wednesday, try lifting weights on Tuesday and Thursday.

- **Time (duration) of workouts.** To build cardiovascular fitness, keep your heart rate within your target range for at least 20 minutes. Strength-training sessions should take 20 to 30 minutes, while flexibility can be increased in just 10 minutes of stretching.

Cool-Down

A **cool-down** is low-level activity that prepares your body to return to a resting state. The cool-down allows your heart rate, breathing, and body temperature to return to normal gradually. It also helps prevent muscle soreness. A cool-down should include five to ten minutes of gentle activity. This is also a good time for stretching.

Tracking Your Progress

MAIN IDEA Track your progress to see how your fitness level increases over time.

One of the rewards of sticking to a physical activity program is seeing your level of fitness improve over time. You may notice that it takes you less time to walk to and from school, for instance, or you may not breathe as hard when climbing stairs.

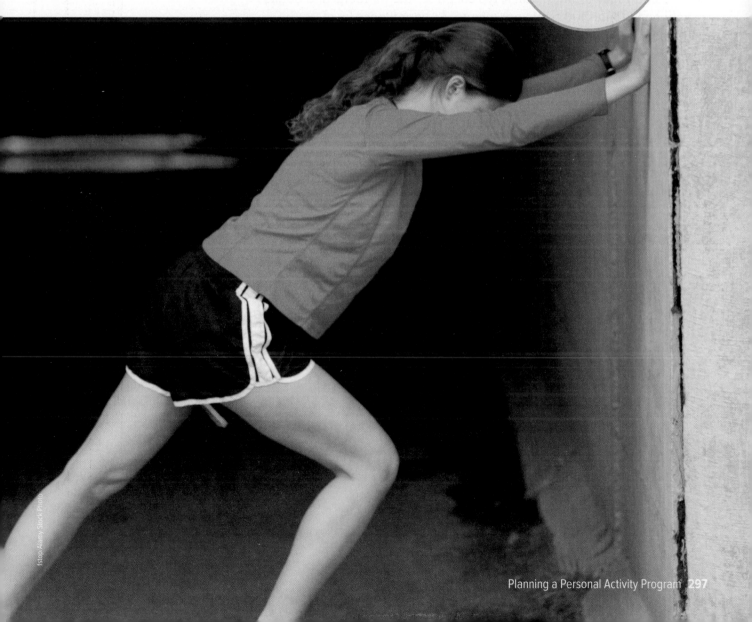

Stretching your muscles helps prevent injuries. **What stage of a workout is the best time for stretching?**

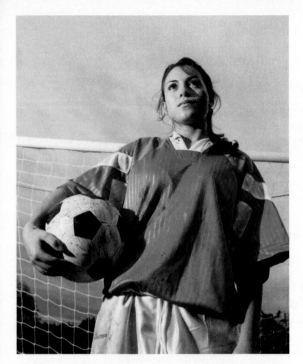

Use a fitness journal, pedometer, or other device to track your progress. List all of your activities, noting how long you work out, how often, and at what level. You'll see a noticeable difference in your fitness level if you stick to your plan for 12 weeks.

Another figure to list in your fitness journal is your **resting heart rate**. This is the number of times your heart beats per minute when you are not active. Before checking your resting heart rate, sit quietly for at least five minutes. Take your pulse for 15 seconds, then multiply the result by four. A typical pulse rate for teens and adults is between 60 and 100 beats per minute. As your fitness level increases, your resting heart rate will drop.

Reading Check

Cause and Effect How does regular exercise affect your resting heart rate?

Fitness Zone

My goal this year is to get in great shape, so I started keeping a journal of what I eat and when I work out. With a journal it's easier to stick with my plan because I know exactly what I have to do. My success has kept me motivated.

Lesson 3 Review

Facts and Vocabulary

1. What personal factors can affect your choice of physical activities?

2. What are the four principles of building fitness?

3. What are the benefits of warming up before exercise and cooling down after exercise?

Thinking Critically

4. **Synthesize.** What activity might you choose if your fitness goals are to increase cardiorespiratory endurance and strengthen your leg and abdominal muscles?

5. **Analyze.** How does where you live affect your choice of activities?

Applying Health Skills

6. **Analyzing Influences.** Draw five columns on a sheet of paper, labeled: "Cost," "Location," "Schedule," "Health," and "Safety." Add examples of how each influence might affect your physical activity choices.

Writing Critically

7. **Narrative.** Write a short story about a teen who designs and begins a fitness plan. List three fitness goals for this teen. Describe the types of activities the teen has chosen.

Fitness Safety and Avoiding Injuries

BIG IDEA It is important to learn how to prevent injuries and respond to them when they occur.

REAL LIFE ISSUES

Preventing Injuries. Children and teens have the highest rates of nonfatal bicycle injuries. Observing safety rules and always wearing a helmet while riding a bicycle will protect your life. *Write a paragraph encouraging a friend to use safety equipment when riding a bicycle.*

After completing the lesson, review and analyze your response to the Real Life Issues question.

Safety First

MAIN IDEA Safety precautions can help you avoid injuries during physical activity.

Regular physical activity keeps you healthy, but it does pose some safety risks. Getting a health screening before you start a physical activity program can identify diseases and disorders that could make some activities unsafe for you. Other ways to protect yourself include:

- using the right safety equipment.
- paying attention to your environment.
- warming up before exercise and cooling down afterwards.
- staying within the areas designated for a given sport or activity.
- following all rules and restrictions.
- avoid overtraining or overuse injuries.
- practicing good sportsmanship.
- getting help immediately if you do become ill or injured.

The Right Equipment

Using the correct equipment can prevent sports injuries. Examples of protective equipment include:

- **Clothing.** Wear well-fitting athletic shoes that are designed for your sport or activity. Wear socks to cushion your feet and keep them dry. Choose comfortable, non-binding clothes that are appropriate for the weather.

BEFORE YOU READ

Create a T-Chart. Make a two-column chart on paper. Label the left column "Risks" and the right column "Prevention." As you read, fill in information about safety risks involved in different physical activities and prevention steps you can take to protect yourself.

Risks	Prevention

Vocabulary
frostbite
hypothermia
overexertion
heat exhaustion
heatstroke
muscle cramps
strains
sprains

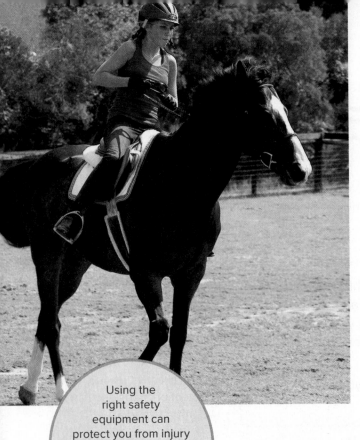

Using the right safety equipment can protect you from injury during physical activity. **What type of safety equipment is required for your favorite sport?**

- **Cycling gear.** For cycling, always wear a helmet that fits you properly. Make sure the helmet is approved by Snell or the American National Standards Institute (ANSI). If you must ride at night, make sure your bike has front and rear reflectors. Also, wear light-colored clothing with reflective patches.

- **Skating gear.** For skating or skateboarding, wear a helmet, knee and elbow pads, gloves, and wrist guards.

- **Male and female protection.** For contact sports, male players should wear a cup to protect the groin. For non-contact sports that involve running, they should wear an athletic supporter. Female players should wear supportive sports bras.

- **Adaptive equipment.** Special adaptive equipment helps players with disabilities take part in a variety of sports, from bowling and golf to skiing.

Watching the Weather

The weather can also affect your safety during exercise. Check weather conditions to decide how to dress for a workout outside. During some weather conditions you should avoid exercising outside. Examples of these conditions include during thunderstorms and blizzards.

Cold-Weather Risks. If you have asthma, always talk to your doctor before beginning to exercise outside during cold weather. Some specific steps that everyone can take to protect yourself in cold weather include the following:

- Dress in layers to stay warm. You can remove layers as you warm up or add more layers as the temperature drops. Adding or removing clothing will help to regulate your body temperature. The Cold-Weather Layering example shows how to layer clothing for warmth. Click on each article of clothing to learn more about it.

- Warm up and cool down, even in cold weather.

- Drink plenty of fluids. Cold air can lead to dehydration, or excessive loss of water from the body.

- Cover your nose and mouth to avoid breathing cold, dry air.

Two particular health risks of cold weather are **frostbite** and **hypothermia**. Frostbite is damage to the skin and tissues caused by extreme cold. It makes the skin pale, hard and numb. To treat frostbite, go to a warm place and thaw the affected areas with warm (not hot) water. As the skin thaws, it will become red and painful. If the frostbite is severe or does not respond to treatment, seek medical help. Frostbite and hypothermia can affect teens living in warmer climates too. If temperatures fall into a range that is extremely cold for the region, remember to dress in layers.

Ed-Imaging

Cold-Weather Layering

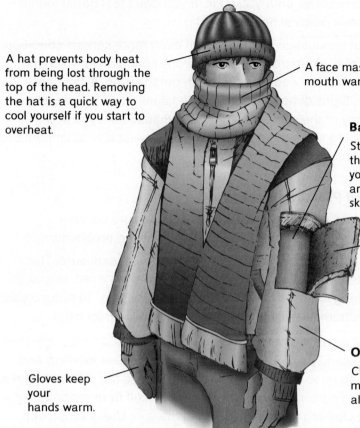

A hat prevents body heat from being lost through the top of the head. Removing the hat is a quick way to cool yourself if you start to overheat.

A face mask or scarf worn over the mouth warms the air you breathe.

Base layer

Start with a thin layer of a material that will pull moisture away from your body. Many synthetic fabrics are specially designed to keep the skin dry.

Insulating layer

The next layer should provide insulation. Wool and synthetic fleece fabrics can help keep you warm even when they are wet.

Outer layer

Choose a waterproof, breathable material that will block wind while allowing moisture to escape.

Gloves keep your hands warm.

Hypothermia is dangerously low body temperature and occurs as a result of **exposure** to extreme cold, submersion in cold water, or wearing wet clothing in cold or windy weather. Hypothermia causes drowsiness, weakness, and confusion. Breathing and heart rate slow down, and shock and heart failure can result. This condition calls for emergency medical help. Try to warm the victim until help arrives.

Hot-Weather Risks. Exercising in hot weather also has risks. Heavy sweating while exercising in hot weather can lead to dehydration. Drinking fluids before, during, and after physical activity can prevent dehydration. If you're exercising during hot weather, you may also need to replace sodium, chloride, and potassium. Sports drinks can help your body replace these elements.

Hot-weather health problems may lead to **overexertion**, or overworking the body. This can cause **heat exhaustion**, a form of physical stress on the body caused by overheating. Its symptoms include:

- heavy sweating.
- cold, clammy skin.
- dizziness, confusion, or fainting.
- a weak, rapid pulse.
- cramps.
- shortness of breath.
- nausea and vomiting.

ACADEMIC VOCABULARY

exposure *(noun)*: the condition of being unprotected

To recover, rest in a shady area, spray or douse yourself with cold water, and blow or fan cool air onto your skin. If you don't feel better within half an hour, seek medical help.

Untreated heat exhaustion can lead to an even more serious condition called **heatstroke**. Heatstroke is a dangerous condition in which the body loses its ability to cool itself through perspiration. It can cause sudden death. Signs of heatstroke include fainting and hot, dry skin, along with many of the symptoms of heat exhaustion. If you see someone showing signs of heatstroke, call for medical help immediately and try to cool the person.

Sun and Wind Protection

Sun and wind can pose a hazard in both hot and cold weather. Exposure to these elements can cause the following problems:

- Windburn is irritation of the skin caused by wind exposure. The skin's protective oil layer is stripped away, leaving it red, dry, and sore. Rubbing lotion into the skin can ease the pain. To reduce your risk of windburn, keep your skin covered and wear lip balm.

- Sunburn is a burning of the skin's outer layers. Mild sunburn makes the skin red and painful. Severe sunburn can cause swelling and blistering. To ease the pain, cool and moisturize the skin and take a mild analgesic pain reliever. To protect yourself from sunburn, wear protective clothing when exercising in the sun. Use a sunscreen with a sun protection factor (SPF) of 15 or more, and reapply it often. Avoid exercising outside when the sun's rays are most intense.

- Skin cancer can result from repeated or prolonged sun exposure. Broad-spectrum sunscreens provide protection by blocking ultraviolet A (UVA) rays, the part of sunlight that leads to skin cancer.

- Eye damage is another health risk that can be caused by exposure to ultraviolet (UV) rays. To protect yourself, wear sunglasses and a broad-brimmed hat in the summer. For winter sports, you may choose UV-absorbing goggles.

Reading Check

Identify Problems and Solutions Name three health problems that can result from exercising in hot weather and explain how to prevent them.

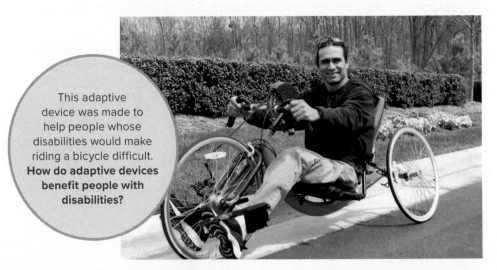

This adaptive device was made to help people whose disabilities would make riding a bicycle difficult. **How do adaptive devices benefit people with disabilities?**

Realistic Reflections

Coping with Injuries

MAIN IDEA You can treat minor sports injuries yourself, but major injuries require professional medical treatment.

Even if you follow safety measures, it is still possible to be injured during exercise. Overuse injuries are common among people who are just beginning a fitness program. Doing more may seem like it will help you achieve your fitness goals faster. Overtraining or overuse, however, can result in injuries that prevent you from reaching your fitness milestones. One common overtraining or overuse condition is **muscle cramps**. When injuries occur, give your body time to heal before resuming your workouts. Minor injuries can generally be treated at home. Try using the P.R.I.C.E. procedure. P.R.I.C.E. stands for Protection, Rest, Ice, Compression, and Elevation:

- **Protect** the affected area with a bandage or splint to prevent further injury.

- **Rest** the muscle or joint for at least a day. Avoid all activities that cause pain or limping. Use crutches to walk if necessary. Keep pressure off the injured area until the pain is gone. Then gradually ease back into using the affected muscle or joint.

- **Ice** the affected area for 10 to 15 minutes at a time, three times a day for two days after the injury. Wrap the ice in a cloth first; do not apply ice directly to your skin. If the joint is still swollen after two days, see your doctor.

- **Compress** the affected area to reduce swelling. An Ace bandage makes a good compress. Wrap it firmly, but not so tightly that you reduce the circulation. If the area feels cold or becomes discolored, loosen the bandage.

- **Elevate** the injured area to keep the swelling down. If possible, keep it raised above the level of your heart.

Minor Injuries

Muscles may become sore after exercise. Applying ice and taking pain relievers can help. Below are some examples of minor injuries related to exercise:

- **Muscle soreness.** Muscles may become sore after exercise. Applying ice and taking pain relievers can help.

- **Blisters.** A blister is a fluid-filled bump caused by friction. Well-fitting shoes and athletic socks can prevent blisters. To treat blisters, cover the blistered area to protect the blisters while they heal. Do not pop them.

- **Muscle cramps.** Cramps can occur when muscles are tired, overworked, or dehydrated. Stretching the affected muscle will usually relieve the cramps.

Reading Check

Explain What are the steps of the P.R.I.C.E. procedure?

● ● ● ● ● ● ● ● ● ●

Myths & Reality

Everyone seems to have a different way of treating injuries, but sometimes, they might be mistaken. What do you think about this myth?

Myth: Putting heat on injuries makes them heal better and faster.

Reality: Placing heat on the injury does not address those problems and may make them worse. Icing an injury will reduce swelling and inflammation.

● ● ● ● ● ● ● ● ● ●

- **Strains.** A strain can result from overstretching and tearing of a muscle. The symptoms of a strain are pain, swelling, and difficulty moving the affected muscle. To reduce the risk of strained muscles, warm up before exercise. Strains can be treated with the P.R.I.C.E. procedure.

- **Sprains.** A sprain is an injury to the ligament around a joint. Sprains causes pain, swelling, and stiffness. Use the P.R.I.C.E. procedure to treat minor sprains. If it hurts to move your joint, or you can't put weight on it, see a doctor.

- **Tendonitis.** Exercise can cause swelling and inflammation in the tendons, the bands of fiber that connect muscles to bones. Treatment may include rest, medication, physical therapy, and in rare cases, surgery.

Major Injuries

Some exercise-related injuries are more serious and require medical care. Here are a few examples of major injuries:

- **Fractures,** or broken bones, cause severe pain, swelling, bruising, and bleeding. If someone has broken a bone, get medical help immediately. Do not move the victim.

The P.R.I.C.E. Procedure

P.R.I.C.E. stands for Protection, Rest, Ice, Compression, and Elevation.

Protect the affected area with a bandage or splint to prevent further injury.

Rest the muscle or joint for at least a day. Avoid all activities that cause pain or limping. Use crutches to walk if necessary. Keep pressure off the injured area until the pain is gone. Then gradually ease back into using the affected muscle or joint.

Ice the affected area for 10 to 15 minutes at a time, three times a day for two days after the injury. Wrap the ice in a cloth first; do not apply ice directly to your skin. If the joint is still swollen after two days, see your doctor.

Compress the affected area to reduce swelling. An Ace bandage makes a good compress. Wrap it firmly, but not so tightly that you reduce the circulation. If the area feels cold or becomes discolored, loosen the bandage.

Elevate the injured area to keep the swelling down. If possible, keep it raised above the level of your heart.

McGraw-Hill Education

- **Dislocations** occur when a bone pops out of its normal position in a joint. The joint will be painful and may appear misshapen. Call for help immediately.

- **Concussion,** an injury to the brain, can result in a severe headache, unconsciousness, or memory loss. A severe concussion can cause brain damage. Signs of brain damage include vomiting, confusion, seizures, or weakness on one side of the body. If any of these symptoms occur, seek medical help immediately.

REAL WORLD CONNECTION

Playing It Safe

Sports and other recreational activities are some of the most common causes of injury among teens. These injuries could be prevented if teens followed guidelines and safety precautions, and used the proper safety equipment for their sport.

Activity: Technology

In groups, choose a sport or recreational activity and conduct an online search. Use reliable online sources such as the Centers for Disease Control and Prevention (CDC) to find injury statistics, precautions for avoiding injuries, and types of protective equipment for this sport. Use your research to create a blog or web page that educates teens about how injuries occur in the sport that your group has chosen, and how to stay safe. Show examples of some protective equipment. Ask for permission to post the group's blog or web page on the school's website.

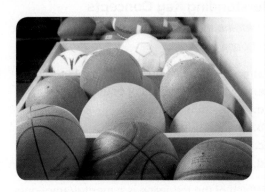

Lesson 4 Review

Facts and Vocabulary

1. What is the purpose of a health screening? How can it prevent injury during physical activity?

2. How should frostbite be treated?

3. Name three symptoms of heat exhaustion.

Thinking Critically

4. **Analyze.** What distinguishes major injuries from minor injuries? How can you use the P.R.I.C.E. procedure to treat minor injuries?

5. **Synthesize.** Suppose you are playing catch with some friends, and one of them falls and injures his ankle. What do you do to treat the injury?

Applying Health Skills

6. **Practicing Healthful Behaviors.** Design a poster that illustrates the risks of sun and wind exposure. Include strategies for protecting yourself from these risks.

Writing Critically

7. **Expository.** Write a script for a one-minute public service announcement that summarizes the importance of using the correct sports equipment. Describe the risks of the injury.

LESSON 1

Vocabulary Review

Use the correct vocabulary term to complete the following statements.

1. _____ is the ability to carry out daily tasks easily.

2. To achieve specific fitness goals, use structured, purposeful physical activity, known as _____.

3. People whose lives include little physical activity can be described as _____.

Understanding Key Concepts

After reading the question or statement, select the correct answer.

4. Stronger muscles and bones, and greater energy, are examples of physical activity's
   a. physical benefits.
   b. mental benefits.
   c. emotional benefits.
   d. social benefits.

5. Which of the following is a mental/emotional benefit of physical activity?
   a. Lower blood pressure
   b. Better balance and coordination
   c. Reduced stress
   d. Forming new friendships

Thinking Critically

After reading the question or statement, write a short answer using complete sentences.

6. **Discuss.** Explain how physical activity can improve your social life.

7. **Identify.** Name two ways to fit physical activity into your daily life.

8. **Synthesize.** Give an example of how the physical, mental/emotional, and social benefits of physical activity are interrelated.

LESSON 2

Vocabulary Review

Choose the correct term in the sentences below.

9. Running a mile without stopping is a sign of good *cardiorespiratory endurance/ muscular endurance.*

10. *Muscular strength/ Flexibility* is the ability to move your body parts through their full range of motion.

11. Sprinting and lifting weights are examples of *aerobic exercise/anaerobic exercise.*

Understanding Key Concepts

After reading the question or statement, select the correct answer.

12. Which of the following is a good test of your cardiorespiratory fitness?
    a. The time it takes to run or walk a mile
    b. How many curl-ups you can do
    c. How heavy a weight you can lift
    d. Whether you can bend over and touch your toes

13. A healthy 30-year-old would have a target heart range between
    a. 60 and 120 beats per minute.
    b. 82 and 133 beats per minute.
    c. 94 and 159 beats per minute.
    d. 101 and 190 beats per minute.

14. Exercises to improve your flexibility are
    a. aerobic exercises.
    b. isometric exercises.
    c. isokinetic exercises.
    d. stretching exercises.

Thinking Critically

After reading the question or statement, write a short answer using complete sentences.

15. **Analyze.** Doing 50 curl-ups each day will improve what elements of fitness? What other activities can improve total fitness?

16. **Compare and Contrast.** Explain the different ways that aerobic and anaerobic exercise affect your body composition.

17. **Analyze.** Is swimming a good way to build bone mass? Why or why not?

LESSON 3

Vocabulary Review

Correct the sentences below by replacing the italicized term with the correct vocabulary term.

18. A *stretch* is gentle activity that prepares the muscles for work.

19. The part of an exercise session when you are exercising at your highest peak is called the *cool-down*.

20. Your *target heart rate* is the number of times your heart beats per minute when you are not active.

Understanding Key Concepts

After reading the question or statement, select the correct answer.

21. To build cardiovascular fitness, perform aerobic exercise at least
    a. twice a week for 20 minutes.
    b. three times a week for 20 minutes.
    c. five times a week for 10 minutes.
    d. one hour per day.

22. Which principle of building fitness involves gradually increasing the demands on your body?
    a. Specificity
    b. Overload
    c. Progression
    d. Regularity

23. If you have time to stretch only once during an exercise session, it's best to do it
    a. before warming up.
    b. after warming up.
    c. in the middle of your workout.
    d. while cooling down.

Thinking Critically

After reading the question or statement, write a short answer using complete sentences.

24. **Predict.** Explain what might happen if a teen builds a fitness plan around exercises that he or she strongly dislikes.

25. **Identify.** What are the four elements of the F.I.T.T. formula? How can the four elements help you become fit?

26. **Analyze.** How does your resting heart rate reflect your level of fitness?

LESSON 4

Vocabulary Review

Choose the correct word in the sentences below.

27. *Overexertion/Heatstroke* is a dangerous condition in which the body loses its ability to cool itself through perspiration.

28. *Frostbite/Hypothermia* is damage to the skin and tissues caused by extreme cold.

29. Injuries to the ligaments around a joint are known as *strains/sprains*.

Understanding Key Concepts

After reading the question or statement, select the correct answer.

30. Drowsiness, weakness, and slowed breathing and heart rate are symptoms of
    a. heat exhaustion.
    b. frostbite.
    c. hypothermia.
    d. concussion.

31. Stretching the affected muscle will usually relieve
   a. muscle cramps.
   b. strains.
   c. sprains.
   d. tendonitis.

32. Which of the following is *not* a major injury?
   a. Fracture
   b. Dislocation
   c. Concussion
   d. Sprain

Thinking Critically

After reading the question or statement, write a short answer using complete sentences.

33. Describe. What safety equipment is required for skating or skateboarding?

34. Explain. Why is it important to protect yourself from the sun during physical activity?

35. Describe. What are the steps in the P.R.I.C.E. procedure?

PROJECT-BASED ASSESSMENT

Staying Informed About Physical Fitness

BACKGROUND

Physical fitness is more than just doing exercise and maintaining a healthy, nutritious diet. Physical fitness requires being informed. Accurate information about the importance of physical activity helps individuals to make well-informed decisions about their health.

TASK

Develop a website for your school showing different activities that students can do to stay fit. Include group, team, and individual activities.

AUDIENCE

Students in your school

PURPOSE

Provide information on physical fitness to your peers.

PROCEDURE

1. Brainstorm and conduct an online search for activities that students can do to stay fit. Be sure to include information about clubs in school that may help with staying fit. You may also want to consider physical fitness for people with disabilities.

2. Divide the tasks among group members. Some members may want to do research, while others may want to help design and create the website.

3. Present the website to your class and ask students to complete a survey using an online survey tool to assess the effectiveness of the website. Also, ask students what other information they would like about physical fitness.

Math Practice

Calculating Distances. Huntsville High's schoolwide olympics will promote physical activity. Races will be run in the gym. For one race, athletes will run one lap around the gym. That distance would be approximately the same as the perimeter of the gym.

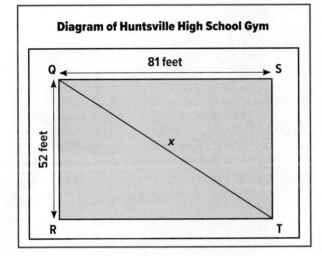

Diagram of Huntsville High School Gym

1. What is the perimeter of the gym?
   a. 1,112 feet
   b. 421 feet
   c. 266 feet
   d. 386 feet

2. One athlete covers about 5 feet every second. If she competed in the race today, approximately how many seconds would it take her to run the one-lap course?
   a. 53 seconds
   b. 55 seconds
   c. 532 seconds
   d. 260 seconds

3. A race across the gym diagonally is represented in the diagram by line x. Line x divides the gym into two congruent right triangles. What is the approximate length, in feet, of line x, the side the two triangles share?
   a. 421.2 feet
   b. 21.60 feet
   c. 133 feet
   d. 96.25 feet

Reading/Writing Practice

Understand and Apply. Read the passage below, and then answer the questions.

On Sunday, 17-year-old Rosa Martinez completed her first marathon. Her time of 2 hours and 45 minutes won't break any records, but she's proud to have finished the race—in her wheelchair. "I lost the use of my legs in a car crash three years ago," says Rosa. "I was really depressed, but getting into wheelchair sports inspired me. I started focusing more on what I could do in my chair than on what I couldn't do." To train for the marathon, Rosa says she did "a lot of aerobic exercises to strengthen my heart and lungs, and a lot of work on my upper body strength." While she's proud of her achievement, Rosa isn't going to rest on her laurels. She's already looking ahead to next year's marathon, and she's determined to beat her time from this year.

1. In the final paragraph, the phrase "rest on her laurels" means
   a. take a break from exercising.
   b. go on to bigger challenges.
   c. keep doing the same activities.
   d. settle for what she's already achieved.

2. Which of the following would make the best title for this passage?
   a. The Winning Spirit
   b. How to Train for a Marathon
   c. Elements of a Fitness Program
   d. Better Wheelchair Designs

3. Describe the physical and mental qualities that make Rosa a successful athlete. How might she apply these qualities to other aspects of her life?

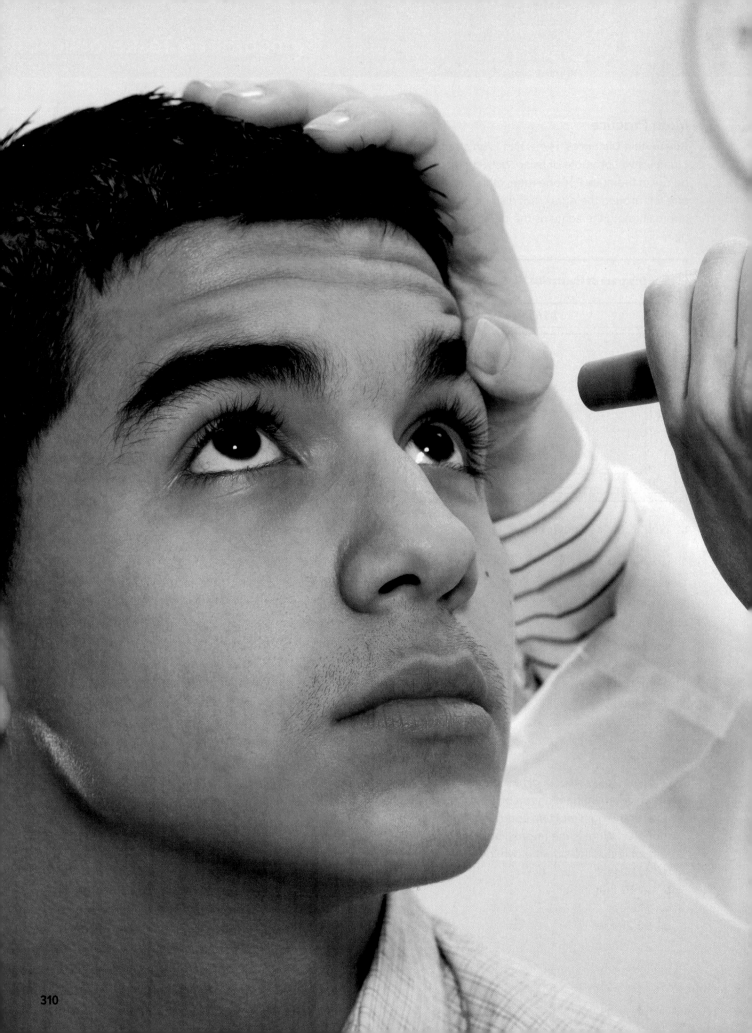

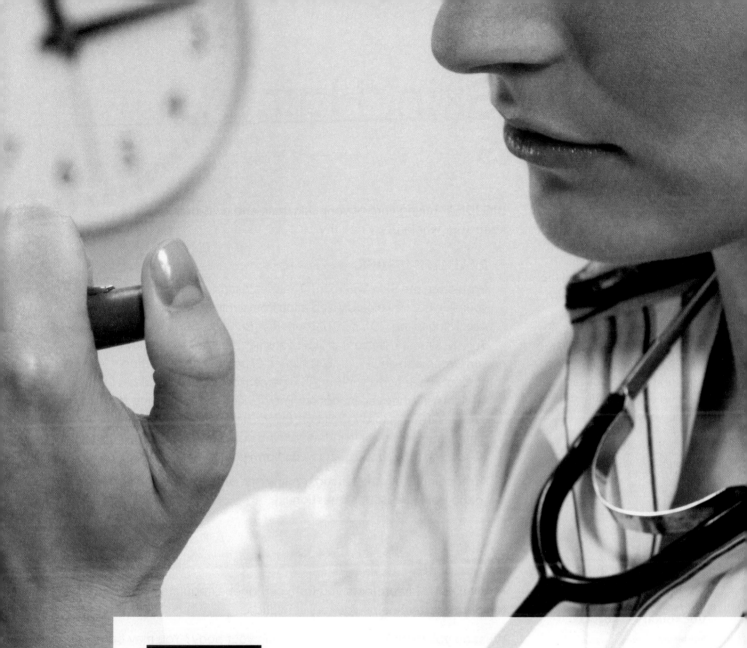

MODULE 13

Personal Health Care

LESSONS

. . . .

1 Healthy Skin, Hair, and Nails

2 Healthy Teeth and Mouth

3 Healthy Eyes and Ears

Healthy Skin, Hair, and Nails

BEFORE YOU READ

Create a Table. Make a three-column table. Label the columns "Tissue," "Structure," and "Function." In the first column, list "Skin," "Hair," and "Nails." In the second column, describe the important structural features of each. In the third column, write the function of each.

Tissue	Structure	Function

Vocabulary

epidermis
dermis
melanin
sebaceous glands
melanoma
hair follicles

● ● ● ● ● ● ● ● ● ● ●

BIG IDEA Taking care of your skin, hair, and nails helps keep your whole body healthy.

REAL LIFE ISSUES

Protecting the Skin You're In. The greatest risks to the health of your skin is ultraviolet (UV) radiation from sunlight and other sources. According to the CDC's 2017 Youth Risk Behavior Surveillance Survey, almost 11 percent of U.S. teens say that they frequently use a sunscreen with an SPF of 15 or higher. 61 percent of high school students have had a sunburn. 5.6 percent of all high school students say they use indoor tanning devices. Indoor tanning also exposes the skin to UV radiation. In fact, half of the states in the U.S. restrict teens from using indoor tanning devices. ***Write a paragraph describing how sun exposure can harm your health.***

After completing the lesson, review and analyze your response to the Real Life Issues question.

Your Skin

MAIN IDEA Skin protects you from pathogens, regulates your body temperature, and helps you feel sensations.

What do you think is the largest organ in your body? You may be surprised to learn that the answer is your skin. The skin consists of two main layers. The **epidermis** is the outer, thinner layer of the skin that is composed of living and dead cells. The **dermis** is the thicker layer of the skin beneath the epidermis that is made up of connective tissue and contains blood vessels and nerves. Cells in the epidermis make substances called lipids, which make your skin waterproof. This waterproofing helps the body maintain a proper balance of water and electrolytes. Other cells produce melanin, a pigment that gives the skin, hair, and iris of the eyes their color—the more melanin that your body produces, the darker the skin. The **melanin** in skin also helps protect the body from harmful ultraviolet (UV) radiation that causes skin cancer.

The dermis is a single thick layer composed of connective tissue, which gives the skin its elastic qualities. **Sebaceous glands**, structures within the skin that produce an oily secretion called sebum, are also found in the dermis. Sebum helps keep skin and hair from drying out. Blood vessels in the dermis supply cells with oxygenated blood and nutrients and help remove wastes from body cells.

Functions of the Skin

The skin performs the following three main functions to keep you healthy:

- **Protection.** The skin protects your internal organs from damage. It also acts as a barrier to prevent pathogens (disease-causing germs, such as viruses and bacteria) from entering your system. If this barrier is broken by a cut or other wound, the skin repairs itself to keep pathogens from entering the body.

- **Temperature control.** If your body temperature begins to drop, the blood vessels in your skin constrict. This reduces the amount of heat loss and helps to maintain body heat. When your body temperature begins to rise, by contrast, the blood vessels dilate. This allows heat to escape through the skin's surface. Sweat glands also help cool the skin by releasing perspiration through ducts to pores on the skin's surface, where it can evaporate.

- **Sensation.** Touch a hot stove, and your hand immediately pulls back. Why? The skin is a major sense organ. Nerve cells in the dermis receive signals from the outside environment. Through these receptors, you can feel sensations such as pressure, pain, heat, and cold.

Reading Check

Explain What are the dermis and epidermis?

The skin is composed of two main layers, the epidermis and the dermis. These two layers are attached to bones and muscles by the subcutaneous layer, a layer of fat and connective tissue located beneath the dermis. **Explain how the skin helps regulate body temperature.**

The Skin's Structure

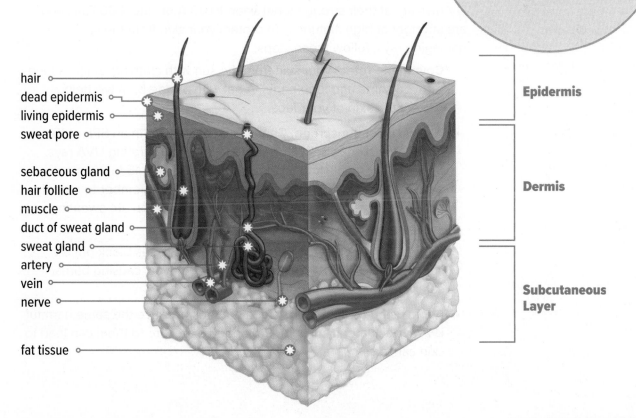

hair
dead epidermis
living epidermis
sweat pore

sebaceous gland
hair follicle
muscle
duct of sweat gland
sweat gland
artery
vein
nerve

fat tissue

Epidermis

Dermis

Subcutaneous Layer

Keeping Your Skin Healthy

MAIN IDEA A daily routine will help keep your skin healthy.

As a teen, one of the most important ways to look and feel your best is to keep your skin healthy. A good skin-care routine includes these steps:

- Wash your face every morning and evening with water and a mild soap.

- Bathe or shower each day to **remove** bacteria that can cause body odor.

- Avoid touching your face with your hands. This can introduce new bacteria to the skin's surface.

- Choose personal skin-care products carefully to avoid irritation and possible allergic reactions. Check with a health care professional before purchasing any skin-care product to make sure it's right for you.

- Eat healthful foods that are rich in vitamins and minerals, especially vitamin A. Milk, green and yellow vegetables, and liver are all good for promoting healthy skin.

UV Protection

Do you love the look of a dark suntan? Many people think that tanned skin looks really healthy. In reality, a suntan is a sign that the skin has been damaged by UV rays. When skin is exposed to UV radiation, it increases its production of melanin. This is the skin's way of trying to protect itself from the UV rays. Prolonged exposure to UV rays can lead to skin cancer.

UV rays are at their strongest between 10:00 A.M. and 4:00 P.M., and are stronger at high altitudes. To protect your skin from the sun's damaging rays, follow these steps:

- **Cover up!** Protect your skin from the sun with clothing, such as long-sleeved shirts and long pants. A hat with a wide brim will help protect the skin of your face.

- **Always wear sunscreen.** Choose a sunscreen with an SPF of 15 or higher that blocks both UVB and the more penetrating UVA rays. Make sure to apply it to all exposed areas of skin 15 to 30 minutes before going outside—even on cloudy days. Remember to reapply sunscreen every 2 hours, or more frequently if you are sweating or in the water.

- **Wear sunglasses.** Make sure that your sunglasses block out UV light. Exposure to UV rays can damage the eyes, causing burns, cataracts, and even blindness.

- **Avoid using tanning beds.** Tanning beds produce the same harmful UV rays as natural sunlight. Prolonged exposure to them can lead to skin cancer.

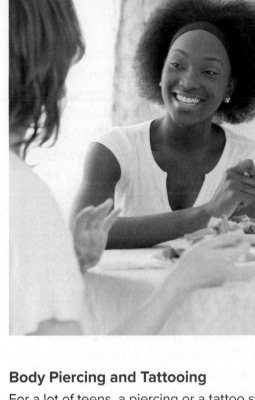

An eating plan rich in vitamin A will promote healthy skin. **Which foods do you enjoy that are a good source of vitamin A?**

Body Piercing and Tattooing

For a lot of teens, a piercing or a tattoo seems like a great way to express their identities. These two forms of body decoration have been around for thousands of years. However, unlike wearing makeup or changing hair color, piercings and tattoos are permanent. Also, both carry potential health risks because they break the physical barrier of the skin. This can allow pathogens to enter the body, resulting in infection. In addition, if the needles used for tattooing are not sterile, they can spread viruses such as hepatitis B, hepatitis C, and HIV. The American Dental Association also warns that oral piercing can damage your mouth and teeth. Finally, the decision to get a tattoo or piercing may impact your social health. These body decorations may look cool to you now, but in the adult world, they may limit your future job opportunities and relationships.

Skin Problems

Many skin problems can affect your self-image, but do not threaten your overall health. Others, however, can be dangerous. Moles, for example, can develop into **melanoma**, a potentially deadly form of skin cancer. Common skin problems include:

- **Acne**. When pores in the skin get clogged, material can build up below the skin surface, causing swollen, red bumps called pimples. Touching and picking at pimples may cause scarring. To prevent acne, keep pores open by washing your face gently twice a day and avoiding oily products or too much makeup. Acne can be treated with over-the-counter products. Extreme cases may require prescription medication.

- **Warts**. These are caused by a virus and are most commonly found on the feet, hands, and face. They can spread through direct contact with another person's wart. Most warts are harmless, but some are annoying or painful. Warts can be removed by a doctor or with over-the-counter treatments.

Reading Check

Describe What are two ways to protect your skin from UV rays?

- **Dermatitis**. This is an itchy rash usually caused by contact with an irritating substance. It usually clears up on its own when the irritant is removed. One form of dermatitis is eczema, which causes scaly and itchy patches on the skin. Keeping the area moist can help reduce the irritation. A doctor may also prescribe medication.

- **Fungal infections**. Ringworm and athlete's foot are two examples of skin infections caused by fungi. They can spread by contact with skin, infected clothing, or public showers. To treat them, keep the area clean and try to use over-the-counter medications.

- **Boils**. These form when **hair follicles**—sacs or cavities that surround the roots of hairs—become infected. The area becomes inflamed, and pus forms. Bursting or squeezing a boil may spread the infection. Treatment can involve draining the pus cleanly and taking antibiotics.

- **Vitiligo (vih-tuh-LY-go)**. In this condition, patches of skin lose melanin and have no pigment. These areas are extremely susceptible to burning when exposed to UV light, so they should always be covered or otherwise protected.

- **Moles**. These are raised, dark bumps on the skin. Most moles are harmless, but some types may develop into melanoma, which can be deadly. Early detection and treatment are critical to controlling the spread of this cancer. Report any changes to a dermatologist.

The ABCD's of Melanoma

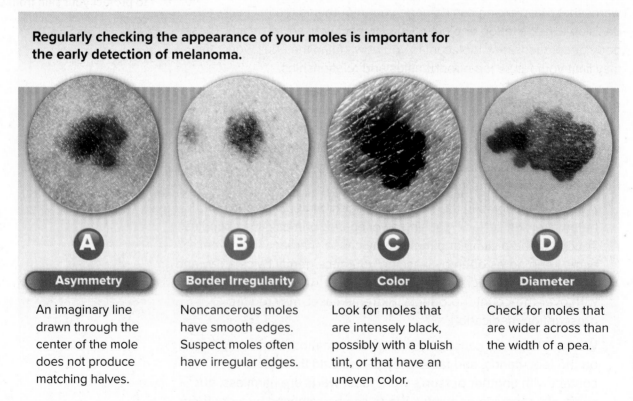

Regularly checking the appearance of your moles is important for the early detection of melanoma.

A Asymmetry

B Border Irregularity

C Color

D Diameter

| An imaginary line drawn through the center of the mole does not produce matching halves. | Noncancerous moles have smooth edges. Suspect moles often have irregular edges. | Look for moles that are intensely black, possibly with a bluish tint, or that have an uneven color. | Check for moles that are wider across than the width of a pea. |

National Cancer Institute (NCI)

Your Hair

MAIN IDEA Your hair protects your skin from UV radiation and helps maintain body heat.

Hair grows on every surface of your skin, except for the palms of your hands and the soles of your feet. You have more than 100,000 hairs on your head alone. Hair helps protect the skin, especially the scalp, from exposure to UV radiation. The eyebrows and eyelashes protect the eyes from dust and other particles. Hair also reduces the amount of heat lost through the skin of the scalp.

Although hair itself is made up of dead cells, it grows from living cells in the skin. To keep your hair looking good, you need to keep these cells healthy with a well-balanced diet. Without proper nutrients, your hair can become thin and dry. Daily brushing keeps dirt from building up and helps distribute the natural oils in your hair evenly. Regular shampooing is also an important part of your hair-care routine. However, it's best to limit the use of harsh chemical treatments—such as dyes, bleach, or permanents—as well as heating irons or hot combs. Overexposure to these can make the hair dry and brittle.

Hair Problems

Normally, the oil produced by your sebaceous glands keeps your hair soft and shiny. If your scalp becomes too dry, it will begin to shed dead skin cells in the form of sticky white flakes, known as *dandruff.* You can treat most cases of dandruff with an over-the-counter dandruff shampoo. If itching or scaling persists, consult a health care professional.

Another problem that can affect the hair is head lice. These tiny, parasitic insects live on the human scalp and feed on blood by biting through the skin. Lice can infect anyone. They are transmitted mainly by head-to-head contact or through objects such as brushes, combs, or hats that an infected person has used. A special medicated shampoo can kill head lice. Washing sheets, pillowcases, combs, and hats with hot water and soap, as well as frequent vacuuming of the home, can help prevent the spread of head lice and make sure that they do not return.

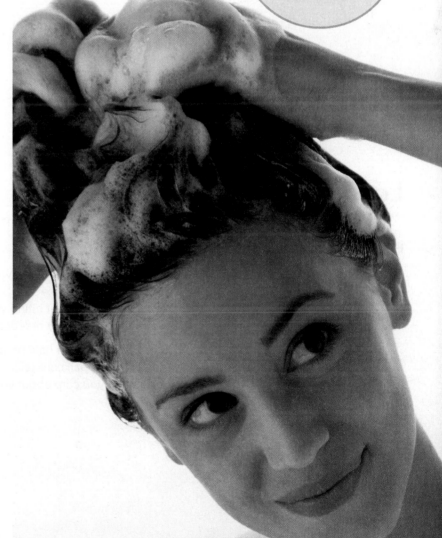

Fitness Zone

Want healthy hair? I guess we all do! My cousin is learning to be a hair stylist. She says that good nutrition and drinking lots of water helps keep your hair healthy. She also says that if your body is healthy and well nourished, your hair will be your shiny crowning glory.

Give your hair daily attention to keep it clean and healthy. **How do you choose hair care products that are right for your hair?**

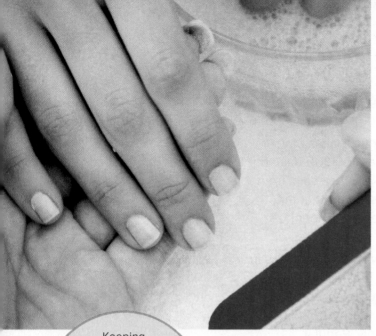

Your Nails

MAIN IDEA Nails help protect your fingers and toes.

Like your hair, your fingernails and toenails are made of closely packed dead cells containing a protein called *keratin*. Cells beneath the root of each nail divide and multiply, causing the nail to grow longer. Your nails protect and support the tissues of your fingers and toes.

Caring for your nails includes keeping them clean and evenly trimmed. This can prevent splitting or hangnails. Use a nail file to shape and smooth the nails, and keep cuticles pushed back. Trim toenails straight across just slightly past the end of the toe to reduce the chances of ingrown nails. Keeping these nails short also reduces the risk of fungal infections under the nails. If such an infection occurs, it can be treated with an antifungal ointment.

A cut, split, or break in the skin around a nail allows pathogens into the body and may lead to infection. Keep the area clean and apply an antibiotic ointment if necessary.

Keeping nails neatly clipped and filed improves your overall appearance. **List three other grooming habits that contribute to a healthy appearance.**

Lesson 1 Review

Facts and Vocabulary

1. Define the terms melanin and hair follicle.

2. Explain the causes of acne. How is acne treated?

3. Identify three viruses that can be transmitted while getting a tattoo.

Thinking Critically

4. **Apply.** Taking care to keep your nails clean and trimmed is important. Why might biting your nails be an unhealthy practice?

5. **Synthesize.** Explain how proper skin, hair, and nail care tells others that you care about your appearance.

Applying Health Skills

6. **Analyzing Influences.** Darla wants an eyebrow piercing because the lead singer in her favorite band has one. A friend offered to do the piercing for free. Write a letter to Darla and point out the influences on her choice. Remind her of the health risks.

Writing Critically

7. **Persuasive.** Write a brief dialogue between two teens. One wants to get a shoulder tattoo. The other explains the health and social risks.

Healthy Teeth and Mouth

BIG IDEA Your teeth and mouth need care to function well and keep you healthy.

┌─ **REAL LIFE ISSUES** ─────────────────

Preventive Health. Maria is afraid that having dental work will be very painful. She avoids going to the dentist, even though she knows that getting her teeth cleaned every six months is important to her health. She has made several appointments, and as the date of the appointment nears, she gets nervous and cancels it. Maria's brother, Juan, overhears her canceling her latest appointment. ***Write a dialogue between Maria and Juan. Juan should try to convince Maria that going to the dentist twice a year is important.***

After completing the lesson, review and analyze your response to the Real Life Issues question.

BEFORE YOU READ

Make an Outline. Use the headings and subheadings in this lesson to make an outline of what you'll learn. Use this type of format to help you organize your notes.

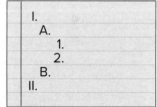

Your Teeth

MAIN IDEA Every tooth has three main parts.

Smile! As you know, a great smile depends on great teeth. Your teeth aren't just for looks, though; they're also important for your overall physical health. You need them to break down foods into pieces that are small enough to easily digest. Teeth also help form the shape and structure of your mouth.

When you were little, you had a set of "baby teeth." These most likely began to fall out when you were around age five and have been replaced by your permanent teeth. Even now, you may not have your last set of permanent molars, known as "wisdom teeth" because they come in right around the time you reach adulthood.

Parts of a Tooth

Each tooth has three main parts: the crown, the neck, and the root. The crown is the visible part of the tooth. It has a protective coating of enamel, a hard substance made of calcium. Beneath the enamel is a layer of connective tissue called *dentin,* which contributes to the shape and hardness of the tooth. Below this, protected by the overlying layers of enamel and dentin, lies the **pulp**, which is the tissue that contains the blood vessels and nerves of a tooth and extends down into the roots.

Vocabulary

pulp
periodontium
plaque
halitosis
periodontal disease
malocclusion

The neck of the tooth is the portion between the crown and the root. Your teeth are surrounded by the **periodontium** (per-ee-oh-DAHN-tee-um), which includes the gum, periodontal ligaments, and the jawbone. These structures support the tooth and hold it in place.

Keeping Your Teeth and Mouth Healthy

MAIN IDEA You can make choices that help keep your teeth and mouth clean and healthy.

The process of keeping your mouth clean and healthy is known as oral hygiene. One important part of oral hygiene is brushing and flossing your teeth to remove **plaque**. Plaque is a combination of bacteria and other particles, such as small bits of food, which adheres to the outside of a tooth. Plaque forms as the bacteria that inhabit your mouth break down the sugars in the foods you eat. They produce an acid that can damage the protective outer enamel of your teeth, forming holes, or cavities. When enough of the enamel is destroyed, bacteria can penetrate the tooth, causing tooth decay. If the decay spreads all the way down to the pulp, the tooth may have to be removed.

Plaque coats your teeth and seals out the saliva that normally protects the teeth from bacteria. Brushing your teeth after eating removes plaque before the bacteria can cause damage. Flossing between your teeth removes plaque from the areas that your toothbrush can't reach. Here are some additional steps you can take to keep your teeth and gums healthy:

- Get regular dental checkups. The dentist, or a dental hygienist, will give your teeth a thorough cleaning and check them for signs of decay. Dentists may also use sealants to protect the teeth from decay.

A protective layer of enamel covers the crown of a tooth. Inside the tooth, blood vessels supply the living tissue with oxygen and nutrients.

Cross Section of a Tooth

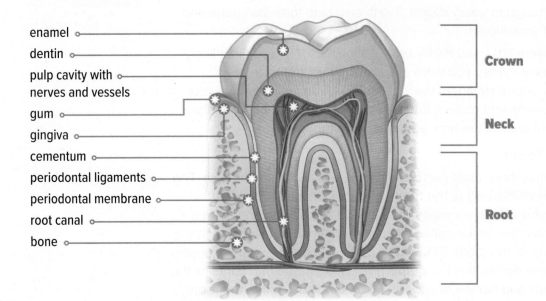

enamel

dentin

pulp cavity with nerves and vessels

gum

gingiva

cementum

periodontal ligaments

periodontal membrane

root canal

bone

Crown

Neck

Root

- See a dentist if your gums bleed when you brush and floss your teeth, if you have a toothache or dry mouth, or if you develop sores on your tongue or the inside of your mouth.

- Eat a well-balanced diet. Include foods containing phosphorus, calcium, and vitamin C, which are all important for healthy teeth. Also, cut down on sugary drinks and snacks.

- Wear a mouth guard to protect your mouth and teeth during contact sports and similar activities.

- Avoid all tobacco products. They stain teeth and cause gums to recede. They also increase the risk of oral cancer (cancers that affect the mouth).

Reading Check

Cause and Effect Describe how plaque leads to tooth decay.

Tooth and Mouth Problems

MAIN IDEA Neglecting your teeth can result in problems.

Cavities are not the only problem that can affect your mouth and teeth. Some oral problems are caused by poor hygiene, others by poorly aligned teeth. Be alert to these common problems:

- **Halitosis**, or bad breath, can be caused by eating certain foods, poor oral hygiene, smoking, bacteria on the tongue, decayed teeth, and gum disease. Fixing this problem involves identifying and correcting the cause.

Reading Check

Describe What are six possible causes of halitosis?

- Gum disease, or **periodontal disease**, is an inflammation of the periodontal structures. It is caused by bacterial infection. When plaque hardens, it builds up to form a hard crust known as *tartar.* This can cause the gums to become irritated and swollen. This early stage of gum disease is called *gingivitis* (jin-jih-VY-tis). If the condition is left untreated, the bone and tissue that support the teeth are destroyed, and teeth can be lost.

- **Malocclusion** (mal-uh-KLOO-zhun), is a misalignment of the upper and lower teeth, or a "bad bite." It can be caused by crowded or extra teeth, thumb sucking, injury, or heredity. If not treated, malocclusion can lead to decay. It can also affect a person's speech and ability to chew.

- Impacted wisdom teeth occur when there is not enough room in the mouth for the final row of molars to come in behind the other teeth. Impacted wisdom teeth may crowd and push on other teeth or become infected. They may need to be removed surgically.

Healthy teeth are important to your overall health. **Explain how healthy teeth protect your health.**

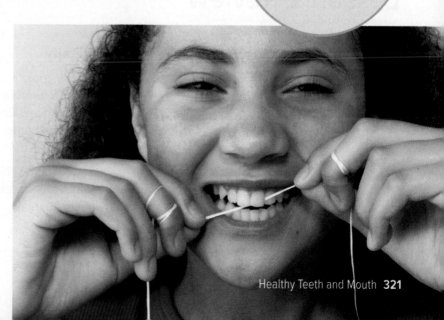

Ken Karp/McGraw-Hill Education

Examining Product Claims

The toothpaste aisle contains products that make many different claims. Some brands of toothpaste whiten teeth, others prevent cavities, some prevent bad breath, and others combine some or all of these claims. How can you tell if these claims are true?

- Check for exaggerated or misleading claims on product labels. Does the label tell you how the product works?

- Determine whether the product is safe. Some tooth whiteners, for example, contain abrasives that may cause gum irritation.

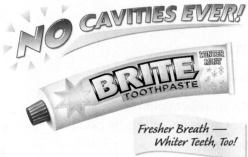

Activity: Technology

Investigate the claims made by various toothpaste manufacturers.

1. Begin by conducting an online search about product claims for toothpaste. A few good places to start are the Food and Drug Administration (FDA), professional dental associations, and nonprofit consumer protection organizations.

2. Find out what these organizations recommend that all toothpastes should do. Which features are important? If the information cannot be located on the websites, you may have to call or e-mail the organizations.

3. Create a multimedia slide presentation based on the information you were able to obtain. During your presentation, be able to cite sources and explain why you think the claims you support are reliable.

Lesson 2 Review

Facts and Vocabulary

1. Define the terms periodontal disease and plaque.

2. Describe the characteristics of the pulp of the tooth.

3. Explain how tooth decay happens.

Thinking Critically

4. **Infer.** Dentists may apply a sealant to children's teeth to protect them from decay. How do you think these sealants work?

5. **Compare and Contrast.** Which layers of the tooth are sensitive, and which are not? Explain.

Applying Health Skills

6. **Accessing Information.** Do research at the library or on the Internet to learn more about what an endodontist does.

Writing Critically

7. **Persuasive.** Write a short letter to a younger brother or sister describing the reasons why it's important to brush and floss teeth regularly.

Healthy Eyes and Ears

BIG IDEA Eyes and ears are sensitive organs that need protective care.

REAL LIFE ISSUES

How Loud Is Too Loud? Noise over 100 decibels can cause hearing damage after more than 15 minutes of unprotected exposure. The chart reveals decibel levels of common sounds. *Write a letter to yourself describing ways that you can reduce your exposure to everyday noises.*

After completing the lesson, review and analyze your response to the Real Life Issues question.

BEFORE YOU READ

Create a K-W-L Chart. Make a three-column chart. In the first column, write what you know about your eyes and ears. In the second column, write what you want to know about them. As you read, fill in the third column describing what you have learned.

K	W	L

Vocabulary

sclera
retina
cornea
auditory ossicles
labyrinth
tinnitus

Your Eyes

MAIN IDEA The eyes and their supporting structures are a complex of parts.

Take a quick look around you. Everything that you see right now is an image being sent to your brain through your eyes. In fact, light signals received by your eyes account for most of the sensory information that your brain receives.

Structurally, your eyes are two balls sitting in bony sockets, called *orbits,* at the front of your skull. A layer of fat cushions each eyeball in its socket. A structure called the *lacrimal gland* produces tears and secretes them into your eyes through ducts. Tears are made of water, salt, mucus, and a substance that protects the eye from infection. Each time you blink, tears move across the surface of your eye. They keep the surface of the eyeball moist and free of foreign particles.

Parts of the Eye

The outermost layer of the eyeball wall, the **sclera** (SKLEHR-uh), the white part of the eye, is composed of tough, fibrous tissue that protects the inner layers of the eye. The sclera is lined by a thin structure called the *choroid* (KOHR-oid). Behind that lies the **retina.** The retina is the inner layer of the eye wall which contains millions of light-sensitive cells called *rods* and *cones.* Rods enable you to see in dim light. Cones function in bright light and allow you to see colors. When light stimulates these cells, a nerve impulse travels to the brain through the *optic nerve,* which is located at the back of the eye.

The Eye

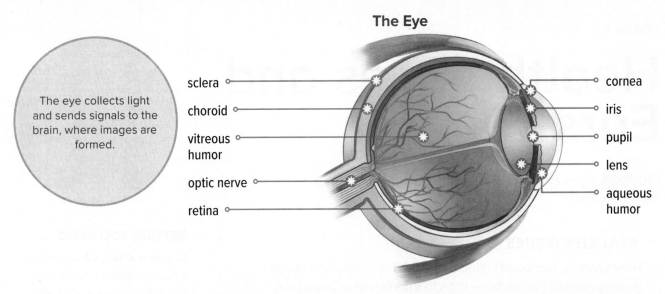

sclera
choroid
vitreous humor
optic nerve
retina

cornea
iris
pupil
lens
aqueous humor

The eye collects light and sends signals to the brain, where images are formed.

• • • • • • • • • • • •

ACADEMIC VOCABULARY

portion (*noun*): a part set off from the whole

• • • • • • • • • • • •

At the front of the eye are the structures that admit and focus light. Light enters the eye through the **cornea**. The cornea is a transparent tissue that bends and focuses light before it enters the lens. Light then passes through the pupil, a hole in the middle of the *iris,* the colored **portion** of the eye. Behind the iris and pupil is the transparent *lens,* which helps refine the focus of images on the retina. The area between the cornea and the lens is filled with a watery fluid called *aqueous humor,* which provides nutrients to the eye. Between the lens and the retina there is a cavity filled with a gelatin-like substance called *vitreous humor.* This helps the eyeball keep its shape and holds the retina in place against the choroid.

Vision

Suppose you're looking at a flower. Light rays bouncing off the flower enter your eye, where they are first focused by the cornea and then refined by the lens to strike against your retina. The light stimulates the rods and cones of the retina, sending nerve impulses into the brain through the optic nerve. The brain translates these nerve impulses into an image that you can recognize as a flower.

• • • • • • • • • • • •

Reading Check

Explain How do light signals become images?

• • • • • • • • • • • •

If you have clear, or 20/20, vision, images form sharply and clearly on your retina. The term 20/20 means that you can stand 20 feet away from an eye chart and read the top eight lines. However, in some cases, the shape of the eye distorts the images formed on the retina, causing either *myopia* (nearsightedness) or *hyperopia* (farsightedness). A nearsighted person can see close-up objects clearly, while distant objects appear fuzzy. Someone with 20/60 vision, for instance, must stand 20 feet away from the eye chart in order to read it as well as a person with normal vision who can read it from 60 feet. For a farsighted person, the problem is reversed; distant objects are clear while close-up ones are blurry.

Keeping Your Eyes Healthy

MAIN IDEA Making healthy choices will keep your eyes healthy.

Many different problems can affect your eyes. One problem not mentioned in the chart is corneal disease. This condition can sometimes be corrected through a corneal transplant, which can restore vision and reduce pain. This is the most commonly performed transplant surgery in the United States.

EYE PROBLEMS

Structural Problems	Cause	Treatment
Nearsightedness (myopia) The inability to see distant objects clearly	May occur naturally; cornea is misshaped, or eye is too long.	Contact lenses, eyeglasses, or laser surgery
Farsightedness (hyperopia) The inability see close objects clearly	May occur naturally; cornea is misshaped, or eye is too short.	Contact lenses, eyeglasses, or laser surgery
Astigmatism Blurred vision	May occur naturally; lens or cornea is misshaped.	Contact lenses, eyeglasses, or surgery
Strabismus Eyes off-center, turned inward or outward	Weak eye muscles	Vision therapy, contact lenses, eyeglasses, or surgery
Detached retina Blurred vision or bright flashes of light	Retina has become detached from the choroid due to injury or aging.	Laser surgery to reattach retina
Disease or Vision Problems	**Cause**	**Treatment**
Infections and Viruses (such as sties, pinkeye, hepatitis) Swelling, irritation, blurred vision, change in sclera color	Pathogens infect the eye or the tissue around the eye.	Medications such as antibiotics may cure infections. No treatment for viruses.
Glaucoma Cloudy, impaired vision, sometimes permanent eye damage	High pressure inside the eye damages the retina and optic nerve.	Laser treatment; early detection helps minimize damage.
Cataracts Foggy vision	Lens becomes cloudy and cannot focus light.	Surgical removal of old lens and replacement with an artificial lens
Macular degeneration Vision loss	Part of the retina opposite the lens deteriorates due to aging.	No cure exists. Treatment is limited.

Fortunately, there are steps you can take to prevent eye problems and keep your eyes healthy. Here are some tips to keep in mind.

- **Follow a well-balanced eating plan.** Include foods that contain vitamin A, such as carrots and sweet potatoes. A deficiency of vitamin A can result in night blindness—the inability to see well in dim light.

- **Protect your eyes.** Wear safety goggles when participating in activities that pose a risk of eye injury, such as working with chemicals in your school's science lab. Keep dirty hands and other objects, such as makeup applicators, away from your eyes to reduce the risk of infection or injury. Wear sunglasses that block UV light. Never look directly into the sun or any other bright light.

- **Rest your eyes regularly.** Take regular breaks when using a computer or reading. Looking up and away every 10 minutes or so reduces eyestrain.

- **Get regular eye exams.** During a routine eye exam, your health care professional can detect and treat eye diseases and other problems while they are still in their early stages.

Eye problems include structural problems, infections, and other conditions, such as glaucoma. **Identify symptoms of an eye infection.**

Reading Check

Describe What are four things you can do to keep your eyes healthy?

Your Ears

MAIN IDEA The inner, middle, and outer ear work together so you can hear.

Generally speaking, the ear can be divided into three main sections, each with its own distinct structures.

- **The Outer Ear.** The outer ear, also known as the *auricle,* is the part of the ear that you can see. Its shape channels sound waves into the *external auditory canal.* The skin of this canal is lined with tiny hairs and glands that produce wax to protect the ear from dust and foreign objects. The canal leads to the eardrum, or tympanic membrane, which serves as a barrier between the outer and middle ear.

- **The Middle Ear.** Directly behind the eardrum are the **auditory ossicles,** which are three small bones linked together that connect the eardrum to the inner ear. These are the three smallest bones in the body. The middle ear is connected to the throat by the eustachian tube. This tube allows pressure to be equalized on both sides of the eardrum when you swallow or yawn.

- **The Inner Ear.** Deep in your ear lies the **labyrinth**, a network of curving passages that can be divided into three main parts. The cochlea, a spiral-shaped canal, is the area of the inner ear responsible for hearing. The other two parts, the vestibule and the semicircular canals, are involved in balance.

Hearing and Balance

Suppose your phone were to ring right now. The ringing would produce a sound wave, which would enter the external auditory canal, causing your eardrum to vibrate. The vibrations in the eardrum would cause fluid in the cochlea to move, stimulating receptor cells in your inner ear. These cells would then send a nerve impulse to the brain, which would interpret the sound to mean, "Someone's calling me!"

At the same time, other receptor cells in the vestibule and semicircular canals would be sending their own messages to the brain about your sense of balance. The tiny hairs in your ear would sense movement. They would then send nerve impulses to the brain, which would make the necessary adjustments to maintain balance.

The ear has two functions: hearing and balance. **Which parts of the ear are involved in hearing?**

The Ear

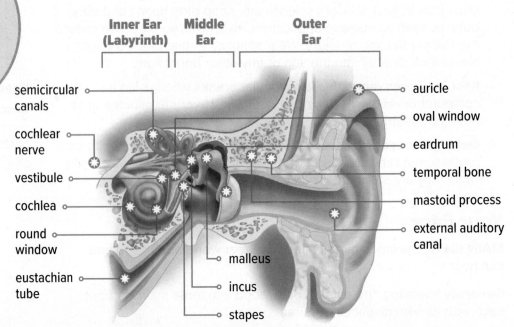

Inner Ear (Labyrinth)   Middle Ear   Outer Ear

semicircular canals
cochlear nerve
vestibule
cochlea
round window
eustachian tube
auricle
oval window
eardrum
temporal bone
mastoid process
external auditory canal
malleus
incus
stapes

Keeping Your Ears Healthy

MAIN IDEA Caring for your ears helps prevent irritation, injury, infection, and damage to the ears, as well as hearing loss.

Your ears are important not just to your physical health, but to your social health as well. If you can't hear clearly, it's harder for you to communicate with others, and communication is the key to good relationships. Here are a few ways to protect your hearing:

- See a health care professional any time you suspect an ear infection. Symptoms of an ear infection include ear pain, a feeling of pressure in the ear, drainage of fluid from the ear, and trouble hearing. Middle ear infections can damage hearing, but they can be treated with antibiotics.

- In cold weather, wear a hat that covers your ears, including the earlobes.

- When playing sports, wear protective gear, such as a batting helmet.

- Keep foreign objects, including cotton swabs, out of the ear canal.

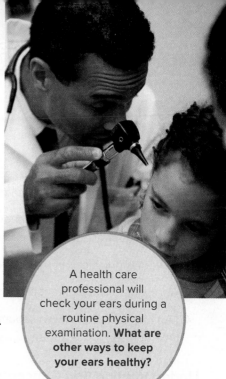

A health care professional will check your ears during a routine physical examination. **What are other ways to keep your ears healthy?**

Preventing Hearing Loss

Exposure to loud noises can lead to temporary or even permanent hearing loss, or deafness, over time. There are two main types of hearing loss. In *conductive hearing loss,* sound waves do not pass from the outer ear to the inner ear. This is usually because of a blockage or injury to the inner ear. For example, middle-ear infections may cause fluid to build up within the middle ear. *Sensorineural hearing loss* may result from a birth defect, exposure to noise, aging, or problems with medications. One type of sensorineural hearing loss is **tinnitus**. Tinnitus is a condition in which a ringing, buzzing, whistling, roaring, hissing, or other sound is heard in the ear in the absence of external sound. To prevent tinnitus, avoid loud music and wear earplugs in excessively noisy environments, such as loud concerts or sporting events. By limiting your exposure to loud noise, you reduce the risk of permanent damage.

Fitness Zone

I love listening to music when I exercise, but I heard that wearing headphones with the volume turned up can cause permanent hearing loss over time. You might also miss warnings, like a car horn. Now I turn down the volume so I can still enjoy my music while protecting my hearing and my safety.

Lesson 3 Review

Facts and Vocabulary

1. Describe how having cataracts affects vision.

2. Define astigmatism.

3. Explain the function of the wax and tiny hairs in the ear canal.

Thinking Critically

4. **Infer.** What are four characteristics that you think good safety goggles should have?

5. **Identify.** What are two common activities that would require hearing protection?

Applying Health Skills

6. **Accessing Information.** Conduct research to learn about community health services for people with vision problems. Make a pamphlet that can be used as a reference on the availability of these community services.

Writing Critically

7. **Persuasive.** Write a script or skit featuring two teens. One teen is urging the other to avoid exposure to loud noises to reduce the risk of hearing impairment.

Vocabulary Review

Correct the sentences below by replacing the italicized term with the correct vocabulary term.

1. The *dermis* is the outer, thinner layer of the skin that is composed of living and dead cells.

2. Sweat is produced in the *sebaceous glands*.

3. *Melanoma* is a pigment in the skin.

4. An oily secretion called sebum is produced by the *dermis*.

Understanding Key Concepts

After reading the question or statement, select the correct answer.

5. Which substance cools the skin?
   a. Sebum
   b. Melanin
   c. Dandruff
   d. Sweat

6. What is the order of the structure of the skin, going from the inner body to the outer body?
   a. Epidermis, dermis, subcutaneous layer
   b. Subcutaneous layer, dermis, epidermis
   c. Dermis, subcutaneous layer, epidermis
   d. Subcutaneous layer, epidermis, dermis

7. Which of the following is a risk from overexposure to UV radiation?
   a. Hepatitis B
   b. Hepatitis C
   c. Skin cancer
   d. HIV

Thinking Critically

After reading the question or statement, write a short answer using complete sentences.

8. **Describe.** Why should you avoid exposure to the sun between 10:00 A.M. and 4:00 P.M.?

9. **Identify.** List some steps you can take to treat acne.

10. **Explain.** How does a balanced diet help you have healthy hair?

11. **Analyze.** What features make a mole on your skin suspicious? What should you do if you have a suspicious mole?

12. **Compare and Contrast.** What are the similarities and differences between moles and warts?

Vocabulary Review

Use the correct vocabulary term to complete the following statements.

13. The _____ is the area immediately around the teeth.

14. The part of the tooth that contains the blood vessels and nerves of a tooth is called the _____.

15. The combination of bacteria and other particles that adhere to the outside of a tooth is called _____.

16. When an inflammation of the periodontal structures occurs, you have (a)-_____.

Understanding Key Concepts

After reading the question or statement, select the correct answer.

17. What component of plaque works on sugars to create acids that cause cavities?
    a. Viruses
    b. Bacteria
    c. Moles
    d. Boils

18. Which minerals are most important for healthy teeth?
    a. Phosphorus and calcium
    b. Iron and magnesium
    c. Iron and phosphorus
    d. Magnesium and calcium

19. What is malocclusion?
    a. Bad breath
    b. A crust that forms from unremoved plaque
    c. A source of acids on teeth
    d. A misalignment of teeth

20. What part of the tooth is the connective layer between the enamel and the pulp?
   a. Dentin
   b. Root canal
   c. Periodontal ligaments
   d. Gum

Thinking Critically

After reading the question or statement, write a short answer using complete sentences.

21. Describe. What are two functions of the teeth?

22. Identify. Why is flossing as important as brushing?

23. Infer. Why should you brush your tongue when you brush your teeth?

24. Predict. If gingivitis is left untreated, it may destroy the bone tissue that supports the tooth. What may happen to the tooth that is supported by the affected bone?

25. Analyze. Why might malocclusion lead to tooth decay?

LESSON 3

Vocabulary Review

Choose the correct term in the sentences below.

26. The *cornea/sclera* is the tough white part of the eye.

27. The *retina/cornea* is the inner layer of the eye wall that contains millions of light-sensitive cells.

28. The *auditory ossicle/labyrinth* is made of three bones that connect the eardrum to the inner ear.

29. *Tinnitus/Auditory ossicle* is a ringing or other sound heard in the ear in the absence of external sound.

Understanding Key Concepts

After reading the question or statement, select the correct answer.

30. When you blink, tears move across the surface of the eyeball to
   a. moisten and clean the eye.
   b. reduce glare from sunlight.
   c. give the eye time to adjust to images.
   d. prevent eyestrain.

31. In which disease does abnormal pressure build up inside the eye?
   a. Cataracts
   b. Macular degeneration
   c. Strabismus
   d. Glaucoma

32. What refines the focus of an image onto the retina?
   a. The lens
   b. The sclera
   c. The cornea
   d. The choroid

33. Which parts of the ear are involved in balance?
   a. Semicircular canals and vestibule
   b. Round window and eustachian tube
   c. Oval window and incus
   d. Temporal bone and cochlea

34. What object is safe to put in your ear?
   a. A cotton-tipped swab
   b. A pair of tweezers
   c. A small brush
   d. None of the above

Thinking Critically

After reading the question or statement, write a short answer using complete sentences.

35. Identify. What can you do now to protect your hearing in the future?

36. Describe. What is the effect of strabismus on the eyes?

37. Infer. Which important structure of the eye has no solid mass? Explain your answer.

38. Analyze. Which kind of hearing loss can result from a buildup of earwax? Explain your answer.

PROJECT-BASED ASSESSMENT

Tattoos and Piercings—Risky Business?

BACKGROUND

Tattoos and body piercing have become popular. Both tattoos and piercings, however, can cause serious health problems if unsanitary needles or methods are used.

TASK

Create an animated video that can be shown on the Internet that illustrates the health risks of getting tattoos or body piercings.

AUDIENCE

Students in your class

PURPOSE

Point out specific health risks associated with either tattoos or body piercings. In your video, show how these health risks can affect one or more areas of the health triangle: physical, mental/emotional, or social health.

PROCEDURE

1. Decide whether your video will be about body piercing or tattoos. Using the information in Module 13, review the health risks of the procedure you selected.

2. Use governmental websites to find more information on the health risks of body piercing or tattoos.

3. Conduct an online search of animated videos to see what themes are constant in every video that should be used in your group's video.

4. Collaborate as a group to create an animated video and decide on the story line and flow of the video.

5. Divide the tasks of creating the video among the members of the group. Every member should have a task to complete.

6. Present your video to your class. Ask for permission to upload your video to the school's website.

Math Practice

Interpret Graphs. Use the graph below of a UV Index for four weeks in Orlando and Jacksonville, Florida to answer questions 1–3.

Ultraviolet Index

The United States uses a UV Index (UVI) that goes from 1 to 11. The higher the number on the UVI, the more intense the exposure to UV rays will be on that day at noon. The bar graph below shows the average UVI for four different weeks for Orlando and Jacksonville.

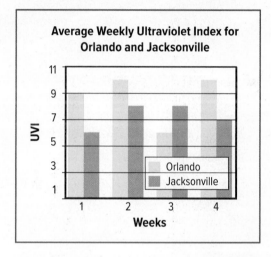

1. Which of the following statements is a correct interpretation of the bar graph above?
   a. The highest UVI for Jacksonville was 10.
   b. The lowest UVI for Orlando was 5.
   c. The mean UVI for Jacksonville was 7.25.
   d. The median UVI for Orlando was 5.50.

2. Which of these measures of central tendency would make Orlando seem to have as high a UVI as possible for the time span shown?
   a. Mean   c. Range
   b. Median   d. Mode

3. What is the mean UVI for Orlando during these four weeks?
   a. 8.50   c. 7.25
   b. 7.0   d. 7.50

Reading/Writing Practice

Understand and Apply. Read the passage below and then answer the questions.

1. *People start exercise programs for many reasons.* **2.** *Some hope to lose weight, while others want to look better.* **3.** *Many people are simply following doctor's orders.* **4.** *But people often find that exercising helps them feel good as well as look good.* **5.** *Here are two simple steps to help you get fit.* **6.** *Schedule your workout in the same way you schedule any important activity or part of your daily life.* **7.** *Morning works best for most people.* **8.** *Some people however, prefer to exercise later in the afternoon.* **9.** *The important thing is to find the best time and stick to it.*

1. Read sentence 6 in the essay. Which revision best supports the organization of the piece?
   a. There are three important things to remember in scheduling a workout.
   b. First, schedule your workout in the same way you schedule any important activity or part of your daily life.
   c. Second, schedule your workout in the same way you schedule any important activity or part of your daily life.
   d. First, it's hard to know where to begin to discuss scheduling workouts.

2. What change in *punctuation* should be made to sentence 8?
   a. Insert a colon after *people*.
   b. Insert a comma after *people*.
   c. Delete the comma after *however*.
   d. Delete the period after *afternoon*.

3. Write a newspaper column that asks and answers three questions from readers of different ages about exercise programs.

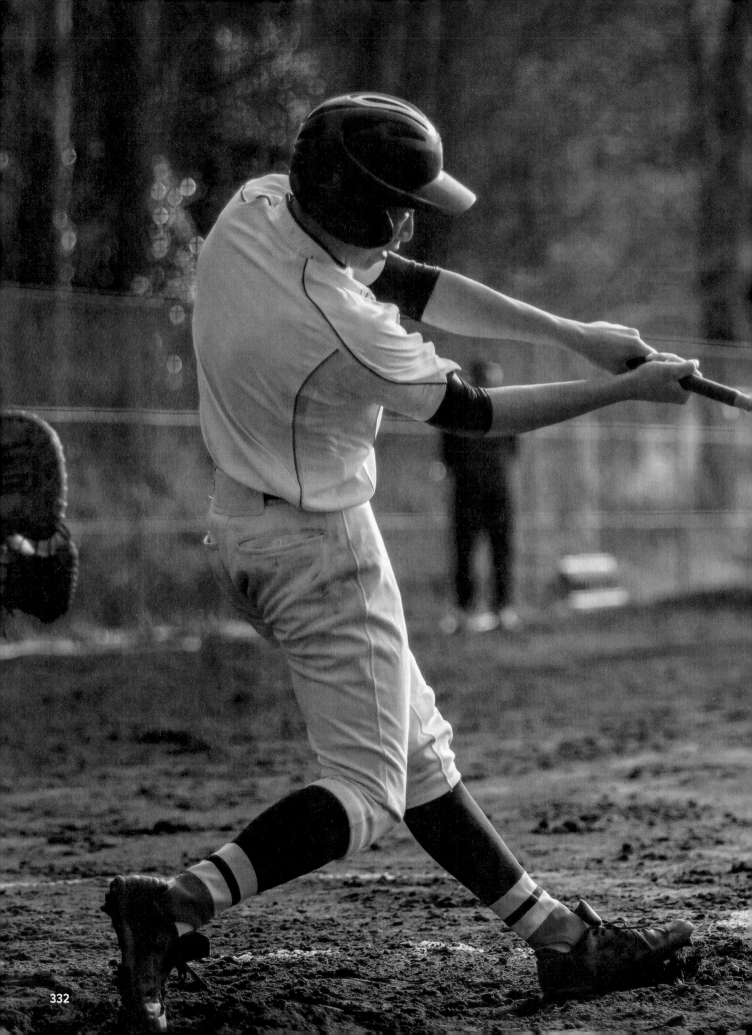

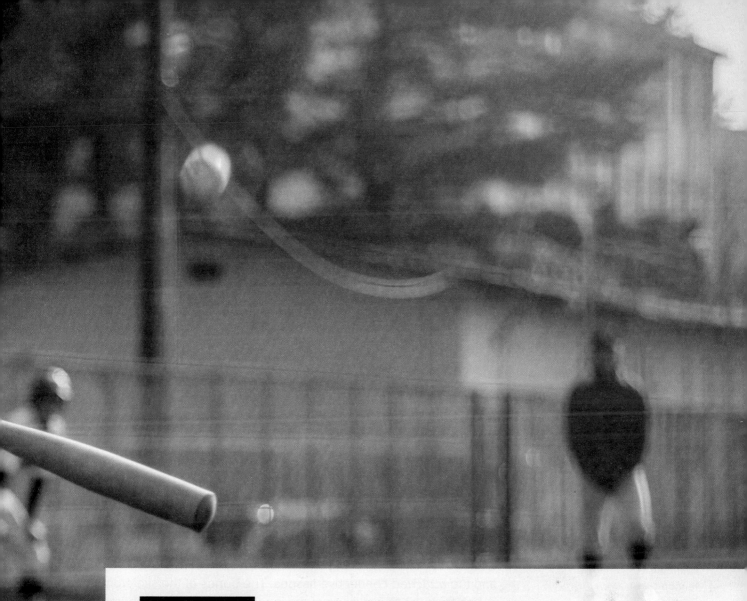

MODULE 14

Skeletal, Muscular, and Nervous Systems

LESSONS

The Skeletal System

BEFORE YOU READ

Create a Table. Make a two-column table. Title the first column "Function" and the second column "Example." Write the functions of the skeletal system as listed in the text. As you read, write in the names of specific bones that perform each function.

Function	Example

Vocabulary

ligament
tendon
cartilage
ossification
fracture
dislocation

BIG IDEA The skeletal system provides a living structure for the body.

REAL LIFE ISSUES

Speaking on Safety. At his school's health fair, David will give a presentation on the importance of using safety equipment when playing sports or getting exercise. His talk will include information on wrist, elbow, and knee pads—for in-line skating or skateboarding. These activities are popular in his neighborhood. However, many teens don't wear protective equipment. *Write a paragraph listing the protective equipment needed for in-line skating and skateboarding, and the benefits of using this equipment.*

After completing the lesson, review and analyze your response to the Real Life Issues question.

How the Skeletal System Works

MAIN IDEA The skeletal system consists of bones and connective tissue.

Do you remember the old song that begins, "The toe bone's connected to the foot bone"? All told, your skeletal system consists of 206 bones and the attached connective tissues. The bones of the skeleton range in size from the tiniest bone of the inner ear (about 0.25 centimeters long) to the longest bone of your thigh. The connective tissues cushion the bones, attach bone to bone, and attach bone to muscle.

The skeletal system has many functions, including:

- providing support for the body.
- protecting internal organs and tissues from damage.
- acting as a framework for attached muscles.
- allowing movement of limbs and digits.
- producing new red and white blood cells.
- storing fat and minerals, such as calcium and phosphorus.

Bones

Your bones are made up of several layers of living tissue. The outer layer is hard, densely packed, compact bone. Beneath that is spongy bone, a less-dense bone with a network of cavities filled with red bone marrow, where blood cells are produced. Some bones also contain yellow bone marrow, a type of connective tissue.

Bones are classified according to their shape. Types include long bones, short bones, flat bones, and irregular bones.

Connective Tissue

Your skeletal system is held together by three types of connective tissue: ligaments, tendons, and cartilage. A **ligament** is a band of fibrous, slightly elastic connective tissue that attaches one bone to another. Ligaments attach to bones to create joints. For example, one ligament connects the two bones of the forearm to each other, forming the pivot joint. **Tendons**, by contrast, connect bones to the muscles that enable them to move. **Cartilage** is a strong, flexible connective tissue that can act as a cushion between two bones to reduce friction. It can also provide a flexible structure for soft parts of the body, such as the outer ear or the tip of the nose. All the body's bones begin as cartilage in a developing embryo. Early in development, the cartilage hardens, a process known as **ossification** (ah-sih-fi h-KAY-shun). Ossification is the process by which bone is formed, renewed, and repaired.

Joints

The point at which two bones meet is called a *joint*. Some joints, such as the ones between the bones of the skull, do not move. Others move in various ways depending on how the bones are connected. Types of flexible joints include ball-and-socket joints, hinge joints, pivot joints, and ellipsoidal joints.

Caring for the Skeletal System

Because your skeletal system supports your entire body, your overall health depends on having healthy bones and joints. There are five main ways to keep your skeletal system healthy:

- Eat a healthful diet. Include foods high in calcium, phosphorus, and vitamin D, which are important for bone health.

- Get regular physical activity. Weight-bearing exercise, such as walking or weight training, stimulates bone cells to increase bone mass, which helps keep your bones strong.

- Have regular medical checkups. During a checkup, your doctor can screen you for skeletal disorders such as scoliosis.

- Wear protective gear during sports to reduce the risk of broken bones.

- When sitting at a desk and working on a computer, maintain good posture. Adjust the height of your chair so that your knees are level with your hips. Your wrists should be straight when you are typing. The computer monitor should be about an arm's length away, directly in front of you.

Bone Structure

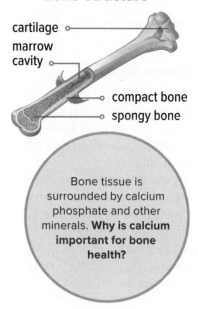

cartilage
marrow cavity
compact bone
spongy bone

Bone tissue is surrounded by calcium phosphate and other minerals. **Why is calcium important for bone health?**

Bone Shapes

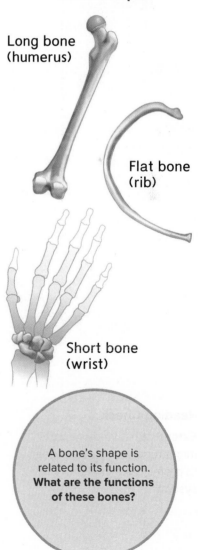

Long bone (humerus)

Flat bone (rib)

Short bone (wrist)

A bone's shape is related to its function. **What are the functions of these bones?**

Understanding Skeletal Problems

MAIN IDEA Injuries and disorders harm the skeletal system.

Problems with the skeletal system can result from poor nutrition, sports injuries, or poor posture. In addition, some degenerative diseases can affect your bones.

When bones weaken and become brittle, osteoporosis occurs. This disease affects millions of older Americans. Bone tissue loss is a natural part of aging, but healthful behaviors during the teen years can reduce your risk of developing osteoporosis later in life.

Eating foods containing calcium, vitamin D, and phosphorus will help bones remain strong and healthy. Regular weight-bearing physical activity, such as walking and weight training, stimulates bone cells to increase bone mass.

Joints

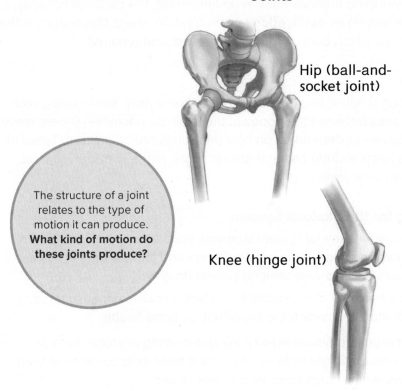

Hip (ball-and-socket joint)

The structure of a joint relates to the type of motion it can produce. **What kind of motion do these joints produce?**

Knee (hinge joint)

Fractures

A break in a bone is called a **fracture**. Fractures can be simple (if the broken end of the bone does not break through the skin) or compound (if it does). Fractures are also classified by the pattern of the break. In a *hairline fracture,* the parts of the bone do not separate. In a *transverse fracture,* the break goes completely across the bone. In a *comminuted fracture* the bone shatters into more than two pieces.

The Skeletal System

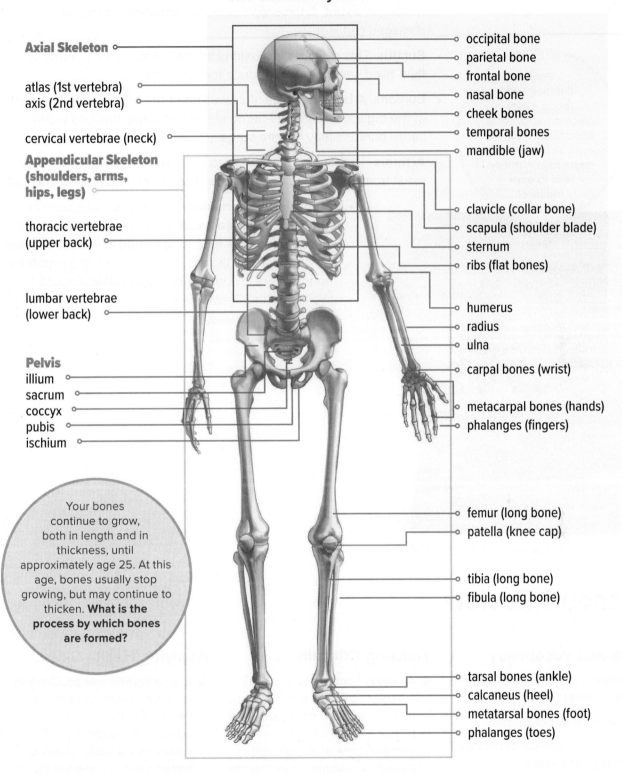

Axial Skeleton

atlas (1st vertebra)
axis (2nd vertebra)

cervical vertebrae (neck)

Appendicular Skeleton (shoulders, arms, hips, legs)

thoracic vertebrae (upper back)

lumbar vertebrae (lower back)

Pelvis
illium
sacrum
coccyx
pubis
ischium

Your bones continue to grow, both in length and in thickness, until approximately age 25. At this age, bones usually stop growing, but may continue to thicken. **What is the process by which bones are formed?**

occipital bone
parietal bone
frontal bone
nasal bone
cheek bones
temporal bones
mandible (jaw)

clavicle (collar bone)
scapula (shoulder blade)
sternum
ribs (flat bones)

humerus
radius
ulna
carpal bones (wrist)

metacarpal bones (hands)
phalanges (fingers)

femur (long bone)
patella (knee cap)

tibia (long bone)
fibula (long bone)

tarsal bones (ankle)
calcaneus (heel)
metatarsal bones (foot)
phalanges (toes)

Injuries to Joints. Joints can suffer injuries as a result of overuse, strain, or disease. Read about each type of joint injury in the list below to learn more about it.

- **Dislocation.** In a dislocation, a bone slips out of place, tearing the ligaments that attach the bone at the joint. A doctor may reset the joint and immobilize it until the ligaments heal.

- **Torn cartilage.** Cartilage may be torn by a sharp blow or severe twisting of a joint. Arthroscopic surgery can remove pieces of the damaged cartilage.

- **Bursitis.** This disorder is a painful inflammation of the *bursae*, or fluid-filled sacs that help reduce friction in joints.

- **Bunions.** A bunion is a painful swelling of the bursa in the first joint of the big toe. Wearing ill-fitting shoes can make bunions worse. Large bunions may require surgery.

- **Arthritis.** The term arthritis refers to inflammation of the joints. It may result from an injury, an autoimmune disease, or natural wear and tear.

- **Repetitive Motion Injury.** Some activities, such as sewing or computer work, may involve repeating the same movements for a long period of time. Over time, this can damage tissues. One example of a repetitive motion injury is *carpal tunnel syndrome*, caused by swelling of the ligaments and tendons in the wrist. It produces numbness, hand weakness, and pain in the thumb and forefinger.

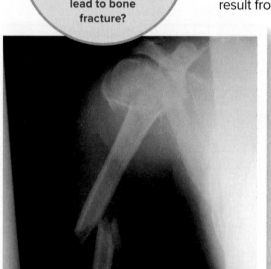

Good nutrition and taking safety precautions can help avoid breaks like the fracture shown here. **How might poor nutrition lead to bone fracture?**

Lesson 1 Review

Facts and Vocabulary

1. Explain how the skeletal system affects other body systems.

2. Describe how bones form.

3. Explain how you can avoid injury to bones and joints.

Thinking Critically

4. **Analyze.** Some people are allergic to lactose, which is found in milk and many other dairy products. How can lactose-sensitive people get enough calcium for maintaining a healthy skeletal system?

5. **Evaluate.** How might behaviors that you practice as a teen affect your skeletal system later in life?

Applying Health Skills

6. **Accessing Information.** Conduct research to learn more about injury prevention related to activities that teens enjoy. Prepare a pamphlet or poster showing teens how they can avoid injuries.

Writing Critically

7. **Descriptive.** Write a paragraph describing three or more ways in which you have made healthy choices to protect your skeletal system this week.

The Muscular System

BIG IDEA The muscular system enables the limbs and other parts of the body to move.

REAL LIFE ISSUES

Friends Get Fit. Both Misaki and Cara are interested in getting fit. Misaki's goal is to eventually join the track team. Cara just wants to improve her muscle tone. They decide to walk to the park near where they live and do a 30 minute run before school three days a week. Each week, they plan to increase the distance they run to improve their fitness level. *Write a paragraph describing some of the benefits of running. Be sure to include benefits for other aspects of health besides muscular health.*

After completing the lesson, review and analyze your response to the Real Life Issues question.

What Muscles Do

MAIN IDEA The muscular system allows for voluntary and involuntary movements.

Like rubber bands, your muscles are elastic: they stretch to allow a wide range of motion. Because of this elasticity, your muscles can move the bones or organs to which they are attached. Every part of your body relies on muscles to allow it to move.

You may think that your muscles are working only when you are doing something active, such as running or catching a ball. Some muscles in your body, however, are always at work. Even when you are asleep, muscles are helping you breathe, making your heart beat, and moving food through your digestive system. These processes are *involuntary:* they occur without your knowing it. At other times—such as when you play the piano, make a dash toward first base, or shoot a basketball— you use muscles that are under conscious, or *voluntary,* control. Your body relies on both voluntary and involuntary muscles to function.

How Muscles Work

MAIN IDEA Muscles consist of long, fibrous cells that shorten and stretch to make every part of your body move.

A muscle is made up of long cells called *muscle fibers*. Major muscles in the body contain hundreds of bundles of these fibers. When signals from your nerves stimulate these bundles, they contract, or shorten. When they relax, the bundles extend, or stretch.

BEFORE YOU READ

Create a K-W-L Chart. Make a three-column chart. In the first column, list what you **k**now about the muscular system. In the second column, list what you **w**ant to know about this topic. As you read, use the third column to summarize what you **l**earned about the topic.

K	W	L

Vocabulary
smooth muscles
skeletal muscles
flexor
extensor
cardiac muscles
tendonitis

Some nerves stimulate many muscle fibers, especially in large muscles such as your calf muscle or your biceps. In other areas, such as your eyes, a single nerve may provide impulses to only two or three muscle fibers.

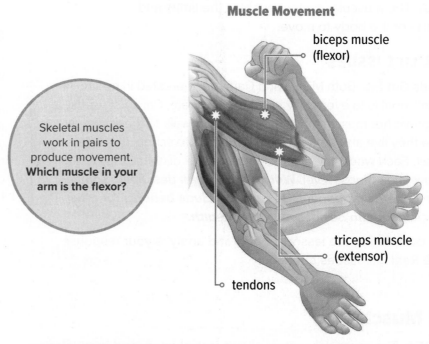

Muscle Movement

biceps muscle (flexor)

triceps muscle (extensor)

tendons

Skeletal muscles work in pairs to produce movement. **Which muscle in your arm is the flexor?**

Types of Muscles

Your body contains three types of muscle tissue: smooth muscle, skeletal muscle, and cardiac muscle.

- **Smooth muscles** are muscles that act on the lining of the body's passageways and hollow internal organs. These muscles can be found in the digestive tract, the urinary bladder, the lining of the blood vessels, and the passageways that lead into the lungs. Smooth muscles are involuntary muscles.

- **Skeletal muscles** are muscles attached to bone that cause body movements. They are made of tissue that has a *striated,* or striped, appearance under a microscope. Most of your muscle tissue is skeletal, and nearly all your skeletal muscles are under voluntary control. Skeletal muscles often work together in pairs to produce motion. One muscle contracts while the other extends. An example of this pair are the biceps and triceps muscles of the upper arm. These muscles work together to bend and straighten your arm at the elbow. The **flexor** is the muscle that closes a joint. In this example, the biceps is the flexor. The **extensor** is the muscle that opens a joint. In this case, the triceps is the extensor. When the biceps contracts, the triceps extends and the joint closes. When the biceps extends, the triceps contracts and the joint opens.

- **Cardiac muscle** is a type of striated muscle that forms the wall of the heart. It is involuntary and is responsible for the beating of your heart. The heart contracts rhythmically about 100,000 times each day to pump blood throughout your body.

Reading Check

Explain What are the two types of striated muscle, and how do they differ?

The Skeletal Muscles

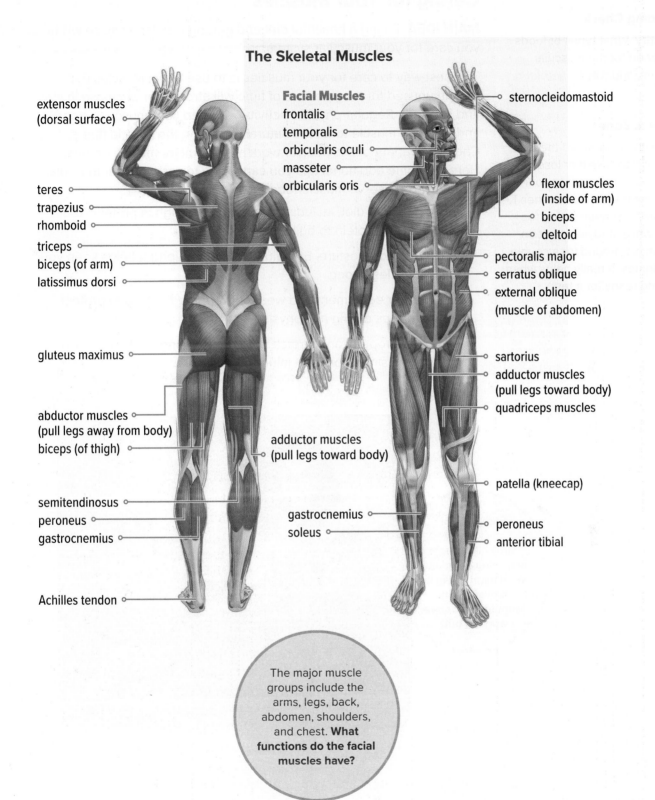

Facial Muscles
- frontalis
- temporalis
- orbicularis oculi
- masseter
- orbicularis oris

extensor muscles (dorsal surface)

teres
trapezius
rhomboid
triceps
biceps (of arm)
latissimus dorsi

gluteus maximus

abductor muscles (pull legs away from body)
biceps (of thigh)

semitendinosus
peroneus
gastrocnemius

Achilles tendon

adductor muscles (pull legs toward body)

gastrocnemius
soleus

sternocleidomastoid

flexor muscles (inside of arm)
biceps
deltoid

pectoralis major
serratus oblique
external oblique (muscle of abdomen)

sartorius
adductor muscles (pull legs toward body)
quadriceps muscles

patella (kneecap)

peroneus
anterior tibial

The major muscle groups include the arms, legs, back, abdomen, shoulders, and chest. **What functions do the facial muscles have?**

Reading Check

Identify What types of foods are good for the muscular system, and why?

Fitness Zone

Have you ever heard the expression "use it or lose it"? That's true for keeping your muscles healthy. Now, when I feel like I've been sitting too long while studying, I get up and move around for a couple of minutes. It really helps when getting ready for a test.

Caring for Your Muscles

MAIN IDEA Eating a healthful diet and getting regular exercise will help you care for your muscular system.

The best way to care for your muscles is to use them. Muscles that remain unused for long periods of time will atrophy, or decrease in size and strength. Regular physical activity will keep your muscles strong and maintain muscle tone, the natural tension in the muscle fibers. Choose a variety of activities to work all your major muscle groups. Here are some additional tips you can follow to care for your muscular system and preserve muscle tone:

- Eat a healthful diet, including foods that are high in protein. Your body needs protein to build muscle tissue.

- Practice good posture. Standing and sitting upright helps keep your back muscles strong.

- Use proper equipment and wear appropriate clothing to protect your muscles during any physical activity.

- Warm up properly and stretch before exercising, and cool down after exercising to prevent injury.

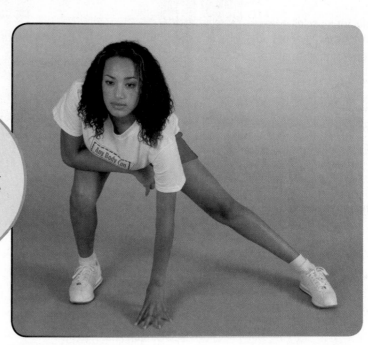

Prepare your muscles by stretching before beginning a workout. **What injuries can be prevented by warming up before working out?**

McGraw-Hill Education

Understanding Muscular Problems

MAIN IDEA Caring for the muscular system can help prevent health problems and injuries.

Have your muscles ever felt sore after some strenuous activity, such as an all-day hike or bike ride? Muscle soreness, although painful, is usually a temporary problem. However, other problems of the muscular system can be more serious. The recovery time will vary according to the type and severity of the injury or disease.

- Bruises are areas of discolored skin that appear after an injury, usually a blow of some kind. The injury causes the blood vessels beneath the skin to rupture and leak, causing swelling, discoloration, and pain. Large bruises can be treated with an ice pack to reduce initial swelling.

- Muscle strains or sprains result when muscles are stretched or partially torn from overexertion. Apply ice to the injury to reduce swelling, and rest the affected area.

- **Tendonitis**, or the inflammation of a tendon, can result from injury, overuse, or the natural effects of aging. Treatment may include ultrasound or anti-inflammatory medicines to reduce pain and swelling.

- Hernias commonly occur in the abdomen as a result of straining to lift a heavy object. Surgery is usually recommended, and may be required, to repair a hernia.

- Muscular dystrophy is an inherited disorder. The disorder gradually destroys the fibers of the skeletal muscles. There is no cure, but with early detection, muscle weakness can be delayed through a regular exercise program.

Reading Check

Compare and Contrast How does muscular dystrophy differ from the other muscular problems listed?

Lesson 2 Review

Facts and Vocabulary

1. Describe the functions of the muscular system.

2. Identify where the smooth muscle is found.

3. Describe the term hernia. Identify one cause for a hernia.

Thinking Critically

4. **Apply.** What muscles are important for playing baseball? How can you protect these muscles from injury?

5. **Analyze.** How can you prevent muscle strains when you are participating in a new physical activity?

Applying Health Skills

6. **Decision Making.** Danielle strained her arm muscle. Her coach says it should heal by the gymnastics meet next week. Danielle wants to go kayaking this weekend. Describe Danielle's decision-making steps.

Writing Critically

7. **Narrative.** Write a story from the point of view of a muscle. Have the muscle describe itself, what it does in the body, how it works, and the care it requires.

The Nervous System

BEFORE YOU READ

Create an Outline. Preview this lesson by scanning the pages. Organize the headings and subheadings into an outline. As you read, fill in the outline with important details.

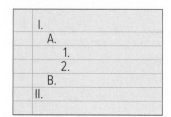

Vocabulary

neurons
cerebrum
cerebellum
brain stem
epilepsy
cerebral palsy

BIG IDEA The nervous system sends messages through the nerves to coordinate all the body's activities.

REAL LIFE ISSUES

Feeling the Heat. It's Petra's turn to clean the stovetop. She remembers that her sister just heated up some milk to make hot chocolate. The electric burner is off, but Petra knows that an unlit burner can still be hot enough to cause a burn. She carefully holds her hand two inches over the burner to feel for heat. It feels cool enough, so she safely wipes down the stove. ***Write a brief journal entry describing the ways you use your sense of touch. How does your sense of touch help you avoid danger?***

After completing the lesson, review and analyze your response to the Real Life Issues question.

How the Nervous System Works

MAIN IDEA The nervous system coordinates all of the activities in the body.

Your brain is sometimes called the body's "command center." If this is true, then the rest of the nervous system could be called the body's communication system because it sends messages back and forth between the command center and all your other organs, tissues, and cells. The nervous system coordinates all your body's activities, from breathing or digesting food to sensing pain and feeling fear.

The nervous system has two main divisions. The central nervous system (CNS) consists of the brain and spinal cord. The peripheral nervous system (PNS) includes all the nerves that branch out from the brain and spinal cord. The PNS gathers information from both inside and outside your body. For example, sensory receptors in the skin can sense pressure, temperature, or pain and transmit this information through the nerves back to the CNS. The CNS interprets the messages it receives and sends back a response.

Understanding Neurons

MAIN IDEA Neurons transmit messages from the brain and spinal cord to the rest of the body.

All your nerves are made up of **neurons**, or nerve cells. They transmit messages to and from the spinal cord and brain. Unlike the other cells in the body, neurons have limited ability to repair damage or replace destroyed cells.

Each neuron consists of three main parts:

- The cell body of a neuron contains the nucleus, which regulates the production of proteins within the cell.

- *Dendrites* are branched structures that extend from the cell body in most neurons. They receive information and transmit impulses toward the cell body.

- *Axons* transmit impulses way from the cell body and toward another neuron, a muscle cell, or a gland.

A nerve impulse begins when a sensory receptor is stimulated. The impulse travels to the CNS and is interpreted with the help of an interneuron. Then an impulse is sent to a muscle cell or gland in response to the stimulus.

The Nerve Impulse

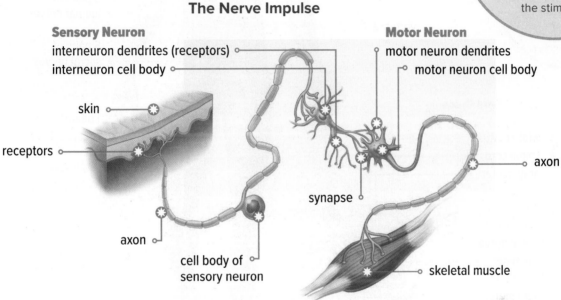

Sensory Neuron
interneuron dendrites (receptors)
interneuron cell body
skin
receptors
axon
cell body of sensory neuron

Motor Neuron
motor neuron dendrites
motor neuron cell body
axon
synapse
skeletal muscle

There are three main types of neurons, each with a different function. *Sensory neurons* carry messages from receptors in the body to the CNS. *Motor neurons* carry messages from the CNS back to the muscles or glands. *Interneurons* communicate with and connect other neurons. The illustration shows how these three types of neurons work together to send a message, called a *nerve impulse*.

The Central Nervous System

MAIN IDEA The central nervous system is made up of the brain and the spinal cord.

The two organs that make up the CNS—the brain and the spinal cord—send and receive impulses to and from all the nerves in the body. The spinal cord is a long column of nerve tissue about the thickness of your index finger. It is surrounded by several **layers** of connective tissue called the *spinal meninges*. The meninges, along with the vertebrae—the bones of the spine—help protect the spinal cord. The spinal cord is also bathed in cerebrospinal fluid that absorbs shock and nourishes the nerve tissue.

Reading Check

Explain How is the cell body important to a nerve cell?

ACADEMIC VOCABULARY

layer *(noun)*: one thickness or fold spread over or under another

The Nervous System

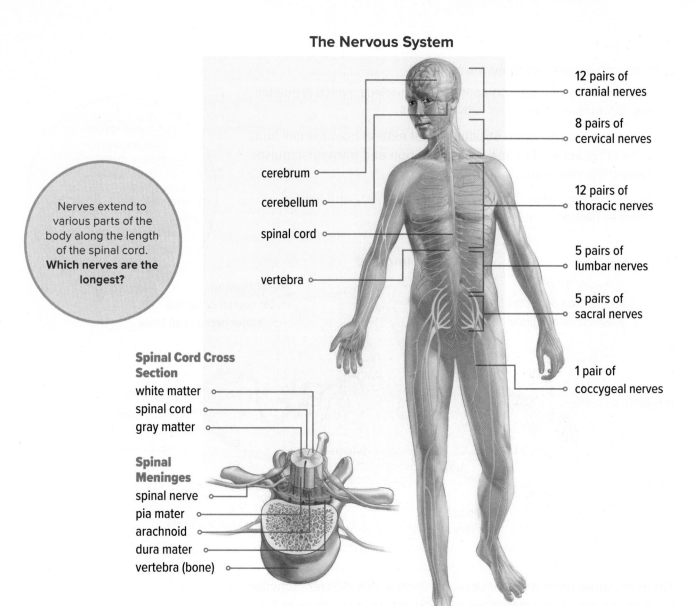

Nerves extend to various parts of the body along the length of the spinal cord. **Which nerves are the longest?**

cerebrum

cerebellum

spinal cord

vertebra

12 pairs of cranial nerves

8 pairs of cervical nerves

12 pairs of thoracic nerves

5 pairs of lumbar nerves

5 pairs of sacral nerves

1 pair of coccygeal nerves

Spinal Cord Cross Section

white matter

spinal cord

gray matter

Spinal Meninges

spinal nerve

pia mater

arachnoid

dura mater

vertebra (bone)

Sections of the Brain

The brain coordinates and controls the activities of the nervous system. Your brain helps you to receive and process messages; to think, remember, reason, and feel emotions; and to coordinate muscle movements. The brain has three main divisions: the cerebrum, the cerebellum, and the brain stem.

The Cerebrum. The **cerebrum** (seh-REE-brum) is the largest and most complex part of the brain. Billions of neurons in the cerebrum are the center of conscious thought, learning, and memory. The cerebrum's right and left sides, or hemispheres, communicate with each other to coordinate movement. The right hemisphere controls the left side of the body, and the left hemisphere controls the right side of the body. The left hemisphere is the center of language, reasoning, and critical thinking skills. The right hemisphere is the center for processing music and art and comprehending spatial relationships.

Each hemisphere has four lobes:

- The frontal lobe controls voluntary movements and has a role in the use of language. The prefrontal areas are thought to be involved with intellect and personality.

- The parietal lobe is involved with sensory information, including feelings of heat, cold, pain, touch, and body position in space.

- The occipital lobe controls the sense of sight.

- The temporal lobe contains the sense of hearing and smell, as well as memory, thought, and judgment.

The Cerebellum. The **cerebellum** (ser-eh-BEL-um) is the second largest part of the brain. It coordinates the movement of skeletal muscles. This area of the brain also continually receives messages from sensory neurons in the inner ear and muscles. It uses this information to maintain the body's posture and balance. Being able to carry out a complex series of muscle movements, such as serving a volleyball or playing the violin, is made possible by the cerebellum.

The Brain Stem. The **brain stem** is a 3-inch-long stalk of nerve cells and fibers that connects the spinal cord to the rest of the brain. Incoming sensory impulses and outgoing motor impulses pass through the brain stem. It has five parts:

- The medulla oblongata regulates heartbeat, respiratory rate, and reflexes such as coughing and sneezing.

- The pons helps regulate breathing and controls the muscles of the eyes and face.

- The midbrain controls eyeball movement, pupil size, and the reflexive response of turning your head.

- The thalamus relays incoming sensory impulses from the eyes, the ears, and from pressure receptors in the skin.

- The hypothalamus regulates body temperature, appetite, sleep, and controls secretions from the pituitary gland, affecting metabolism, sexual development, and emotions.

The Brain

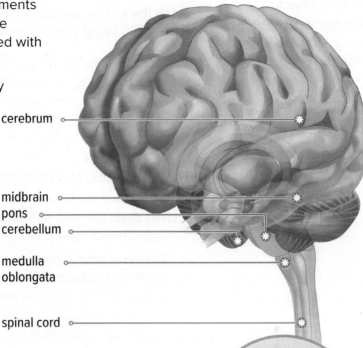

cerebrum

midbrain
pons
cerebellum

medulla
oblongata

spinal cord

The brain coordinates all activities of the body. **What part of the brain coordinates muscle movements?**

- - - - - - - - - - -

Reading Check

Describe What are the three sections of the brain, and what is the function of each?

- - - - - - - - - - -

The Peripheral Nervous System

MAIN IDEA The peripheral nervous system is made up of the nerves that are not in the brain and spinal cord.

The peripheral nervous system (PNS) carries messages between the CNS and every part of the body. It keeps the CNS informed about changes that take place within the body, as well as sensory information received from outside the body. The PNS is made up of two subsystems: the *autonomic nervous system* and the *somatic nervous system.*

The Autonomic Nervous System

The *autonomic nervous system* controls involuntary body functions, such as digestion and heart rate. It consists of a network of nerves divided into two main parts.

- The sympathetic nervous system kicks in when you are startled, sending messages that cause your heart rate to increase. Blood vessels in your muscles dilate, allowing greater blood flow. This is the "fight-or-flight" response that prepares you to react to a dangerous situation. It is an example of a *reflex,* the body's spontaneous response to a stimulus. One of the most familiar reflexes is the knee-jerk response that happens when the doctor taps the ligament below your knee during a physical exam.

- The parasympathetic nervous system opposes the action of the sympathetic nervous system by slowing body functions. During periods of rest, it slows your heartbeat, relaxes your blood vessels, and lowers your blood pressure to conserve energy. The parasympathetic nervous system also stimulates production of saliva and stomach secretions to promote the digestion of food.

The Somatic Nervous System

The *somatic nervous system* deals with voluntary body responses—that is, the ones that are under your control. Its sensory neurons send messages from the eyes, ears, nose, and tongue to the CNS. Its motor neurons transfer impulses from the CNS to the skeletal muscles.

Reflexes can prevent injuries such as a burn from a hot stove.

How Your Reflexes Work

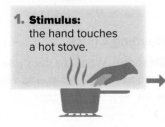

1. Stimulus: the hand touches a hot stove.

2. The sensory neuron contacts a connecting neuron in the spinal cord.

3. The connecting neuron contacts a motor neuron that sends an impulse to the muscles.

4. The nerve impulse finally reaches the brain.

5. Reflex: the muscles respond by pulling the hand away from the stove.

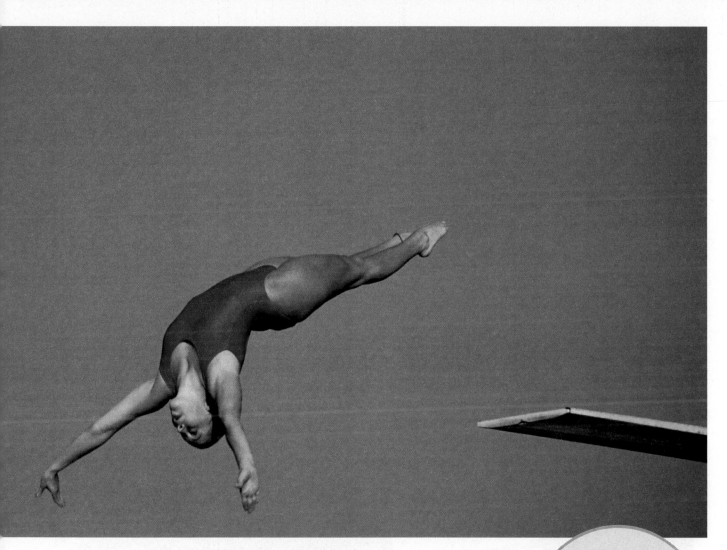

Caring for Your Nervous System

MAIN IDEA Making healthful choices can protect your nervous system from injury.

One of the most important ways to care for your nervous system is to protect your head and spine from injury. There are several ways to do this:

- Always wear a safety belt when driving or riding in a motor vehicle.

- Wear a helmet and other protective gear for riding a bicycle, motorcycle, or other open vehicle, or when playing contact sports.

- When swimming, always check the depth of water before diving. Never dive headfirst into shallow water or into water where you cannot see the bottom.

Other ways to care for your nervous system are the same as for other body systems. They include eating a well-balanced diet, exercising regularly, and getting enough sleep. Also, avoid drugs and alcohol, which can permanently damage nerve cells.

Safe behaviors, such as diving only when you know the depth of the water, can reduce your risk of head and spinal injuries. **What other behaviors can protect you from head or spinal injury?**

Problems of the Nervous System

Many types of illness and injury can affect the nervous system. Some nervous system problems include:

- **Headaches.** Headaches can have many causes, including muscle tension, eyestrain, exposure to harmful fumes, a sinus infection, dehydration, or food allergies. Migraines are recurrent headaches that may be accompanied by sensitivity to light.

- **Head injuries.** Each year, 435,000 American children and teens sustain brain injuries. Types of head injuries include concussion and contusion (bruising of the brain tissue that causes swelling). A head injury can cause temporary loss of consciousness or even long-term unconsciousness, known as a *coma*. A coma generally results from major trauma.

- **Spinal injuries.** Injuries of the spinal cord require medical care. Swelling of the spinal cord or the tissue around it can result in temporary loss of nerve function. Without treatment, the nerve damage can become permanent. If the spinal cord is completely severed, it results in paralysis, an inability to move part of the body.

Multiple sclerosis is an autoimmune disease, often resulting in impaired mobility. **What kinds of activities can you enjoy with someone who has limited voluntary muscle control?**

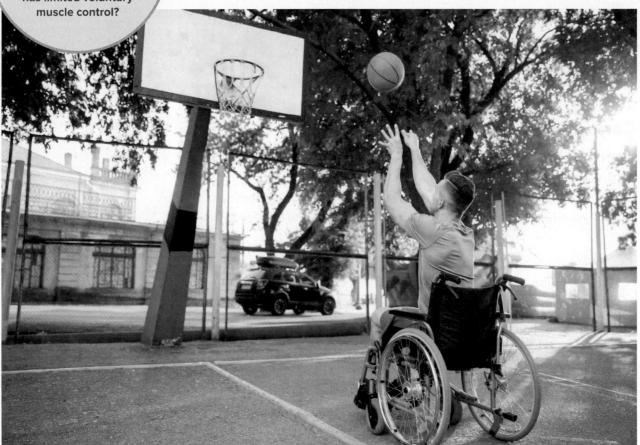

- **Meningitis.** Meningitis is an inflammation of the spinal and cranial meninges caused by a bacterial or viral infection. Symptoms include fever, headache, sensitivity to light and sound, and neck stiffness. This disease is very serious and can be deadly. Anyone with symptoms of meningitis should seek medical attention right away.

- **Degenerative diseases.** Some nervous system diseases are degenerative, meaning that they occur over time as cells break down. Examples include multiple sclerosis, Parkinson's disease, and Alzheimer's.

- **Epilepsy.** This is a disorder of the nervous system that is characterized by recurrent seizures—sudden episodes of uncontrolled electrical activity in the brain. Epilepsy can result from brain damage at birth, infections, head injury, or exposure to toxins. People with epilepsy may be able to control their seizures with medication.

- **Cerebral palsy.** This refers to a group of neurological disorders that are the result of damage to the brain before, during, or just after birth or in early childhood. Physical therapy and medication can help patients cope with this disorder.

Character Check

When you understand the effects a nervous system disease can have, you can find ways to help others through a difficult time. Offering your companionship; reading aloud; or helping with small tasks such as letter writing, watering plants, grocery shopping, or meal delivery are meaningful ways to help those who are disabled.

Lesson 3 Review

Facts and Vocabulary

1. Identify where the nucleus of a neuron is located.

2. Describe how a reflex can prevent injury.

3. List two causes of nervous system diseases and disorders.

Thinking Critically

4. **Analyze.** After sustaining a head injury, a patient is having trouble comprehending spatial relationships and controlling the left side of her body. What part of the brain might be damaged?

5. **Compare.** How are the functions of the autonomic nervous system and the somatic nervous system different?

Applying Health Skills

6. **Accessing Information.** Write a one-page report on current research into helping people with degenerative nervous system disorders, such as Parkinson's disease, multiple sclerosis, or Alzheimer's. Why are these diseases so difficult to treat?

Writing Critically

7. **Expository.** Write a paragraph describing what happens during a reflex action.

LESSON 1

Vocabulary Review

Use the correct vocabulary term to complete the following statements.

1. _____ is the connective tissue that can act as a cushion between two bones.

2. A fibrous cord called a(n) _____ attaches muscle to bone.

3. A lateral curvature of the spine is called _____.

4. The process by which bone is formed is called _____.

Understanding Key Concepts

After reading the question or statement, select the correct answer.

5. Which of the following is *not* a function of the skeletal system?
   a. Storing minerals and fats
   b. Producing red blood cells
   c. Responding to external stimuli
   d. Protecting internal tissues and organs

6. Which of the following is a condition that involves a progressive loss of bone tissue?
   a. Arthritis
   b. Osteoporosis
   c. Repetitive motion injury
   d. Scoliosis

7. In a hairline fracture,
   a. the break is completely across the bone.
   b. the two parts of the bone do not separate.
   c. the bone shatters into more than two pieces.
   d. one part of the bone protrudes through the skin.

Thinking Critically

After reading the question or statement, write a short answer using complete sentences.

8. **Contrast.** Contrast the shape of the skull bones with the shape of the arm bones, and relate these shapes to their different functions.

9. **Evaluate.** How are tendons and ligaments important for movement?

10. **Analyze.** How can non-rigorous activities, such as typing or sewing, lead to skeletal system injuries?

11. **Apply.** What kinds of protective gear can prevent injuries to the skeletal system?

12. **Analyze.** How will behaviors you practice during your teen years affect your chances of getting osteoporosis later in life?

LESSON 2

Vocabulary Review

Choose the correct word in the sentences below.

13. A(n) *flexor/extensor* is a muscle that closes a joint.

14. *Smooth/Cardiac* muscle is striated muscle in the heart.

15. All *smooth/skeletal* muscles are under involuntary control.

16. *Tendinitis/Hernia* results when an organ protrudes through an area of weak muscle.

17. A tendon problem resulting from overuse, injury, or natural aging is *tendinitis/hernia*.

Understanding Key Concepts

After reading the question or statement, select the correct answer.

18. Which type of muscle is *not* striated?
    a. Cardiac
    b. Extensor
    c. Flexor
    d. Smooth

19. Where is smooth muscle found?
    a. In the digestive tract
    b. In the walls of the heart
    c. In the triceps and biceps of the arms
    d. In the muscles controlling finger movement

20. How can you improve muscle tone?
  a. Practicing good posture
  b. Getting regular physical exercise
  c. Wearing safety equipment
  d. Eating fruits and vegetables

21. What problem of the muscular system is an inherited disorder?
  a. Hernia
  b. Muscle sprain
  c. Muscular dystrophy
  d. Tendinitis

Thinking Critically

After reading the question or statement, write a short answer using complete sentences.

22. Connect. What are some ways that the muscular system works together with other body systems?

23. Infer. Consider an injury to a muscle in the thigh. Why might it cause pain when straightening the leg, but not when bending the leg?

24. Apply. Why might it be important for the children of a person with muscular dystrophy to be screened for the disease?

25. Apply. How can strengthening muscles prevent injury?

LESSON 3

Vocabulary Review

Use the correct vocabulary term to complete the following statements.

26. The _____ coordinates the movement of skeletal muscles.

27. The _____ is the center of conscious thought.

28. Several important involuntary functions, such as breathing and heartbeat, are controlled by _____.

29. _____ is a disorder that is characterized by recurrent seizures.

30. A group of neurological disorders resulting from damage to the brain at birth is called _____.

Understanding Key Concepts

After reading the question or statement, select the correct answer.

31. Which of the following is *not* a part of the brain stem?
  a. Cerebellum
  b. Medulla oblongata
  c. Midbrain
  d. Thalamus

32. What can result from a spinal cord injury?
  a. Concussion
  b. Contusion
  c. Epilepsy
  d. Paralysis

33. Which disease or disorder is *not* degenerative?
  a. Alzheimer's disease
  b. Cerebral palsy
  c. Multiple sclerosis
  d. Parkinson's disease

34. What disease or disorder is characterized by sudden episodes of electrical activity in the brain?
  a. Alzheimer's disease
  b. Cerebral palsy
  c. Epilepsy
  d. Parkinson's disease

Thinking Critically

After reading the question or statement, write a short answer using complete sentences.

35. Analyze. How do the central nervous system and peripheral nervous system work together during the motor response to a stimulus?

36. Infer. How does the nervous system protect the brain and spinal cord?

37. Compare. Explain the difference between axons and dendrites.

38. Infer. Why might the symptoms of a degenerative disease of the nervous system be difficult to treat?

39. Describe. What might happen in the nervous system and muscles when a person is surprised by a sudden loud sound like a fire alarm going off nearby?

40. Explain. Why is it important to wear protective gear and to check the depth of water before diving?

PROJECT-BASED ASSESSMENT

Sleep and Your Brain

BACKGROUND

Getting enough sleep means more than resting your body. It's also a time when your brain prepares for the next day. To function at its best, your brain needs to go through five cycles while you sleep. If you don't get enough sleep, both your body and brain won't function at their best the next day.

TASK

Create a podcast describing the importance of sleep to brain functioning.

AUDIENCE

Students in your class

PURPOSE

Help explain the importance of sleep in re-energizing the brain.

PROCEDURE

1. Review the information on the nervous system in Module 14.

2. Conduct research online to learn about the importance of sleep to brain functions.

3. Create a podcast lasting two or three minutes on why the brain needs sleep. Also, using an online survey tool, develop a survey for classmates to fill out on the effectiveness of your podcast.

4. Play the podcast for your class.

5. Ask students to complete the survey to learn if they have any additional questions about why the brain needs sleep. The survey should also assess whether your podcast was effective.

Math Practice

Interpret Tables. A diet high in calcium and vitamin D can help prevent bone loss or osteoporosis. The table below shows the amount of calcium and vitamin D needed each day for different age groups. Use the table to answer Questions 1–3.

DAILY NEED FOR CALCIUM AND VITAMIN D		
Age Group	Calcium	Vitamin D
0 to 6 months	210 mg	200 IU
7 to 12 months	270 mg	200 IU
1 to 3 years	500 mg	200 IU
4 to 8 years	800 mg	200 IU
9 to 18 years	1,300 mg	200 IU
19 to 50 years	1,000 mg	200 IU
51 to 70 years	1,200 mg	400 IU
Over 70 years	1,200 mg	600 IU

Adapted from *"What Is Osteoporosis?"* National Institutes of Health, Osteoporosis and Related Bone Diseases-National Resource Center, March 2006.

1. What is the difference between the vitamin D daily need for babies, under 12 months, and the daily amount of vitamin D for people over 70?
   a. 200 IU
   b. 400 IU
   c. 600 IU
   d. 800 IU

2. Between which two age groups is there a decrease in the amount of calcium needed?
   a. 0 to 6 months and 7 to 12 months
   b. 4 to 8 years and 9 to 18 years
   c. 9 to 18 years and 19 to 50 years
   d. 19 to 50 years and 51 to 70 years

3. Which group needs the most calcium daily?
   a. 0 to 6 months
   b. 9 to 18 years
   c. Over 50 years
   d. Over 70 years

Reading/Writing Practice

Understand and Apply. Read the passage below, and then answer the questions.

Each year in the United States, 10,000 new cases of spinal cord injury are reported. These injuries may result from sports or recreational activities, motor vehicle crashes, falls, physical assaults, and gunshot wounds. Spinal injuries may result in paralysis, or the loss of muscle function and feeling in part of the body. An injury to the upper part of the spinal cord may result in **quadriplegia,** *or paralysis of both upper and lower limbs.* **Paraplegia,** *paralysis of both lower limbs, is caused by an injury lower on the spinal column. Researchers are looking for ways to cure paralysis. Electrical sensors and stimulators can help quadriplegic victims flex their limbs. Possible cures include removal of scar tissue and transplantation of cells that promote nerve growth.*

1. What was the author's purpose?
   a. To explain how to cure paralysis
   b. To persuade people to wear helmets
   c. To describe the effects of spinal injuries
   d. To describe different types of paralysis

2. Which sentence best represents the main idea of the second paragraph?
   a. Paralysis can be cured.
   b. There are different degrees of paralysis.
   c. Paralysis can result from accidents.
   d. Paralysis cannot be cured.

3. Write a paragraph persuading a friend to wear a safety belt while riding in a motor vehicle. Provide details about spinal cord injuries to support your main points.

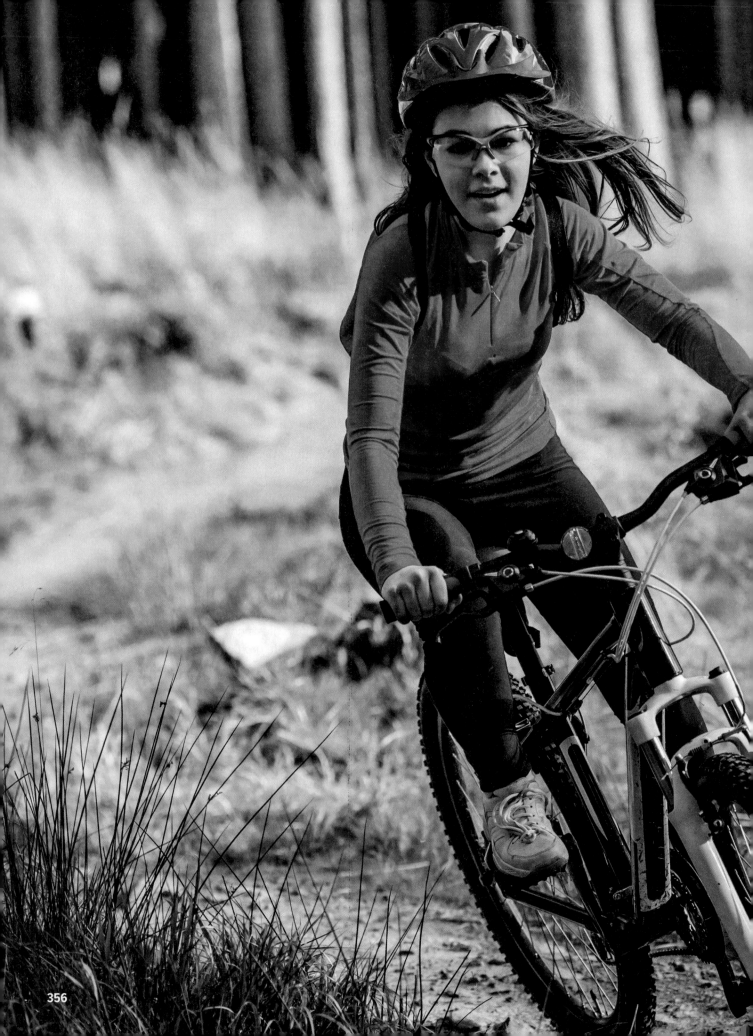

MODULE 15

Cardiovascular, Respiratory, and Digestive Systems

LESSONS

The Cardiovascular and Lymphatic Systems

. . . .

BEFORE YOU READ

Create a T Chart. As you read, list the problems of the cardiovascular and lymphatic systems on the left side, under the label "Problems." List preventive health behaviors that can help reduce these problems on the right side, under the label "Prevention."

Problems	Prevention

Vocabulary

plasma
hemoglobin
pathogen
platelets
capillaries
lymph
blood pressure

. . . .

BIG IDEA The cardiovascular system moves blood through the body, while the lymphatic system circulates lymph throughout the body.

REAL LIFE ISSUES

The Beat Goes On. Marcos hears the announcement for the boys' 100-yard dash. His pulse quickens. This is it—the moment he's been training for all year. He gets into the starting position. At the sound of the starter pistol, he takes off. His legs are pumping, his lungs are burning, and his heart is racing as he crosses the finish line. He smiles, as the cheers of the crowd affirm that he has won. *Write a persuasive paragraph that explains to a younger person why it's important to practice behaviors that keep your heart healthy.*

After completing the lesson, review and analyze your response to the Real Life Issues question.

Blood Circulation

MAIN IDEA The cardiovascular system provides nutrients and oxygen, carries away wastes, and helps fight disease.

When you're exercising hard, like Marcos in the Real Life Issues story, you can feel your heart pounding. At other times, your heartbeat is less noticeable, but it is always there. Even when you're asleep, your heart is working, pumping blood to every cell in your body. Blood reaches your cells through a network of blood vessels that would stretch over 60,000 miles if they were all laid end to end. That's enough to circle Earth almost two and a half times.

Together, your heart and blood vessels form your cardiovascular system. This system is responsible for many important tasks:

- Carrying oxygen from the lungs to your body's cells

- Absorbing nutrients from food and delivering them to body cells

- Carrying carbon dioxide, a waste gas, from your cells back to your lungs to be exhaled

- Delivering other waste products to the kidneys for removal from the body

- Carrying the white blood cells that fight disease

The Heart

The circulation of your blood depends on the steady beating of your heart. The heart is a muscle containing four chambers. The two top chambers are called the *atria.* The lower chambers are the *ventricles.* A wall of tissue, the *septum,* separates the two sides of the heart. Between the atrium and ventricle on each side is a valve that allows blood to flow through the chambers.

At the top of the right atrium is an area of muscle that acts as a pacemaker for the heart. Electrical impulses stimulate the atria to **contract**, forcing blood into the ventricles. These electrical impulses travel through the heart to an area between the two ventricles. There they stimulate the muscle of the ventricles to contract, pumping blood out of the heart.

ACADEMIC VOCABULARY

contract *(verb)*: to draw together

Pulmonary Circulation

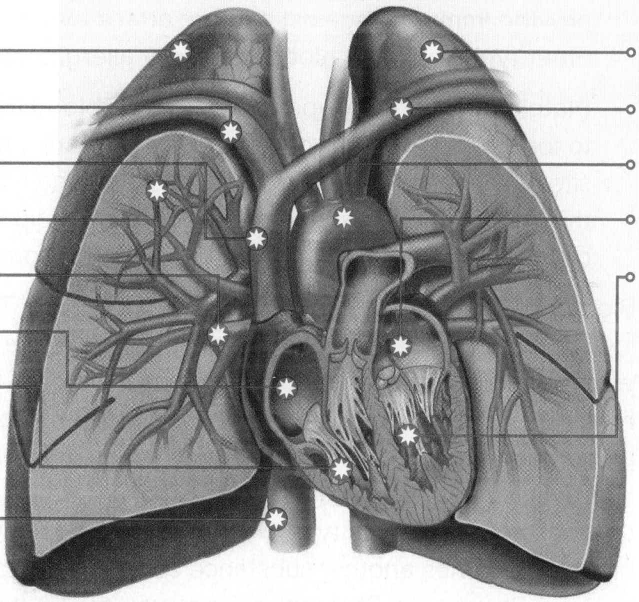

right lung
pulmonary artery
superior vena cava
capillaries
pulmonary veins
right atrium
right ventricle
inferior vena cava
left lung
pulmonary artery
aorta
left atrium
left ventricle

Pulmonary circulation is the transfer of blood between the heart and the lungs.

The two sides of the heart are responsible for two different jobs. The right side carries out the *pulmonary circulation*—the process by which blood moves between the heart and the lungs. Blood that has lost oxygen and picked-up carbon dioxide and waste enters the right side of the heart and is pumped out to the lungs, where it picks up fresh oxygen. From the lungs, the oxygen-rich blood returns to the left side of the heart and is circulated again through the body. This process is called *systemic circulation.*

Blood

The whole purpose of the heart is to circulate blood, which delivers oxygen, hormones, and nutrients to the cells and carries away wastes. Blood is made up of four components:

- **Plasma.** This is the fluid that contains other parts of the blood. About 55 percent of your blood's total volume consists of plasma. This fluid is mostly water, but it also contains nutrients, proteins, salt, and hormones.

- **Red blood cells.** These cells make up about 40 percent of normal blood. They contain **hemoglobin,** which is the oxygen-carrying protein in blood. The iron in hemoglobin binds with oxygen in the lungs and releases oxygen in the body's tissues. There, the hemoglobin combines with carbon dioxide, which is carried from the cells to the lungs.

- **White blood cells.** These cells protect the body against infection. Some white blood cells surround and ingest **pathogens—** microorganisms that cause disease. Others produce antibodies that provide immunity against a future attack by the same pathogen. Still other types of white blood cells fight allergic reactions.

- **Platelets.** These are types of cells in the blood that cause blood clots to form. When the wall of a blood vessel tears, platelets collect at the site. They release chemicals that stimulate the blood to produce small thread-like fibers that trap nearby cells and help to form a clot. The clot blocks the flow of blood and dries out to form a scab.

Blood can also contain substances called *antigens.* The types of antigens in your blood determine your blood type. If you have the A or B antigen, your blood will be type A or type B. If you have both antigens, you are type AB, and if you have neither, you are type O. People cannot receive blood from other people whose blood carries different antigens. However, everyone can receive type O blood, which has no antigens. For this reason, people with type O blood are called *universal donors.* Most blood also carries another substance called the *Rh factor.* If your blood contains Rh, you are *Rh positive;* if not, you are *Rh negative.*

Blood Vessels

There are three main types of blood vessels: arteries, capillaries, and veins.

- Arteries branch into progressively smaller vessels called *arterioles.* These, in turn, deliver blood to capillaries.

- **Capillaries** are small vessels that carry blood from arterioles and to small vessels called venules, which empty into veins. Capillaries form a vast network throughout tissues and organs in the body, reaching almost all body cells. The capillaries also play a role in controlling body temperature. Capillaries near the skin's surface can dilate, allowing heat to escape through the skin. They can also constrict to reduce heat loss if body temperature drops below normal.

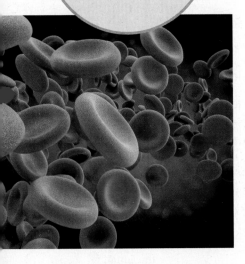

Millions of each type of blood cell can be found in just 1 milliliter of blood. **What is the main role of red blood cells?**

Phoniamai Photo/Shutterstock

- Veins have thinner and less elastic walls than those of the arteries. However, they are still strong enough to withstand the pressure exerted by blood flowing through them. The body's largest veins, the upper and lower *vena cava,* carry oxygen-depleted blood to the right atrium of the heart. Pulmonary veins carry oxygenated blood from the lungs to the left atrium. Many veins throughout the body, especially those in the legs, have valves that help prevent the backflow of blood as it is pumped back to the heart. Surrounding muscles also help move blood through the veins by putting pressure on the veins each time they contract.

A network of arteries, veins, and capillaries moves blood throughout the body, providing cells with oxygen and nutrients as well as removing wastes.

The Cardiovascular System

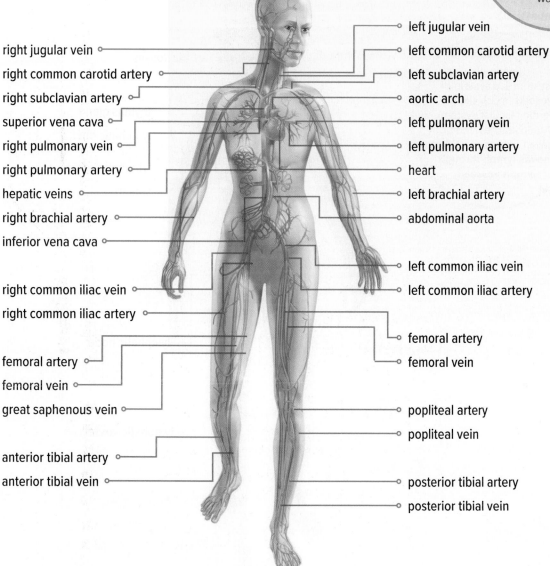

right jugular vein

right common carotid artery

right subclavian artery

superior vena cava

right pulmonary vein

right pulmonary artery

hepatic veins

right brachial artery

inferior vena cava

right common iliac vein

right common iliac artery

femoral artery

femoral vein

great saphenous vein

anterior tibial artery

anterior tibial vein

left jugular vein

left common carotid artery

left subclavian artery

aortic arch

left pulmonary vein

left pulmonary artery

heart

left brachial artery

abdominal aorta

left common iliac vein

left common iliac artery

femoral artery

femoral vein

popliteal artery

popliteal vein

posterior tibial artery

posterior tibial vein

Lymph Circulation

MAIN IDEA The lymphatic system helps fight infection and provides immunity to disease.

The lymphatic system consists of a network of vessels and tissues that move and filter **lymph**, which is the clear fluid that fills the spaces around body cells. Like plasma, lymph contains water and proteins. It also contains fats and specialized white blood cells called *lymphocytes*. Like the white blood cells in the blood, these cells protect the body against pathogens. There are two types of lymphocytes: B cells and T cells:

- **B cells.** These cells multiply when they come in contact with a pathogen. Some of the new B cells produce antibodies that fight the pathogen. Other B cells create an immune response to prevent a second attack of the same disease.

Reading Check

Compare and Contrast How are the cardiovascular and lymphatic systems similar? How are they different?

Lymphatic System

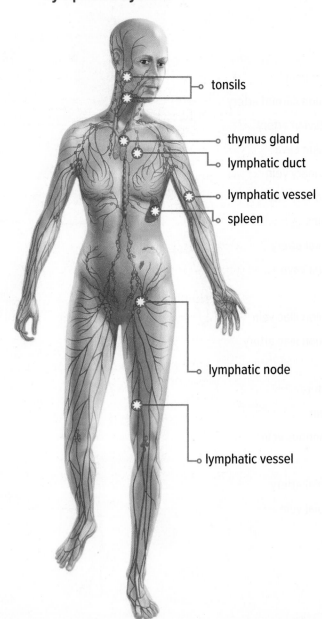

The lymphatic system is a system of vessels, much like the cardiovascular system, that helps protect the body against pathogens. **What moves lymph through lymph vessels?**

- tonsils
- thymus gland
- lymphatic duct
- lymphatic vessel
- spleen
- lymphatic node
- lymphatic vessel

- **T cells.** These cells also multiply and enlarge when they come in contact with a pathogen. There are two main types of T cells: killer cells and helper cells. Killer T cells release toxins that prevent infection from spreading. Helper T cells activate the B cells and the killer T cells. They also control the body's immune system.

Smooth muscles surrounding the walls of lymph vessels, helped by surrounding skeletal muscles, contract to move lymph toward the heart. Two large lymphatic ducts empty lymph into veins close to the heart, returning the fluid to the blood. Lymph within the lymph vessels is filtered by small bean-shaped organs called *lymph nodes*. White blood cells within the lymph nodes trap and destroy pathogens. The lymphatic system also includes larger organs and tissues—such as the spleen, thymus gland, tonsils, adenoids, and appendix—that help protect the body from infection.

Maintaining Your Circulatory Health

MAIN IDEA Healthy habits can protect the health of the cardiovascular and lymphatic systems.

Many problems with the cardiovascular and lymphatic systems first appear later in life. However, the choices you make while you are young can reduce your risk for these problems. Here are a few healthful behaviors that should become regular habits:

- Eat a well-balanced diet.
- Maintain a healthy weight.
- Get regular aerobic exercise—at least 30 minutes three or four times a week.
- Avoid tobacco use and secondhand smoke.
- Avoid illegal drug use.
- Get regular medical checkups.

Blood Pressure

Maintaining pressure in the cardiovascular system is important for proper blood circulation. When the ventricles of the heart contract, they create pressure in the arteries. As blood is forced into the arteries, arterial walls stretch under the increased pressure. When the ventricles relax and refill with blood, arterial pressure decreases. **Blood pressure** is a measure of the amount of force that the blood places on the walls of blood vessels, particularly large arteries, as it is pumped through the body.

● ● ● ● ● ● ● ● ● ● ●

Reading Check

Cause and Effect What cardiovascular disorder can be avoided through diet?

● ● ● ● ● ● ● ● ● ● ●

A blood pressure reading includes two numbers. The first number, called *systolic pressure*, indicates the maximum pressure reached in your blood vessels as your heart contracts. The second, or bottom, number is *diastolic pressure*. This is the pressure at its lowest point when the ventricles relax. The normal range for blood pressure is anywhere below 120/80, although exercise and stress can raise this number temporarily. A blood pressure reading above 140/90 is considered high and places a strain on the heart.

Cardiovascular System Problems

Some problems that affect the cardiovascular system are inherited. Others may result from illness, diet, or aging. Cardiovascular disorders can have a wide range of effects and treatments. Read about each disorder in the list below to learn more.

- **Congenital heart defects.** A congenital heart defect is a condition of the heart that is present at birth. One example is a septal defect—a hole in the septum that allows oxygenated blood to mix with oxygen-depleted blood. Congenital heart defects may occur if a baby's mother suffers from poor health during pregnancy. In some cases, medication and possibly surgery can repair the affected portion of the heart. In severe cases, a heart transplant may be performed. The donor heart must match the tissue and blood type of the patient. Even so, the recipient must take drugs for the remainder of his or her life to prevent the body from rejecting the donated heart.

- **Heart murmurs.** A heart murmur may be caused by a hole in the heart or a leaking or malfunctioning valve.

- **Varicose veins.** This condition occurs when the valves in veins do not close tightly enough to prevent backflow of the blood.

- **Anemia.** The blood of a person with anemia cannot carry as much oxygen as it should. It may occur because there are too few red blood cells or because those cells have low concentrations of hemoglobin. The most common cause is iron deficiency.

- **Hemophilia.** In this inherited disorder, the blood does not clot properly. Bruising and uncontrolled bleeding may occur spontaneously or as a result of an injury. Treatment for hemophilia includes injections to introduce the missing clotting proteins into the blood.

- **Leukemia.** This is a form of cancer in which white blood cells are produced excessively and abnormally. The person becomes susceptible to infection, severe anemia, and possibly uncontrolled bleeding. Chemotherapy, radiation, and bone marrow transplant are all treatment options.

Lymphatic System Problems

Disorders of the lymphatic system can range from mild to life threatening. They may be caused by infection or heredity. Read about each lymphatic disorder to learn more.

- **Tonsillitis.** This is an infection of the tonsils, two organs that help reduce the number of pathogens entering the body through the respiratory system. It is often treated with antibiotics, or surgery for chronic cases.

- **Immune deficiency.** If the immune system becomes weakened, it can no longer protect the body against infection. Immune deficiency can result from a congenital condition in which the body cannot make specialized white blood cells, limiting protection against infection. Other causes include HIV, chemotherapy, and sometimes aging.

- **Hodgkin's Disease.** Also called Hodgkin's lymphoma, this type of cancer affects the tissue found in the lymph nodes and the spleen. Early detection and treatment is essential for recovery. Treatment may include removal of lymph nodes, radiation, or chemotherapy.

Reading Check

Apply What is the connection between the immune system and HIV?

Fitness Zone

I heard that antioxidants provide protection against conditions such as heart disease and cancer. They might even slow down the aging process. I read that researchers at Tufts University in Boston recommend these seven foods in your daily diet: prunes, raisins, blueberries, blackberries, kale, strawberries, and spinach. I should be able to eat at least one of those each day.

Lesson 1 Review

Facts and Vocabulary

1. Describe why the cardiovascular system is important to overall health.

2. List three behaviors that will help prevent high blood pressure.

3. Explain what blood pressure numbers measure.

Thinking Critically

4. **Infer.** Why are people with type O blood called "universal donors"?

5. **Apply.** Why might lymph nodes become the main site of the body's response to an infection?

Applying Health Skills

6. **Advocacy.** Find out more about heart disease and how to prevent it. What foods and physical activities promote heart health? Design a website that promotes heart-healthy behaviors.

Writing Critically

7. **Expository.** Write a paragraph describing three healthy choices you have made to maintain your cardiovascular and lymphatic health.

The Respiratory System

BEFORE YOU READ

Prepare Note Cards. On separate index cards, list the various organs of the respiratory system. On the reverse side of each card, write the function of the organ.

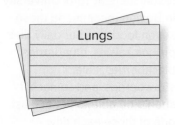

Lungs

Vocabulary

trachea
bronchi
diaphragm
asthma
tuberculosis
emphysema

• • • • • • • • • • •

Reading Check

Explain In what structures does gas exchange take place?

BIG IDEA The respiratory system provides oxygen to the blood and removes carbon dioxide from the body.

> ### REAL LIFE ISSUES
>
> **Respiratory Problems.** Asthma is a common problem for young people. According to statistics from the CDC, among those ages 0–17, 11 percent of males, and 7.8 percent of females have asthma. Among those ages 18 and over, 5.7 of males and 9.7 of females have asthma. ***Write a paragraph describing what you think causes asthma and triggers asthma attacks.***
>
> After completing the lesson, review and analyze your response to the Real Life Issues question.

The Process of Respiration

MAIN IDEA The respiratory system provides oxygen to the blood and removes carbon dioxide from the body.

Take a deep breath. You can feel your lungs expanding slightly as they fill with air, and deflating again as you exhale. But do you ever think about what your body is doing with that air?

Your respiratory system removes carbon dioxide from the body and supplies it with fresh oxygen. Respiration is a two-part process. In *external respiration,* oxygen drawn from outside the body moves from the lungs into the blood, and carbon dioxide moves from the blood into the lungs, where it can be removed from the body. In *internal respiration,* the blood transfers oxygen to the body's cells and picks up carbon dioxide. This continual exchange of gases is essential for survival. Your body relies on oxygen to fuel the brain and to metabolize food for energy.

Your Lungs

The structure of the lungs can be compared to the structure of a branching tree. Air moves into the lungs through the **trachea** (TRAY-kee-uh), or the windpipe. The trachea branches out into two **bronchi** (BRAHN-ky), the main airways that reach into each lung. The airways grow smaller as they branch out deeper into the lungs. A network of tubes called *bronchioles* draws air down into microscopic structures called *alveoli.* These are thin-walled air sacs covered with capillaries. Gas exchange takes place as oxygen and carbon dioxide pass across the thin walls of the capillaries and alveoli.

How You Breathe

Your lungs automatically fill with air and are emptied in a rhythmic way. This rhythm changes with your level of activity. You've probably noticed that when you do aerobic exercise, such as running or brisk walking, you tend to breathe faster than when you're sitting still. Breathing is regulated by the brain, which sends impulses to stimulate the muscles involved in respiration. This process provides your body with the oxygen it needs to keep going. It also removes carbon dioxide from the lungs. The lungs are found within the chest cavity and are protected by the ribs. In the base of the chest cavity is the **diaphragm** (DY-uh-fram), a muscle that separates the chest from the abdominal cavity.

When you inhale, your diaphragm and the muscles between your ribs contract. This causes your chest cavity and lungs to **expand**. The pressure inside your lungs is lower than the pressure outside your body, so air naturally flows into your lungs to equalize the pressure. As you exhale, these same muscles relax and your chest cavity deflates. Pressure inside your lungs is higher, so air naturally flows out of your lungs to the lower-pressure area outside.

ACADEMIC VOCABULARY

expand *(verb)*: to open up

The lungs are the principal organs of the respiratory system. **Which structures in the diagram are also parts of the cardiovascular system?**

The Respiratory System

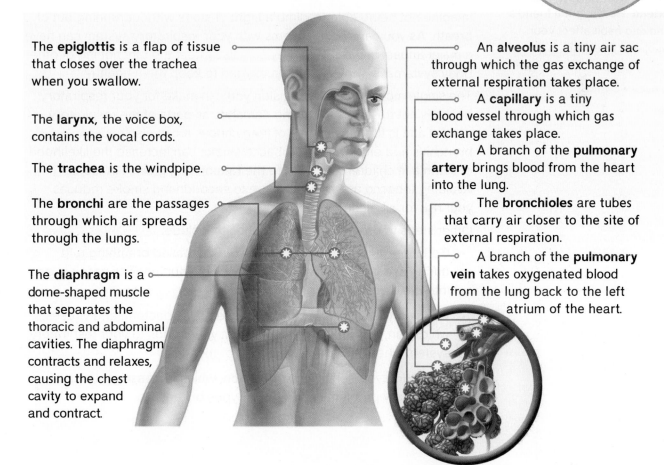

The **epiglottis** is a flap of tissue that closes over the trachea when you swallow.

The **larynx**, the voice box, contains the vocal cords.

The **trachea** is the windpipe.

The **bronchi** are the passages through which air spreads through the lungs.

The **diaphragm** is a dome-shaped muscle that separates the thoracic and abdominal cavities. The diaphragm contracts and relaxes, causing the chest cavity to expand and contract.

An **alveolus** is a tiny air sac through which the gas exchange of external respiration takes place.

A **capillary** is a tiny blood vessel through which gas exchange takes place.

A branch of the **pulmonary artery** brings blood from the heart into the lung.

The **bronchioles** are tubes that carry air closer to the site of external respiration.

A branch of the **pulmonary vein** takes oxygenated blood from the lung back to the left atrium of the heart.

Air enters and exits your body through the nose and mouth. The membranes of the nose are lined with hairlike structures, called *cilia,* and with cells that produce mucus. The cilia and mucus work together to filter out foreign particles, such as dust, bacteria, and viruses. The air is also warmed and moistened as it passes through your nose and mouth. The air then moves into the *pharynx,* or throat. Next it passes through the *larynx,* or voice box. The larynx contains the vocal cords, two bands of tissue that produce sound when air forced between them causes them to vibrate. From there, air moves into the *trachea,* or windpipe. The tissue that lines the trachea also has mucus and cilia to trap particles and prevent them from making their way into your lungs.

One other structure is not directly involved in respiration, but it still plays an important role in the respiratory system. This is the *epiglottis,* a flap of tissue located above the larynx. It folds down to close off the entrance to the larynx and trachea when you swallow. This is an involuntary action that keeps food or drink from entering the respiratory system. If you eat too quickly or laugh while eating, your food may get past the epiglottis and "go down the wrong pipe." This will stimulate the cough reflex to force the material out of your respiratory system.

Maintaining Your Respiratory Health

MAIN IDEA Caring for your lungs can prevent many respiratory disorders.

Imagine not being able to climb a flight of stairs without running out of breath. As you can see, problems with your respiratory system can have a major impact on your life. They can also affect the functioning of other body systems, which depend on oxygen to keep them healthy.

The single most important decision you can make for your respiratory health is not to smoke. Smoking damages all parts of the respiratory system and is the main cause of lung cancer. It can also cause bronchitis and emphysema. Tobacco smoke can increase the likelihood of asthma in children and reduce the rate of lung growth in teens. Avoiding tobacco use and exposure to secondhand smoke reduces your risk for all these problems.

Other steps to promote respiratory health include:

- Getting regular physical activity. Your increased breathing rate during exercise improves the capacity of your lungs to pass oxygen into the blood.

- Washing your hands regularly. This removes bacteria and viruses, which can easily be transmitted from your hands to your respiratory system when you touch your nose or mouth.

- Protecting yourself from air pollution, which increases the risk of respiratory problems and certain types of cancers.

Reading Check

Extend How might a friend's smoking habit affect your respiratory health?

Respiratory System Problems

MAIN IDEA Problems of the respiratory system can be mild, such as a cold, or serious and even life threatening.

If you're like most people, you've had a cold or influenza ("the flu") at some point in your life. These infections of the upper respiratory system are common and usually mild. However, other respiratory disorders can be much more serious. Some can cause permanent damage to the lung tissue, preventing the proper transfer of air in the alveoli. If the damage is severe, a lung transplant may be the only treatment. A deceased donor may provide one or both lungs. Recent medical advances have enabled living donors to provide a portion of one lung to a recipient. The list below includes some examples of respiratory infections, ranging from mild to severe.

- **Sinusitis.** This is an inflammation of the tissues that line the sinuses (air-filled cavities above the nasal passages and throat). It can result from allergies or infection. Symptoms include nasal congestion, headache, and fever. Treatment includes nasal decongestant drops or sprays and, for a bacterial infection, antibiotics.

- **Bronchitis.** This is an inflammation of the bronchi caused by infection or exposure to irritants such as tobacco smoke or air pollution. The membranes that line the bronchi produce excessive amounts of mucus, blocking the airways. This leads to symptoms such as coughing, wheezing, and shortness of breath, which worsen with physical activity. Treatment includes avoiding exposure to the irritant and taking antibiotics if appropriate.

- **Asthma** (AZ-muh). This is an inflammatory condition in which the trachea, bronchi, and bronchioles become narrowed, causing difficulty breathing. It can affect both adults and children. During an asthma attack, the smooth muscles of the airway contract involuntarily, causing chest tightness and breathing difficulty. Acute asthma attacks can be relieved with an inhaler that dispenses medication to dilate, or widen, the airways.

- **Pneumonia.** This is an inflammation of the lungs commonly caused by a bacterial or viral infection. In one common type of pneumonia, the alveoli swell and become clogged with mucus, decreasing the amount of gas exchange. Symptoms include cough, fever, chills, and chest pain. Bacterial pneumonia is treated with antibiotics.

An inhaler can relieve an asthma attack. Long-term treatment of asthma includes using medication that reduces inflammation and avoiding substances that can trigger an attack, such as pollen, dust, animal dander, and tobacco smoke. **Why is it important for an asthmatic person to avoid air pollution?**

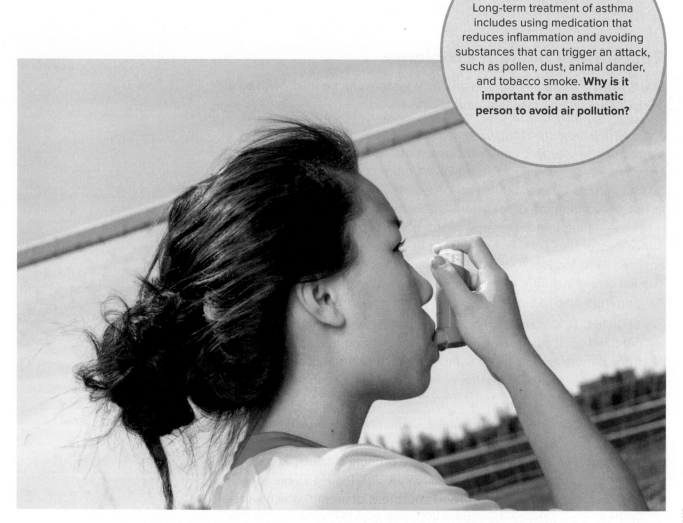

- **Tuberculosis (TB).** TB is a contagious bacterial infection that usually affects the lungs. It may show no symptoms for many years. This happens because when a person becomes infected with TB, the immune system surrounds the infected area and isolates it. However, if the immune system is weakened by illness or age, the infection can become active. During this active stage, symptoms include cough, fever, fatigue, and weight loss. Treatment includes antibiotics and hospitalization.

- **Emphysema.** This is a disease that progressively destroys the walls of the alveoli. It is almost always caused by smoking. Its symptoms include a chronic cough and breathing difficulty. Although these symptoms can be treated, the tissue damage is permanent.

Reading Check

Explain Why can you get tuberculosis from someone who doesn't show any symptoms of the disease?

Myths & Reality

Do you or one of your friends have asthma? Think about its effects on daily life and consider this myth about asthma.

Myth: A person can grow out of asthma.

Reality: A person cannot grow out of asthma. For about half of children with asthma, the condition becomes inactive during the teen years. In adulthood, though, asthma symptoms can return.

Lesson 2 Review

Facts and Vocabulary

1. Describe what causes the lungs to fill with air.

2. Identify which problems of the respiratory system might be caused by smoking.

3. Describe how handwashing can protect the respiratory system.

Thinking Critically

4. **Compare.** How do internal respiration and external respiration differ?

5. **Apply.** A friend wants to quit smoking. You notice that just walking to school with you leaves her breathing hard. How can you encourage her to quit smoking?

Applying Health Skills

6. **Communication Skills.** Imagine you have a close family member who bicycles to work on major streets during rush hour. During this time, air pollution is at its worst, and a cyclist inhales a lot of it. Write a dialogue in which you encourage the family member to consider the negative effects of this practice. Explain the problems that can result.

Writing Critically

7. **Expository.** Write a paragraph explaining how oxygen and carbon dioxide are exchanged through the respiratory system.

The Digestive System

BEFORE YOU READ

Create a Chart. Make a three-column chart like the one below. In the first column, list the organs of the digestive system. In the second, describe the function of each organ. In the third, list behaviors that contribute to the health of each organ.

Digestive organ	What it does	How to keep healthy

Vocabulary

mastication
peristalsis
gastric juices
bile
peptic ulcer
appendicitis

ACADEMIC VOCABULARY

involve *(verb)*: to require as a necessary accompaniment

BIG IDEA The digestive system provides nutrients and energy for your body through the digestion of food.

REAL LIFE ISSUES

Fast-Food Folly. Joey has been looking forward to lunch with his uncle at their favorite fast-food restaurant. Once they are seated, Joey orders a double burger, a side of cheese fries, and a giant-size soda. They share a banana split for dessert. Soon after eating, Joey feels bloated and queasy. Later that afternoon, he feels tired, even though he hasn't done any physical activity. Even after a quick nap in front of the television, he still doesn't feel good. Joey wonders if it has something to do with his lunch. *Write a description of a time when the food you ate affected the way you felt afterward. Describe how your energy level was affected.*

After completing the lesson, review and analyze your response to the Real Life Issues question.

What Happens During Digestion

MAIN IDEA In digestion, foods are broken down and absorbed as nourishment or eliminated as waste.

What was the last thing you had to eat? Depending on when you ate it, that food may be sitting in your stomach right now, or it may be making its way through your body to provide nourishment to your cells. Food is your body's fuel source, but before your body can use it, it needs to be broken down into smaller nutrients that can be absorbed into the blood. This is the job of your digestive system. It can be divided into three main processes:

- Digestion is the mechanical and chemical breakdown of foods within the stomach and intestines for use by the body's cells.

- Absorption is the passage of digested food from the digestive tract into the bloodstream.

- Elimination is the expulsion of undigested food or waste from the body.

The Digestive Organs

MAIN IDEA The digestive system consists of the mouth, esophagus, stomach, and intestines.

Digestion **involves** two processes. The mechanical process involves chewing, mashing, and breaking food down. The chemical process involves secretions produced by digestive organs.

The Digestive System

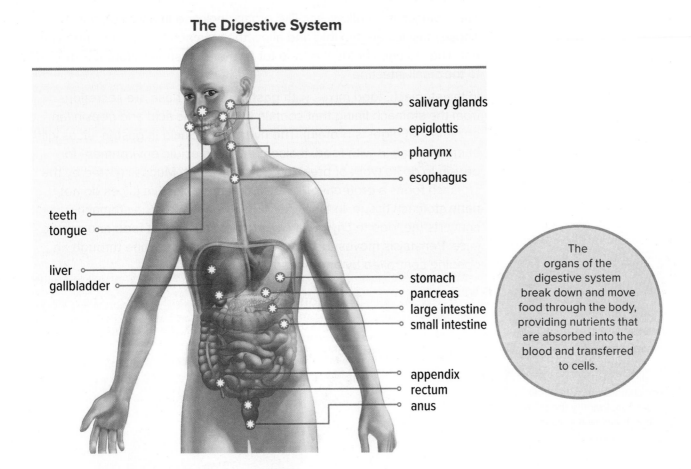

salivary glands
epiglottis
pharynx
esophagus

teeth
tongue

liver
gallbladder

stomach
pancreas
large intestine
small intestine

appendix
rectum
anus

> The organs of the digestive system break down and move food through the body, providing nutrients that are absorbed into the blood and transferred to cells.

The Mouth

The process of digestion begins in the mouth. The teeth break down the food you eat into smaller pieces. **Mastication** is the process of chewing, which prepares food to be swallowed. The tongue prepares chewed food for swallowing by shaping it. The salivary glands also do their part by producing digestive juices. Saliva contains an enzyme that begins to break down the sugars and starches in food into smaller particles. As you chew your food, two other structures help make sure that it goes down into the stomach where it belongs. The *uvula,* a small flap of tissue at the back of the mouth, prevents food from entering the nasal passages. The *epiglottis,* tissue covering the throat, prevents food from entering the respiratory system.

The Esophagus

When food is swallowed, it enters the esophagus. This is a muscular tube about 10 inches long that connects the pharynx, or throat, to the stomach. Food is moved through the esophagus, stomach, and intestine through a process called **peristalsis**. Peristalsis is a series of involuntary muscle contractions that moves food through the digestive tract. It begins as soon as food is swallowed. At the end of the esophagus, a circular muscle called a *sphincter* allows food to enter the stomach.

The Stomach

The stomach is a hollow, sac-like organ enclosed in a wall of muscles. These muscles are flexible and allow the stomach to expand when you eat. The stomach holds the food for further digestion before it is moved to the small intestine.

In the stomach, food mixes with **gastric juices**. These are secretions from the stomach lining that contain hydrochloric acid and pepsin (an enzyme that digests protein). The hydrochloric acid in gastric juices kills bacteria taken in with food. It also creates an acidic environment for pepsin to do its work of breaking down proteins. Mucus created by the stomach forms a protective lining so that the digestive juices do not harm stomach tissue. In time, the digestive action of the stomach converts the food to *chyme,* a creamy, fluid mixture of food and gastric juice. Peristalsis moves the chyme into the small intestine through an opening controlled by another sphincter muscle.

The Stomach

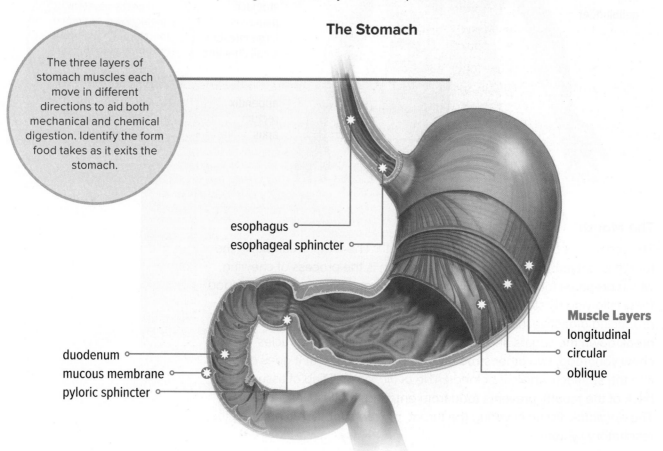

The three layers of stomach muscles each move in different directions to aid both mechanical and chemical digestion. Identify the form food takes as it exits the stomach.

esophagus
esophageal sphincter

duodenum
mucous membrane
pyloric sphincter

Muscle Layers
longitudinal
circular
oblique

The Pancreas, Liver, and Gallbladder

When chyme enters the small intestine, it contains partially digested carbohydrates and proteins and undigested fats. The juices of two other digestive organs mix with the chyme to continue breaking it down. The pancreas produces enzymes that break down the carbohydrates, fats, and proteins in food. Glands in the wall of the intestine produce other enzymes that help this process.

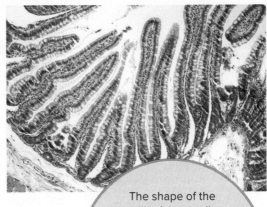

The liver produces another digestive juice—**bile**, a yellow-green, bitter fluid important in the breakdown and absorption of fats. Bile is stored in the gallbladder between meals. At mealtimes, it is secreted from the gallbladder into the bile duct to reach the intestine, where it mixes with the fats in food. Bile acids dissolve the fats into the watery contents of the intestines. After the fat is dissolved, it can be digested by the other enzymes in the small intestine.

The Small and Large Intestines

The small intestine is 20 to 23 feet in length and 1 inch in diameter. The *duodenum* is the upper part of the small intestine. Here partially digested food mixes with digestive juices secreted from the small intestine, liver, and pancreas. Then the broken-down mixture continues into the lower part of the small intestine, where about 90 percent of all nutrients are absorbed. The inner wall of the small intestine contains millions of fingerlike projections called *villi*. The villi are lined with capillaries that absorb the nutrients.

The undigested parts of the food—including liquid and fiber, or roughage—move by peristalsis into the large intestine, or *colon*. The large intestine is about 2.5 inches in diameter and 5 to 6 feet in length. Its function is to absorb water, vitamins, and salts, and to eliminate waste.

The shape of the villi of the small intestine gives them a large surface area to maximize the amount of nutrients they can absorb. **Where do nutrients go once they are absorbed by the small intestine?**

Reading Check

Interpret What are the differences between the small and large intestines?

The Digestive System

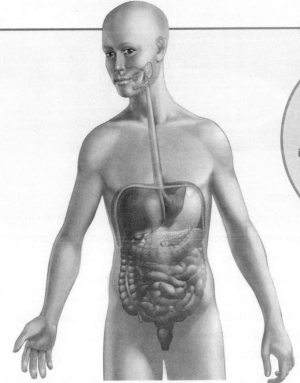

The organs of the digestive system break down and move food through the body, providing nutrients that are absorbed into the blood and transferred to cells. **Describe how nutrients in food are transferred to the body's cells.**

Digestive Problems

MAIN IDEA Digestive problems range from indigestion to conditions that require immediate medical attention.

Taking care of your digestive system begins with the foods you eat—and the way you eat them. To maintain your digestive health, eat a variety of low-fat, high-fiber foods and drink plenty of water. Wash your hands before eating to keep harmful germs from entering your digestive system. Eat slowly and chew your food thoroughly. Finally, to keep yourself from overeating, avoid using food as a way to deal with your emotions.

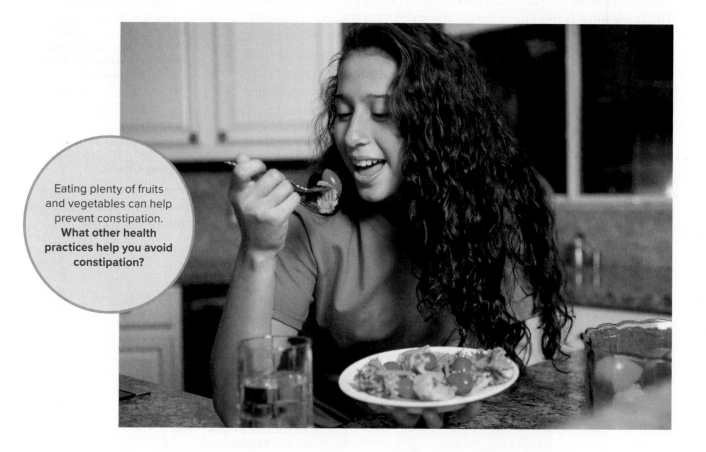

Eating plenty of fruits and vegetables can help prevent constipation. **What other health practices help you avoid constipation?**

Functional Problems

The functioning of the digestive system may be affected by illness, stress, or eating a particular food. Read about each functional problem in the list below to learn more.

- **Indigestion.** Indigestion is a feeling of discomfort in the upper abdomen, sometimes accompanied by gas and nausea. It can be caused by eating too much food, eating food too quickly, or eating spicy or high-fat foods. Stress and certain stomach disorders can also cause indigestion.

- **Constipation.** Constipation causes your feces to become dry and hard, making bowel movements difficult. It can be caused by not drinking enough water or not consuming enough fiber to move wastes through the digestive system.

- **Heartburn.** Heartburn is a burning sensation in the center of the chest that may rise up to the throat. It results from acid reflux, or the backflow of stomach acid into the esophagus. Using tobacco, alcohol, and aspirin, or eating spicy or greasy foods, can cause heartburn.

- **Gas.** The breakdown of food naturally produces gas. Excessive gas can result in cramps or an uncomfortable feeling of fullness in the abdomen.

- **Nausea.** Nausea is the feeling of discomfort that sometimes precedes vomiting. Motion sickness, pregnancy, pathogens, some medications, and dehydration can cause nausea.

- **Diarrhea.** Diarrhea is the frequent passage of watery feces. It can be caused by bacterial or viral infections, some medications, a change in eating style, overeating, emotional turmoil, or nutritional deficiencies. Diarrhea can result in dehydration.

Structural Problems

The seriousness of structural problems in the digestive system can vary. Some problems are temporary or easily treated, while others are serious and require immediate medical attention.

- **Tooth decay** may make it difficult to chew food thoroughly. Brushing and flossing teeth daily can prevent tooth decay, and regular medical checkups can catch the problem early.

- **Lactose intolerance** results from an inability to digest lactose, a type of sugar found in milk and other dairy products. Symptoms include abdominal cramps, bloating, gas, and diarrhea. People who are lactose intolerant do not produce enough *lactase,* the enzyme that breaks down lactose. They may choose soy products as an alternative to milk or dairy products.

- **Hemorrhoids** are veins in the rectum and anus that may become swollen and inflamed. Hemorrhoids may occur with constipation, during pregnancy, and after childbirth. Signs of hemorrhoids include itching, pain, and bleeding.

- **Gastritis** is an inflammation of the mucous membrane that lines the stomach. Increased production of stomach acid, alcohol or tobacco use, bacterial or viral infections, and some medications can cause gastritis. Symptoms include pain, indigestion, decreased appetite, and nausea and vomiting.

- **Colitis** is the inflammation of the large intestine, or colon. It may be caused by bacterial or viral infections. Symptoms can include fever, abdominal pain, and diarrhea that may contain blood.

- **Crohn's disease** causes inflammation of the lining of the digestive tract. Symptoms include diarrhea, weight loss, fever, and abdominal pain. The cause is not known, but seems to be associated with immune system problems.

- **Peptic ulcers** are sores in the lining of the digestive tract. They can be caused by a bacterial infection or the overuse of aspirin. Common symptoms include abdominal pain that worsens when the stomach is empty, nausea, and vomiting. Ulcers can cause stomach bleeding.

• • • • • • • • • • • •

Reading Check

Compare Which structural problems of the digestive system can result from bacterial infection?

• • • • • • • • • • • •

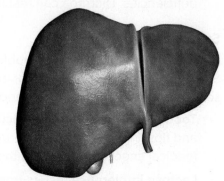

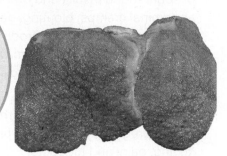

I've heard all kinds of advice about how many meals a day you should eat. Everyone seems to have a different opinion about whether it's best to have three large meals a day or five or six small ones. Eating can help speed up your metabolism so you burn more calories, so eating smaller meals throughout the day can keep your body's engine revved up. Still, it's really a personal decision based on what works best for you.

- **Gallstones** form when cholesterol in bile crystallizes. Gallstones can block the bile duct between the gallbladder and the small intestine. Symptoms of a blockage include pain in the upper right portion of the abdomen, nausea, vomiting, and fever.

- **Appendicitis** is an inflammation of the appendix. It can be caused by a blockage or bacterial infection of the appendix. Symptoms include pain in the lower right abdomen and a fever. Decreased appetite, nausea, and vomiting can also occur. The appendix may burst, spreading infection throughout the abdomen, which can lead to death.

- **Colon cancer** is the second leading cause of cancer death in the United States. It usually develops in the lowest part of the colon, near the rectum. Any bleeding from the rectum should be checked by a medical professional. A low-fat, high-fiber eating plan decreases the risk of colon cancer.

- **Cirrhosis,** or scarring of the liver tissue, is caused by prolonged, heavy alcohol use. Cirrhosis can lead to liver failure and may cause death.

Severe damage to the liver from cirrhosis may require a liver transplant. **What are the causes of cirrhosis?**

Lesson 3 Review

Facts and Vocabulary

1. Describe the functions of the digestive system that take place in the small intestine.

2. Describe the actions that cause food to move through the digestive tract.

3. Name three behaviors that help prevent indigestion.

Thinking Critically

4. **Evaluate.** What happens to the nutrients in food as it passes through the digestive system?

5. **Apply.** Create a menu with a full day of meals that you can serve to a friend who has lactose intolerance. Make sure that the menu you prepare contains foods high in calcium.

Applying Health Skills

6. **Advocacy.** Write a script for a play for elementary or middle school student on the importance of taking care of their teeth to protect their digestive systems.

Writing Critically

7. **Narrative.** Write a story from the point of view of a piece of food. Have the food describe its path through the digestive system, describing the function of each of the organs it meets.

The Excretory System

BIG IDEA The excretory system removes wastes from the body.

REAL LIFE ISSUES

The Artificial Kidney. Wendy is driving her grandfather, who has type 2 diabetes, home from the clinic. After his kidneys failed last year, Wendy's grandfather has been going to the clinic for dialysis. The first time Wendy picked him up, it looked as if he was giving blood, except the blood goes into a machine instead of a plastic bag. The machine acts like a real kidney, filtering wastes from the blood before returning the blood to her grandfather's body. ***Write a letter to yourself describing ways you can reduce your risk for type 2 diabetes and prevent kidney failure.***

After completing the lesson, review and analyze your response to the Real Life Issues question.

BEFORE YOU READ

Create an Outline. Preview this lesson by scanning the pages. Then organize the headings and subheadings into an outline. As you read, fill in the outline with important details.

I.		
	A.	
		1.
		2.
	B.	
II.		

Vocabulary

nephrons
ureters
urethra
cystitis
urethritis
hemodialysis

How Excretion Works

MAIN IDEA The excretory system uses several organs to remove all types of wastes from the body.

Every day, while your body is digesting food, it is also producing wastes in the form of solids, liquids, and gases. These wastes must be removed to keep the body functioning well. The process of removing wastes from the body is called *excretion*.

Many parts of other body systems also play a role in excretion. For example, the lungs, which are part of the respiratory system, also remove waste gases—carbon dioxide—from the body when you exhale. Your skin also removes body wastes when you sweat. The main purpose of sweat is to cool the body, but it also removes excess water and salts through the pores. Sweating too much, however, can cause dehydration.

Solid wastes produced by the digestive system are eliminated through the large intestine. Bacteria living in the large intestine convert the undigested food material into a semi-solid mass called *feces*. The liver, in addition to its role in the digestive system, helps remove certain toxins from the blood. It is the first organ to receive the chemicals absorbed from the small intestine. The liver processes materials such as drugs, alcohol, and some cellular waste products, and excretes them into bile.

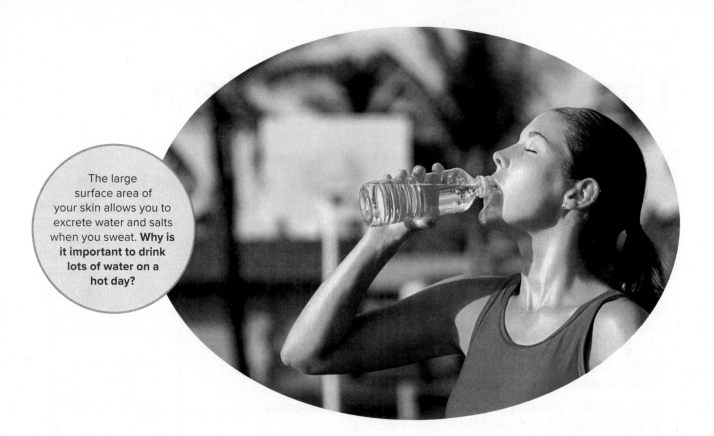

The large surface area of your skin allows you to excrete water and salts when you sweat. **Why is it important to drink lots of water on a hot day?**

ACADEMIC VOCABULARY

monitor *(verb)*: to watch or keep track of

The Urinary System

Some of the organs involved in excretion form a system of their own: the urinary system. This system consists of the kidneys, bladder, ureters, and urethra. Its main function is to filter waste and extra fluid from the blood. The liquid waste material excreted from the body is called *urine*. It consists of water and body wastes that contain nitrogen.

The Kidneys. Your kidneys are bean-shaped organs about the size of a fist. They are located near the middle of the back, just below the rib cage, one on each side. The kidneys remove waste products from the blood through tiny filtering units called **nephrons** (NEH-frahnz). Nephrons are the functional units of the kidneys. Each kidney contains more than a million nephrons. Each nephron consists of a ball of small blood capillaries, called a *glomerulus,* attached to a small renal tubule that acts as a filtering funnel.

The kidneys **monitor** the body's acid-base and water balances. Then they adjust the amount of salts, water, and other materials excreted. This meets the body's needs to maintain proper balance. The pituitary gland aids the kidneys by releasing *antidiuretic hormone* (ADH) when the body becomes dehydrated. This causes thirst and allows the kidneys to balance the body's fluid levels.

The Ureters. From the kidneys, urine travels to the bladder through the **ureters**. Ureters are tubes that connect the kidneys to the bladder. Each ureter is about 8 to 10 inches long. Muscles in the ureter walls tighten and relax to force urine down and away from the kidneys. Urine is passed from the ureters to the bladder about every 15 seconds.

The Bladder and Urethra. The bladder is a hollow muscular organ located in the pelvic cavity. It is held in place by the pelvic bones and by ligaments attached to other organs. The bladder can store about 2 cups of urine comfortably for two to five hours. Sphincter muscles keep urine from leaking. The sphincter muscles close tightly like a rubber band around the opening of the bladder into the **urethra** (yur-EE-thruh). The Urethra is the tube that leads from the bladder to the outside of the body.

Reading Check

Explain What vital body function do the kidneys provide?

The Kidney

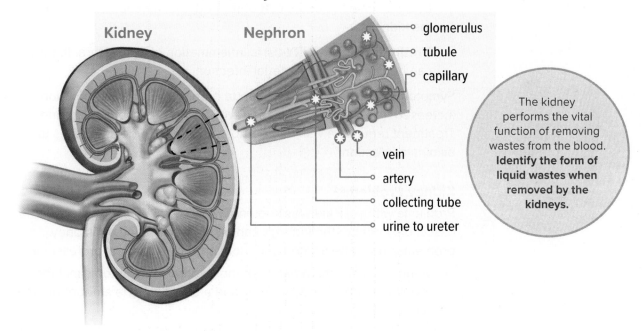

Kidney   Nephron   glomerulus
          tubule
          capillary

vein
artery
collecting tube
urine to ureter

The kidney performs the vital function of removing wastes from the blood. **Identify the form of liquid wastes when removed by the kidneys.**

Maintaining Your Excretory Health

MAIN IDEA Healthful behaviors will keep your excretory system healthy.

You depend on your excretory system to remove wastes from the body that could be toxic. To take care of this important system, practice these healthy behaviors:

- Drink enough water. Your body needs about 9 to 13 cups of water each day to function properly. Some of this water can come from the foods you eat. Drink water with meals and any time you feel thirsty, and remember to drink extra when you exercise.

- Limit your intake of caffeine and soft drinks, which can increase the amount of water lost through urination.

- Follow a well-balanced eating plan.

- Practice good hygiene to eliminate harmful bacteria that could cause infection.

- Get regular medical checkups. Tell your health care provider about any changes in bowel habits and in the frequency or urination or the color or odor of urine.

Reading Check

Infer Why is it better to drink water rather than soft drinks when you are dehydrated?

Excretory System Problems

MAIN IDEA Excretory system problems commonly result from infection or blockage.

Disorders of the excretory system can have several different causes, including infection, blockage of urine, or natural aging. Two common disorders of the urinary system are cystitis and urethritis.

- **Cystitis** (sis-TY-tis) is inflammation of the bladder, most often caused by a bacterial infection. Left untreated, the infection can spread to the kidneys.

- **Urethritis** (yur-eh-THRY-tis) is inflammation of the urethra. It, too, can be caused by a bacterial infection.

Symptoms of both conditions include burning pain during urination, increased frequency of urination, fever, and possibly blood in urine. Treatment requires a visit to a doctor and may include antibiotics to eliminate infection.

Kidney Problems

Problems with your kidneys should always be taken seriously. In some cases, disorders of the kidneys can be life threatening. All kidney problems should be treated and monitored by a medical professional.

- Nephritis is an inflammation of the nephrons. Symptoms include fever, swelling of body tissues, and a change in the amount of urine produced.

- Kidney stones are formed when salts in the urine can crystallize into solid lumps called stones. If a kidney stone moves into the ureter, it causes pain and may block the passage of urine. Smaller stones may be able to pass through the ureter on their own and exit the body through the urethra. Larger stones can be broken up using shock waves so that they can pass out of the body. In some cases, surgery is needed to break up the stones.

- Uremia is a serious condition in which the kidneys do not filter the blood enough, causing abnormally high levels of nitrogen waste products to remain in the bloodstream. These wastes are poisonous to body cells and can cause tissue damage or death if allowed to accumulate.

Kidney Failure

In some cases, the kidneys may completely lose their ability to function. Kidney failure can be result from infection, decreased blood flow, or diseases that damage kidney tissue. There are three ways to treat this life-threatening condition:

- **Hemodialysis** (HEE-moh-dy-AL-uh-sis) is a technique in which an artificial kidney machine filters and removes waste products from the blood. This process takes three to five hours and is done three to four times per week, usually in a clinical setting.

- **Peritoneal dialysis** uses the *peritoneum*, a thin membrane that surrounds the digestive organs, to filter the blood. Substances that promote the removal of toxins enter into the abdomen through the catheter and are drained after filtration is complete.

- **Kidney transplant** involves the replacement of a nonfunctioning kidney with a healthy kidney from an organ donor. The donor allows a healthy organ to be removed from his or her body and surgically placed into a patient who needs it.

Other organs that can be transplanted from living donors include part of the liver and a lobe of a lung. As a result of a transplant, the recipient's health and quality of life improve. They can resume normal activities, and their life span increases. When a transplanted organ comes from a living donor, the recipient is removed from the national transplant waiting list. Some people cannot find a match to a living donor. Removing a recipient from the waiting list increases the possibility that other people on the list will receive a donation from a recently deceased donor.

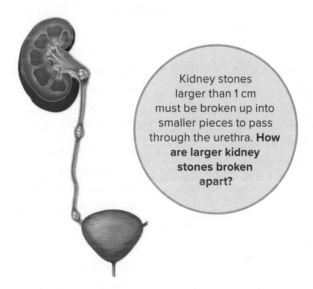

Kidney stones larger than 1 cm must be broken up into smaller pieces to pass through the urethra. **How are larger kidney stones broken apart?**

Lesson 4 Review

Facts and Vocabulary

1. Describe the main function of the excretory system. What organs are part of it?

2. Describe how the ureter, a urethra, and urethritis are different.

3. Explain how you can prevent cystitis and urethritis.

Thinking Critically

4. **Evaluate.** What might pain during urination indicate? What should you recommend to a friend who experiences this?

5. **Analyze.** Why is it possible to donate a kidney and survive?

Applying Health Skills

6. **Analyzing Influences.** List the health behaviors that will help teens avoid problems that can affect the urinary system.

Writing Critically

7. **Comparative.** Write a brief paragraph comparing the way a kidney works and the way a hemodialysis machine works.

Vocabulary Review

Use the correct vocabulary term to complete the following statements.

1. _____ is the fluid in which other parts of the blood are suspended.

2. _____ are types of cells in the blood that cause blood clots to form.

3. A measure of the force that blood places on the walls of blood vessels as it is pumped through the body is called _____.

Understanding Key Concepts

After reading the question or statement, select the correct answer.

4. Which of the following is *not* a function of the cardiovascular system?
   a. Getting oxygen from air
   b. Producing red and white blood cells
   c. Removing carbon dioxide from the body
   d. Fighting disease by attacking infections

5. Congenital heart defects
   a. are present at birth.
   b. result from poor diet.
   c. affect mainly older people.
   d. can be prevented with regular exercise.

Thinking Critically

After reading the question or statement, write a short answer using complete sentences.

6. **Describe.** Describe and give examples of each type of blood vessel.

7. **Explain.** Explain how blood replaces oxygen with carbon dioxide.

8. **Analyze.** Why is early detection of high blood pressure important?

9. **Contrast.** Explain the difference between anemia and hemophilia.

Vocabulary Review

Choose the correct word in the sentences below.

10. The *trachea/bronchi* deliver air to and from the lungs.

11. The *diaphragm/trachea* is a muscle that changes the shape of the lungs.

12. In a(n) *bronchitis/asthma* attack, smooth muscles involuntarily contract and cause chest tightness.

Understanding Key Concepts

After reading the question or statement, select the correct answer.

13. Which of the following structures is the smallest?
    a. Bronchioles
    b. Diaphragm
    c. Lungs
    d. Trachea

14. Which behavior is *least* likely to prevent respiratory system problems?
    a. Smoking tobacco
    b. Washing your hands
    c. Getting regular exercise
    d. Eating fruits and vegetables

15. What problem of the respiratory system is almost always caused by smoking?
    a. Bronchitis   c. Pneumonia
    b. Emphysema   d. Tuberculosis

Thinking Critically

After reading the question or statement, write a short answer using complete sentences.

16. **Describe.** Describe the main function of the respiratory system.

17. **Analyze.** How might increased lung capacity benefit your health?

18. **Describe.** What is sinusitis? What causes it?

19. **Apply.** Why is it important for a person with asthma to avoid known allergens?

LESSON 3

Vocabulary Review

Use the correct vocabulary term to complete the following statements.

20. _____ is the series of muscle contractions that moves food through the digestive tract.

21. The stomach lining secretes _____, which contain hydrochloric acid and pepsin.

22. A(n) _____ is a sore in the lining of the digestive tract that can be caused by bacterial infection.

Understanding Key Concepts

After reading the question or statement, select the correct answer.

23. Which of the following is *not* one of the main functions of the digestive system?
    a. Absorption
    b. Digestion
    c. Elimination
    d. Circulation

24. Which substance is secreted by the liver?
    a. Bile
    b. Chyme
    c. Hydrochloric acid
    d. Mucus

25. Which of these tasks is *not* a function of the stomach?
    a. Storing food
    b. Moving food into the small intestine
    c. Absorbing nutrients from food
    d. Mixing food with gastric juices

26. Which of the following disorders involves a sensitivity to a sugar found in milk and other dairy products?
    a. Cirrhosis
    b. Gastritis
    c. Lactose intolerance
    d. Tooth decay

Thinking Critically

After reading the question or statement, write a short answer using complete sentences.

27. **Describe.** Describe how peristalsis moves food through the digestive tract.

28. **Connect.** What parts of foods do hydrochloric acid, pepsin, and bile work on?

29. **Contrast.** How are the roles of the small intestine and large intestine different?

30. **Analyze.** Why is it important to drink plenty of water when you have diarrhea or constipation?

LESSON 4

Vocabulary Review

Choose the correct word in the sentences below.

31. In *hemodialysis/urethritis,* a machine removes waste products from the blood.

32. The *ureters/nephrons* are the parts of the kidneys that filter blood.

33. The *ureter/urethra* carries urine from the bladder to the outside of the body.

34. *Cystitis/Urethritis* is an inflammation of the bladder caused by bacterial infection.

Understanding Key Concepts

After reading the question or statement, select the correct answer.

35. What role does skin play in excretion?
   a. Eliminating solid wastes
   b. Removing carbon dioxide
   c. Removing excess water and salts
   d. Breaking down toxic chemicals

36. Which of the following is *not* a recommended way to maintain the health of the excretory system?
   a. Having regular medical checkups, and reporting problems to your doctor
   b. Practicing good hygiene and personal health care
   c. Increasing your intake of caffeine and soft drinks
   d. Drinking eight 8-ounce glasses of milk each day

37. What problem of the urinary system could require hemodialysis?
   a. Cystitis
   b. Kidney failure
   c. Kidney stones
   d. Nephritis

Thinking Critically

After reading the question or statement, write a short answer using complete sentences.

38. **Infer.** Why might ingesting an unhealthful substance such as alcohol harm the liver first before any other organ?

39. **Analyze.** How does practicing good hygiene maintain the health of the urinary system?

40. **Apply.** Why is it important to address even mild cases of cystitis and urethritis?

41. **Infer.** Why might a patient choose a kidney transplant over hemodialysis?

PROJECT-BASED ASSESSMENT

Create a True/False Test

BACKGROUND

Everyone is familiar with tests. Tests measure your readiness to tackle a new topic or your mastery of a topic. One form of test question is true/false. These questions make a statement that must be judged to be either true or false, based on your knowledge of the topic.

TASK

Using a free online survey tool, write a 15-question true/false survey to learn what your classmates know about organ transplants.

AUDIENCE

Students in your class

PURPOSE

Accurately and fairly test your classmates' knowledge of organ transplants.

PROCEDURE

1. Review examples of true/false test questions provided by your teacher.

2. Conduct an Internet search to find information on organ transplants.

3. As a group, create the 15 questions for the online survey. Each member of the group should have input on the questions. Make sure you cover each section of the module. Consider creating questions that refer to diagrams or illustrations in the text.

4. Review your questions and prepare an answer key and scoring instructions for the survey.

5. Ask students to take the survey and tally the results. Present the results to your class for discussion.

Math Practice

Interpret Graphs. The bar graph below shows the percentages of high school students who were physically active for at least 60 minutes a day on 5 or more days a week. Use the graph to answer Questions 1–3.

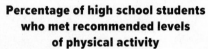

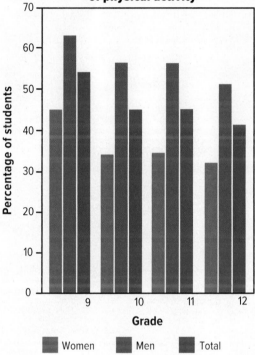

Percentage of high school students who met recommended levels of physical activity

Legend: Women | Men | Total

Adapted from: "Youth Risk Behavior Surveillance"; Centers for Disease Control and Prevention, June 2018.

1. Which grade level had the lowest levels of physical activity for females?
   a. 9th grade   c. 11th grade
   b. 10th grade   d. 12th grade

2. At which grade level did at least half of the total students meet the currently recommended levels of physical activity?
   a. 9th grade   c. 12th grade
   b. 10th grade   d. None

3. Write a paragraph describing your general conclusion from the bar graph.

Reading/Writing Practice

Understand and Apply. Read the passage below, and then answer the questions.

1. Have you ever heard of the influenza epidemic of 1918–1919? 2. Many people died worldwide. 3. In the United States, nearly 800,000 people died. 4. That's more than the number of Americans who died in World War I, World War II, and the Korea and Vietnam wars combined. 5. Influenza viruses still exist. 6. Why doesn't the flu kill as many people today? 7. People in the health-care industry today know that they need to tell flu patients some things about how to feel better. 8. One of the most important treatments is simple—drink liquids. 9. People with the flu should drink lots of water, juice, and clear soups.

1. Which sentence below could be added after sentence 5 to support the first paragraph?
   a. Sick people should not drink liquids.
   b. Washing your hands often is important.
   c. Everyone can learn to wash their hands.
   d. You've probably had the flu yourself.

2. Which revision of sentence 7 is the most coherent and focused?
   a. Doctors and nurses need to know how to talk to sick people.
   b. Follow these logical and new rules of flu treatment to be safe.
   c. Health care professionals understand better how to treat the flu.
   d. To keep you safe from catching the flu, follow simple, new steps.

3. Create a poster using familiar children's book characters, words, and pictures to teach young flu patients to drink lots of liquids.

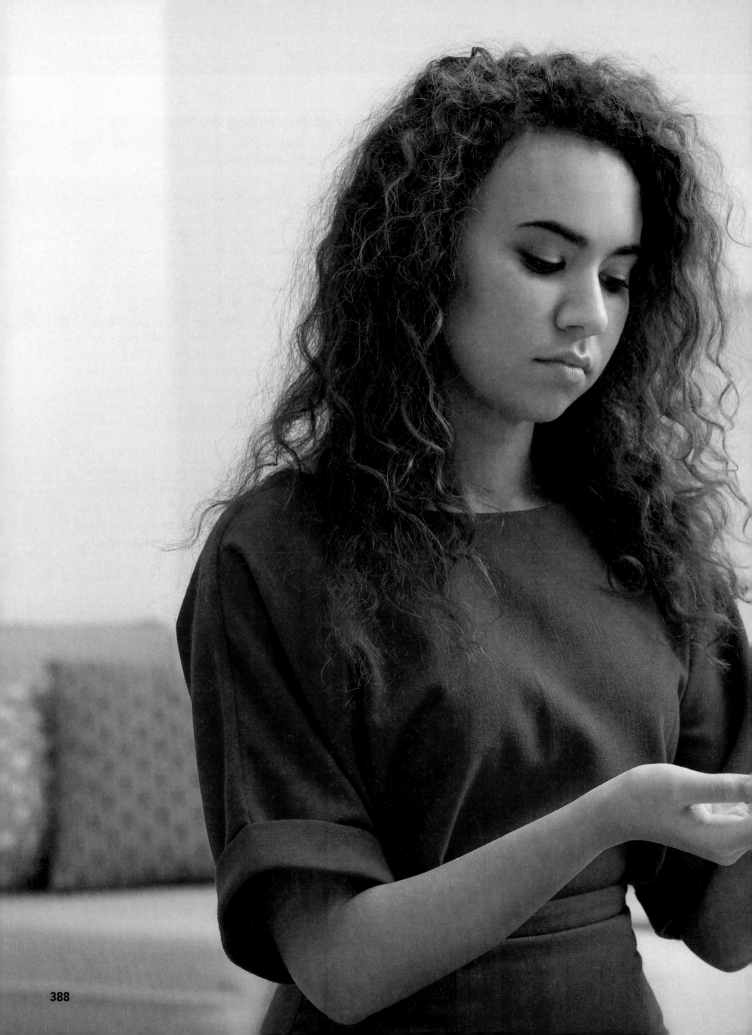

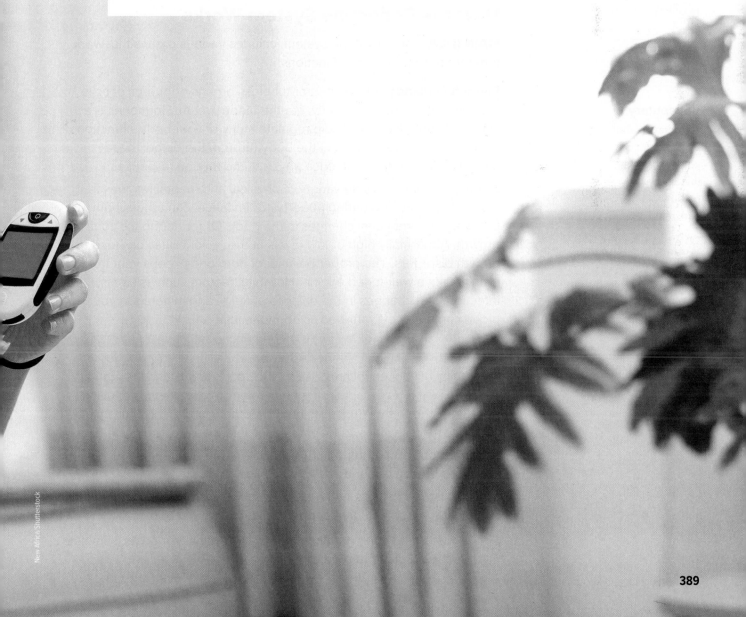

MODULE 16

Endocrine and Reproductive Health

LESSONS

The Endocrine System

BEFORE YOU READ

Create Flashcards. Write the name of each endocrine gland on the front side of a blank index card. Write the function of each on the reverse side. When you have completed the lesson, partner with a friend and use the cards to check your knowledge.

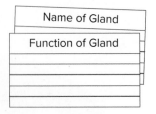

Name of Gland

Function of Gland

Vocabulary

endocrine glands
pituitary gland
adrenal glands
thyroid gland
parathyroid glands
pancreas

BIG IDEA Your body's endocrine system sends and receives chemical messages that control many body functions.

REAL LIFE ISSUES

A Close Call. Emily and Laura are walking home at dusk. Right after they step into the crosswalk, a car suddenly rounds the corner from behind them. Both girls dash forward to get out of the way. Emily yells at the driver to watch out. A few minutes later, Laura says her heart is still racing. *In a short essay, describe what your body feels like in a situation when you are suddenly startled or frightened.*

After completing the lesson, review and analyze your response to the Real Life Issues question.

How the Endocrine System Works

MAIN IDEA The endocrine system includes various organs that work together to regulate body functions.

Endocrine glands are ductless or tubeless organs or groups of cells that secrete hormones directly into the bloodstream. Hormones are chemical substances that help regulate many of your body's functions. Carried to their destination in the body through the blood, these chemical messengers influence physical and mental responses.

Hormones control a wide variety of physical and mental responses. Hormones produced during puberty, for instance, can trigger both physical and emotional changes in the body. Other hormones control growth. Abnormally high or low levels of these hormones can lead to growth disorders. The proper balance of hormones keeps your body running like a well-tuned engine. However, factors such as stress, infection, and changes in the balance of fluids and minerals in your blood can throw off your body's hormone levels.

The Pituitary: The Master Gland

If you think of your endocrine system as a sports team, then the **pituitary gland** is like the team captain. It is often referred to as the master gland because it controls the functions of all the other glands. The pituitary gland has three main sections, or lobes: anterior, intermediate, and posterior.

Anterior Lobe. The anterior, or front, lobe of the pituitary gland produces these hormones:

- *Somatotropic,* or *growth hormone,* stimulates normal body growth and development by altering chemical activity in body cells.

- *Thyroid-stimulating hormone* (TSH), as its name suggests, stimulates the thyroid gland to produce hormones.

- *Adrenocorticotropic hormone* (ACTH) stimulates production of hormones in the adrenal glands.

- *Follicle-stimulating hormone* (FSH) and *luteinizing hormone* (LH) stimulate production of all other sex hormones. The anterior lobe secretes these two hormones during adolescence. They control the growth, development, and functions of the gonads, another name for the ovaries and testes. In females, FSH stimulates cells in the ovary to produce *estrogen,* a female sex hormone that triggers the development of ova, or egg cells. LH is responsible for ovulation and stimulates ovarian cells to produce *progesterone,* another female sex hormone. (Another hormone, *prolactin,* stimulates milk production after a woman has given birth.) In males, LH stimulates cells in the testes to produce the male hormone *testosterone.* FSH controls the production of sperm.

Intermediate Lobe. The **intermediate**, or middle, lobe of the pituitary secretes *melanocyte-stimulating hormone* (MSH), which controls the production of pigments in the skin.

Posterior Lobe. The posterior, or rear, lobe of the pituitary secretes *antidiuretic hormone* (ADH). This regulates the balance of water in the body. ADH also produces oxytocin, which stimulates the smooth muscles in the uterus during pregnancy. This stimulation causes the contractions that enable the baby to be born.

The Adrenal Glands

The **adrenal glands** help the body deal with stress and respond to emergencies. Your adrenal glands are located just above your kidneys. Each gland has two parts. The *adrenal cortex* secretes a hormone that controls the amount of sodium excreted in urine and maintains blood volume and blood pressure. It also secretes hormones that help your body digest fats, proteins, and carbohydrates. These hormones play several other roles in the body, as well. They influence the body's response to stress. They are also involved in both the immune response and sexual function.

The smaller, inner region of each adrenal gland, known as the *adrenal medulla,* is controlled by the hypothalamus and the autonomic nervous system. It secretes the hormones *epinephrine* (also called adrenaline) and *norepinephrine.* Epinephrine is the main hormone involved in the stress response. It increases your heartbeat and respiration. It also raises blood pressure and suppresses the digestive process.

Other Glands

Your body contains many other glands, each with its own particular function. The *hypothalamus* is the part of the brain that links the endocrine system with the nervous system. If your pituitary gland can be considered the captain of the endocrine "team," the hypothalamus is like the coach. It stimulates the pituitary gland to produce hormones.

Reading Check

Explain What are the functions of the thyroid gland and the parathyroid glands?

The Endocrine System

Hypothalamus The hypothalamus links the endocrine system and the nervous system and stimulates the pituitary gland to secrete hormones.

Pineal gland The pineal gland secretes the hormone *melatonin*, which is thought to affect the onset of puberty, and regulates sleep cycles.

Pituitary gland The **pituitary gland** *regulates and controls the activities of all other endocrine glands.*

Thymus The thymus regulates development of the immune system.

Adrenal glands These glands produce hormones that regulate the body's salt and water balance. Secretions from the adrenal cortex and the adrenal medulla stimulate several important body functions and control the body's emergency response.

Pancreas The **pancreas** is *a gland that serves both the digestive and the endocrine systems.* As an endocrine gland, it secretes two hormones—glucagon and insulin—that regulate the level of glucose in the blood.

Thyroid The **thyroid gland** *produces hormones that regulate metabolism, body heat, and bone growth.* It produces thyroxine, which regulates the way cells release energy from nutrients.

Parathyroid glands The **parathyroid glands** *produce a hormone that regulates the body's balance of calcium and phosphorus.*

Testes The testes are the male reproductive glands that produce sperm for fertilization.

Ovaries The ovaries are the female reproductive glands that produce the egg cells. The testes and ovaries control the development of secondary sex characteristics during puberty. You'll learn more about how the testes and ovaries play a role in reproduction in Lessons 2 and 3.

The glands of the endocrine system are located throughout the body. Each gland has a particular function. **Describe the function of the thymus?**

Reading Check

Identify What are three ways you can care for your endocrine system?

Maintaining Your Endocrine Health

MAIN IDEA To keep your endocrine system working at its peak, you need to follow sound health practices.

Your endocrine health is directly related to your overall health. You can support your endocrine system by following these tips:

- Eat balanced meals to make sure that you get the nutrients you need.

- Engage in regular physical activity to keep your body strong.

- Use stress-management techniques.

- Get enough sleep. Adequate sleep is important for endocrine health. Teens generally need 8½ to 9 hours of sleep every night.

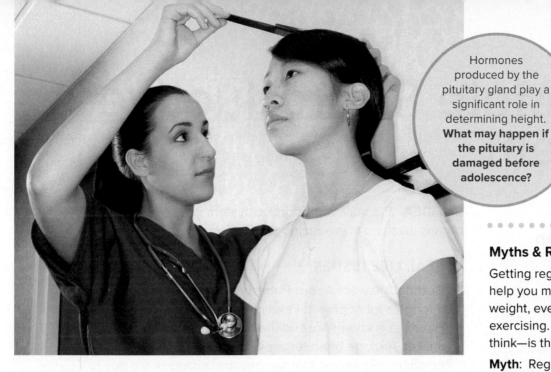

Hormones produced by the pituitary gland play a significant role in determining height. **What may happen if the pituitary is damaged before adolescence?**

Myths & Reality

Getting regular exercise can help you maintain a healthy weight, even when you're not exercising. What do you think—is this a myth or reality?

Myth: Regular exercise helps maintain a healthy weight.

Reality: Exercising for more than 30 minutes at a pace that raises the heart rate will speed up the metabolism. When the metabolism speeds up, you burn more calories, which can help you maintain a healthy weight.

• Have regular medical checkups. Some hormonal disorders have symptoms you may not notice or recognize. A health care professional can perform tests to determine whether your endocrine function is normal.

Certain endocrine disorders can have lifelong effects on your health. Factors such as stress, infection, and changes in the balance of fluid and minerals in your blood can cause hormone levels to fluctuate. In many cases, these situations will correct themselves. However, serious problems—including diabetes mellitus, hypothyroidism, hyperthyroidism, goiter, or overproduction of adrenal hormones—may require medical treatment.

Lesson 1 Review

Facts and Vocabulary

1. Define the term hormones.

2. Name the hormone that stimulates normal growth and development.

3. Name the gland that helps regulate the chemicals that control sleep.

Thinking Critically

4. **Infer.** Why do the hormones FSH and LH have different effects in men and women?

5. **Apply.** If the water in your body is not properly balanced, what endocrine gland (or part of a gland) may be malfunctioning?

Applying Health Skills

6. **Self-Management.** Sleep keeps the endocrine system healthy. For one week, log the number of hours you sleep each night. At the end of the week, calculate your average. Create a plan to get the appropriate amount of sleep each night.

Writing Critically

7. **Persuasive.** Write a script for a public service announcement reminding teens that everyone grows at a different rate. Include information about normal growth and genetic influences.

Thinkstock/Getty Images

The Male Reproductive System

BEFORE YOU READ

Create a Flow Chart. As you read, sketch the path that sperm take through each of the male reproductive organs.

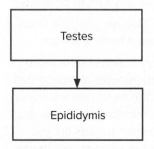

Vocabulary

sperm
testosterone
testes
scrotum
penis
semen
inguinal hernia
sterility

Fitness Zone

It's really important to me to succeed in whatever I set out to do. I know I need to take care of myself and keep in shape, even when I'm not feeling up to it. I am going out for track this year so I will be motivated to run every day. I know if I choose a sport I really like, I won't give up.

BIG IDEA The male reproductive system is a series of organs involved in producing children.

REAL LIFE ISSUES

Getting Answers About Puberty. Jackson has been going through a lot of physical and mental/emotional changes lately. His voice is changing, and the hair above his lip is becoming thicker. Also, he often feels as if he is not in control of his emotions. He knows that the physical changes are due to puberty, but wonders why his emotions are so strong. He's worried about his health, but feels embarrassed to talk to someone about his concerns. *Write a letter to Jackson offering suggestions on what questions to ask, and advice on getting help from a trusted male adult or his doctor.*

After completing the lesson, review and analyze your response to the Real Life Issues question.

How Male Reproduction Works

MAIN IDEA The male reproductive system includes both external and internal organs that, with the help of hormones, allow physically mature males to produce children.

The male reproductive system has two main functions; it produces and stores the male reproductive cells, or **sperm**, and it transfers sperm to the female's body during sexual intercourse. During the early teen years, usually between the ages of 12 and 15, the male reproductive system reaches maturity. At that time, hormones produced by the pituitary gland stimulate the production of **testosterone**, which is the male sex hormone. This hormone results in physical changes that signal maturity. The shoulders grow broader, muscles become more developed, facial and other body hair forms, and the voice becomes deeper. Testosterone also controls the production of sperm. After puberty begins, a physically mature male is capable of producing sperm for the rest of his life.

External Reproductive Organs

A male's external reproductive organs include the testes, the penis, and the scrotum. The **testes**, also called testicles, are two small glands that secrete testosterone and produce sperm. They are located in the **scrotum**, an external skin sac. The **penis** is a tube-shaped organ that extends from the trunk of the body just above the testes. The penis is composed of spongy tissue that contains many blood vessels. When blood flow to the penis increases, it becomes enlarged and erect, causing an erection. Erections are normal body functions that occur more easily and more frequently during puberty. They can occur for no reason.

When the penis becomes erect, **semen** can be ejected from the body. Semen is a thick fluid containing sperm and other secretions from the male reproductive system. The process that makes this possible is *ejaculation,* a series of muscular contractions that can occur at the height of sexual arousal. Ejaculation during sexual intercourse can transmit semen into a woman's body so that *fertilization*—the joining of a male sperm cell and a female egg cell—can occur. Ejaculation can also occur during sleep, an occurrence known as a *nocturnal emission.* During adolescence, nocturnal emissions are normal and common. They relieve the buildup of pressure that occurs as a male begins to produce sperm during puberty.

At birth, the tip of the penis is covered by a thin, loose skin called the *foreskin.* Some parents of male children choose to have the foreskin surgically removed, a process known as *circumcision.* This procedure is usually chosen for cultural or religious reasons. Circumcision changes the appearance of the penis, but it does not interfere with a male's ability to have intercourse or to father children.

Sperm cannot live in temperatures higher than the normal body temperature of 98.6 degrees Fahrenheit. The scrotum protects sperm by keeping the testes slightly below the normal body temperature. When body temperature rises, muscles attached to the scrotum relax. This causes the testicles to lower away from the body. If body temperature lowers, the muscles tighten, moving the testes closer to the body for warmth. Tight clothing that holds the testes too close to the body may interfere with sperm production.

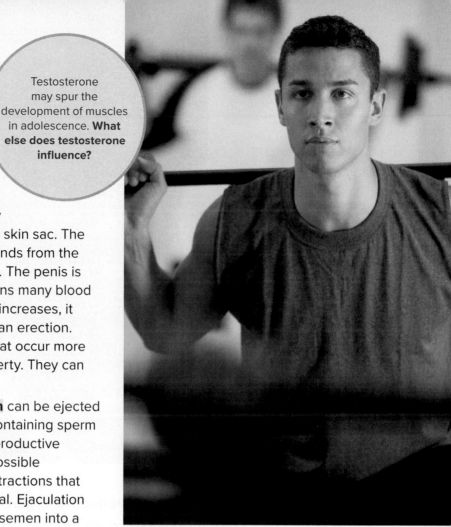

Testosterone may spur the development of muscles in adolescence. **What else does testosterone influence?**

Reading Check

Explain How does fertilization occur?

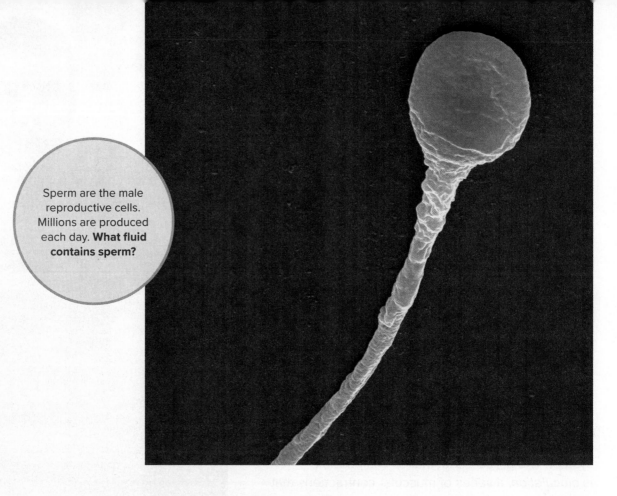

Sperm are the male reproductive cells. Millions are produced each day. **What fluid contains sperm?**

Internal Reproductive Organs

Although sperm are produced in the testes, which are suspended outside the body, they must travel through several structures within the body before they are released. These include the epididymis, the vas deferens, the seminal vesicles, the urethra, and the prostate and Cowper's glands.

Maintaining Reproductive Health

MAIN IDEA Male reproductive health involves care and monitoring throughout a male's lifetime.

As with any other body system, the male reproductive system needs care. Here are some important guidelines to follow.

- **Practice good personal hygiene.** Males should shower or bathe daily, thoroughly cleaning the penis and scrotum. Uncircumcised males should take care to wash under the foreskin.

- **Wear protective equipment.** Use a protective cup or athletic supporter during physical activity to shield the external reproductive organs.

- **Practice abstinence.** Abstaining from sexual activity will prevent exposure to sexually transmitted diseases (STDs), also known as sexually transmitted infections (STIs).

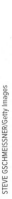

- **Perform regular self-examinations.** Check the scrotum and testicles monthly for signs of cancer. Report any change to a physician. Even though lumps do not always mean cancer is present, it is still important to check them out as early as possible. Early detection usually leads to successful treatment.

- **Get regular checkups.** All males should have regular checkups by a physician every 12 to 18 months. If an abnormality is found, the patient will be referred to a urologist, who specializes in care and problems of the male reproductive system.

Reading Check

Identify How does practicing abstinence help protect the reproductive system?

The internal structures of the male reproductive system work together to promote the delivery of sperm. **Name which part of the male reproductive system is also part of the urinary system.**

Male Reproductive System

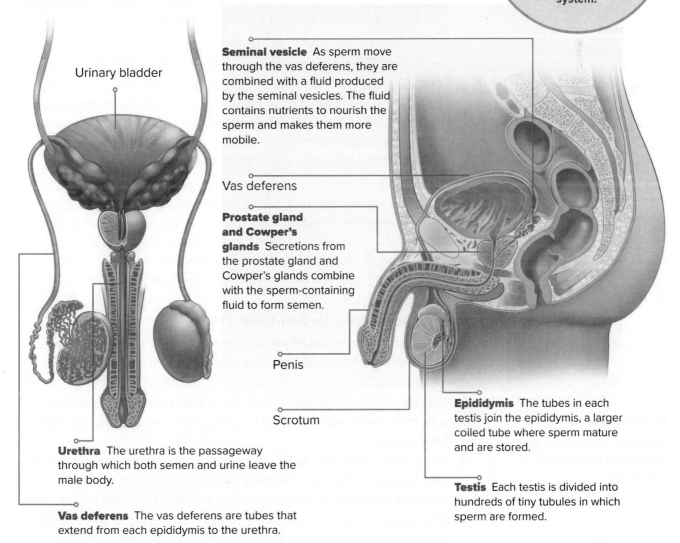

Urinary bladder

Seminal vesicle As sperm move through the vas deferens, they are combined with a fluid produced by the seminal vesicles. The fluid contains nutrients to nourish the sperm and makes them more mobile.

Vas deferens

Prostate gland and Cowper's glands Secretions from the prostate gland and Cowper's glands combine with the sperm-containing fluid to form semen.

Penis

Scrotum

Epididymis The tubes in each testis join the epididymis, a larger coiled tube where sperm mature and are stored.

Testis Each testis is divided into hundreds of tiny tubules in which sperm are formed.

Urethra The urethra is the passageway through which both semen and urine leave the male body.

Vas deferens The vas deferens are tubes that extend from each epididymis to the urethra.

Male Reproductive System Problems

MAIN IDEA The organs of the male reproductive system can be affected by both functional and structural problems.

Some problems of the male reproductive system are described below. Males should watch out for the signs of these problems, as well as signs of infection from STDs:

- **Inguinal (in-gwi-nuhl) hernia.** An inguinal hernia occurs when part of the intestines push through a tear in the abdominal wall. The tear may result from straining the abdominal muscles or from lifting heavy objects. Symptoms include a lump in the groin near the thigh, pain in the groin, or blockage of the intestine. Surgery can repair an inguinal hernia.

- **Sterility.** This is the inability to reproduce. It can occur when the body produces too few sperm or sperm of poor quality. Exposure to X-rays or other radiation, lead, and other toxic chemicals can lead to sterility. Other causes include hormonal imbalances, mumps contracted during adulthood, or using certain medications or drugs such as anabolic steroids. Some STDs can also cause sterility.

- **Testicular cancer.** This type of cancer can affect males of any age. However, in almost half of all cases, testicular cancer is diagnosed in males between the ages of 20 and 34, according to the American Cancer Society. With early detection, most testicular cancer is treatable through surgery, radiation, or chemotherapy.

- **Enlarged prostate.** The prostate gland can become enlarged as a result of age, an infection, or, most seriously, a tumor. A prostate exam is recommended for men starting at the age of 50. For men who have a higher risk of developing cancer, health care professionals may recommend the exams start at an earlier age. Early detection of prostate cancer increases survival rates.

How to Do a Testicular Self-Exam (TSE)

The American Cancer Society recommends that all males perform a self-exam once a month to check for signs of testicular cancer. Follow these steps:

1. Standing in front of a mirror, look for swelling. Examine each testicle with both hands. Roll the testicle gently between the thumbs and forefingers.

2. Cancerous lumps are usually found on the side of the testicle but can also appear on the front. Find the epididymis, the soft tube-like structure behind each testicle, so that you won't mistake it for a lump.

3. Most lumps are not cancerous. If you do find a lump or experience pain or swelling, however, consult a health care professional.

Reading Check

Describe What steps are involved in a testicular self-exam?

TSE Awareness Campaign

To raise awareness of the importance of performing a monthly testicular self-exam (TSE), you will work with a group to develop an awareness program. Perform an online search to find facts such as risk factors and other facts about testicular cancer.

Activity: Technology

Gather the information that was obtained from the online searches and what has been learned from the text and organize into groups of three or four students. As a group, create a podcast that has both audio and visual components for a public service announcement. Groups should work together to make sure that the campaign presents consistent information featuring the same key points.

1. Create a public service announcement script, blog, or podcast that raises awareness of TSE.
2. Create slides for a multimedia presentation about the warning signs of testicular cancer. Ask for permission to place the podcast and the multimedia presentation on the school's website.
3. Present the group's podcast and multimedia presentation to your class.

Lesson 2 Review

Facts and Vocabulary

1. Sperm cannot survive at body temperature. How does the body protect sperm from heat?
2. What is sterility?
3. What are the vas deferens?

Thinking Critically

4. **Infer.** How might giving a mumps vaccine to a boy help protect his reproductive health later?
5. **Compare and Contrast.** How might a man's reproductive health concerns change at different periods of his life?
6. **Distinguish.** What is the difference between semen and sperm?

Applying Health Skills

7. **Practicing Healthful Behaviors.** Describe some behaviors that can help males maintain their reproductive health.

Writing Critically

8. **Persuasive.** Write an article persuading males of the need for protective equipment during football and other sports. Describe how shoulder pads, knee pads, and protective cups help prevent injury.

The Female Reproductive System

BEFORE YOU READ

Create a T-Chart. Set up a T-chart like the one pictured below to organize information about the parts of the female reproductive system and their functions.

Part	Function

Vocabulary

eggs
ovaries
uterus
ovulation
fallopian tubes
vagina
cervix
menstruation

BIG IDEA The female reproductive system matures at puberty and enables women to reproduce.

REAL LIFE ISSUES

Being Teased. Jody and her friend Sandra decide to try out for the girls' basketball team at school. Later, however, Sandra tells Jody that she has changed her mind. Sandra is embarrassed to shower and change in the locker room because she's developing at a slower pace than most of the other girls. Some of the girls have teased her and she feels self-conscious. *Write a supportive note to Sandra telling her that all girls mature at various rates. Be sure your note respects Sandra as she is and encourages her to understand she is not alone.*

After completing the lesson, review and analyze your response to the Real Life Issues question.

Female Reproductive Organs

MAIN IDEA The organs of the female reproductive system enable pregnancy to occur as soon as monthly ovulation begins.

The female reproductive system produces female sex hormones and stores the **eggs**, also known as the female gametes or *ova* (singular: *ovum*). Eggs are stored in the female sex glands, called **ovaries**. Ovaries are located on either side of the **uterus**. The uterus is the hollow, muscular, pear-shaped organ that nourishes and protects a fertilized ovum until birth. The ovaries do not produce eggs continuously, the way the male testes produce sperm. Instead, all the egg cells in the female body—more than 400,000 of them—are present at birth. At puberty, the pituitary gland releases hormones that cause these ova to mature, and **ovulation** begins. Ovulation is the process of releasing a mature ovum into the fallopian tube each month.

Each month, a mature ovum is released from an ovary into one of the two **fallopian tubes**. These are a pair of tubes with fingerlike projections that draw in the ovum. Muscular contractions in the fallopian tubes, along with the motions of tiny, hairlike structures called *cilia,* move the ovum along through the tube. In the fallopian tube, the egg may encounter sperm from a male. Sperm can enter the female reproductive system through a muscular, elastic passageway that extends from the uterus to the outside of the body, called the **vagina**. If this happens, fertilization can occur. A single sperm cell unites with the ovum, producing a single, complete cell called

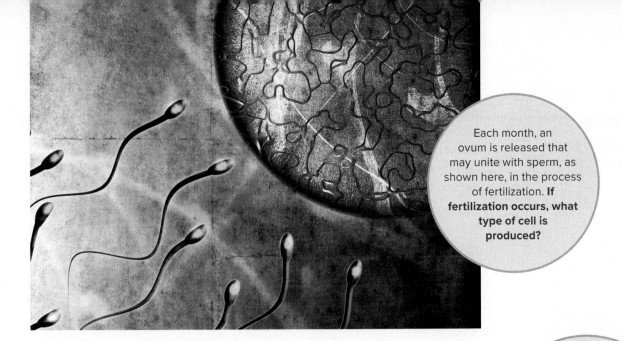

Each month, an ovum is released that may unite with sperm, as shown here, in the process of fertilization. **If fertilization occurs, what type of cell is produced?**

a *zygote.* The zygote continues down the fallopian tube and enters the uterus, where it attaches itself to the uterine wall. There, it develops into a *fetus,* which will remain in the uterus until birth.

The female reproductive system produces egg cells called ova, and each month provides a place for a fertilized ovum to grow. **Name which part of the female reproductive system contains the ova.**

Female Reproductive System

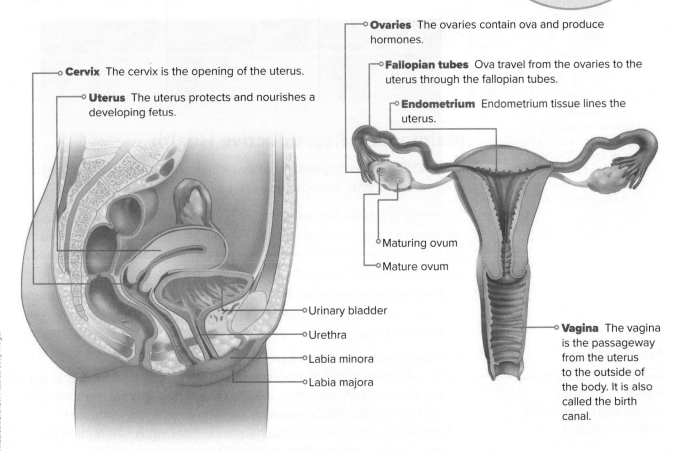

Cervix The cervix is the opening of the uterus.

Uterus The uterus protects and nourishes a developing fetus.

Ovaries The ovaries contain ova and produce hormones.

Fallopian tubes Ova travel from the ovaries to the uterus through the fallopian tubes.

Endometrium Endometrium tissue lines the uterus.

Maturing ovum

Mature ovum

Urinary bladder

Urethra

Labia minora

Labia majora

Vagina The vagina is the passageway from the uterus to the outside of the body. It is also called the birth canal.

Reading Check

Describe How does the uterine wall prepare for the zygote?

Menstruation

After a female reaches physical maturity, the uterus prepares each month for possible pregnancy. The walls of the uterus thicken with blood to nourish the zygote as it grows. If pregnancy doesn't occur, the thickened lining of the uterus, called the *endometrium,* breaks down into blood, tissue, and fluids. The endometrium tissues pass through the cervix, which is the opening to the uterus, and into the vagina.

During the cycle of **menstruation**, which is the shedding of the uterine lining, females wear sanitary pads or tampons to absorb the blood flow.

Most females begin menstruating between the ages of 10 and 15. The menstrual cycle may be irregular at first. As a female matures, it usually becomes more predictable. Endocrine hormones control this cycle, but poor nutrition, stress, excessive exercise, low body weight, and illness may disrupt it. Menstruation occurs each month from puberty until *menopause,* the end of the reproductive years. Most women reach menopause between the ages of 45 and 55 years.

The Menstrual Cycle

Days 1–8	Days 9–13	Day 14	Days 15–28
The cycle begins with the first day of menstruation.	The hormones FSH and LH cause an egg to mature in one of the ovaries.	Ovulation occurs and the mature egg is released into one of the fallopian tubes.	The egg travels through the fallopian tube to the uterus. If the egg is not fertilized, the cycle starts again.

A woman's menstrual cycle is approximately 28 days long. **Identify what happens halfway through the menstrual cycle.**

Maintaining Reproductive Health

MAIN IDEA Good hygiene, monthly breast self-exams, and abstinence from sexual activity promote good female reproductive health.

The same practices that keep the whole body healthy—such as good nutrition and regular physical activity—will also promote the health of the female reproductive system. In addition, a few other practices will keep this body system working at its best.

- **Practice good hygiene.** It is especially important to shower or bathe daily and change tampons or sanitary pads every few hours during the menstrual period.

- **Have regular medical exams.** Regular medical exams for adult females should include a test called a Pap smear, which checks for the presence of cancerous cells on the cervix. Women past middle age should also have regular mammograms to test for breast cancer. Report any pain, discharge, or other signs of infection to your health care provider as soon as possible.

Reading Check

Describe What are three important steps for maintaining reproductive health in females?

- **Practice abstinence.** Abstaining from sexual activity will protect you from unplanned pregnancy and STDs.

Breast Self-Exam

Breast cancer is the most common type of cancer (not counting skin cancers) for women in the United States. It is also one of the deadliest cancers for women, second only to lung cancer in number of deaths per year. The best way to survive breast cancer is to catch the disease early. The American Cancer Society recommends that females examine their breasts once a month, right after their menstrual period, when breasts are not tender. Follow these steps:

1. Lie down with a pillow under your right shoulder. Put your right arm behind your head. Place the three middle finger pads of your left hand on your right breast. Move your fingers in a circular motion, pressing first with light, then medium, then firm pressure. Feel for any lumps or thickening in the breast. Follow this process in an up-and-down path over the breast. Be sure to check all the breast tissue, from the underarm edge to the middle of the chest bone and from the collarbone to the ribs. Repeat the process using your right hand on your left breast.

2. Stand in front of a mirror with your hands pressed firmly on your hips. Inspect your breasts for *any* changes in size, shape, or appearance. Look for dimpling, rash, puckering or scaliness of the skin or nipple, or discharge.

3. Next, raise your arms over your head, palms pressed together, and look for any visible changes in the breasts.

4. Finally, examine your underarms with your arms only slightly raised so you can more easily feel these areas.

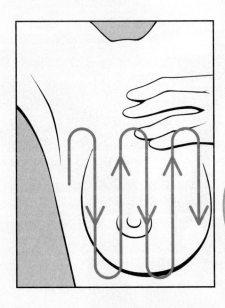

In a vertical pattern, check from the underarm to the chest bone, and from the collarbone to the ribs. **Describe the steps involved in a breast self-exam.**

Breast Self-Exam

Female Reproductive System Problems

MAIN IDEA Several disorders can affect the female reproductive system, and some can lead to infertility.

Some problems of the female reproductive system, such as menstrual cramps and premenstrual syndrome, are common. Others, such as toxic shock syndrome, are uncommon. Some disorders can result in *infertility,* an inability to bear children.

- **Menstrual cramps.** This can sometimes occur at the beginning of a menstrual period. Light exercise or applying a heating pad to the abdominal area may help relieve cramps. If cramps are severe, a health care professional may recommend an over-the-counter or prescription medicine.

- **Premenstrual syndrome (PMS).** This is a disorder caused by hormonal changes. Symptoms may include anxiety, irritability, bloating, weight gain, depression, mood swings, and fatigue. Regular physical activity and good nutrition may ease these symptoms.

- **Toxic shock syndrome (TSS).** This is a rare but serious bacterial infection that affects the immune system and liver. It can be fatal. Symptoms include fever, vomiting, diarrhea, rash, red eyes, dizziness, and muscle aches. To reduce TSS risk, use tampons with the lowest absorbency and change them often. If symptoms occur, see a doctor.

Annual gynecological exams by a healthcare professional are an important part of maintaining a healthy reproductive system.

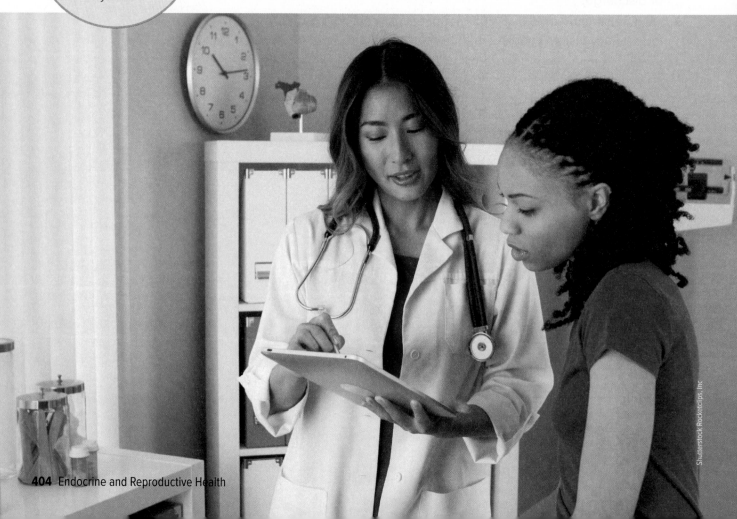

Shutterstock.Rocketclips, Inc

- **Endometriosis.** This occurs when uterine tissue grows in the ovaries, fallopian tubes, or the lining of the pelvic cavity.

- **Sexually transmitted diseases (STDs).** These may damage the female reproductive system. Untreated STDs, such as gonorrhea and chlamydia, are associated with pelvic inflammatory disease (PID) and may cause infertility. Abstinence from sexual activity is the only guaranteed way to avoid STDs.

- **Vaginitis.** This results in discharge, odor, pain, itching, or burning. Two common forms of vaginitis are *candida* (yeast infection) and bacterial vaginosis.

- **Ovarian cysts.** These are fluid-filled sacs on the ovary. Small, noncancerous cysts may disappear on their own. Larger cysts may have to be removed surgically.

- **Reproductive system cancers.** These may affect the cervix, uterus, or ovaries. Regular exams are important for early detection and treatment. Early sexual activity and STDs such as human papillomavirus (HPV) increase the risk of cervical cancer. The FDA has approved a vaccine that prevents infection from four strains of HPV.

Lesson 3 Review

Facts and Vocabulary

1. What is the function of the uterus?

2. Distinguish between ova, ovaries, and ovulation.

3. Identify a kind of cancer of the female reproductive system that is linked to a sexually transmitted disease (STD).

Thinking Critically

4. **Distinguish.** What is the difference between menstrual cramps and PMS?

5. **Infer.** Why do blocked fallopian tubes often result in infertility?

Applying Health Skills

6. **Advocacy.** Create a brochure that educates females about ways to promote reproductive health. Include preventive care such as hygiene, mammograms, and Pap smears.

Writing Critically

7. **Persuasive.** Some students in Mrs. Garcia's class are uncomfortable learning about the reproductive system of the opposite gender. Write a persuasive letter explaining why this education is important.

Vocabulary Review

Correct the sentences below by replacing the italicized term with the correct vocabulary term.

1. The *hypothalamus* produces hormones that regulate metabolism, body heat, and bone growth.

2. The *adrenal glands* regulate calcium.

3. The *thymus* regulates and controls the activities of all other endocrine glands.

Understanding Key Concepts

After reading the question or statement, select the correct answer.

4. What is the main role of the pituitary gland?
   a. Controls sleep
   b. Helps digestion
   c. Regulates other endocrine glands
   d. Adjusts water balance

5. Which gland is involved with the release of epinephrine?
   a. Thyroid
   b. Adrenal glands
   c. Pineal gland
   d. Thymus

Thinking Critically

After reading the question or statement, write a short answer using complete sentences.

6. **Infer.** What might happen if the adrenal glands stop regulating the body's salt and water balance?

7. **Analyze.** If you suddenly began having trouble sleeping, how might the pineal gland be involved?

8. **Infer.** Epinephrine helps you respond to dangerous situations. Why might it help to stop digesting food if you are in danger?

9. **Analyze.** What would happen if scientists applied luteinizing hormone to a female's ovary cells and to a male's testes cells?

10. **Compare and Contrast.** Discuss similarities and differences of the adrenal cortex and adrenal medulla.

Vocabulary Review

Use the correct vocabulary term to complete the following statements.

11. The _____ is the skin sac that holds the testes.

12. _____ is a thick fluid containing sperm from the male reproductive system.

13. The inability to produce children is called _____.

Understanding Key Concepts

After reading the question or statement, select the correct answer.

14. What is an inguinal hernia?
   a. A separation where part of the intestine pushes into the abdominal wall
   b. The inability to reproduce
   c. A type of cancer affecting the prostate
   d. An STD

15. How often should males conduct a testicular self-exam?
   a. Once a day
   b. Once a week
   c. Once a month
   d. Once a year

16. Where are sperm formed?
   a. In the urethra
   b. In the epididymis
   c. In the penis
   d. In the testes

17. What is the passageway through which both semen and urine leave the body?
   a. The urethra
   b. The testes
   c. The seminal vesicles
   d. The epididymis

Thinking Critically

After reading the question or statement, write a short answer using complete sentences.

18. **Analyze.** How does the scrotum respond to temperature, and for what purpose?

19. **Identify.** Where are you most likely to find a cancerous lump on a testicle?

20. **Infer.** What should a male infer if he begins to develop facial hair?

21. **Compare and Contrast.** How are testicular cancer and prostate cancer different?

22. **Infer.** Why is it important to see a health care provider right away if a testicular lump is discovered?

LESSON 3

Vocabulary Review

Choose the correct term in the sentences below.

23. The *ovaries/fallopian tubes* produce hormones.

24. *Menstruation/Ovulation* is the process of releasing a mature ovum into the fallopian tube each month.

25. The *cervix/uterus* is the hollow, muscular, pear-shaped organ inside a female's body.

26. *Toxic shock syndrome/Premenstrual syndrome* is a rare but serious bacterial infection.

Understanding Key Concepts

After reading the question or statement, select the correct answer.

27. What type of disease, if left untreated, is associated with pelvic inflammatory disease?
    a. STDs
    b. Vaginitis
    c. Ovarian cancer
    d. Ovarian cysts

28. What is the opening to the uterus called?
    a. Ovum
    b. Bladder
    c. Endometrium
    d. Cervix

29. What happens to the uterine wall as it prepares for a zygote?
    a. The wall shrinks.
    b. The wall dissolves.
    c. The wall thickens.
    d. The wall sheds skin cells.

30. How many ova mature each month in a female reproductive system?
    a. 1
    b. 100
    c. 400,000
    d. Millions

Thinking Critically

After reading the question or statement, write a short answer using complete sentences.

31. **Infer.** Charlotte and her friend Karen are the same age. Charlotte has started menstruating, but Karen has not. What could be the cause?

32. **Explain.** How can practicing healthful behaviors help a female maintain a healthy reproductive system and even prevent some infertility problems later in life?

33. **Analyze.** Why is it important for females to conduct a breast exam after a menstrual period ends?

34. **Synthesize.** How can good hygiene help prevent toxic shock syndrome?

PROJECT-BASED ASSESSMENT

Care of the Reproductive System

BACKGROUND

When it comes to serious health issues, teens often think, "It can't happen to me." Teens are not immune to developing serious health problems, such as those that can affect the male or female reproductive systems. For this project, small groups of students will create a multimedia presentation providing teens with information on how to prevent reproductive health problems.

TASK

Create a multimedia presentation that illustrates a problem of the reproductive system. (If you are female, select a problem of the female reproductive system; if you are male, choose a problem of the male reproductive system.)

AUDIENCE

Students in your school and community

PURPOSE

Help teens become better informed about how to prevent problems related to the male and female reproductive systems.

PROCEDURE

1. Review the student text and choose a particular problem related to the male or female reproductive system.

2. Research the problem online. Identify the cause, symptoms, and treatments (historical and present-day), as well as methods by which the occurrence of the problem could be reduced.

3. Search through approved websites to find suitable illustrations and video clips.

4. As a group, organize the relevant information and illustrations to create an informative and attractive multimedia presentation.

5. Present your presentation to your class. Ask for permission to possibly place the presentation on your school's website.

Math Practice

Reading Tables. The time between fertilization of an egg by a sperm and birth is a known as a *gestation period.* This amount of time varies from organism to organism. The table gives the average gestation periods (in days) for several different types of animals.

Animal	Gestation Period
Hamster	16.5 days
Ferret	42 days
Coyote	63 days
Lion	108 days
Human	267 days
Horse	337 days
Camel	406 days

1. What is the median of the gestation periods in the table?
   a. 108 days
   b. 177 days
   c. 389.5 days
   d. There is no median because all the numbers are different.

2. The actual gestation period can be stated as a range of days. For a human, that range is from 250 to 285 days. If the value in the table is the average gestation period, the value is the
   a. median.
   b. mode.
   c. mean.
   d. first quartile.

3. Compare the size of each animal listed to its gestation period. Predict the relative gestation period of a rhinoceros. Explain your prediction.

Reading/Writing Practice

Understand and Apply. Read the passage below, and then answer the questions.

Gigantism is a problem of the endocrine system caused when the pituitary gland secretes too much growth hormone during childhood before the bones have completed their growth cycle. As a result, the body's long bones become overdeveloped. The person grows to an abnormally tall height. This very rare disorder can be the result of a tumor in the pituitary gland. A related disorder, acromegaly (ak-roh-MEG-uh-lee), occurs when the production of growth hormone continues after the normal growth cycle has ended. People with acromegaly experience abnormal growth of bones in the face, hands, feet, and skull.

1. Which outline best represents the passage?
   a. Gigantism
      a. Famous Giants
      b. Symptoms
   b. Endocrine Problems
      a. Gigantism
      b. Excessive Growth Hormone
   c. Growth Disorders
      a. Gigantism
      b. Acromegaly
   d. Functions of the Pituitary Gland
      a. Growth Hormone Production
      b. Sex Hormone Production

2. In which type of publication would this passage most likely appear?
   a. Encyclopedia
   b. Fictional novel
   c. Letter from a doctor
   d. A pamphlet

3. Write a short story about a person with gigantism. Give details about the disorder.

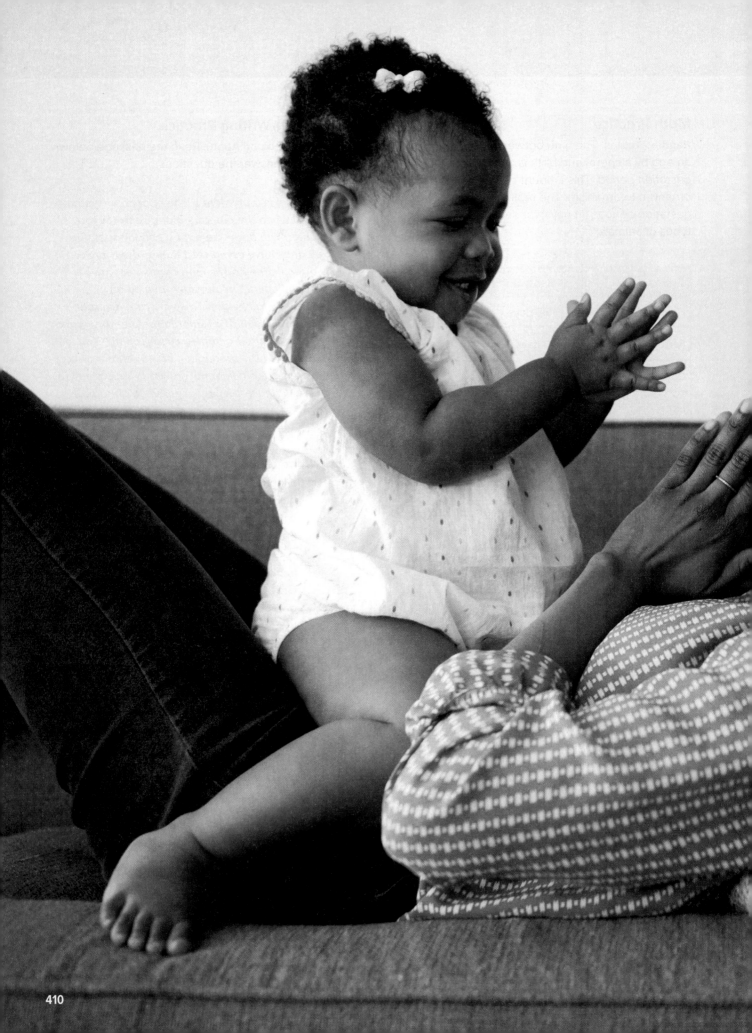

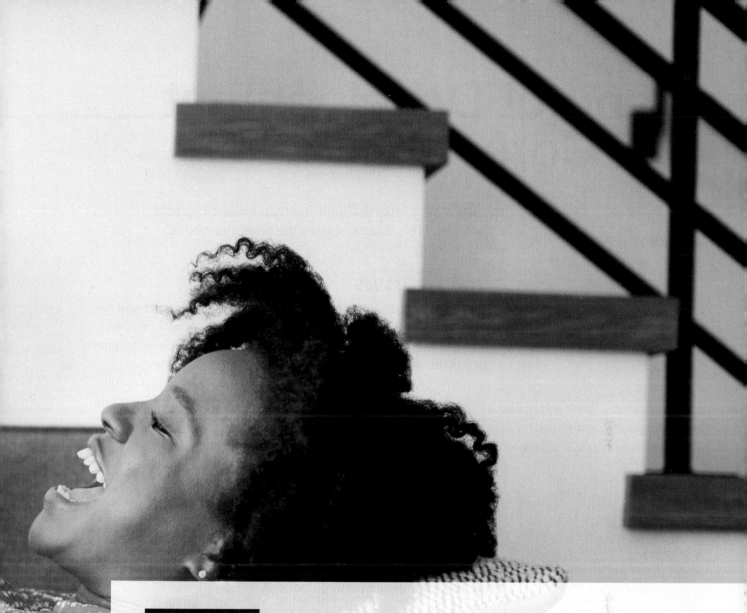

The Beginning of the Life Cycle

LESSONS

1 Prenatal Development and Care

2 Heredity and Genetics

3 Birth Through Childhood

monkeybusinessimages/Getty Images

Prenatal Development and Care

Create a Table. Make a two-column table. Label the first column "Things to Avoid." Label the second column "Things to Do." Fill in the table as you read the lesson.

Things to Avoid	Things to Do

Vocabulary

fertilization
implantation
embryo
fetus
prenatal care
fetal alcohol syndrome

BIG IDEA As a fetus develops during pregnancy, special care needs to be taken to ensure the fetus and mother remain healthy.

REAL LIFE ISSUES

Eating for Two. Amanda's older sister, Linda, is pregnant and has moved back home while her husband is overseas on a military assignment. Amanda's health class is starting a lesson on healthy pregnancies. Their mother says that good nutrition is very important for a healthy pregnancy, so they decide to plan menus that will be healthy for Linda and her growing baby. *Create a one-day menu and a shopping list that could help Amanda and her mother plan meals to keep Linda healthy during her pregnancy.*

After completing the lesson, review and analyze your response to the Real Life Issues question.

The Very Beginning

MAIN IDEA A single cell, formed from one egg and one sperm, can grow into a complex human being.

The human body begins as a single microscopic cell called a *zygote,* which forms as a result of **fertilization**. Fertilization, also known as *conception,* is the union of a male sperm cell and a female egg cell. As the zygote travels through the fallopian tube, it begins to divide. By the time it reaches the uterus, it has become a cluster of cells. Within a few days, **implantation** occurs. This is the process by which the zygote attaches to the uterine wall.

After about two weeks, the zygote has become an **embryo** (EM-bree-oh), a cluster of cells that develops between the third and eighth week of pregnancy. In most cases, fertilization results in one embryo. However, sometimes multiple embryos are formed, resulting in *multiple births*—twins, triplets, or quadruplets. Identical twins result from a single zygote that splits into two separate embryos. These twins are always of the same gender and have identical physical traits. Fraternal twins occur when two eggs are released at the same time and are fertilized by two different sperm. Fraternal twins can be of different genders, and they are no more likely to look the same than any other siblings.

Implantation

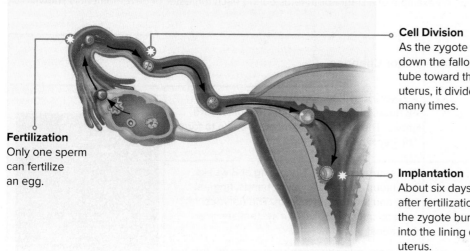

Cell Division
As the zygote travels down the fallopian tube toward the uterus, it divides many times.

Fertilization
Only one sperm can fertilize an egg.

Implantation
About six days after fertilization, the zygote burrows into the lining of the uterus.

Fertilization and implantation occur after an egg is released from the ovary. **Explain how long it takes after fertilization before implantation takes place.**

The Growing Embryo

The cells of an embryo continue to divide as it grows. **Eventually,** three layers of tissue are formed. Over time, these layers develop into various body systems. One layer becomes the respiratory and digestive systems. The second develops into muscles, bones, blood vessels, and skin. The third layer forms the nervous system, sense organs, and mouth.

Meanwhile, several important structures form outside the embryo. A thin, fluid-filled membrane, known as the *amniotic sac,* surrounds and protects the developing embryo. At the same time, the walls of the uterus become lined with thick, blood-rich tissue, called the *placenta,* which nourishes the embryo. The fetus is connected to the placenta through a ropelike structure called the *umbilical cord.*

During pregnancy, the blood supply of the mother and the developing embryo are kept separate. Oxygen and nutrients pass from the mother's blood to the embryo through the umbilical cord. Wastes from the embryo pass into the mother's blood. These wastes are excreted from the mother's body along with her own body wastes. Substances that are harmful to the fetus can also pass through the umbilical cord. If a pregnant female uses tobacco, alcohol, or other drugs, these substances can cross the placenta and harm the developing embryo.

The time from conception to the birth of a baby is usually about 280 days, or nine months. The nine months are divided into three *trimesters* of three months each. Starting around the middle of the first trimester—about eight weeks after conception—the embryo is known as a **fetus** (FEE-tuhs).

ACADEMIC VOCABULARY

eventually *(adverb)*: at an unspecified later time

Reading Check

Describe What are some of the changes that occur during the second trimester?

STAGES OF EMBRYONIC AND FETAL DEVELOPMENT

Fetal development occurs over nine months. The nine months are divided into three trimesters, lasting three months each. An example of a single birth fetus during each trimester of development is shown below.

First Trimester (0 to 14 weeks)	Major Changes	
0–2 weeks	A zygote may float freely in the uterus for 48 hours before implanting. The spinal cord grows. The brain, ears, and arms begin to form. The heart begins to beat.	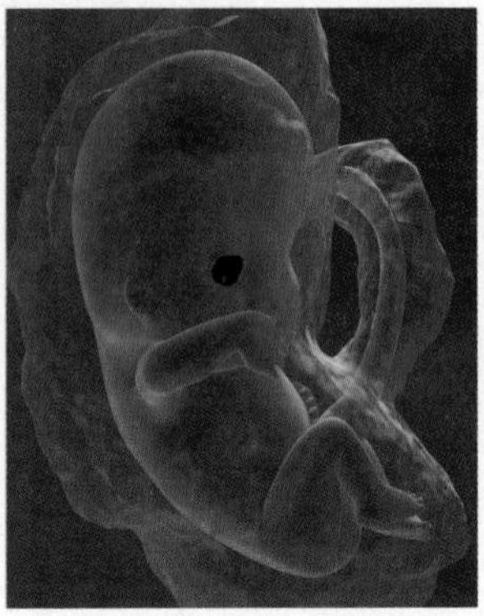
3–8 weeks	The embryo is about 1 inch long at 8 weeks. The mouth, nostrils, eyelids, hands, fingers, feet, and toes begin to form. The nervous system and cardiovascular system are functional.	
9–14 weeks	The fetus develops a human profile. Sex organs, eyelids, fingernails, and toenails develop. By week 12 it can make crying motions and may suck its thumb.	
Second Trimester (15 to 28 weeks)	Major Changes	
15–20 weeks	The fetus can blink its eyes and becomes more active. The body begins to grow, growth of the head slows and the limbs reach full proportion. Eyebrows and eyelashes develop.	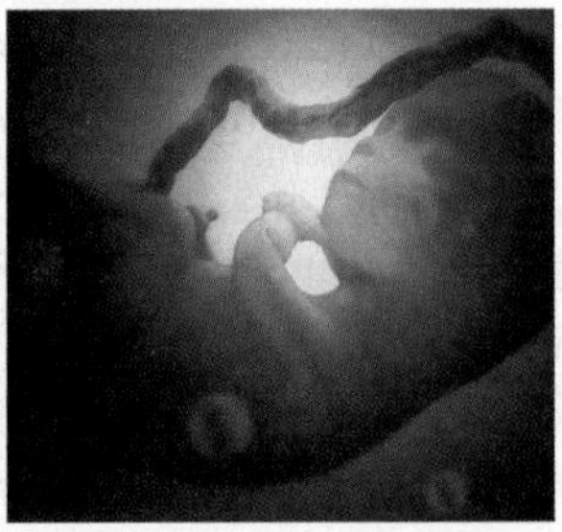
21–28 weeks	The fetus can hear conversations and has a regular cycle of waking and sleeping. Weight increases rapidly. The fetus is about 12 inches long and weighs a little more than 1 pound. The fetus may survive if born after 24 weeks, but will require special medical care.	
Third Trimester (29 weeks to birth)	Major Changes	
29–40 weeks	The fetus uses all five senses and begins to pass water from the bladder. Brain scans have shown that some fetuses dream during their periods of sleep in the eighth and ninth months of development. Approximately 266 days after conception, the baby weighs 6 to 9 pounds and is ready to be born.	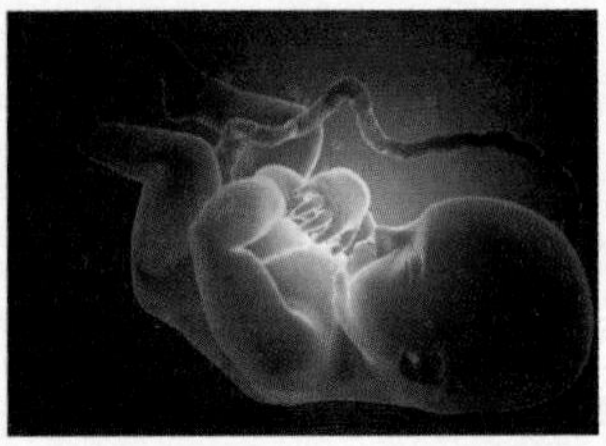

A Healthy Pregnancy

MAIN IDEA A pregnant female can maintain the health of her fetus in many different ways.

As soon as a woman learns that she is pregnant, she should begin **prenatal (pree-NAY-tuhl) care** to protect her health and the health of her growing baby. This type of care refers to the steps that a pregnant female can take to provide for her own health and the health of her baby. She will need to see a doctor regularly throughout her pregnancy to make sure she gets proper care and advice. The doctor can also perform tests on the fetus to make sure it is developing normally.

What to Eat While Pregnant

Have you ever heard a pregnant woman say that she is "eating for two"? In a way, it's true: an unborn baby receives all its nourishment from the mother. However, a pregnant female does not really need to consume twice as much food to feed herself and the fetus. In most cases, an additional 300 calories a day are enough to achieve a healthy weight gain during pregnancy. A female who was at a healthy weight before pregnancy can expect to gain between 25 and 35 pounds. Gaining too little weight may result in a small, undeveloped baby. Gaining too much can result in an early delivery. Extra weight can also harm the mother. It increases her risk of developing high blood pressure, diabetes, and varicose veins.

Pregnant females should follow the guidelines in MyPlate for a healthy, balanced diet. In addition, they are encouraged to take prenatal vitamins. This will ensure that they get enough of several important nutrients, such as:

- Calcium, which helps build strong bones and teeth, healthy nerves, and muscles. It is also important for developing heart rhythm.

- Protein, which helps form muscle and other tissue.

- Iron, which makes red blood cells and supplies oxygen to cells.

- Vitamin A, which helps in the growth of cells and bones and in eye development.

- Vitamin B complex, which aids in forming the nervous system.

- Folic acid, critical in development of the neural tube, which contains the nervous system. It is recommended that all females of childbearing age consume 400 micrograms of folic acid daily. Women who are pregnant are advised to consume 600 mg of folate daily.

During pregnancy, good nutrition and rest keep both the mother and the developing child healthy. **Why are healthy snacks important to fetal development?**

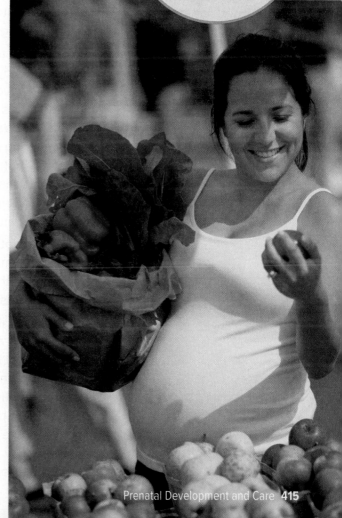

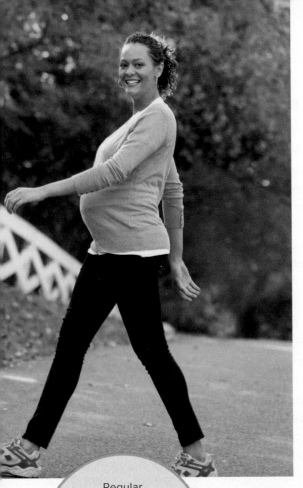

Regular exercise is an important part of a healthy pregnancy. **How can regular physical activity help the health of a pregnant female and the fetus?**

Fitness During Pregnancy

Physical activity can help a female maintain a healthy weight during pregnancy. Toward the end of the pregnancy, however, it may become more difficult to maintain a fitness program. Before starting any exercise program, an expectant mother should discuss it with her health care provider.

Avoiding Harmful Substances

Food and oxygen aren't the only things that a fetus can absorb through the mother's blood. The umbilical cord can also transmit harmful substances, such as tobacco, alcohol, and other drugs. For this reason, an expectant mother should take care to avoid substances that can harm her and the fetus.

Tobacco. Smoking and using other tobacco products during pregnancy is harmful to the fetus. It is estimated that smoking accounts for up to 30 percent of low-birth-weight babies, 14 percent of premature births, and 10 percent of all infant deaths. Studies suggest that smoking during pregnancy may also affect growth, mental development, and behavior after a child is born. Secondhand smoke from other people's cigarettes can also be harmful. Research by the American Lung Association shows that pregnant females who are exposed repeatedly to secondhand smoke increase their risk of having a low-birth-weight baby.

Alcohol. When an expectant mother uses alcohol, so does her developing baby. Alcohol passes through the umbilical cord to the fetus. Its body, however, breaks down alcohol more slowly than the mother's body does. This means that alcohol reaches a higher concentration in the fetus' bloodstream and stays there for a longer period of time. Drinking during pregnancy can result in a severe disorder known as **fetal alcohol syndrome**, or FAS. This is a group of alcohol-related birth defects that includes both physical and mental problems. Infants born with FAS may have learning, memory, and attention problems, as well as visual and hearing impairments.

Drugs. Prescription or over-the-counter medications that are safe to take at other times may not be safe to use during pregnancy. They might cause harm to the developing fetus. A pregnant female should not take any medications during pregnancy without consulting her doctor first.

The use of any illegal drugs poses a health risk to both the mother and the fetus. Drug abuse can harm the mother's health and make her less able to support the pregnancy. Drugs can also harm the development of the fetus. Infants born to mothers who use drugs may not grow at the same rate as other infants. They may also have respiratory or cardiovascular problems, mental impairments, or birth defects. In some cases, drug use may lead to premature birth or miscarriage. A final risk is that the baby may be born addicted to the same drugs the mother used during pregnancy.

Ariel Skelley/Blend Images/Getty Images

Hazards in the Environment. Many common substances found in the environment can be hazardous to a fetus. Pregnant women should always use caution when using household chemicals. They should read cleaning-product labels carefully, wear gloves, and work in a well-ventilated area. They should also take particular care to avoid these substances:

- **Lead.** Exposure to lead has been linked to miscarriage, low birth weight, mental disabilities, and behavior problems in children. Lead may be found in paint in houses built before 1978, as well as in some glassware and dinnerware.

- **Mercury.** Some types of fish, including tilefish, shark, swordfish, and king mackerel, are known to contain higher than average levels of mercury. Women should avoid eating these fish during pregnancy.

- **Smog.** Medical studies have linked air pollution with birth defects, low birth weight, premature birth, stillbirth, and infant death. The period of greatest risk is the second month of pregnancy, when the organs are developing.

- **Radiation.** Ionizing radiation, such as that found in X-rays, can affect growth and cause mental disabilities.

Activities such as painting or using lead-based products should be avoided or done carefully during pregnancy. **Why is it important to keep a room well-ventilated while painting?**

Complications of Pregnancy

MAIN IDEA A pregnancy may have an unexpected outcome.

If you ask an expectant couple whether they're hoping for a boy or a girl, they will probably say, "Either, as long as it's healthy." Most pregnancies result in the birth of a healthy baby. About 70 percent of all babies are born through a vaginal delivery. However, complications in a pregnancy may make it necessary for the mother to have a *cesarean delivery.* This procedure involves delivering the baby through an incision in the mother's abdomen.

Complications during pregnancy can also cause a pregnant woman to go into labor too early. If a baby is born at least three weeks before the due date, the birth is said to be *premature.* Sometimes, serious complications may cause a woman to go into labor before the twentieth week of pregnancy, when the fetus is not developed enough to survive. This is known as a *miscarriage.* If a fetus dies in the womb and is delivered after the twentieth week of pregnancy, the birth is called a *stillbirth.* Miscarriages and stillbirths may result from medical problems, but the risk of them increases greatly if a mother uses tobacco or drugs during pregnancy.

Easy Production/Image Source

Medical complications can affect the expectant mother as well as the fetus. *Gestational hypertension,* or high blood pressure during pregnancy, may occur after the twentieth week of pregnancy. A severe form of this is *preeclampsia.* Symptoms include high blood pressure, swelling, and large amounts of protein in the urine. Preeclampsia can prevent the placenta from getting enough blood to nourish the fetus. Treatment involves reducing blood pressure through bed rest or medication. Hospitalization may be necessary.

An *ectopic pregnancy* results when a zygote implants not in the uterus but in the fallopian tube, abdomen, ovary, or cervix. This makes it impossible for the fetus to receive nourishment and grow. An ectopic pregnancy cannot lead to the birth of a healthy baby. It is also the number one cause of death in women during the first trimester of pregnancy.

Proper prenatal care can reduce the risk and severity of problems during pregnancy. During a prenatal examination, a doctor may be able to identify medical problems with the mother and fetus before the birth. In some cases, the baby may receive medical care, or even surgery, while still in the womb.

The birth of a healthy baby is a joyous event. **What steps can pregnant women take to help ensure a healthy pregnancy and delivery?**

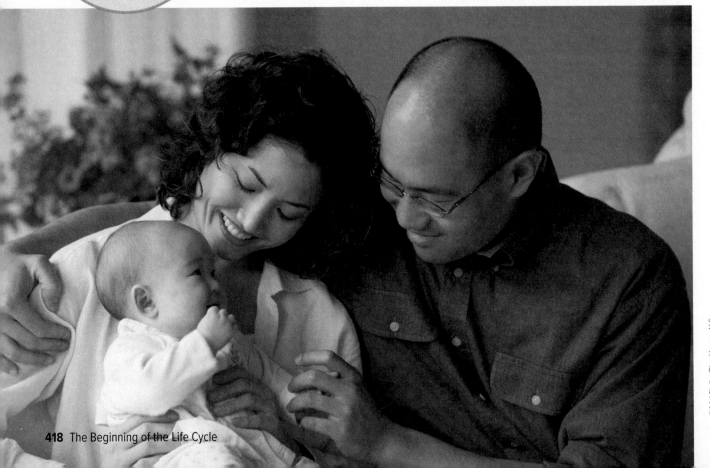

Childbirth and Perinatal Care

MAIN IDEA The birth of a baby takes place in three stages: labor, delivery, and afterbirth.

Expectant parents must decide where the birth will take place. Most births occur in hospital maternity wards staffed by nurses and doctors, with medical equipment to handle complications. Other options include birthing centers or home births, which offer a more comfortable environment. A health professional called a *midwife,* rather than a doctor, may attend births in these settings.

As the birth approaches, the fetus becomes more crowded in the uterus. The birth itself occurs in three stages:

- **Stage 1: Labor.** Muscle contractions begin in the uterus. Gradually, these contractions become regular, stronger, and closer together. This causes the cervix—the opening to the uterus—to dilate, or widen.

- **Stage 2: Delivery.** Once the cervix is fully dilated, the baby passes through the birth canal and emerges from the mother's body. The baby takes its first breath and cries to clear its lungs of amniotic fluid.

- **Stage 3: Afterbirth.** The placenta is still attached to the baby by the umbilical cord. Contractions, although weaker, will continue until the placenta (now called the *afterbirth*) is pushed from the mother's body.

The first seven days after delivery is a part of the perinatal period. The perinatal period begins at week 23 of a pregnancy and ends seven full days after birth. Nursing begins during the perinatal period and can begin as soon as the baby is born.

Lesson 1 Review

Facts and Vocabulary

1. Describe an *embryo* and a *fetus*.

2. What is the difference between identical and fraternal twins?

3. What is the relationship between the placenta and the umbilical cord?

Thinking Critically

4. **Evaluate.** How is the diet of a pregnant female important to her growing fetus?

5. **Cause and Effect.** What are some of the risks that may occur if a pregnant female uses tobacco, alcohol, or drugs during her pregnancy?

Applying Health Skills

6. **Accessing Information.** Research library or Internet resources to learn more about gestational hypertension. Explain the warning signs and the need for proper treatment.

Writing Critically

7. **Persuasive.** Write a short essay from the point of view of a fetus persuading its mother to eat healthy foods during pregnancy.

Heredity and Genetics

BEFORE YOU READ

Make an Outline. Use the headings of this lesson to make an outline of what you'll read. Use a format like the one below to help you organize your notes.

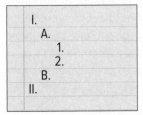

Vocabulary

genes
chromosomes
DNA
genetic disorders
amniocentesis
chorionic villi sampling (CVS)
gene therapy

. . . .

BIG IDEA Certain traits, such as eye and hair color, come from both of your parents.

REAL LIFE ISSUES

The Same Genes. Casey's friend Sean has asked him to pick up Sean's brother, Jason, at the bus stop and give him a ride back to school. Casey is glad to help out, but he has never met Jason and isn't sure he'll recognize him. He is surprised when he gets to the bus stop and spots a boy who looks almost exactly like his friend. *Write a paragraph describing two related people you know, or have seen, that share common traits.*

After completing the lesson, review and analyze your response to the Real Life Issues question.

Heredity

MAIN IDEA Heredity is the passing of physical traits from parents to their children.

Has anyone ever said you have your father's nose or your mother's smile? Each one of us inherits traits from our parents, including hair color, eye color, and even the shape of our earlobes. These traits are passed down through **genes**, which are the basic units of heredity.

Most of the cells in the human body contain a nucleus, which is the cell's control center. Inside the nucleus is a set of **chromosomes** (KROH-muh-sohmz). These thread-like structures within the nucleus of a cell carry the codes for inherited traits. Each chromosome, in turn, is made up of genes, which are arranged in pairs, one from each parent. Genes and chromosomes are made of **DNA**, short for *deoxyribonucleic* (dee-AHK-see-ry-boh-noo-KLEE-ik) *acid.* All living things contain DNA, but each individual's DNA is different. DNA is made up of a long sequence of chemical building blocks strung together in pairs to form two twisted strands. These building blocks spell out the genetic code, just as letters on a page might spell out a recipe. In fact, in a way, your unique DNA sequence *is* a recipe for making a complete copy of you. No one else has exactly the same DNA pattern as you—unless you happen to have an identical twin.

DNA determines all the physical characteristics you have, from your eye color to the amount of curl in your hair. However, some of the traits you inherit can also be influenced by environment. For example, height is an inherited trait, but poor nutrition may limit a person's growth during childhood. The environment can also affect traits such as body weight and the tendency to develop certain diseases, such as diabetes.

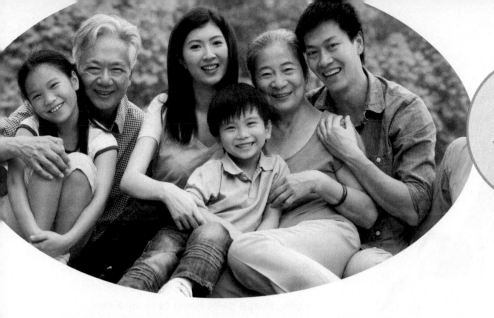

Family members often share similar physical traits. **What determines your physical traits?**

Genetics and Fetal Development

MAIN IDEA Chromosomes from a sperm and an egg unite to carry the hereditary traits from parents.

The process of passing down traits from parent to child through genes is known as *genetics.* To understand how genetics works, you need to know that most human cells have 46 chromosomes, or 23 pairs. However, egg and sperm cells have only half that number—23 individual chromosomes. When an egg and a sperm unite during fertilization, they produce a zygote with 46 chromosomes, 23 from each parent. These chromosomes carry the genes of the parents, which are passed down to the child.

The zygote then begins to divide repeatedly, ultimately forming a complete human body. Before each cell division, each chromosome in the nucleus of the cells copies itself, producing two sets of the 46 chromosomes. When the cell divides, these two sets of chromosomes separate, with one set going to each of the two new cells. This means that each one of the trillions of cells in your body contains an exact copy of the 46 chromosomes you received from your parents.

Dominant and Recessive Traits

If all traits are passed down through genes, then you may wonder how it is that two parents with brown eyes can have a child with blue eyes. The answer is that some genes are *dominant,* while others are *recessive.* Each trait is determined by at least one pair of genes. However, if one gene in that pair is dominant and one is recessive, then the trait for the dominant gene is the one that will appear. The gene for brown eyes, for example, is dominant. This means that if a child receives two genes for eye color, one for brown eyes and one for blue eyes, the child will have brown eyes. The only way for a child to have blue eyes is to inherit a recessive gene for blue eyes from each parent.

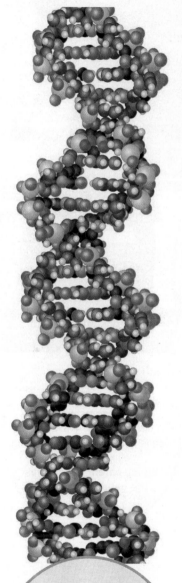

DNA, like this double helix, look like a long, twisted ladder. Nitrogen bases make up the rungs of this ladder. **What determines your own personal genetic code?**

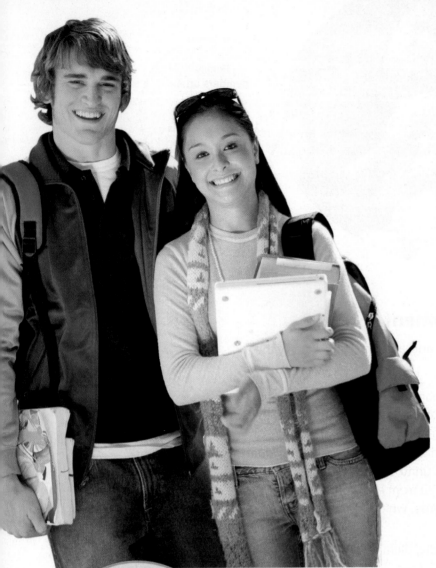

Genes and Sex

Out of your 23 pairs of chromosomes, one pair, known as the *sex chromosomes,* determines your sex. Females have two chromosomes that look exactly alike; these are called X chromosomes: Males, on the other hand, have two different chromosomes, an X chromosome and a shorter one called a Y chromosome.

Since egg and sperm cells contain only half as many chromosomes as other cells, these cells have only one sex chromosome each. Because females have only X chromosomes, every egg cell in a female's body contains a single X chromosome. Sperm, because they come from a male, can contain either an X or a Y chromosome. Thus, the sperm from the male determines the sex of the child. If the sperm cell that fertilizes an egg carries an X chromosome, the child will be a girl. If it has a Y chromosome, the child will be a boy.

Genetic Disorders

MAIN IDEA Genetic disorders are caused by defects in genes.

The body cells of a male have both an X chromosome and a Y chromosome. The body cells of a female have two X chromosomes. **Which parent determines the gender of a child, and why?**

Sometimes, one of the genes a person inherits may contain a mutation, or abnormality. In many cases, the mutation will have little or no effect on the person. Some genetic mutations, however, can produce birth defects. Others can increase the person's likelihood of developing a disease. Some **genetic disorders**, which are disorders caused by defects in genes, are apparent at birth. Others may not show up until later in life.

Most genetic disorders cannot be cured, but some can be treated. For this reason, it is important to know as early as possible whether a child has any genetic disorders. Two technologies used to test for genetic disorders before birth are **amniocentesis** (am-nee-oh-sen-TEE-sis) and **chorionic villi sampling** (kor-ee-ON-ik VIL-eye) (CVS).

Amniocentesis is a procedure in which a syringe is inserted through a pregnant female's abdominal wall to remove a sample of the amniotic fluid surrounding the developing fetus. Doctors examine the chromosomes in fetal cells for genetic abnormalities. This test is performed 16 to 20 weeks after fertilization.

Chorionic villi sampling, or CVS, is a procedure in which a small piece of membrane is removed from the chorion, a layer of tissue that develops into the placenta. The tissue can be examined for genetic disorders or to determine the age and gender of the fetus. The procedure is done around the eighth week of fetal development.

It is also possible to test a child for genetic disorders after birth. For example, many states require that all newborns be tested for phenylketonuria (PKU). If PKU is diagnosed soon after birth, a baby's diet can be altered to stop possible complications caused by this genetic disorder.

Battling Genetic Diseases

MAIN IDEA Research is ongoing to correct genetic diseases.

In 1990, researchers working on the Human Genome Project began to identify all of the genes in human DNA. By 2003, they had identified individual genes that are linked to more than 1,800 diseases. This information was an important first step in learning more about genetic diseases. With it, scientists have gained a greater understanding of how diseases progress. They have also learned how to identify people who may be susceptible to genetic diseases or disorders. Having a faulty gene, however, does *not* guarantee that the person will get the disease.

Some genetic disorders occur when an individual is missing a functioning gene, without which it cannot produce some of the substances it needs. Scientists have begun to experiment with **gene therapy** as a way to correct these disorders. Gene therapy is the process of inserting normal genes into human cells to correct genetic disorders. The idea behind gene therapy is that once a defective gene is replaced with a normal gene, the cells can then begin producing the normal gene. At this time, gene therapy is only experimental.

COMMON HUMAN GENETIC DISORDERS	
Disorder	**Characteristics**
Sickle-cell anemia	Red blood cells have a sickle shape and clump together; may result in severe joint and abdominal pain, weakness, kidney disease, restricted blood flow
Tay-Sachs disease	Destruction of nervous system; blindness; paralysis; death during early childhood
Cystic fibrosis	Mucus clogs many organs, including lungs, liver, and pancreas; nutritional problems; serious respiratory infections and congestion
Down syndrome	Varying degrees of mental disability, short stature, round face with upper eyelids that cover inner corners of the eyes
Hemophilia	Failure of blood to clot

This table shows some disorders that can be caused by genetic mutations. **Describe two characteristics displayed by a person with Down Syndrome.**

Reading Check

Cause and Effect What happens when a defective gene is replaced by a normal one?

Fitness Zone

I see ads for workout equipment that promise to give me washboard abs, to melt off the fat, or to tone my body in just two minutes a day. Those promises are too good to be true. We are born with our bodies, and we can only make the most of what we've got. The best way to get fit is to set goals, eat healthy, and exercise to get into shape.

Genetic Counseling

Genetic research has resulted in many ways to diagnose and treat genetic diseases. Families of children with genetic disorders can see a genetic counselor to learn about possible treatments. Genetic counselors rely on a complete family medical history. They use this information to educate families about their risks for certain diseases and guide them through their options for treatment.

Genetically Engineered Drugs

Scientists have also begun experimenting with *genetic engineering,* or placing parts of DNA from one organism into another. Instead of inserting a disease-treating gene directly into a human being, scientists can place it into another organism. This causes that organism to produce substances that can be used to treat human diseases and disorders. Genetic engineering has already resulted in some vaccines that can prevent disease.

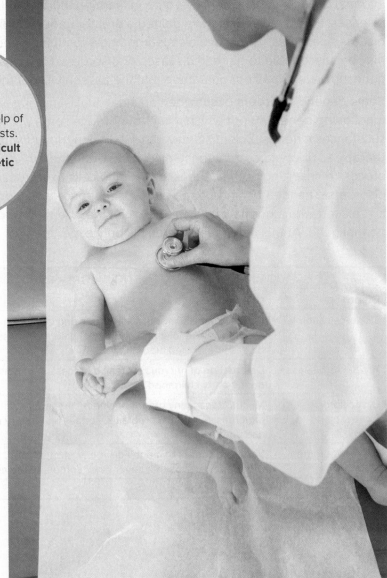

Newborns can be checked for certain genetic disorders with the help of some very simple tests. **Why might it be difficult to diagnose a genetic disorder early in life?**

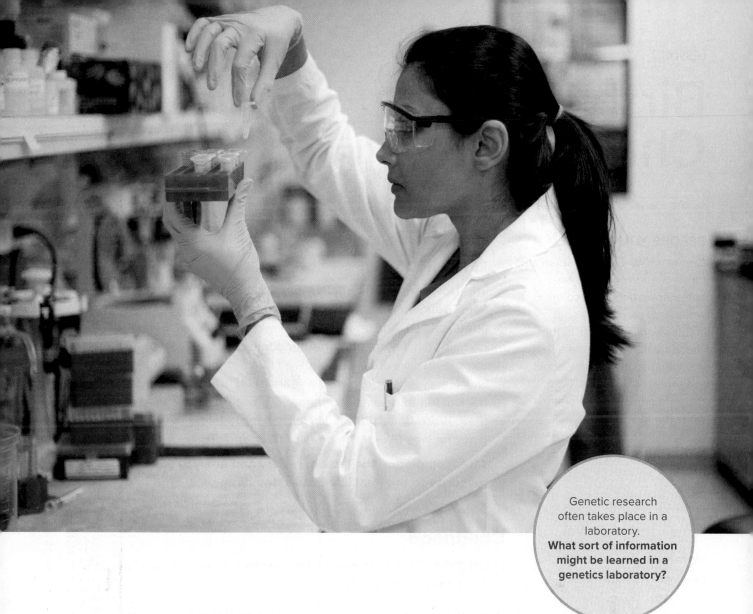

Genetic research often takes place in a laboratory. **What sort of information might be learned in a genetics laboratory?**

Lesson 2 Review

Facts and Vocabulary

1. Define the terms *chromosomes* and *genes*.

2. How many chromosomes are found in most human cells? How many are found in egg and sperm cells?

3. Identify the difference between the chromosomes of a male and the chromosomes of a female.

Thinking Critically

4. **Evaluate.** When might a pregnant woman consider having CVS?

5. **Interpret.** The gene for brown hair is dominant, while the gene for blond hair is recessive. What genes might a brown-haired person have?

Applying Health Skills

6. **Accessing Information.** Use library or Internet resources to learn more about genetic research. Explain how this technology can prevent disease, and how it can impact personal, family, and community health.

Writing Critically

7. **Descriptive.** Write a short essay describing how genetic counseling and gene therapy might change someone's life.

Heredity and Genetics **425**

Birth Through Childhood

BEFORE YOU READ

Create a K-W-L Chart. Make a three-column chart like the one below. In the first column, write what you know about infancy and childhood. In the second column, write what you would want to know about this topic. As you read, fill in the third column describing what you have learned.

K	W	L

Vocabulary

developmental tasks
autonomy
scoliosis

. . . .

BIG IDEA Infancy and childhood are times of great changes and growth.

REAL LIFE ISSUES

Trip Down Memory Lane. Henry and his parents are going to a family reunion. He's looking forward to seeing his grandparents, aunts, uncles, and cousins who live in other states. Earlier today he helped his mom put together some photo albums to take on the trip. At one point, she showed him a photo of a young boy. It was Henry when he was five years old. This made him think back to when he was younger and how he has changed since then. *Write three entries in Henry's diary as he remembers what he was like at the ages of 5, 8, and 10.*

After completing the lesson, review and analyze your response to the Real Life Issues question.

Childhood

MAIN IDEA Each child passes through four stages of development during infancy and childhood.

Right now, as an adolescent, you are going through major changes—physical, mental/emotional, and social. However, these are not the first major changes you have gone through in your life, and they will not be the last. Our lives can be divided up into eight developmental stages, and each has its own set of **developmental tasks**. These are events that need to happen in order for a person to continue growing toward becoming a healthy, mature adult. You have already gone through the first four of these stages, from infancy through late childhood.

Infancy

Infancy, the first twelve months of your life, is the time of fastest growth in a person's life. It is also a time of learning. Infants have many new skills to master: sitting up, opening and closing their hands, eating solid food, crawling, and possibly walking a few steps. One of an infant's biggest challenges is beginning to learn about speech. During the first year, an infant may begin to associate certain sounds with certain objects and to imitate new word sounds.

Infants also develop emotionally and socially. They experience basic emotions, and they show strong likes and dislikes. They also begin to smile as a way to express happiness. Infants feel a desire for companionship. They enjoy the company of other children, and they also form a strong attachment to their parents. At the same time, they become anxious in the presence of strangers.

Early Childhood

During early childhood (ages one to three), children begin to take pride in their accomplishments. They become eager to try new tasks and learn new things. Parents are encouraged to let their children try new things and test their abilities. This helps young children develop the confidence to control their own bodies, impulses, and environment, also known as a sense of **autonomy**.

During this period, children master both physical and mental skills. Young children can walk well and pick up objects without losing their balance. They can throw balls overhead, but not very accurately. They can also draw recognizable pictures. Emotionally, they show affection and a desire for approval. They may wish to help adults, but they also begin to show defiance and disagreement. They also begin to be bothered by fears. Socially, children at this stage first begin to learn how to play in groups with others—though sometimes they may try to boss the other children.

Middle Childhood

During middle childhood (ages four to six), children become more independent. They can dress and undress themselves and eat with utensils. They also gain self-confidence and become eager to explore the larger world. However, they still crave praise and approval. Socially, children at this age learn to initiate play rather than follow the lead of others. They become more outgoing and talkative, and they begin forming friendships. At the same time, they may have a strong desire to do things their own way. Children at this stage must be taught to recognize emotions and practice expressing them in appropriate ways.

Late Childhood

In late childhood (ages 7 to 12), school becomes an important part of a child's life. Children learn to get along with their peers and form deeper friendships. They may also experience peer pressure more strongly. Their relationships with parents change as they become more self-aware. A child at this age begins to develop a sense of competence and to recognize his or her unique personality traits. Children this age also become aware of dangers in the world. They begin to face moral decisions and develop a conscience. School-age children may become sensitive about their body image, especially as puberty may begin at this age.

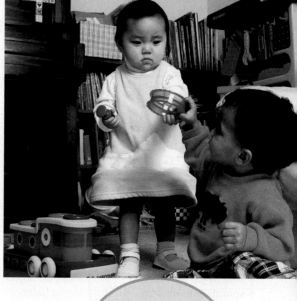

Infants learn to trust and depend on others. **What do infants learn during the infancy stage of development?**

Reading Check

Infer How can a parent help a child develop a sense of autonomy?

Stages of Infancy and Childhood

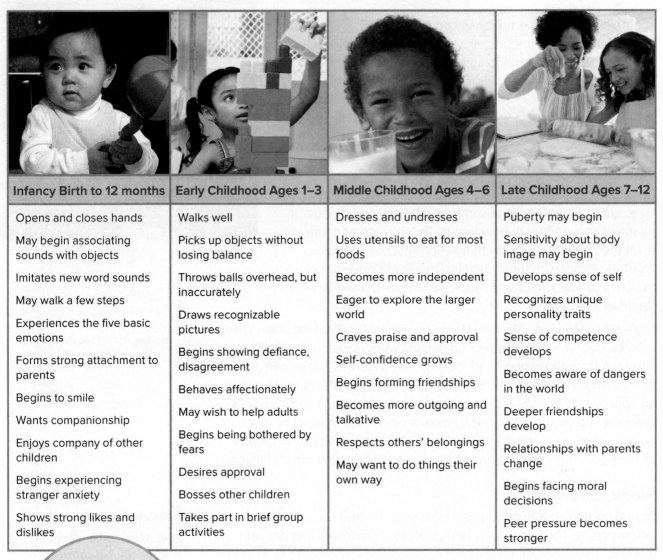

Infancy Birth to 12 months	Early Childhood Ages 1–3	Middle Childhood Ages 4–6	Late Childhood Ages 7–12
Opens and closes hands	Walks well	Dresses and undresses	Puberty may begin
May begin associating sounds with objects	Picks up objects without losing balance	Uses utensils to eat for most foods	Sensitivity about body image may begin
Imitates new word sounds	Throws balls overhead, but inaccurately	Becomes more independent	Develops sense of self
May walk a few steps	Draws recognizable pictures	Eager to explore the larger world	Recognizes unique personality traits
Experiences the five basic emotions	Begins showing defiance, disagreement	Craves praise and approval	Sense of competence develops
Forms strong attachment to parents	Behaves affectionately	Self-confidence grows	Becomes aware of dangers in the world
Begins to smile	May wish to help adults	Begins forming friendships	Deeper friendships develop
Wants companionship	Begins being bothered by fears	Becomes more outgoing and talkative	Relationships with parents change
Enjoys company of other children	Desires approval	Respects others' belongings	Begins facing moral decisions
Begins experiencing stranger anxiety	Bosses other children	May want to do things their own way	Peer pressure becomes stronger
Shows strong likes and dislikes	Takes part in brief group activities		

Each stage of development is associated with a developmental task that involves a person's relationship with other people.

Childhood Health Screenings

MAIN IDEA Many screening tests are performed in childhood to monitor the health and growth of a child.

To make sure they stay healthy throughout childhood, children need to receive regular checkups from a doctor. During these checkups, they will receive immunizations against disease. They will also be screened for problems that can affect their ability to grow, learn, and develop. These screenings include:

- **Vision tests.** Nearly one in every four school-aged children in the United States has a vision problem. The American Academy of Ophthalmology recommends that children receive vision screenings throughout childhood, starting at birth. However, many children never receive a vision screening until they reach age 18. To prevent this problem, some schools now provide regular vision screenings for students.

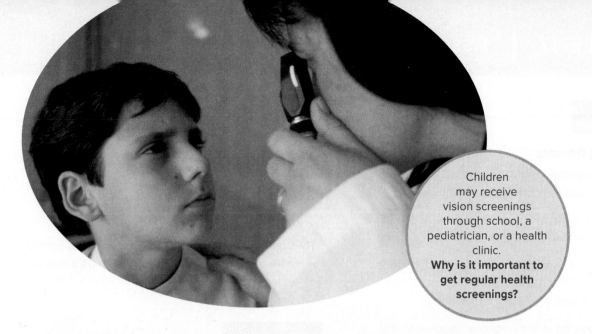

Children may receive vision screenings through school, a pediatrician, or a health clinic. **Why is it important to get regular health screenings?**

- **Hearing tests.** Hearing impairment, like vision problems, can affect a child's ability to learn. Two or three out of every 1,000 children in the United States are born with a hearing impairment severe enough to affect their language development. Some states require that infants be screened for hearing loss. Again, some school districts may provide screenings for students to identify hearing impairments.

- **Screening for scoliosis.** Scoliosis is an abnormal lateral, or side-to-side, curvature of the spine. This condition may begin in childhood and go unnoticed until the child reaches adolescence. The exact cause of scoliosis is unknown, but it is more common in girls. Many middle schools have developed screening methods to check students for scoliosis.

- **Other tests.** Children are tested for lead poisoning yearly until age four. Blood pressure screenings begin after age three. Children with a family history of cholesterol problems or anemia may also be screened for these conditions.

Reading Check

Explain Why are students screened for vision and hearing?

Character Check

When a child feels understood and has physical and emotional needs taken care of, he or she will thrive. Take the time to listen attentively and show that you care whenever you have a chance to help a toddler or young child. Think of ways you demonstrate caring with younger siblings of other children.

Lesson 3 Review

Facts and Vocabulary

1. What are some *developmental tasks* children learn in early childhood?

2. What is an important part of a child's life during late childhood?

3. What is *scoliosis?*

Thinking Critically

4. **Evaluate.** How can positive parenting affect the autonomy and independence of a child?

5. **Analyze.** What is the result when a parent allows a child autonomy?

Applying Health Skills

6. **Accessing Information.** Research library or Internet resources to learn more about vision and hearing screenings. Explain how these screenings could prevent problems later in life.

Writing Critically

7. **Descriptive.** Write a short essay about the changes a child will face from early childhood to late childhood.

Vocabulary Review

Correct the sentences below by replacing the italicized term with the correct vocabulary term.

1. A(n) *fetus* is a cluster of cells that develops between the third and eighth week of pregnancy.

2. *Fetal alcohol syndrome* refers to the steps that a pregnant female can take to provide for her own health and the health of her baby.

3. The process by which a zygote attaches to the uterine wall is called *fertilization*.

Understanding Key Concepts

After reading the question or statement, select the correct answer.

4. Which of the following nutrients helps form the nervous system of an embryo?
   a. Calcium
   b. Vitamin A
   c. Folic acid
   d. Iron

5. Exposure to which of the following may cause birth defects in the second month of pregnancy?
   a. Lead
   b. Mercury
   c. Radiation
   d. Smog

6. What is the result when a zygote implants in the fallopian tube or ovary?
   a. Preeclampsia
   b. Ectopic pregnancy
   c. Miscarriage
   d. Stillbirth

Thinking Critically

After reading the question or statement, write a short answer using complete sentences.

7. **Analyze.** What is the role of prenatal care in protecting the health of the mother and the fetus?

8. **Evaluate.** What should parents consider when choosing a childbirth method?

9. **Explain.** How can drinking alcohol during pregnancy damage a fetus?

10. **Analyze.** What is the result if one healthy zygote splits into two?

11. **Compare and Contrast.** What are the similarities and differences between preeclampsia and an ectopic pregnancy?

Vocabulary Review

Use the correct vocabulary term to complete the following statements.

12. _____ are the basic units of heredity.

13. The process of inserting normal genes into human cells to correct genetic disorders is called _____.

14. Disorders caused by a defect in genes are called _____.

Understanding Key Concepts

After reading the question or statement, select the correct answer.

15. How many chromosomes do most human cells have?
   a. 12
   b. 23
   c. 46
   d. 69

16. Where are chromosomes located?
   a. Within the DNA molecule
   b. In genes
   c. In the nucleus of a cell
   d. Outside a cell

17. What is the chemical compound that makes up genetic material?
   a. Genes
   b. DNA
   c. Chromosomes
   d. Genetic code

Thinking Critically

After reading the question or statement, write a short answer using complete sentences.

18. **Explain.** How does genetics play a role in fetal development?

19. **Synthesize.** How might a disorder like sickle-cell anemia be traced to its origin?

20. **Infer.** Why would a brown-eyed parent and a blue-eyed parent have a brown-eyed child?

21. **Predict.** What would a pregnant female expect to find out after having an amniocentesis?

LESSON 3

Vocabulary Review

Use the correct vocabulary term to complete the following statements.

22. The confidence that you can control your own body, impulses, and environment is called _____.

23. _____ are events that need to happen for a person to continue growing toward being a healthy, mature adult.

24. The abnormal lateral curvature of the spine is known as _____.

Understanding Key Concepts

After reading the question or statement, select the correct answer.

25. Which of the following is the time of fastest growth in a person's life?
    a. Infancy
    b. Early childhood
    c. Middle childhood
    d. Late childhood

26. Which of the following may lead to low self-esteem in children?
    a. Overprotective parents
    b. Parents who encourage questions
    c. Parents who encourage autonomy
    d. Attentive parents

27. Which group is more likely to be diagnosed with scoliosis?
    a. Boys
    b. Infants
    c. Girls
    d. Preschoolers

28. Which of the following can impact a child's development?
    a. Vision impairments
    b. Hearing impairments
    c. Social factors
    d. All of the above

Thinking Critically

After reading the question or statement, write a short answer using complete sentences.

29. **Analyze.** What developmental tasks are involved as friendships and school become especially important during late childhood?

30. **Infer.** What might happen to a child who is constantly scolded for making a mess or for getting in the way?

31. **Infer.** If a parent is overprotective and does not let a child explore his surroundings, what may happen?

32. **Explain.** Why do most states require that students be screened for hearing and vision problems?

PROJECT-BASED ASSESSMENT

Genes Count

BACKGROUND

In 1962, James Watson, Francis Crick, and Maurice Wilkins received a Nobel Prize for their explanation of the chemical structure of DNA. Since then, our knowledge of genetics has increased rapidly. In 1992, research turned to human genome sequencing to identify the location of hundreds of thousands of human genes. (The term *genome* means the genetic material of an organism.)

TASK

Conduct research online to learn the accomplishments of the Human Genome Project. Develop a multimedia slide presentation based on your findings.

AUDIENCE

Students in your class

PURPOSE

Understand the progress that has been made in recent years by the Human Genome Project.

PROCEDURE

1. Use a variety of online resources to learn the progress of the Human Genome Project and to identify recent advances in genetic research.

2. Based on your findings, create the slides for your presentation.

3. Include information on genetic maps, summarize the progress that has been made to identify genes that cause specific genetic disorders, and describe how genetic counseling and genetic engineering are used.

4. Compile your notes and create your multimedia presentation. Assign part of the presentation to each member of your group.

5. Be sure to use several images for your presentation.

6. Present your presentation to your class.

Math Practice

Interpret Graphs. The pie chart below shows the number of weeks in a typical 40-week pregnancy designated for each trimester. Use the pie chart to answer questions 1–3.

Stages of Pregnancy

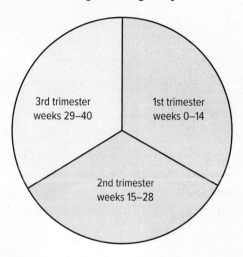

3rd trimester
weeks 29–40

1st trimester
weeks 0–14

2nd trimester
weeks 15–28

1. According to the information in the pie chart, what percentage of duration of the pregnancy makes up the first trimester?
   a. 14%
   c. 35%
   b. 30%
   d. 40%

2. The term *zygote* describes the fertilized egg in the first two weeks after conception. For what percentage of a typical 40-week pregnancy is the developing human called a zygote?
   a. 2%
   c. 14%
   b. 5%
   d. 35%

3. A baby is born early, after only 36 weeks of pregnancy. What percentage of the typical 40-week pregnancy did the baby complete?
   a. 10%
   c. 90%
   b. 36%
   d. 96%

Reading/Writing Practice

Understand and Apply. Read the passage below, and then answer the questions.

Jean Piaget (1896–1980) was the first theorist to study how children learn. Piaget analyzed facts about the way children develop cognitive abilities. He also conducted studies on the way children develop thinking skills. One of Piaget's famous studies used pieces of candy to test children's discriminative abilities. Piaget placed equal numbers of the candy into two lines. He spread one line farther apart than the other line. The two- to three-year-olds tested saw that the rows had the same amount of candies, while the three- to four-year-olds tested believed the longer row had more candies. Piaget's test showed that during this stage of development, three to four year olds temporarily lose their ability to problem solve.

1. What is a *theorist*?
   a. A person who solves a problem
   b. A person who writes a story
   c. A person who analyzes a set of facts
   d. A person who uses a large vocabulary

2. The word *discriminative*, used in paragraph two, means which of the following?
   a. Objective
   b. Distinguish
   c. Prejudice
   d. Judicious

3. Considering Piaget's test, why do you think children between ages three to four temporarily lose the ability to solve?

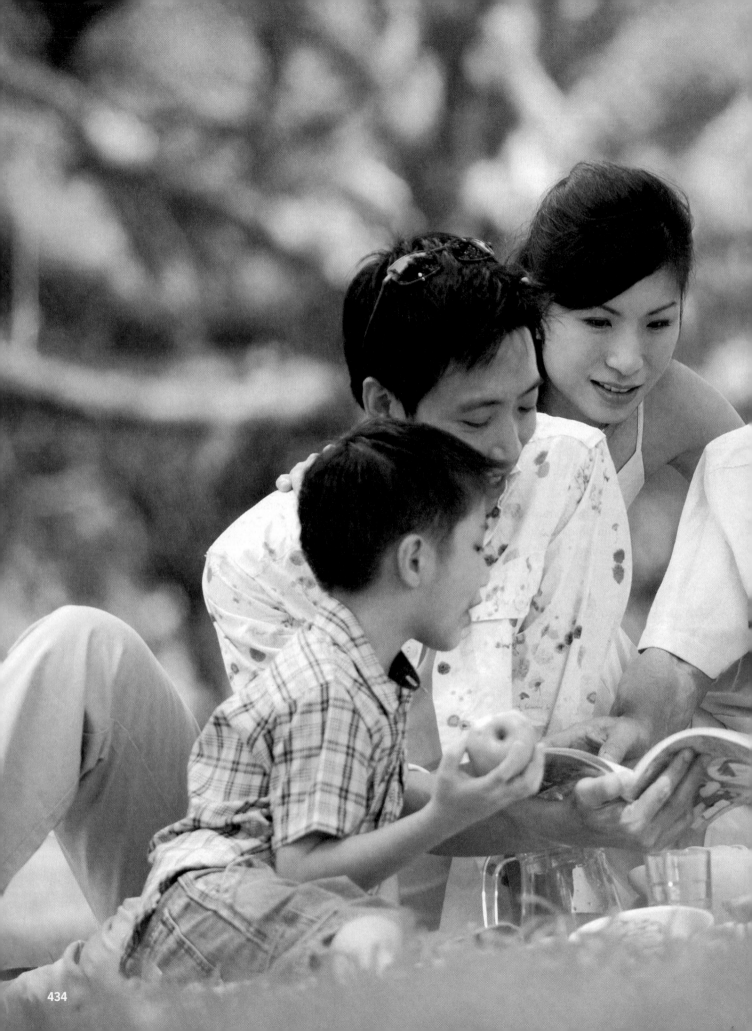

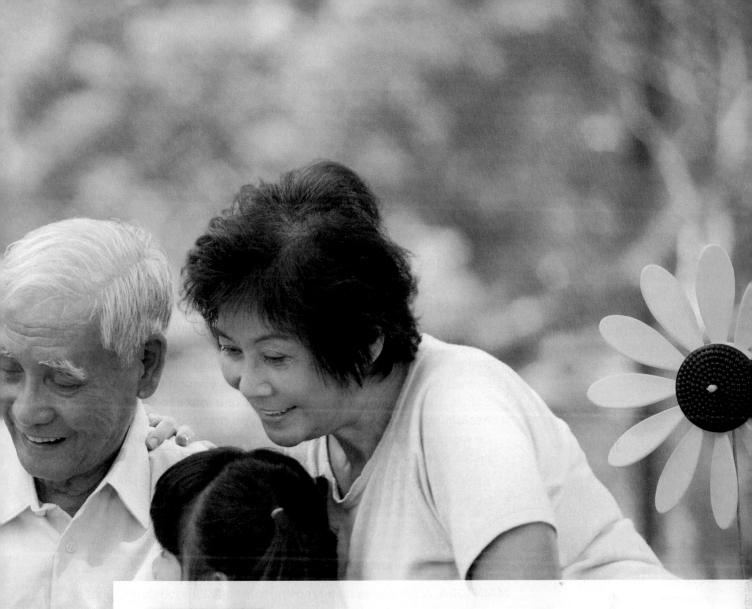

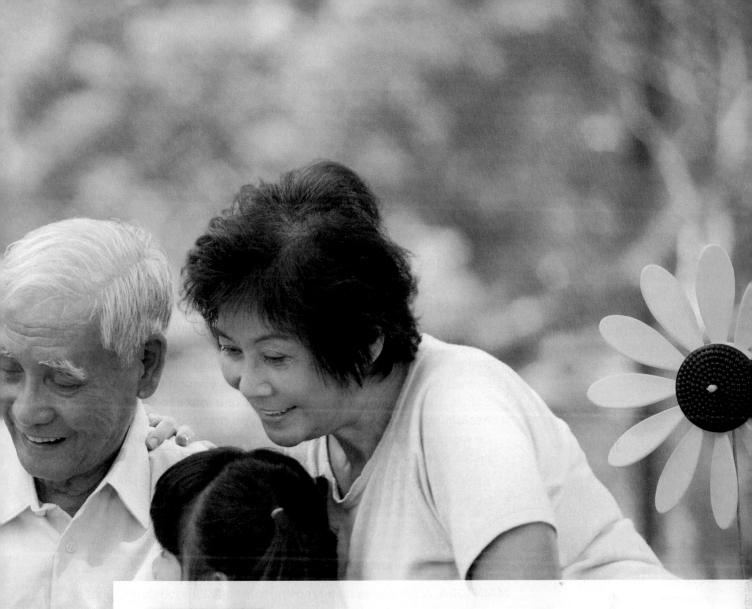

MODULE 18

The Life Cycle Continues

LESSONS

1 Changes During Adolescence

2 Adulthood, Marriage, and Parenthood

3 Health Through the Life Cycle

435

Changes During Adolescence

BEFORE YOU READ

Create an Outline. Preview this lesson by scanning the pages. Then, organize the headings and subheadings into an outline. As you read, fill in the outline with important details.

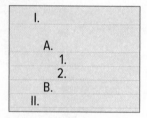

Vocabulary

adolescence
puberty
cognition

BIG IDEA Adolescence begins with puberty, as a person starts to mature physically, emotionally, and mentally.

REAL LIFE ISSUES

Puberty Differs from Person to Person. Two fraternal twins, Seth and Claire, are not as close as they used to be. Lately, they have not been spending much time together. Claire is experiencing the physical, social, and mental/emotional changes that come with puberty, but Seth is not. Nothing has changed for him yet and he wonders if there is something wrong with him. Seth is feeling confused and scared. *Write a letter to Seth, explaining some of the reasons why you think Seth should not be worried about developing at a different pace than his sister. Reassure him that there is no need for concern.*

After completing the lesson, review and analyze your response to the Real Life Issues question.

Puberty: A Time of Changes

MAIN IDEA Adolescents begin moving toward adulthood during puberty.

Adolescence, the period between childhood and adulthood, is a time of many challenges and changes. Physical growth is one of the most noticeable changes during this period. Teens grow taller, their voices change, and their bodies begin to fill out. After infancy, adolescence is the fastest period of growth in a person's life. It is also a time of great change in your mental, emotional, and social life.

The physical changes of adolescence mark the onset of **puberty**. Puberty is the time when a person begins to develop certain traits of adults. Puberty usually begins sometime between the ages of 12 and 18. These changes are triggered by *hormones.* These are chemical substances produced by glands that help regulate many of the body's functions. The hormones involved in the changes of puberty include the male hormone testosterone and the female hormones estrogen and progesterone.

Physical Changes

One of the most important and **significant** body changes that takes place during puberty is the development of *sex characteristics*. These are the distinctive traits related to a person's gender. Of course, this does not mean that it is impossible to tell boys and girls apart before puberty.

ACADEMIC VOCABULARY

significant *(adjective)*: having meaning

Starting from birth, children have the *primary sex characteristics,* or reproductive organs, associated with their gender. However, their reproductive systems do not mature until puberty. This is the age when the reproductive cells, or *gametes,* begin to develop. In males, the testes begin producing *sperm,* the male gametes. In females, the *eggs,* or *ova,* are already present in the body at puberty; in fact, all the eggs a female's body will ever produce are present from birth. However, puberty is the point at which the eggs begin to mature and ovulation begins. The onset of these changes indicates sexual maturity—that is, the physical ability to reproduce. However, being physically able to have a child is not the same as being ready to become a parent. That also requires a level of emotional maturity that most teens have not yet reached.

As their reproductive systems mature, teens also begin to develop other physical characteristics of their gender that are not directly related to reproduction. These are the *secondary sex characteristics.* Each teen develops these characteristics at his or her own rate. Some teens begin to look like adults well before their friends do. Others take a much longer time to change. This means that in any group of teens, there will be a variety of body sizes and shapes.

You may have started going through puberty already, and you may feel uncomfortable about the way your body is changing. It may help to remember that what you are experiencing is normal. Every teen goes through these changes, and they will resolve themselves in time.

In females:

- Breasts develop
- Waistline narrows
- Hips widen
- Body fat increases
- Menstruation starts

In males:

- Facial hair appears
- Voice deepens
- Shoulders broaden
- Muscles develop
- Hairline begins to recede

In both:

- Body hair appears
- All permanent teeth grow in
- Perspiration increases

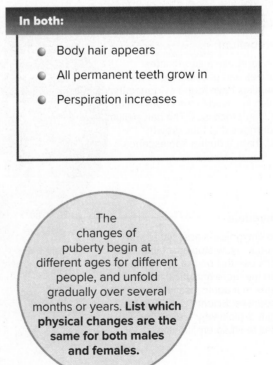

The changes of puberty begin at different ages for different people, and unfold gradually over several months or years. **List which physical changes are the same for both males and females.**

Mental and Emotional Changes

The physical changes of adolescence are easy to see. However, although you can't see it, your brain is changing at this age as well. By age six, your brain had already reached 95 percent of the size it will be in adulthood. However, your cerebrum, the largest part of your brain, is continuing to develop during adolescence, increasing your memory and **cognition**. Cognition is the ability to reason and think out abstract solutions. Other parts of your brain are undergoing changes as well.

A child sees only a limited number of solutions to a problem. Adolescents, by contrast, become increasingly capable of solving problems in more complex ways. During adolescence, you will learn to:

- anticipate the consequences of a particular action.
- think logically.
- understand different points of view.

Adolescence is a time of emotional change as well. As a teen, you may begin to look outward to try to understand yourself and your place in society. Most adolescents begin to search for meaning, personal values, and a sense of self. The emotional exploration you do during your teen years will help you find your place in the world as an adult.

Over the past 25 years, neuroscientists have discovered a great deal about the human brain. Recent imaging techniques have enabled scientists to examine the brains of people throughout their life spans—including the teen years.

Cerebellum

The cerebellum coordinates muscles and physical movement. Scientists have found evidence that it is also involved in the coordination of thinking processes. The cerebellum undergoes dramatic growth and change during adolescence.

Amygdala

The amygdala is associated with emotion. New studies indicate that teens use this part of the brain, rather than the more analytical frontal cortex that adults use in emotional responses. Scientists believe this might explain why teens sometimes react so emotionally.

Frontal Cortex

The frontal cortex is responsible for planning, strategizing, impulse control, and reasoning. The area undergoes a growth spurt when a child is 11 to 12 years of age. This is followed by a growth period, during which new nerve connections form.

Corpus Callosum

The corpus callosum connects the two sides of the brain. It is thought to be involved in creativity and problem solving. Research suggests that it grows and changes significantly during adolescence.

Social Changes

Your social life also changes quite a bit during adolescence. Friends play a big part in a teen's social experience. At this time of your life, your school and outside activities may be introducing you to new friends, including people of other cultural and social backgrounds. Getting to know people with diverse backgrounds can enrich your life by teaching you about cultures and ethnic groups that are different from your own.

Some of your friends may also have different values from you. This may lead you to challenge your own ideas about what is right and wrong. It's okay to explore new ideas, but ultimately, you are the one who must decide what you believe in. Responsible decision-making skills will help you stand by your beliefs if a friend asks you to do something that goes against your personal values.

Accomplishments in Adolescence

MAIN IDEA Adolescents will develop independence, find their identity, and establish their personal values.

You are probably aware that the physical, mental/emotional, and social changes that teens experience do not happen separately. These changes are all related, and teens often have to deal with many issues at the same time. This makes adolescence a wonderful, but often difficult, time of life.

Reading Check

Describe How does a person change emotionally during adolescence?

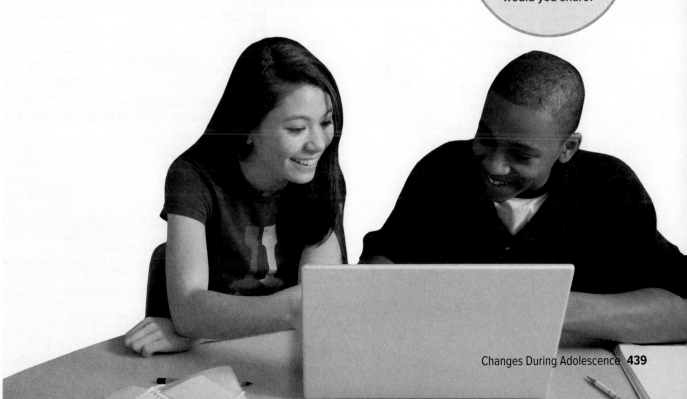

Friends from different cultural backgrounds share their traditions and cultural interests. **What traditions or interests would you share?**

Digital Vision/Getty Images

As you mature during adolescence, you will perform a series of specific developmental tasks. These will be an important part of your transition to adulthood. Some of these tasks include achieving emotional independence from your parents, developing your identity, and adopting a system of personal values. You will also begin to establish career goals. You will learn that adopting healthful, responsible behaviors can help you achieve those goals. Each item in the list below will help you learn about the various developmental tasks that you are facing. Then evaluate your progress by asking yourself the question at the end of each description.

- **Emotional and Psychological Independence.** During adolescence, you may find yourself moving back and forth between wanting independence and wanting the security of your family. During this time, you are developing confidence and building your self-esteem as you begin to make more decisions on your own. Having ongoing, open communication with your parents or guardians can be an advantage during your teen years. This gives you a way to seek advice and feedback about the decisions you need to make. Your parents can help you learn problem-solving skills by discussing and explaining situations, rules, and reasons in the decision-making process. They can also help you by modeling good decision-making through their own behavior. Being independent and being close to your family is not an either-or decision. Your can rely on your family's support and guidance, even as you become more emotionally and socially independent. *In what ways are you a different person than you were two years ago?*

Teens begin to make decisions about their future and goals at this stage of their lives. **What are your vocational goals?**

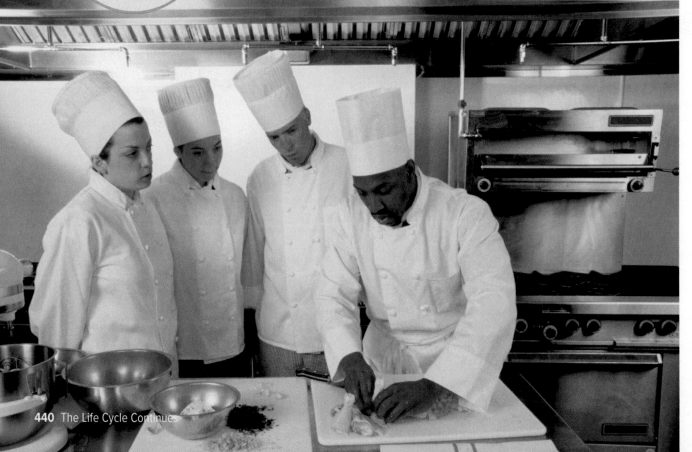

- **Personal Value System.** When you were a young child, your parents or guardians provided rules about appropriate and inappropriate behavior. These rules helped lay the foundation for your value system. Now, as a teen, you will begin to assess your values when they differ from the values expressed by your peers and others. In some cases, you will decide to hold firm to your existing values; in others, you may find that your values change as you learn more about the world around you. However, the core ethical values of trustworthiness, respect, responsibility, loyalty, caring, and citizenship will never let you down. *Have you begun to establish personal beliefs and values that enhance your health and well-being? Are you acting in ways that support those standards?*

- **Vocational Goals.** The teen years are a time to begin identifying your vocational goals, or career goals, for the future. You do not need to decide right now what you want to do for a living, but you will find it helpful to start thinking about what kind of work would be most satisfying for you. As you explore the possibilities open to you and develop new interests, you may discover that some of these interests can lead you to a career. *Have you set long-term goals and identified steps to reach those goals?*

- **Control Over Behaviors.** As a teen, you must face decisions every day about whether to engage in risky behaviors that could harm your health. Consider your values, as well as your short-term and long-term goals. This will give you a firm basis for making healthful decisions and avoiding risky situations. *Identify two recent events that challenged you to show emotional maturity and avoid a risky behavior.*

Reading Check

Identify What are your vocational goals for the future?

Fitness Zone

I make hundreds of choices every day. From the time I get up until I go to sleep, I choose what to wear, what to eat, and what friends to hang out with. I also see how all these choices can have either a positive or negative impact on my health. That's why one of my easiest choices is working out and eating healthy foods. After all, I deserve the best.

Lesson 1 Review

Facts and Vocabulary

1. Define the terms *adolescence* and *puberty*.

2. What are the reproductive cells of females called? What are those of males called?

3. What are some secondary sex characteristics of males that develop during puberty?

Thinking Critically

4. **Infer.** How does the fact that the cerebrum is still developing during adolescence explain some teenage behavior?

5. **Explain.** During which time frame does adolescent development typically occur?

Applying Health Skills

6. **Refusal Skills.** At times, your peers might encourage you to do something that you know is wrong. Write a scenario describing how you would handle such a situation.

Writing Critically

7. **Persuasive.** Your friend is being asked to participate in an activity that you think is unsafe and unwise. Write a short letter suggesting why you think this is a mistake and how to get out of it. Be encouraging and supportive, but suggest alternatives.

Adulthood, Marriage, and Parenthood

BEFORE YOU READ

Create a K-W-L Chart. Make a three-column chart like the one below. In the first column, write what you **k**now about parenthood. In the second column, write what you **w**ant to know about this topic. As you read, fill in the third column describing what you have **l**earned.

K	W	L

Vocabulary

physical maturity
emotional maturity
commitment
adoption
unconditional love

Reading Check

Infer What positive events may happen during middle adulthood?

BIG IDEA During adulthood, individuals may choose to get married and become parents.

REAL LIFE ISSUES

Wedding Bells? Lily's older sister, Maya, will graduate from college at the end of the year. Maya confides in Lily that she and her boyfriend are thinking about getting married as soon as they graduate. Lily likes Maya's boyfriend, but has learned in her health class that marriage is a very big step. *Write a letter from Lily to Maya, explaining what she thinks marriage involves and why it's an important step that requires a lot of thought.*

After completing the lesson, review and analyze your response to the Real Life Issues question.

Adulthood

MAIN IDEA Adulthood is reached when both physical maturity and emotional maturity are achieved.

Most people reach **physical maturity**, the state at which the physical body and all its organs are fully developed, in late adolescence or their early twenties. Being physically mature does not make you an adult, however. To be an adult, you need to develop emotionally as well. **Emotional maturity** is the state at which the mental and emotional capabilities of an individual are fully developed. Emotionally healthy individuals have positive values and goals. They are able to give and receive love, have the ability to face reality and deal with it, and have the capacity to learn from life experiences. Relationships with peers, family, and friends can have a positive effect on a person's physical and emotional health.

The adult years are made up of three different stages: young adulthood, middle adulthood, and late adulthood. Each stage is marked by a particular goal involving a person's relationships with others. Read about each of the three stages to learn more about this stage and the accomplishments that go with it.

- **Young Adulthood.** This stage lasts from approximately 19 to 40 years of age. The goal of this stage is to develop intimacy. During young adulthood, people work on developing close personal relationships with others. Many people choose to get married and start a family during this stage. Physical changes that occur during this period include changes in vision and decreased sensitivity in hearing. Hair may start to thin and turn gray. Fertility also decreases.

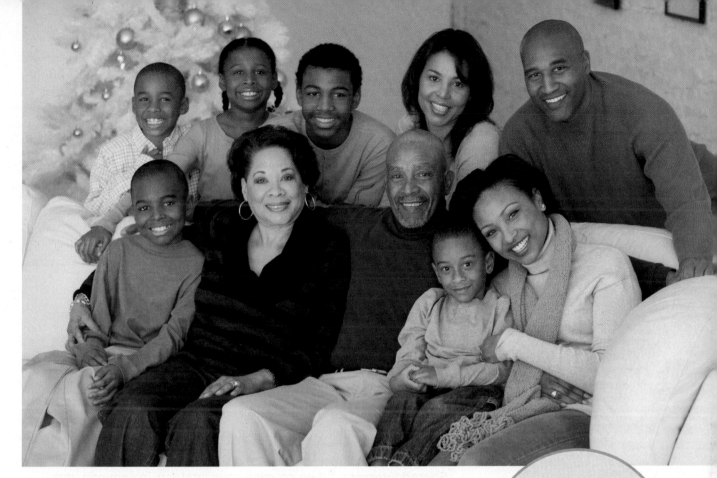

- **Middle Adulthood.** This stage occurs from about the ages of 40 and 65. The goal at this time of life is to make a meaningful contribution to society. People in this stage look outside themselves and care for others through such activities as work, volunteering, or caring for grandchildren.

- **Late Adulthood.** This stage lasts from around age 65 until death. The goal of a person in this stage of life is to feel a sense of satisfaction with the life he or she has lived. People in this stage try to understand and appreciate the meaning and purpose of their lives.

Your extended family may include aunts, uncles, and grandparents, as well as your parents and brothers or sisters. **Which members of your extended family do you enjoy a close relationship with?**

Marriage

MAIN IDEA Marriage is a commitment to share your life with another person.

Most people marry because they fall in love and are ready to enter into a lasting, intimate relationship. Married couples share togetherness and support each other in hard times as well as in good times.

Deciding to Marry

There are important differences between a dating relationship and a marriage. When two people agree that marriage may be in their future, their relationship becomes more serious, and they make a deeper **commitment**—a promise or a pledge—to each other. From that point on, they must consider the long-term consequences of all their decisions.

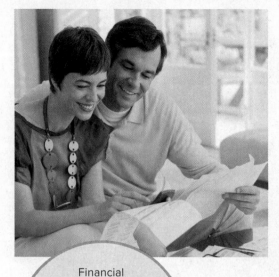

Financial concerns are a common problem that married couples face. **What can this couple do to make sure that finances do not become a problem in their relationship?**

• • • • • • • • • • • •

ACADEMIC VOCABULARY

conflict *(noun)*: Any disagreement, struggle, or fight.

• • • • • • • • • • • •

They evaluate their decisions, not just for themselves, but for each other as well. This joint decision-making should start with the decision to marry itself. If either partner has any doubts or questions about the other's reasons for marrying, the couple should explore and resolve these questions before they say, "I do."

Successful Marriages

Making a commitment to each other is only the first step in a successful marriage. *Marital adjustment*—how well a person adjusts to a marriage and to a spouse—also depends on the following factors:

- **Communication.** Couples need to be able to share their feelings and to express their needs and concerns to each other. Good communication skills are essential to building and maintaining a healthy marriage.

- **Emotional maturity.** Emotionally mature partners try to understand each other's needs and are willing to compromise. They don't always think of themselves first; they consider what is best for them as a couple.

- **Shared interests.** When couples have interests in common, they spend more time together, which strengthens the marriage.

- **Shared values.** Since married couples must make decisions together, it helps for them to draw on similar values. Couples will work together best when they agree on the importance of good health, spirituality, ethical standards, family, and friendships.

Resolving Conflict in Marriage

Even in the strongest marriages, conflicts will arise sometimes, because no two people can agree on everything all the time. Possible causes of **conflict** in a marriage include:

- differences in spending and saving habits.
- conflicting loyalties involving family and friends.
- lack of communication.
- lack of intimacy.
- jealousy, infidelity, or lack of attention.
- decisions about having children and arranging child care.
- abusive tendencies or attitudes.

Strong couples will learn to recognize the causes of their conflicts and to resolve them in ways that strengthen the relationship. When partners trust, respect, and care for each other, they will try to settle their conflicts fairly, without damaging the self-esteem of either partner. Good communication and conflict-resolution skills can help reduce the impact of conflict on a marriage. In some cases, couples may need the help of a counselor to settle marital differences.

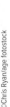

©Chris Ryan/age fotostock

Teen Marriage

Some people begin talking about marriage at a young age. However, many teens do not have the level of emotional maturity needed to deal with the problems and decisions of a marriage. Most teens are still struggling to find their own identities and set goals for the future. It's unlikely that they have had enough life experience to get a clear idea of their own life path or what they need from a marriage partner. Teens who get married may soon discover that the responsibilities of a marriage are interfering with their personal freedom and their educational or career goals. Financial pressures can add stress to the marriage. Marriage difficulties may arise as the novelty wears off. Because of all these reasons, teens must recognize the level of commitment needed to make a marriage work. Between 50 to 60 percent of marriages involving teens end in divorce, many of them in the first few years. That's one of the reasons that most states have laws forbidding people under 18 to make this important and lasting decision without parental permission.

Reading Check

Identify What are three issues that often cause problems in a marriage?

Parenthood

MAIN IDEA Parenthood is a great responsibility.

Many married couples decide to start a family together. For many, this means going through pregnancy and childbirth. Other couples choose **adoption** or become the legal guardians of foster children. Most parents find raising a child to be a rewarding experience, and they take great joy in loving and caring for their children.

However, with all its rewards, raising a child is also challenging. Prospective parents need to understand how their lifestyle will change as a result of having or adopting a child. Parenthood is a major responsibility, and it continues for many years. Parents must provide protection, food, clothing, shelter, education, and medical care for their children. They also need to care for them emotionally. This involves providing guidance, instilling values, setting limits, and providing unconditional love.

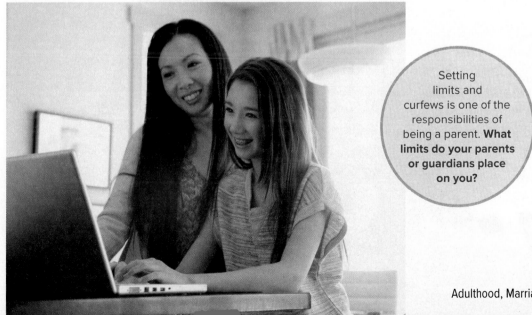

©Hero/Corbis/Glow Images

Setting limits and curfews is one of the responsibilities of being a parent. **What limits do your parents or guardians place on you?**

Providing Guidance

Parents need to guide and protect their children, but they also need to help them learn to make their own decisions. Involved parents will teach children to take responsibility for their own successes and failures. They will also encourage their children and help them develop a sense of pride in their accomplishments. Watching children learn to get along with others and solve problems on their own is a satisfying experience for a parent.

Members of the extended family, such as grandparents, can also play an important role in teaching children. By interacting together in a mature, loving, and caring manner, they can provide good role models for children in their future relationships.

Instilling Values

Values, as you have learned, are the beliefs and standards of conduct that guide the way people live. One of a parent's biggest jobs is to help their children develop a strong value system. Values can guide children in their decisions and help them resist harmful influences in their lives. They promote good character and help children grow to become happy, productive, and mature adults.

Setting Limits

Part of a parent's responsibility is setting limits. When children are young, they do not have the knowledge and skills they need to make sound decisions. Parents must make rules to control their behavior and protect their health and safety. These may include rules about bedtime, eating habits, and television exposure. Over time, the limits on children's behavior will change as they become able to handle more responsibility. However, teens will still have limits on their behavior, such as curfews and rules about the use of the family car.

Reading Check

Explain How do limits change as a child grows older?

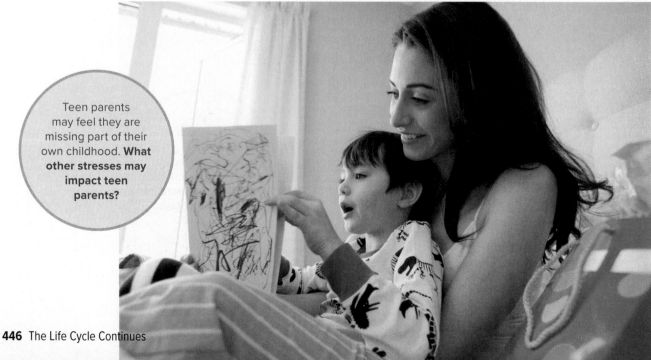

Teen parents may feel they are missing part of their own childhood. **What other stresses may impact teen parents?**

©Hero/Corbis/Glow Images

Giving Unconditional Love

Although parents must know when to say no to their children, they must also know when to say yes. One question that should always be answered with a yes is, "Do you love me?" A parent's **unconditional love** meets one of a child's most basic needs: the need to love and be loved. It is love without limitations or quantifications. On Maslow's hierarchy of needs, this is just one step up from the basic physical needs for food, shelter, and safety.

Teen Parenthood

Becoming a parent is challenging at any stage of life. It is even more so when the parents are teenagers. Although parenthood is very rewarding, it also requires maturity. This is why some teens who become pregnant choose to put their babies up for adoption. Those who choose to raise the child themselves must be prepared to deal with the consequences of teen parenthood, such as:

- financial difficulties.
- emotional stress.
- limitations on social and personal life.
- restrictions on educational and career plans.

Some states, such as California, have a Safely Surrendered Baby Law that allows parents to surrender custody of an infant at a safe site, such as a hospital or fire station, within three days after birth. These laws can help teens who are not ready for parenthood to give up a child safely.

Fitness Zone

Every summer I visit my grandparents. They have a habit of sharing a mid-afternoon snack. My grandmother calls it "sweets for my sweetie." Their snack is always something healthy, like a cut-up apple drizzled with chocolate or butterscotch syrup. My grandparents are both in good shape, so I guess it works.

Lesson 2 Review

Facts and Vocabulary

1. Distinguish between *physical maturity* and *emotional maturity*.

2. How do the goals of young adulthood differ from the goals of middle adulthood?

3. Which factors determine how well a person will adjust to marriage?

Thinking Critically

4. **Predict.** What are some factors that may cause conflict, even in a good marriage?

5. **Identify.** What is a parent giving a child by offering unconditional love?

Applying Health Skills

6. **Accessing Information.** Use print or online resources to research the legal rights and responsibilities of teen parents. Compare and contrast these rights with the rights of adult parents.

Writing Critically

7. **Expository.** Write a short essay explaining the disadvantages of marrying during the teen years.

Health Through the Life Cycle

BEFORE YOU READ

Create a Table. Make a two-column table. Label the first column "Middle Adulthood." Label the second column "Late Adulthood." Fill in the major milestones for each stage as you read the lesson.

Middle Adulthood	Late Adulthood

Vocabulary

transitions
empty-nest syndrome

BIG IDEA Middle and late adulthood are times of contribution and reflection.

REAL LIFE ISSUES

Where Did They Go? Anna's grandmother lives less than a mile from Anna and her family. Anna visits her grandmother twice a week on her way home from school. Her grandmother lives alone, and Anna worries that she is lonely. Anna's grandfather died two years ago. Anna has learned in school that writing down your feelings is a good way to begin dealing with them. *Write a scenario between Anna and her grandmother in which Anna encourages her grandmother to write about her feelings.*

After completing the lesson, review and analyze your response to the Real Life Issues question.

Middle Adulthood

MAIN IDEA Many changes occur during middle adulthood.

Middle adulthood is the period of life from around age 40 to 65. These years are full of **transitions**, or critical changes that occur at all stages of life. Many of these changes relate to personal or family events. These may include a child's graduation, the arrival of the first grandchild, achievement of a satisfying career goal, or recognition of an individual's contribution to the community. Adults in middle life also face a variety of other changes in their physical, mental/emotional, and social health.

Physical Transitions

As you have learned, physical change doesn't stop when adolescence ends; it continues—though at a somewhat slower rate—throughout the life cycle. The physical changes of middle adulthood are related to the onset of aging. For instance, females enter *menopause,* or the end of ovulation and menstruation, between the ages of 45 and 55. After this point, a female can no longer become pregnant.

Research indicates that most people who practiced healthful behaviors in their youth, such as weight management, healthy eating, and regular physical activity, stay healthier as they age. One healthful habit that offers significant benefit to most adults is strength training. This type of exercise helps older adults increase muscle mass, preserve bone density, and protect their major joints from injury.

Mental Transitions

You may have heard the saying "You can't teach an old dog new tricks," which suggests that it isn't possible to learn new skills later in life. However, nothing could be farther from the truth. In fact, learning can and should be a lifelong pursuit. During midlife, many adults begin new careers, return to school, and learn new hobbies. Continuing to learn is one way to remain mentally healthy during middle adulthood. Adults can also stimulate their brains with activities such as solving puzzles, reading, and playing strategy games. Mental activities like these strengthen the brain just as physical exercise strengthens the body.

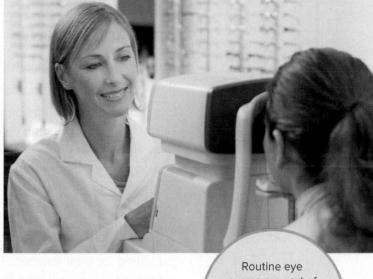

Routine eye exams are part of staying healthy at any age. **How are the lives of middle adults changing?**

Emotional Transitions

The emotional transitions people experience in middle adulthood are similar in some ways to those of adolescence. By this time in life, most people can take pride in their personal accomplishments. However, they may also experience disappointments. Adults at this stage are often said to be going through a "midlife crisis." This means that they feel uncertain about whether they have met their goals, feel loved and valued, and have made a positive difference in the lives of others. Questions like these can be painful, but their effect can also be healthy. They may lead people to try new activities, explore new goals, and form deeper connections with the world around them.

Reading Check

Explain How can skills developed in adolescence help you in middle adulthood?

Social Transitions

Most social transitions during middle adulthood are related to the family. For example, people at this stage of life must often cope with the death of a parent. They may also experience **empty-nest syndrome** as their children grow up and leave home. This is the feeling of sadness or loneliness that accompanies seeing children leave home and enter adulthood.

People who maintain healthy relationships with family and friends have an easier time adjusting to these changes. For many people, middle adulthood is a time to apply their talents and life experiences to community programs. They may pursue new interests and make new friends. Developing good social skills earlier in life can help ease the transitions of middle adulthood.

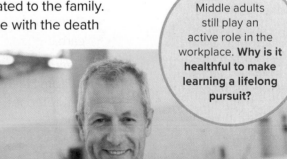

Middle adults still play an active role in the workplace. **Why is it healthful to make learning a lifelong pursuit?**

Late Adulthood

MAIN IDEA People in late adulthood may reflect on their lives and accomplishments.

Late adulthood typically begins after age 65. At this stage of life, people begin to spend less time looking ahead to the future and more time looking back on the lives they have lived. Older adults may take satisfaction in reviewing the events of their lives and their achievements. Those who have lived their lives with integrity, or a firm adherence to a moral code, will probably be able to feel a sense of fulfillment. For example, those who have made family a high priority in their lives will feel satisfied in knowing that they have done a good job providing for their families. Those who have remained committed to a system of values will take pride in feeling that they have stood by their ideals. Older adults who can look back without regret and take pride in their accomplishments will be happy and fulfilled in their later years.

Health Concerns

Each phase of adulthood has its own unique set of health concerns. Older adults need to be aware of several conditions related to aging:

- Eyesight changes with age. At this stage of life, adults may have difficulty bringing images into focus. Many older adults need glasses for reading.

- Hearing may decline, especially for people who have been exposed to loud sounds regularly throughout their lives.

- Muscles and joints may be affected by conditions such as arthritis. Arthritis affects nearly half of all people over age 65.

- Bones may become brittle and more likely to break. This condition, called *osteoporosis,* can affect anyone, but it is most common in older women.

- Teeth and gums can become decayed and diseased without proper care.

- Heart disease affects many older adults. It can result from heredity or from lifestyle factors, such as inactivity and a diet too high in saturated fat.

- Cancer is more common in older adults. Regular screenings for certain cancers are recommended starting in middle adulthood.

Although these problems are common, new scientific breakthroughs are making them easier to detect, treat, and in some cases, prevent. New methods of disease prevention, such as better nutrition, have made a significant difference in the lives of older adults. Today, more people than ever are remaining healthy well into late adulthood.

Many older adults enjoy active lives. **Why is older adulthood such a rewarding time for many?**

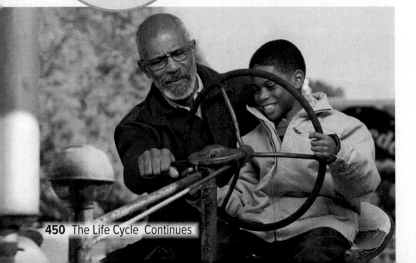

Public Health Policies and Programs

Advances in disease detection, prevention, and treatment have allowed older adults to maintain independent and satisfying lives. However, paying for health care can be a problem for those who no longer have employer-sponsored health insurance. Medicare is a public health program that assists adults over 65 years of age with health care needs. (A related program, called Medicaid, helps those with low income and limited resources.)

Better health care is available today, and people can expect to live longer after retirement. For this reason, financial planning is essential. The Social Security system was created in 1935. It serves as a "safety net" to ensure that older adults have some money to live on during retirement. This program provides benefits to people with disabilities, as well as older adults. However, most retired adults will need an additional source of income.

Some companies provide retirement benefits, such as pensions. Most workers must still plan ahead by saving for retirement. Personal or company-sponsored long-term savings plans can make this process easier. These savings funds, in conjunction with Social Security benefits, have helped reduce the poverty rate among older adults. Many are finding that, after a lifetime of practicing healthful behaviors, the years after retirement are fulfilling and rewarding.

Reading Check

Identify What programs help people in late adulthood?

Character Check

Many older adults enjoy active, vital lives and often possess insights based on their varied experience. Try to draw upon their wisdom and knowledge by seeking their advice. List ways you can show respect to older adults and ways you think their knowledge might benefit you in your health decisions.

Lesson 3 Review

Facts and Vocabulary

1. What is *empty-nest syndrome*?

2. What are some examples of activities older adults can participate in to remain mentally active?

3. What sort of physical changes do females in middle adulthood experience?

Thinking Critically

4. **Infer.** Why is it so important today for adults to plan financially for retirement?

5. **Identify.** How have changes in nutrition and health care changed the lives of older adults?

Applying Health Skills

6. **Accessing Information.** Research library or Internet resources to learn about the Social Security system. Identify problems that may arise with this system in the not-so-distant future. Share what you learn in the form of an informational poster or pamphlet.

Writing Critically

7. **Descriptive.** Write a short essay explaining the emotional transitions one may have in middle adulthood.

Vocabulary Review

Use the correct vocabulary term to complete the following statements.

1. The period of time between childhood and adulthood is called _____.

2. The time when a person begins to develop certain traits of adults is called _____.

3. The ability to reason and think out abstract solutions is called _____.

4. Chemical substances called _____ help regulate the body's many functions.

Understanding Key Concepts

After reading the question or statement, select the correct answer.

5. Assessing your own values when they might be different than the values of your peers shows that you are developing which of the following?
   a. Personal value system
   b. Emotional independence
   c. Vocational goals
   d. Self-control

6. Which is not an example of a vocational goal?
   a. Entering trade school
   b. Entering college
   c. Learning to repair automobiles
   d. Passing the science test tomorrow

7. Which is the term for the development of certain traits of adults of your gender?
   a. Adolescence
   b. Emotional maturity
   c. Puberty
   d. Physical maturity

Thinking Critically

After reading the question or statement, write a short answer using complete sentences.

8. **Describe.** Describe the characteristics of a good friend.

9. **Extend.** Not everyone develops at the same rate. What does this mean?

10. **Analyze.** How can parents or guardians make the transition to emotional independence easier for teens?

11. **Infer.** What sort of decisions might you make that could be potentially risky?

12. **Synthesize.** How will the values you developed earlier in life impact you as you go through the stages of development?

Vocabulary Review

Correct the sentences below by replacing the italicized term with the correct vocabulary term.

13. *Emotional maturity* is the point at which the body and its organs are developed.

14. Children learn to make decisions about behavior when adults aren't present as they become more *physically mature*.

15. Giving love to a child without question in all situations is called *commitment*.

16. Legally taking someone else's child to raise as your own is known as *integrity*.

Understanding Key Concepts

After reading the question or statement, select the correct answer.

17. Which is a responsibility of parenthood?
   a. Instilling values
   b. Setting limits
   c. Giving unconditional love
   d. All of the above

18. In a marriage, the partners don't always think of themselves first. Rather, they consider what is best for the relationship. What is this known as?
   a. Communication
   b. Emotional maturity
   c. Physical maturity
   d. Values and interests

19. Setting limits can help children become which of the following?
- **a.** Self-directed
- **b.** Physically mature
- **c.** Emotionally mature
- **d.** Committed

20. Which is the stage at which the physical body and all its organs are fully developed?
- **a.** Physical maturity
- **b.** Emotional maturity
- **c.** Marital adjustment
- **d.** Commitment

Thinking Critically

After reading the question or statement, write a short answer using complete sentences.

21. Describe. What happens in the three stages of development during the adult years?

22. Analyze. What should a couple consider before entering into marriage?

23. Describe. What particular challenges do teens who get married face?

24. Analyze. What are the different ways a couple may start a family?

LESSON 3

Vocabulary Review

Use the correct vocabulary term to complete the following statements.

25. The middle adult years are often full of _____, critical changes that occur at all stages of life.

26. When their children grow up and leave home, middle adults may suffer from _____.

27. People in late adulthood may reflect on whether they lived their lives according to their moral code, or with _____.

Understanding Key Concepts

After reading the question or statement, select the correct answer.

28. Which provides financial assistance to older adults, as well as disabled individuals?
- **a.** Social Security
- **b.** Medicare
- **c.** Medicaid
- **d.** None of the above

29. What is a social and mental/emotional change that middle and older adults experience?
- **a.** Sadness and loneliness when their children move away
- **b.** Pride in having met personal goals
- **c.** The opportunity to pursue talents and interests
- **d.** All of the above

30. Arthritis may affect which of the following during late adulthood?
- **a.** Heart
- **b.** Eyesight and hearing
- **c.** Teeth and gums
- **d.** Joints

31. What is a potential benefit of strength training in later life?
- **a.** Preserving bone density
- **b.** Improving sleep habits
- **c.** Improving mental sharpness
- **d.** Maintaining a healthy weight

Thinking Critically

After reading the question or statement, write a short answer using complete sentences.

32. Assess. What role have computers played in changing the lives of people in late adulthood?

33. Synthesize. What is a midlife crisis?

34. Predict. How might a person deal with empty-nest syndrome?

PROJECT-BASED ASSESSMENT

The Journey Ahead

BACKGROUND

During adolescence, many changes and transitions occur. Many teens feel the need to begin expressing more independence from their parents. They also begin showing more interest in developing close relationships with other teens. The teen years can be difficult because of these changes and uncertainties.

TASK

Collaborate in groups to develop a podcast aimed at middle school students. Each student will play the role of an expert and discuss one developmental task. The goal is to reassure younger students about the changes they will soon experience.

AUDIENCE

Middle school students

PURPOSE

Analyze the changes that teens experience. Reassure younger students that these changes are normal.

PROCEDURE

1. Review the sections in the chapter describing developmental changes experienced by teens.

2. Select one developmental change that teens commonly experience.

3. Conduct research online on that developmental task using reliable sources.

4. Discuss your findings with the group. Decide on a theme for the podcast. One student will play the role of moderator, and the other students will provide information on a developmental task.

5. Practice presenting the podcast. Make a recording of your podcast, or perform it live for a group of middle school students.

Math Practice

Interpret Graphs. From information she gathered at the public library, Marsha made the following bar graph that shows the number of people of each age group in her town last year. Use the graph to answer Questions 1–3.

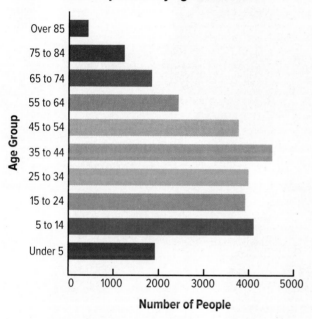

Town Population by Age Last Year

1. Which age group made up the greatest percentage of Marsha's town population last year?
   a. Under 5
   b. 5 to 14
   c. 35 to 44
   d. Over 85

2. Approximately how many people were below the age of 35?
   a. 4,000
   b. 4,500
   c. 14,000
   d. 18,500

3. If the town's total population was approximately 28,100, what percentage of the population was 15 to 24 years of age?
   a. 14%
   b. 24%
   c. 40%
   d. 50%

Reading/Writing Practice

Understand and Apply. Read the passage below, and then answer the questions.

> **1.** Teenagers are working in greater numbers than ever before. **2.** Some choose jobs in fields they feel strongly about, like conservation or recycling. **3.** They might join the parks department to plant trees. **4.** Teenagers interested in working with younger children can work in community centers or tutor students after school. **5.** Many teens work in their own neighborhoods, doing yard work. **6.** Studies show that teens are successful workers. **7.** They relate well to other teens, as well as to older adults. **8.** Most teenage workers find a pleasant surprise—they like their jobs more than they expected to. **9.** Many teens make lasting friendships on the job. **10.** They also learn new skills related to their future career and educational choices.

1. Which detail below supports the idea that teenagers are successful in the workforce?
   a. Many teen have entered the workforce.
   b. Many join the parks department.
   c. Some teens work in conservation jobs.
   d. They relate well to other teens and to older adults.

2. The writer wants to add the following detail to this passage: Some teenagers—girls and boys—babysit neighborhood children.
   Based on the organization of this piece, after which number should this detail be added?
   a. Sentence 1
   b. Sentence 4
   c. Sentence 6
   d. Sentence 7

3. Write an essay giving examples of why you think teens can contribute in the workplace.

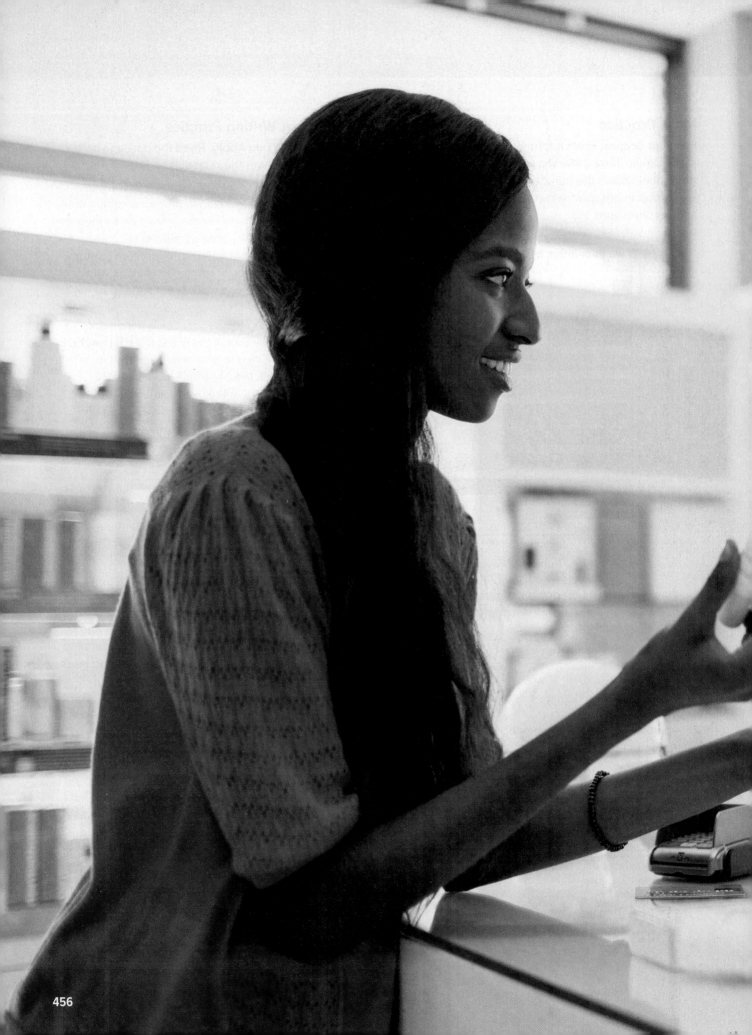

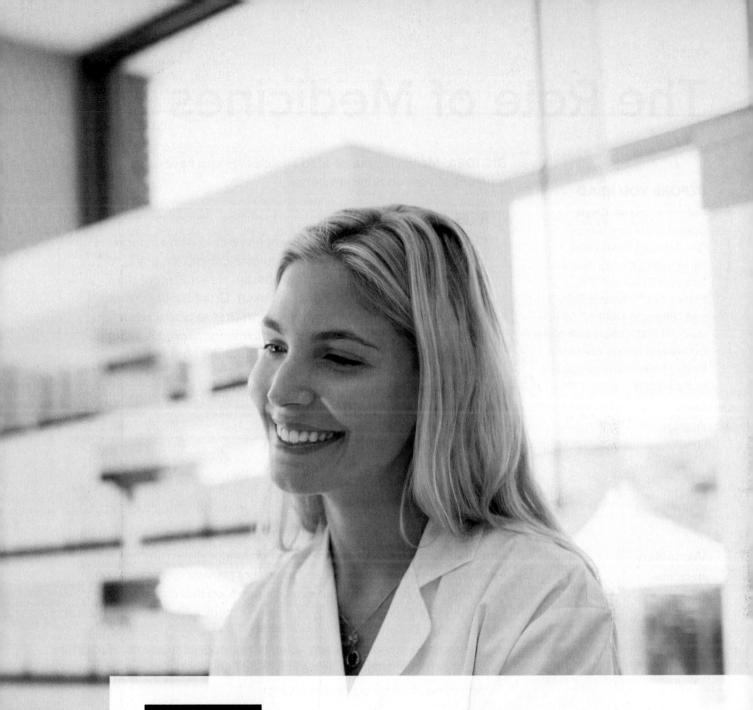

Medicines and Drugs

LESSONS

1 The Role of Medicines

2 Using Medicines Safely

The Role of Medicines

• • • • • • • • • • • •

BEFORE YOU READ

Create a Cluster Chart.
Draw a circle and label it "Medicines." Create four surrounding circles labeled "Prevent Disease," "Fight Pathogens," "Relieve Pain," and "Promote Health." As you read, fill in the chart with more circles and details about the kinds of medicines discussed in the lesson.

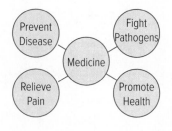

Vocabulary

medicines
drugs
vaccine
side effects
additive interaction
synergistic effect
antagonistic interaction

• • • • • • • • • • • •

BIG IDEA Medicines are divided into classes and have different effects on different people.

REAL LIFE ISSUES

Choosing Medicines Wisely. Grant has a cold with a cough and runny nose. He checks the medicine cabinet for any cold medications that will help him feel better. He finds more than one type of cold medicine in the cabinet. Grant is not sure which one he should take. *Write a paragraph that explains what Grant should look for in a cold medicine; for example, what symptoms he wants to relieve, how much he should take, and how many hours a dose will last.*

After completing the lesson, review and analyze your response to the Real Life Issues question.

Types of Medicines

MAIN IDEA Medicines are classified based on how they work in your body.

People use medicines to help restore their health when they are ill. **Medicines** are drugs that are used to treat or prevent diseases or other conditions. **Drugs** are substances other than food that change the structure or function of the body or mind. All medicines are drugs, but not all drugs are medicines. Drugs are effective in treating illness when taken as directed by a physician or according to the label instructions. Medicines that treat or prevent illness can be classified into four broad categories:

- Medicines that help prevent disease
- Medicines that fight pathogens
- Medicines that relieve pain and other symptoms
- Medicines that manage chronic conditions, help maintain or restore health, and regulate body's systems

Preventing Disease

Vaccines and antitoxins are two types of medicines used for preventing disease. Vaccines are a preparation that prevents a person from contracting a specific disease. Today, about 95 percent of children receive vaccines to protect them against childhood diseases. Vaccines contain dead or weakened versions of the pathogens that cause a particular disease. When injected into your body, they stimulate your immune system to produce antibodies that fight those pathogens. Your body also produces memory

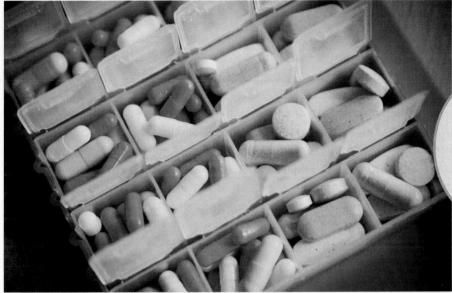

Many types of medications are available. **What was the last medication that you used, and for what purpose did you use it?**

cells that recall how to make these antibodies. This provides you with long-lasting protection against these specific pathogens. The protection from some vaccines, however, fades over time. The vaccine for tetanus, for example, must be given periodically to stay effective. For other vaccines, such as those that prevent the flu, a new version of the vaccine is required every year.

Antitoxins prevent disease in a different way. They help **neutralize** the effects of toxins, or harmful substances, which are produced by certain bacteria. Antitoxins are usually produced by injecting animals with safe amounts of a specific toxin. This stimulates the animal's immune system to produce antibodies. These antibodies can then be given to humans to protect them against the same toxin.

Fighting Pathogens

There are several types of medicines that fight pathogens. *Antibiotics* work against disease-causing organisms called *bacteria*. Other types of medicines fight different pathogens, such as viruses and fungi.

Antibiotics. Antibiotics, such as penicillin, work in one of two ways. They either kill harmful bacteria in the body or prevent them from reproducing. When antibiotics were first introduced, they were considered miracle drugs because they saved so many lives. However, antibiotics can also have harmful side effects. These may include nausea, stomach pain, or allergic reactions. Tell your doctor if you experience any negative side effects when using an antibiotic, or if you know that you are allergic to an antibiotic.

Another problem with antibiotics is that they can lose their effectiveness. This happens because the bacteria have adapted to the drug over time. One reason this happens is because patients sometimes do not finish taking their full prescriptions. If you do not finish taking all of a prescription, you may not kill all the bacteria in your body. The remaining bacteria may develop a resistance, or immunity, to treatment. Resistant bacteria may also develop when antibiotics are overused or are used inappropriately.

ACADEMIC VOCABULARY

neutralize *(verb)*: to counteract the effect of

Antivirals and Antifungals. Antibiotics are effective only against bacteria. They cannot cure illnesses caused by viruses. However, other drugs, called *antivirals,* are available to treat some viral illnesses, such as the flu. These medicines can suppress a virus, but do not kill it. For example, if you take an antiviral medicine for cold sores or fever blisters, you will still have the virus that causes these sores in your body. This means that the symptoms may still flare up from time to time after they have been gone for a while. Also, like bacteria, viruses can develop a resistance to medications. Fungi are another type of pathogen that can infect the body. Antifungals can suppress or kill the fungi that cause certain conditions, such as athlete's foot and ringworm.

Relieving Pain

The most commonly used medicines of all are *analgesics,* or pain relievers. Analgesics range from relatively mild drugs, such as aspirin, to strong narcotics, such as opium-based morphine and codeine. Some analgesics can be used to fight *inflammation,* or swelling accompanied by pain and redness.

Aspirin is one of the most common analgesics. It is used for reducing fever as well as relieving pain. Although it is a widely used drug, it can cause problems, such as stomach upset, dizziness, and ringing in the ears. In addition, children who take aspirin when they have a fever are at risk of developing Reye's syndrome. This is a potentially life-threatening illness of the brain and liver. For that reason, aspirin should not be given to anyone under the age of 20 unless directed by a physician. Another medicine, called *acetaminophen,* is recommended for relieving pain in children. This drug or an alternative called *ibuprofen* can also help people who are sensitive to aspirin.

Pain Reliever Dependence. Certain types of medicines that relieve pain can be addictive. This means that patients who use these drugs can become physically or psychologically dependent on them. Such medicines, usually called *narcotics,* require a doctor's prescription.

Managing Chronic Conditions

Some medicines are used to treat chronic (long-term) conditions, such as allergies or depression. In most cases, these medicines cannot cure the condition permanently. However, by taking these drugs regularly, people with chronic diseases can relieve their symptoms and achieve a higher level of wellness.

Allergy Medicines. Antihistamines reduce allergy symptoms such as sneezing, itchy or watery eyes, and runny nose. They work by blocking the chemicals released by the immune system that cause an allergic response. The most powerful antihistamine of all is called *epinephrine*. Many people who are allergic to peanuts or bee stings can develop severe symptoms very suddenly. For them, an allergic reaction can be deadly. People who have such severe allergies often get a prescription from their doctor to carry an injector containing a single dose of epinephrine. They can use it to give themselves a shot of the drug, which slows down or stops the allergic reaction.

Reading Check

Describe Explain how vaccines prevent a person from getting a disease.

Body-Regulating Medicines. Some medicines work by keeping the body's chemistry in balance. For example, people with diabetes use insulin to regulate the amount of sugar in their blood. Asthma sufferers may take medicines every day to control their symptoms and prevent attacks. Other medicines are used to regulate the cardiovascular system. Some control blood pressure, while others can steady an irregular heartbeat.

Antidepressant and Antipsychotic Medicines. Medications can also help people suffering from mental illnesses. Drugs called *mood stabilizers,* for instance, are often used in the treatment of mood disorders, depression, and schizophrenia. Proper medication can help people with these disorders live healthy lives. However, they may need to continue using the medicines on a lifelong basis. Even if they feel better, they should not stop taking them without consulting their doctor first. In fact, you should follow this rule for any prescribed medicine.

Cancer Treatments. Some medicines can be used to treat cancer. *Chemotherapy* uses chemicals to kill fast-growing cancer cells. *Immunotherapy,* or biological therapy, uses the body's immune system to fight the cancer cells. However, these medicines can also destroy healthy cells. As a result, cancer-fighting drugs often have serious side effects. Other medicines can help treat these side effects.

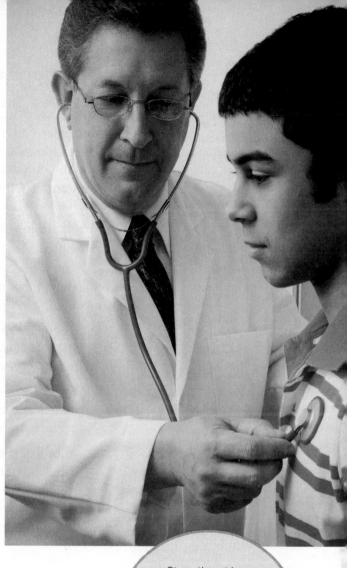

Strep throat is a bacterial infection that is treated with antibiotics prescribed by a doctor. **Why is it important to take all of the antibiotics a doctor prescribes, even if you are feeling better?**

Taking Medications

MAIN IDEA Medicines enter the body in a variety of ways.

Medicines can be delivered to the body in many ways:

- Oral medicines are taken by mouth in the form of tablets, capsules, or liquids. These medicines pass through the digestive system into the bloodstream.

- Topical medicines are applied to the skin. Creams, lotions, and transdermal skin patches are examples.

- Inhaled medicines, such as those used for asthma, are delivered in a fine mist or powder.

- Injected medicines are delivered through a shot that goes directly into the bloodstream.

How a medicine is taken can depend on its purpose. It also depends on how it can do its job most quickly, effectively, and safely. It is important to follow the instructions on the label when using any medicine, regardless of its form.

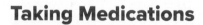

Blend Images/SuperStock

• • • • • • • • • • • •

Reading Check

Describe Give two reasons
that a person would take a
body-regulating medicine.

• • • • • • • • • • • •

Reactions to Medications

MAIN IDEA The effect of medicine depends on many factors.

Medicines can affect the body in a variety of ways. In some cases, they may cause **side effects**. A side effect is a reaction to medicine other than the one that was intended. Some side effects are mild, such as drowsiness. Others can be more severe or even life threatening.

Medicine Interactions

When two or more medicines are taken together, or when a medication is taken with certain foods, the combination may have a different effect than when the medicine is taken alone. Types of medicine interactions include the following:

- **Additive interaction** occurs when medicines work together in a positive way. For example, an anti-inflammatory and a muscle relaxant may be prescribed to treat joint pain.

- **Synergistic effect**—the interaction of two or more medicines that results in a greater effect than when each medicine is taken alone— occurs when one medicine increases the strength of another.

- **Antagonistic interaction** occurs when the effect of one medicine is canceled or reduced when taken with another medicine. For example, someone who receives an organ transplant must take anti-rejection medicines. If the person is diabetic and takes insulin, the anti-rejection medicine may decrease the effectiveness of the insulin.

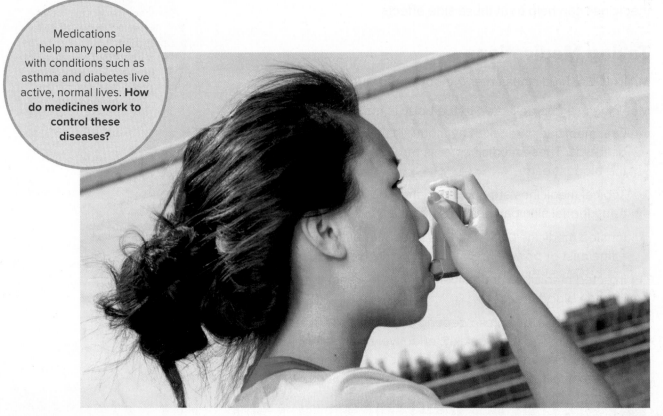

Medications help many people with conditions such as asthma and diabetes live active, normal lives. **How do medicines work to control these diseases?**

Louis-Paul St-Onge/Getty Images

Tolerance and Withdrawal

When a person takes a medication for a long period of time, the body may become used to its effects. It develops a *tolerance* for the medicine, needing larger and larger doses to produce the same effect. However, in some cases a person may experience "reverse tolerance," needing less of the medicine to feel its effects.

After a while, a person's body can become dependent on a medicine. If this happens, the person will go through *withdrawal* when he or she stops using the medicine. Symptoms of withdrawal can include nervousness, insomnia, severe headaches, vomiting, chills, and cramps. These symptoms will gradually ease over time. If you experience withdrawal after using a medicine, talk to your health care provider.

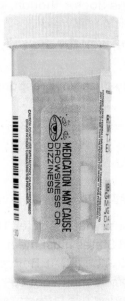

Medicine labels include important information about possible side effects and interactions. **Why is it important to read this information before you take the medicine?**

Myths & Reality

Have you ever taken medicine to treat pain or illness? Consider the truth behind this myth about medicine.

Myth: A person with a serious illness should put off taking painkillers for as long as possible.

Reality: Putting off taking a painkiller until pain is almost unbearable could make managing the pain more difficult.

Lesson 1 Review

Facts and Vocabulary

1. Define the term *medicine* and the term *drugs*.

2. Identify the types of medicines that fight pathogens. What types of medicines prevent disease?

3. Compare a *synergistic effect* with an *antagonistic interaction*.

Thinking Critically

4. **Analyze.** Why are vaccines given to children at a young age?

5. **Evaluate.** Explain why people should not stop taking prescribed medications without talking to their doctor.

Applying Health Skills

6. **Accessing Information.** Use reliable online resources to find information on new and experimental drugs. Write a paragraph evaluating one of the drugs, and list the reasons why you think the information is reliable.

Writing Critically

7. **Descriptive.** Write a paragraph describing why it's important to take a medicine as your doctor prescribed.

Using Medicines Safely

• • • • • • • • • • •

BEFORE YOU READ

Create a T-Chart. Make a two-column chart like the one below. Label one column "Prescriptions" and the other column "OTCs." As you read, fill in the first column with information about prescription medicines. Fill in the second column with information about over-the-counter (OTC) medicines.

Prescriptions	OTCs

Vocabulary

prescription medicines
over-the-counter (OTC) medicines
medicine misuse
medicine abuse
drug overdose

• • • • • • • • • • • • •

BIG IDEA Medicines are safe only if they are used for the intended purpose and according to the directions on the label.

REAL LIFE ISSUES

Safety First. Monica is on the swim team and has an earache. She visits her doctor, who prescribes an antibiotic. Monica is supposed to take the medicine for ten days. Her friend Amy, who is also on the swim team, thinks she may have an ear infection, too. Amy doesn't want to go to the doctor, though, so she asks Monica if she can share her medicine. *Write a dialogue in which Monica explains to Amy why she doesn't think she should share her medication.*

After completing the lesson, review and analyze your response to the Real Life Issues question.

Standards for Medicines

MAIN IDEA Medicines are regulated to make them safe.

When you take a medicine, how can you be sure that it is safe? The answer is that all new medicines in the United States must meet standards set by the Food and Drug Administration (FDA). Before approving a drug for use, the FDA receives information about a medicine's chemical composition and its intended use, effects, and possible side effects. All new medicines must go through at least three clinical trials before they are approved. During a clinical trial, the drug is tested on human volunteers. They are monitored to determine how effective the drug is and whether it has any harmful side effects.

In some cases, people with life-threatening illnesses are allowed to use the drug even if it hasn't completed clinical trials. Such usage is referred to as *experimental*. Patients are given experimental drugs only after clinical trials show that the drugs are safe and may be effective in treating their illnesses.

Unlike medicines, herbal and dietary supplements are not under FDA control. They do not go through the same testing procedures or meet the same strict standards for safety and effectiveness. Many people believe that herbal supplements are safe because they are advertised as "natural." However, even natural compounds can have harmful side effects or interactions. You should check with your health care provider before taking a supplement, just as you would with any other medicine.

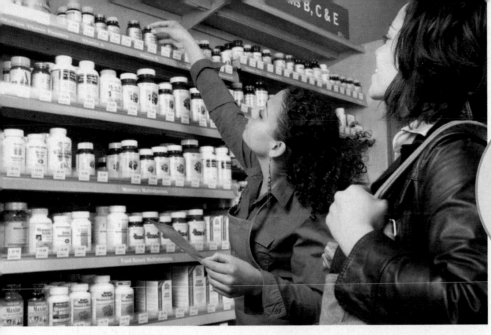

Medicines are regulated by the FDA, but herbal supplements are not. **Explain whether herbal supplements are safer than medicines.**

Blend Images/SuperStock

Prescription Medicines

Prescription medicines are medicines that are dispensed only with the written approval of a licensed physician or nurse practitioner. Only a licensed pharmacist can dispense prescription medicines. A single prescription provides only the amount of medicine needed to treat your condition. If you need more, your health care provider must approve a refill. Only the person whose name appears on the label is allowed to use a prescription medicine.

Over-the-Counter Medicines

Over-the-counter (OTC) medicines, or medicines you can buy without a doctor's prescription, are available without a prescription. You can buy OTC medicines at drugstores and supermarkets. The FDA considers these medicines to be safe as long as they are used as the label directs. However, all medicines can harm you if you do not follow the directions properly.

While all OTC medicines are available without a prescription, the distribution of some OTC medicines is controlled. For example, cold medicines that contain pseudoephedrine must be kept behind the pharmacy counter. This ingredient can be used to make highly addictive, illegal drugs.

Medicine Labels

The FDA requires that all prescription and OTC medicine labels contain information telling consumers how to use the medicine safely and effectively. OTC medicine labels contain information on active and inactive ingredients, the medicines purpose, warnings, conditions, possible side effects, and the expiration date. Prescription medicine labels must include the same information, as well as:

- the patient's name.
- the name of the doctor who prescribed the medicine.

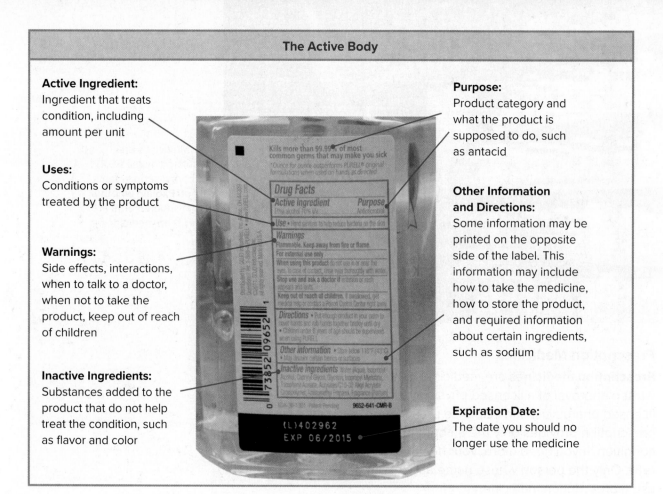

Active Ingredient:
Ingredient that treats condition, including amount per unit

Uses:
Conditions or symptoms treated by the product

Warnings:
Side effects, interactions, when to talk to a doctor, when not to take the product, keep out of reach of children

Inactive Ingredients:
Substances added to the product that do not help treat the condition, such as flavor and color

Purpose:
Product category and what the product is supposed to do, such as antacid

Other Information and Directions:
Some information may be printed on the opposite side of the label. This information may include how to take the medicine, how to store the product, and required information about certain ingredients, such as sodium

Expiration Date:
The date you should no longer use the medicine

- the name and address of the pharmacy that dispensed the medicine.

- the number of refills allowed.

- any special instructions for taking the medicine.

Reading Check

Describe How would you obtain a prescription medicine?

Medicine Misuse

MAIN IDEA Taking medicines unnecessarily or without following the label instructions is dangerous.

Most teens—96 percent—use medicines correctly. This is fortunate, because **medicine misuse** can be dangerous in more than one way. Medicine misuse involves using a medicine in ways other than the intended use. At best, it will only prevent you from getting the full benefits of a medicine. At worst, it can seriously harm your health. Examples of medicine misuse include:

- Failing to follow the instructions on the label

- Giving your prescription medicine to someone else, or taking another person's medicine

- Taking too much or too little of a medication

- Taking a medicine for a longer or shorter period than prescribed or recommended

- Stopping the use of a medicine without informing your health care provider

- Mixing medicines without the knowledge or approval of your health care provider

Medicine Abuse

Some teens have the mistaken idea that prescription and OTC medicines are safer than illegal drugs. In fact, **medicine abuse** is both dangerous and illegal. Medicine abuse involves intentionally taking medications for non-medical reasons. Teens may abuse medicines for the following reasons:

- To lose weight. A healthy diet and exercise are the safest way to maintain a healthy weight.

- To stay awake while studying. Getting plenty of sleep and managing your time wisely will help you study effectively.

- To fit in with peers. A dangerous trend is the practice of having "pill parties," where teens mix whatever OTC and prescription medicines are available.

Using a medicine that was prescribed to someone else is also medicine abuse. Medicines are prescribed for a specific person to treat a specific illness. Using someone else's medicine, even if you think you have the same illness, is illegal and unsafe.

One danger of medicine misuse is **drug overdose**—a strong, sometimes fatal reaction to taking a large amount of a drug. Misusing medicines can also lead to addiction. Never use a medicine other than how it is prescribed or intended.

Reading Check

List What are some ways that teens might misuse medicines?

Lesson 2 Review

Facts and Vocabulary

1. How do *prescription medicines* differ from *OTC medicines*?

2. List four pieces of information that must be on an OTC medicine label. Describe the purpose of each piece of information.

3. What is *medicine misuse*? How does it differ from *medicine abuse*?

Thinking Critically

4. **Analyze.** Why does the FDA regulate medicines and the information on medicine labels?

5. **Evaluate.** What are three ways you can avoid medicine abuse?

Applying Health Skills

6. **Advocacy.** Create a bookmark that gives information on the importance of correct medicine use.

Writing Critically

7. **Expository.** Create a script for a commercial or PSA that explains how people can use their health care providers, pharmacists, and medicine labels to ensure that they are using their medicines properly.

Vocabulary Review

Correct the sentences below by replacing the italicized term with the correct vocabulary term.

1. A(n) *drug* is the interaction of two or more medications that results in a greater effect than when each medicine is taken alone.

2. People may experience *synergistic effects* while taking a medicine, which are effects that are not intended.

3. *Antagonistic interactions* are used to treat or prevent disease, and are dangerous when mixed with alcohol.

4. A(n) *side effect* occurs when medicines work together in a positive way.

5. A(n) *additive interaction* is a substance other than food that changes the structure or function of the body or mind.

Understanding Key Concepts

After reading the question or statement, select the correct answer.

6. A vaccine for polio will do which of the following?
   a. Causes the body to make antibodies to fight polio
   b. Causes people to develop the polio disease
   c. Protects the body against the measles virus
   d. Protects people against polio for a short time

7. What type of medicine might your doctor prescribe if you have an ear infection caused by bacteria?
   a. Antifungal
   b. Antitoxin
   c. Antiviral
   d. Antibiotic

8. What type of medicine might your doctor prescribe if you have the flu?
   a. Antitoxin
   b. Antibiotic
   c. Antiviral
   d. Antifungal

9. Why would you take an antihistamine?
   a. To cure an allergy
   b. To relieve allergy symptoms
   c. To slow an allergic reaction
   d. To build immunity

10. If a person takes two medicines at the same time and one is less effective than when taken alone, what is this called?
   a. Additive interaction
   b. Antagonistic interaction
   c. Side effect
   d. Synergistic effect

11. What type of medication is aspirin?
   a. Analgesic
   b. Antiviral
   c. Antihistamine
   d. Antibiotic

Thinking Critically

After reading the question or statement, write a short answer using complete sentences.

12. **Analyze.** How do bacteria become resistant to certain types of antibiotics?

13. **Evaluate.** Why do narcotic pain relievers require a doctor's prescription?

14. **Describe.** How can medication help people with mental illness?

15. **Compare.** Why might taking a medicine orally rather than taking a medicine topically help a person?

16. **Explain.** What can result if a person takes a medication for a long period of time?

17. **Evaluate.** Anne does not like the side effects of the prescription medicine she is taking. Why should she talk to her doctor before she stops taking the medicine?

18. **Describe.** How does a vaccine work? Can a vaccine help cure disease? If so, how?

19. **Explain.** What is the difference between a synergistic effect and an antagonistic effect when taking medicines?

Vocabulary Review

Use the correct vocabulary term to complete the following statements.

20. Medicines that you can buy without a doctor's prescription are called _____.

21. If you take a large amount of a medicine, you could have a life-threatening reaction known as a(n) _____.

22. Intentionally taking medicines for nonmedical reasons is known as _____.

23. Medicines that are available only with the recommendation of a doctor, and are dispensed only by a licensed pharmacist are called _____.

24. Failing to follow the instructions on or included with a medicine package is an example of _____.

Understanding Key Concepts

After reading the question or statement, select the correct answer.

25. Which does not describe a prescription medication?
  a. Only a specified amount is distributed.
  b. Written approval is required.
  c. It should be taken only by the person it is prescribed to.
  d. It can be purchased without a doctor's recommendation.

26. Which must have proven safety and effectiveness before being sold?
  a. Prescription medicines
  b. Herb-based diet pills
  c. Protein shake drink mix
  d. Vitamins

27. Which of the following information is not on an OTC medicine label?
  a. The directions for taking the medicine
  b. The expiration date
  c. The inactive ingredients in the medicine
  d. The name of the pharmacy

28. Which of the following is a way a person could misuse a medicine?
  a. Taking only half of the prescription with your doctor's approval
  b. Saving half of an antibiotic prescription in case you get sick later
  c. Following the instructions on the medicine label
  d. Taking two medicines at the same time, as directed by a doctor

29. Why might teens abuse medicines?
  a. They take medicine only as prescribed by a doctor.
  b. They do not like the side effects of a certain medicine.
  c. They believe the medicine may help them study longer.
  d. They think the medicine is hard to obtain.

30. Which is *not* a risk of abusing medicines?
  a. Addiction
  b. Death from heart failure
  c. Paranoia
  d. Taking too little medicine

31. Which of the following organizations tests and approves all prescription medicines before they are sold to the public?
  a. the Centers for Disease Control and Prevention
  b. the U.S. Department of Agriculture
  c. the Food and Drug Administration
  d. the Consumer Product Safety Commission

Thinking Critically

After reading the question or statement, write a short answer using complete sentences.

32. Explain. Why should you talk to your doctor before taking herbal supplements?

33. Analyze. Why does the FDA limit the distribution of certain OTC medicines?

34. Explain. Why should you always read the label before taking a medicine?

35. Evaluate. How do the FDA guidelines for approving medicines protect the health of the public?

36. Discuss. How can taking medicines not prescribed to you, or mixing medicines, harm your health?

PROJECT-BASED ASSESSMENT

Explaining Vaccines

BACKGROUND

Your body's immune system has the ability to recognize and destroy bacteria and viruses. It remembers features of these pathogens to fight them. By exposing your immune system to parts of a pathogen, or a pathogen that has been altered so it cannot hurt you, a vaccine allows your body to prepare for that pathogen if you become infected.

TASK

Create an online cartoon that explains to young children how vaccines work.

AUDIENCE

Students in grades 1 through 3

PURPOSE

Explain why vaccines work, and how important they are in maintaining your health.

PROCEDURE

1. Review the text and write notes describing some basic facts about vaccines.

2. Conduct an online search to learn how the body's immune system works. Find answers to these questions: How do vaccines prepare the body to fight pathogens? How do vaccines and antitoxins fight disease?

3. Search for online cartoons that are geared to children in grades 1 through 3 to see the different styles and formats that you might use.

4. Create and organize your cartoon. Use words and pictures that clearly show how vaccines work.

5. Present your cartoon to your class or, if possible, to students in grades 1 through 3.

Math Practice

Interpret Graphs. The table below shows the percentages of nonmedical use of psychotherapeutics among 12- to 17-year-olds. Use the table to answer Questions 1–3.

Non-Medical Use of Psychotherapeutics Among 12- to 17-Year-Olds	Past Year		Past Month	
	1999	2000	1999	2000
Any Psycho-therapeutic*	7.1%	7.1%	2.9%	3.0%
Pain Relievers	5.5%	5.4%	2.1%	2.3%
Tranquilizers	1.6%	1.6%	0.5%	0.5%
Sedatives	0.5%	0.5%	0.2%	0.2%
Stimulants**	2.1%	2.4%	0.7%	0.8%

* Denotes the non-medical use of any prescription-type pain reliever, tranquilizer, stimulant, or sedative; does not include over-the-counter drugs.

** Includes methamphetamine

Source: U.S. Department of Health and Human Services, Substance Abuse and Mental Health Services Administration, NHSDA

1. Of the 12,000 students surveyed in 1999, how many of them have never used any psychotherapeutic drugs in the past year?
   a. 10,000
   b. 11,148
   c. 852
   d. 967

2. After reviewing the chart above, determine the mean, median, and mode of the 2000 data.

3. On one line graph, show the trend, both annually and monthly, of prescription drug abuse in 1999.

Reading/Writing Practice

Understand and Apply. Read the passage below, and then answer the questions .

Aspirin was first introduced by a German company in 1899. Centuries earlier, people used similar chemicals to ease pain and reduce fever. The ancient Greeks used a bitter powder extracted from the bark of willow trees to treat pain. In the 1700s, physicians treated patients with another willow-derived substance that was later discovered to be the chemical salicin.

By the mid-1800s, European pharmacists used an acid form of salicin to treat arthritis. However, patients who took salicylic acid would often suffer from a painful side effect: a severe upset stomach. With the introduction of the milder aspirin, many patients experienced pain relief with fewer stomach problems.

1. What was the author's purpose in writing this piece?
   a. To list the dosages of aspirin
   b. To describe the types of pain relievers
   c. To explain how aspirin works
   d. To tell how aspirin products are used

2. Which sentence best represents the main idea of the second paragraph?
   a. Arthritis causes pain and swelling.
   b. Salicylic acid relieves pain, but can irritate the digestive tract.
   c. European pharmacists tend to prescribe painkillers other than aspirin.
   d. Older aspirin-like products caused stomach irritation.

3. Write a pamphlet that outlines the importance of following a doctor's instructions when taking medicines.

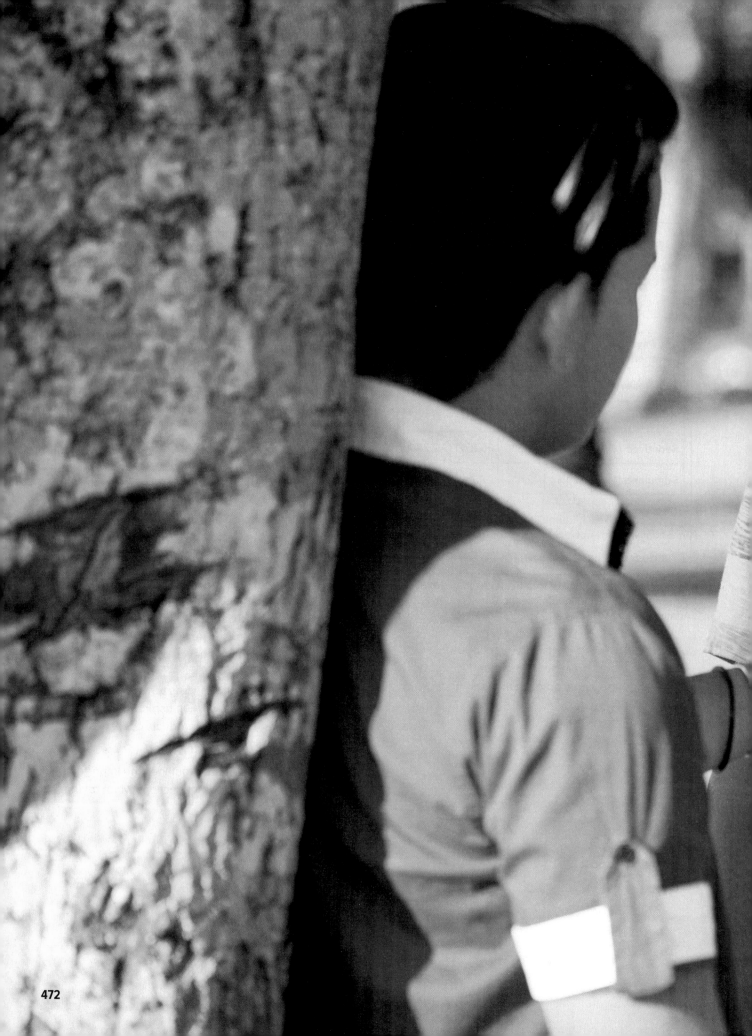

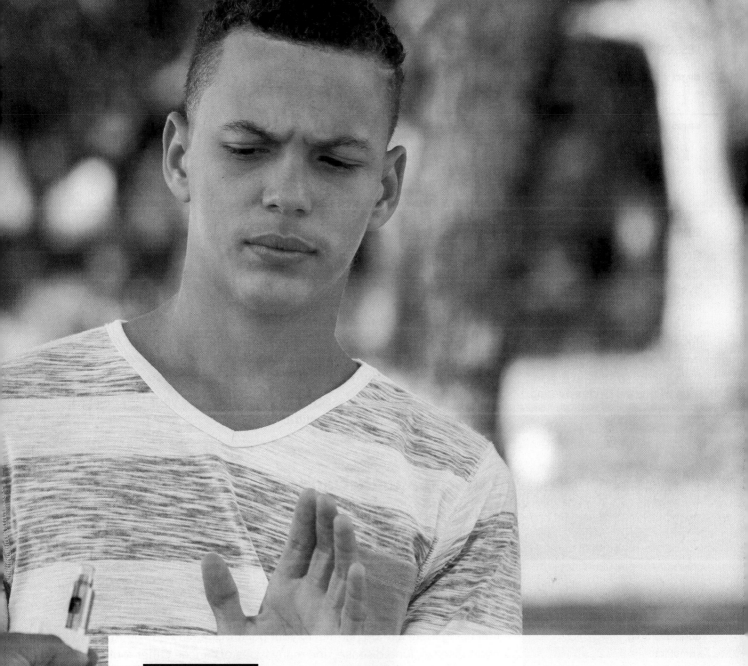

MODULE 20

Tobacco

LESSONS

1 The Health Risks of Tobacco Use

2 Choosing to Live Tobacco-Free

3 Promoting a Smoke-Free Environment

The Health Risks of Tobacco Use

....

BEFORE YOU READ

Create a Venn Diagram. Draw a Venn diagram that has two overlapping circles. Label one circle "Tobacco Smoke" and the other circle "Smokeless Tobacco." Write the risks of each in the circles. Put the risks shared by both in the area where the circles overlap.

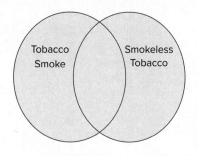

Vocabulary

nicotine
addictive drug
stimulant
carcinogen
tar
carbon monoxide
smokeless tobacco
leukoplakia

....

BIG IDEA The chemicals in all tobacco products harm your body.

REAL LIFE ISSUES

Dangers of Tobacco Use. Teens who decide to start using tobacco can harm their health both now and in the future. Over 6.4 million children who are alive today will eventually die of smoking-related diseases. *Considering what you already know about tobacco use, write a letter expressing your feelings to a close friend or relative who has begun using tobacco.*

After completing the lesson, review and analyze your response to the Real Life Issues question.

Tobacco and Its Dangers

MAIN IDEA All forms of tobacco contain chemicals that are dangerous to your health.

Advertisements for tobacco products often feature healthy, attractive people. Ads like these send the message that using tobacco has no health consequences. However, just one look at a package of cigarettes is enough to tell you this isn't true. Tobacco products display labels warning that using them can be harmful to your health. Smoking has been linked to heart disease, lung disease, and many types of cancer. Other forms of tobacco use, including chewing and dipping tobacco, can also cause health problems. Medical studies have shown that tobacco use is the leading cause of preventable death and disability in the United States.

More than 80 percent of adult smokers started smoking before they were 21 years old. Though, it is illegal for anyone under the age of 21 to purchase or use tobacco. Most teens who start smoking think that they can just quit whenever they want to. The reality is that quitting is very difficult. It's much easier to avoid tobacco use now than to quit later.

Nicotine

The reason tobacco users find it so hard to quit is **nicotine**, which is the drug found in tobacco leaves. This substance, found in all tobacco products, is an **addictive drug**, or a substance that causes physiological or psychological dependence. Nicotine is a **stimulant**, a drug that increases the action of the central nervous system, the heart, and other organs. However, it is only one of many harmful substances found in tobacco.

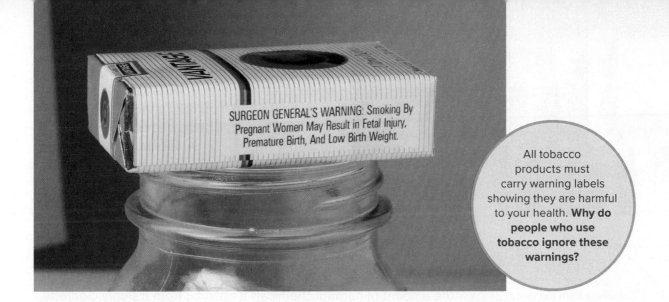

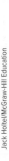
All tobacco products must carry warning labels showing they are harmful to your health. **Why do people who use tobacco ignore these warnings?**

Poisonous Substances in Tobacco Smoke

Tobacco isn't just an addictive drug. It is toxic as well. Tobacco is a **carcinogen**, which is a cancer-causing substance, and it contains a variety of poisonous substances. These include **tar**, **carbon monoxide**, and other poisonous compounds found in products such as paint, rat poison, and toilet cleaner.

Tar. Tar is a thick, sticky, dark fluid produced when tobacco burns. The tar in tobacco smoke damages a smoker's respiratory system in several ways. It paralyzes and destroys cilia, the tiny hair-like structures that line the upper airways and protect the body against infection. Tar also destroys the alveoli, or air sacs. These air sacs absorb oxygen and rid the body of carbon dioxide. Finally, tar damages lung tissue and reduces lung function. Smokers are susceptible to lung problems such as bronchitis, pneumonia, emphysema, and lung cancer. They are also at a higher risk for heart disease and other cancers. According to the CDC, more people in the United States die from lung cancer than any other type of cancer.

Carbon monoxide. Carbon monoxide is a colorless, odorless, and poisonous gas. It is another poison found in cigarette smoke. The body absorbs this gas more easily than oxygen. Exposure to carbon dioxide starves the body's cells and tissues of oxygen. It can also lead to problems with blood circulation. These include heart disease, high blood pressure, and hardening of the arteries.

Pipes, Cigars, and Smokeless Tobacco

When you think about the dangers of tobacco use, you may think mainly of cigarette smoking. However, other forms of tobacco are just as harmful. Cigars, for example, contain significantly more nicotine than cigarettes and also produce more tar and carbon monoxide. A single cigar can contain as much nicotine as an entire pack of cigarettes. Pipe and cigar smokers are at an increased risk for cancers of the lips, mouth, throat, larynx, lungs, and esophagus.

Reading Check

Identify List three harmful substances in tobacco smoke.

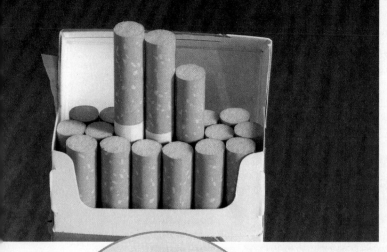

Cigarette filters do not protect smokers from the more than 50 carcinogens, including cyanide and arsenic, which are in tobacco products. The filters themselves contain poisonous chemicals such as those used in insecticides, paint, toilet cleaner, antifreeze, and explosives. **How can you warn others about the risks of using tobacco products?**

Some people believe that **smokeless tobacco**, which is tobacco that is sniffed through the nose, held in the mouth, or chewed, is safer to use than cigarettes because no smoke is inhaled. However, smokeless (or "spit") tobacco products are not a safe alternative to smoking. The nicotine and carcinogens in these products simply enter the body in a different way. Instead of entering the lungs, they are absorbed into the blood through the mucous membranes in the mouth or through the digestive tract. In fact, using smokeless tobacco can expose the body to nearly three times the amount of harmful chemicals it absorbs from a single cigarette. That's because the exposure to chemicals in smokeless tobacco often lasts three times as long.

Smokeless tobacco also poses some additional health risks. Using it can irritate the sensitive tissues of the mouth, causing a condition called **leukoplakia** (loo-koh-PLAY-kee-uh). Leukoplakia causes thickened, white, leathery-looking spots on the inside of the mouth that can develop into oral cancer. Smokeless tobacco also causes cancers of the mouth, throat, larynx, esophagus, stomach, and pancreas. A person who chews eight to ten plugs of tobacco each day takes in the same amount of nicotine as a smoker who smokes two packs of cigarettes a day. Smokeless tobacco is as addictive as smoked tobacco. This makes quitting just as difficult as it is for a smoker.

Electronic Cigarettes

Electronic cigarettes, or e-cigarettes, are a nicotine delivery system. The devices, also called vaping devices, may look like a cigarette, a phone, or a USB drive. They operate using a battery.

Advertisers promote e-cigarettes as being a healthier choice for smokers. They also say that e-cigarettes pose no health risks to non-smokers because the devices produce no tobacco smoke. The advertising of these products can be misleading. For example, e-cigarettes deliver nicotine to the user. Nicotine is addictive.

Additionally, advertisers claim that e-cigarettes are not harmful to others who are nearby. However, the devices do create a water-based vapor. That vapor emitted by e-cigarettes contains many of the same harmful chemicals that are found in tobacco smoke. Many of these chemicals have been linked to cancer. A person who does not use e-cigarettes, but is near someone using one of the devices, is exposed to those cancer-causing chemicals.

Because of the health consequences of e-cigarette use, many states in the U.S. have banned the sale of e-cigarettes to minors. According to a report published by the CDC in 2012, e-cigarette use among teens is low. Less than 7 percent of high school students say they have tried an e-cigarette.

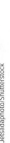

Harmful Effects of Tobacco Use

MAIN IDEA Tobacco use causes both short-term and long-term damage to your body and has other costs as well.

Health officials have been warning the public about the dangers of tobacco use for several **decades**. In some cases, these health risks are not limited to the user. If a pregnant female smokes, for example, she risks the health of her fetus, as well as her own. Women who smoke during pregnancy risk giving birth to infants with low birth weight and other health problems.

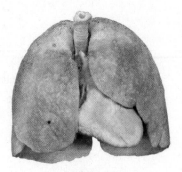

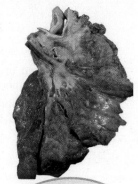

Short-Term Health Effects

Some of the damage tobacco does to the body starts with the very first puff, chew, or sniff. Short-term effects of tobacco use include the following:

- **Brain chemistry changes.** The addictive properties of nicotine cause the body to crave more of the drug. The user may experience withdrawal symptoms, such as headaches, nervousness, and trembling, as soon as 30 minutes after the last tobacco use.

- **Respiration and heart rate increase.** Breathing during physical activity becomes difficult, and endurance decreases. The nicotine in tobacco may cause an irregular heart rate.

- **The sense of taste is dulled and appetite decreases.** Tobacco users often lose much of their ability to enjoy food.

- **Users have bad breath, yellowed teeth, and smelly hair, skin, and clothes.** If tobacco use continues for any length of time, these unattractive effects can become permanent.

Smokers cause severe damage to their lungs. Compare the healthy lung (top) with the one damaged by tobacco smoke (bottom). **How do tar and the other substances in tobacco smoke affect the respiratory system and its ability to function?**

Long-Term Effects

Over time, tobacco use can damage many body systems. People who are exposed to others' tobacco smoke can also suffer many health problems. Some of the long-term effects of tobacco use are:

- **Chronic bronchitis.** Over time, tobacco use can damage the cilia in the bronchi until they become useless. This leads to a buildup of tar in the lungs. The user develops a chronic cough and excessive mucus secretion.

- **Emphysema.** Tobacco smoke destroys the tiny air sacs in the lungs. They become less elastic, making it difficult for the lungs to absorb oxygen. A person with advanced emphysema uses up to 80 percent of his energy just to breathe.

- **Lung cancer.** When the cilia in the bronchi have been destroyed, the lungs cannot expel excess mucus. As a result, cancerous cells can multiply, block the bronchi, and move to the lungs. Nearly 90 percent of lung cancer deaths are caused by smoking.

ACADEMIC VOCABULARY

decade *(noun)*: a group or set of ten

Reading Check

Describe Name two ways in which the long-term health of tobacco users will suffer.

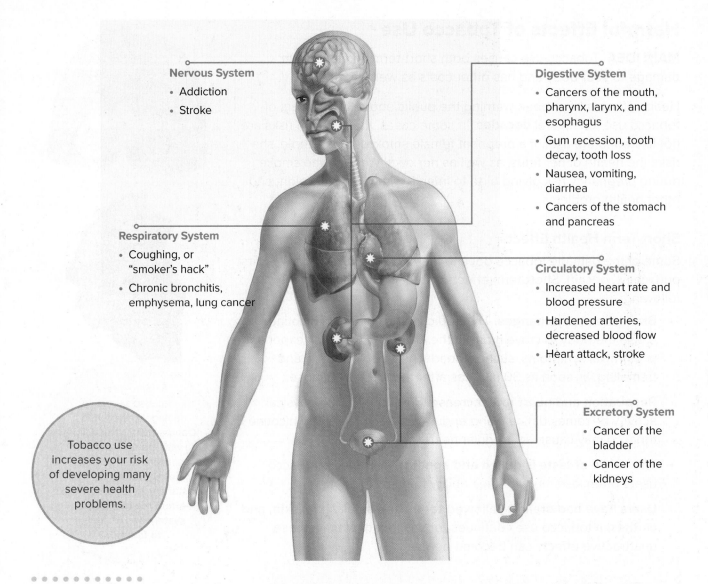

Nervous System

- Addiction
- Stroke

Digestive System

- Cancers of the mouth, pharynx, larynx, and esophagus
- Gum recession, tooth decay, tooth loss
- Nausea, vomiting, diarrhea
- Cancers of the stomach and pancreas

Respiratory System

- Coughing, or "smoker's hack"
- Chronic bronchitis, emphysema, lung cancer

Circulatory System

- Increased heart rate and blood pressure
- Hardened arteries, decreased blood flow
- Heart attack, stroke

Excretory System

- Cancer of the bladder
- Cancer of the kidneys

Tobacco use increases your risk of developing many severe health problems.

Myths & Reality

Most people know that smoking is not a healthy habit. What do you think about smoking? Does this fact change your mind?

Myth: Air pollution outside is much more harmful than environmental tobacco smoke (ETS) indoors.

Reality: The risk a person has for developing cancer from carcinogens in ETS is 100 times greater than the risk of developing cancer from carcinogens in the air outside.

- **Coronary heart disease and stroke.** Nicotine contracts the blood vessels, cutting down blood flow to the body's limbs. Nicotine also contributes to plaque buildup in the blood vessels. This can lead to a condition called *arteriosclerosis,* or hardened arteries. The arteries may become clogged, increasing the risk of heart attack and stroke. Smokers are at a greater risk for developing heart disease than nonsmokers.

- **Weakened immune system.** Long-term tobacco use weakens the immune system, leaving the body more vulnerable to disease.

Health Risks of Tobacco

Latoya knows that tobacco use causes serious health problems. She wants to encourage her friends to avoid tobacco use. She does an online search to learn more about the health effects of tobacco use. Latoya decides to search websites such as the CDC and the National Cancer Institute (NCI) to find statistics about tobacco-related deaths.

Using the CDC and NCI websites, along with other reliable and safe websites, conduct an Internet search to learn more about tobacco use among teens. Search for the following information:

1. How many teens begin smoking each year?

2. How can tobacco use affect a teen's physical health?

3. What impact can tobacco use have on a teen's mental/emotional and social health?

Once your research is complete, create a webpage urging teens who use tobacco to quit. Include information urging teens who have never used tobacco not to start the habit.

Other Consequences of Tobacco Use

Tobacco use has other costs in addition to its health risks. Some of these costs are measured in dollars. A person smoking one pack of cigarettes a day will spend about $3,561 a year on the habit. In addition, when smokers miss work due to tobacco-related illnesses, the entire economy suffers. Tobacco-related illness costs the United States about $193 billion each year.

For minors, tobacco use can have legal consequences as well. Purchasing and using tobacco is illegal for those under the age of 21. Selling tobacco products to individuals under the age of 21 is illegal. Students who use tobacco products on school property risk being suspended or expelled.

Lesson 1 Review

Facts and Vocabulary

1. Define the term *addictive drug*. What is the addictive drug in tobacco?

2. List three types of toxic substances found in cigarette smoke. Why are these substances harmful?

3. Explain four ways using tobacco immediately affects your body.

Thinking Critically

4. **Identify.** What are three ways in which tobacco use affects the respiratory system?

5. **Analyze.** In addition to protecting your health, explain reasons you should not use any form of tobacco.

Applying Health Skills

6. **Advocacy.** Write an editorial for a newspaper that encourages people to quit using tobacco products, and explain the long-term effects of tobacco use on the body.

Writing Critically

7. **Persuasive.** Create a pamphlet raising awareness of the health risks of tobacco use. Include information on the long-term effects of tobacco use.

Choosing to Live Tobacco-Free

BEFORE YOU READ

Create a T-Chart. Make a two-column chart like the one below. Label one column "Start" and the other column "Quit." Fill in the first column with reasons why teens start using tobacco. Fill in the second column with reasons why tobacco users want to quit using tobacco.

Start	Quit

Vocabulary

nicotine withdrawal
nicotine substitute
tobacco cessation program

BIG IDEA Avoiding tobacco use will bring lifelong health benefits.

REAL LIFE ISSUES

Quitting Smoking. Juan started smoking a year ago. Now he doesn't like the hold that tobacco has on him, so he has decided to quit. However, it's been harder than he thought it would be. His friends Joe and Pamela would like to help Juan become tobacco-free, but they aren't sure how. *Write a short essay explaining how Juan's friends can encourage him to quit and support his efforts.*

After completing the lesson, review and analyze your response to the Real Life Issues question.

Teens and Tobacco

MAIN IDEA Today, fewer teens are becoming tobacco users.

The number of nonsmokers in the United States, including teens, is on the rise. Knowing about the health risks of tobacco use influences many teens to stay tobacco-free. However, teens also face other influences, such as tobacco company advertisements. As a result, some teens decide to begin using tobacco.

Why Some Teens Use Tobacco

Teens start smoking for many reasons. Many times, teens are influenced to try tobacco products by movies, TV, and advertisements. Media images may convince teens that tobacco use is glamorous. Some teens falsely believe that smoking will help them control their weight or cope with stress. Others think that smoking will make them seem mature and independent.

The truth is exactly the opposite. Smokers harm their physical appearance. They develop bad breath, yellow teeth, and smelly hair. Smoking reduces the body's capacity for physical activity, so it can actually lead to weight gain. The health problems caused by tobacco use and nicotine dependency can increase stress levels. Finally, rather than making people independent, tobacco use makes them dependent on an addictive drug.

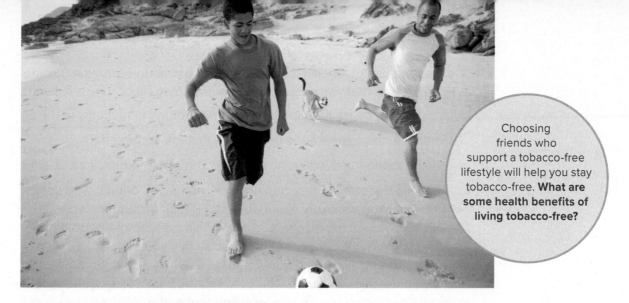

Choosing friends who support a tobacco-free lifestyle will help you stay tobacco-free. **What are some health benefits of living tobacco-free?**

Reduced Tobacco Use Among Teens

More teens than ever are recognizing the health risks of tobacco use and steering clear of tobacco products. The CDC reports that 82 percent of high school students nationwide do not smoke. Several factors have contributed to this trend:

- **Tobacco legislation.** It is illegal for anyone under the age of 21 to purchase and use tobacco products in the United States. In spite of this law, however, tobacco companies used to market their products heavily to teens. In 1998, tobacco companies reached a legal settlement with 46 state governments that limits tobacco advertising aimed at young people. Tobacco companies are also required to fund ads that discourage young people from smoking.

- **No-smoking policies.** Legislation has limited smoking in public places and businesses.

- **Family values.** Teens whose parents avoid tobacco are more likely to abstain from tobacco use themselves.

- **Positive peer pressure.** Teens who do not smoke act as healthy role models for other teens.

- **Understanding of health risks.** More teens today understand that tobacco use can lead to diseases such as heart disease, cancer, and respiratory problems.

Benefits of Living Tobacco-Free

MAIN IDEA Today, fewer teens are becoming tobacco users.

Choosing to avoid tobacco use is probably the best single thing you can do for your health. By avoiding tobacco use, you can affect both your short- and long-term goals. Some of the short-term goals that you might meet by avoiding tobacco use include:

- Performing better at sports or fitness activities.

- Avoiding smoker's breath, yellow teeth and fingers, and having a tobacco smell.

- Retaining your sense of taste and smell.

Fitness Zone

I hate the smell of cigarette smoke. It reminds me that my grandfather has emphysema. He coughs and struggles to breathe all the time. When he was my age, he ran track and played football. Smoking made it hard for him to breathe, so he stopped being active. I don't ever plan to smoke because I've seen what it did to my grandfather's health.

Reading Check

Explain Why has tobacco use decreased among teens?

Alistair Berg/Digital Vision/Getty Images

Choosing to Live Tobacco-Free **481**

Avoiding the use of tobacco can also impact your long-term goals. Some long-term goals that you might achieve by avoiding tobacco use include:

- Maintaining heart and lung health throughout your lifetime.
- Reducing the appearance of wrinkles that age a person.
- Saving money that would be spent buying tobacco products.

Choosing to be tobacco-free has physical, mental/emotional, and social benefits, too. You will likely maintain better health throughout your lifetime by avoiding tobacco use. You will gain a sense of freedom from knowing you are not dependent on an addictive substance. You will have less stress because you do not need to worry about the physical, financial, or legal costs of tobacco use. You will have more confidence in social situations because you look and feel better. Also, you will know that you can go anywhere freely without having to worry about where and when you will be able to smoke.

Strategies for Avoiding Tobacco

The best way to avoid the dangers of tobacco products is never to start using them. Here are a few strategies that can help you stick to the decision to live tobacco-free:

- **Identify and resist marketing tactics.** Recognize that some content on social media that shows young adults using tobacco in fun situations is actually promotional material sponsored by tobacco or *e-cigarette* companies. Some *e-cigarette* companies are offering small scholarships to college students for writing an essay about the possible benefits of using *e-cigarettes*. In doing this, the companies get their links listed on university financial aid websites. Understanding that these materials are an external influence that you can ignore can help you lead a tobacco-free life.

- **Surround yourself with positive influences.** Choose friends who do not use tobacco. Being around people who share your health-related values and beliefs will strengthen your commitment to lead a tobacco-free life.

- **Reduce peer pressure.** Stay away from situations where tobacco products may be used. This will reduce your chances of facing pressure to use tobacco.

- **Be prepared with refusal skills.** Practice in advance what you will say if someone offers you tobacco. Be assertive, and leave the situation if the pressure continues. Be confident and stand up for your healthful choices.

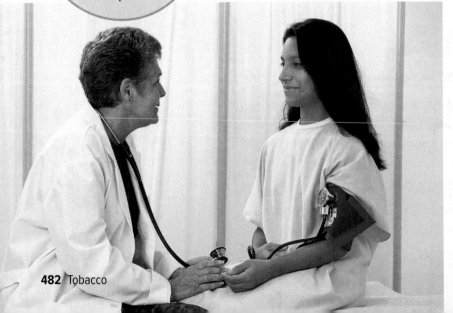

Health care professionals can help tobacco users find the resources they need to successfully quit using tobacco. **Why is it difficult for people to quit?**

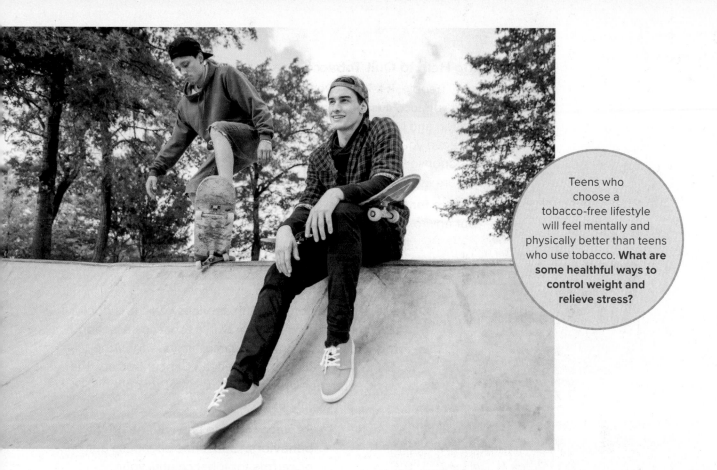

Teens who choose a tobacco-free lifestyle will feel mentally and physically better than teens who use tobacco. **What are some healthful ways to control weight and relieve stress?**

Oneinchpunch/Shutterstock.com

Quitting Tobacco Use

MAIN IDEA There are good reasons for quitting tobacco use.

Teens who use tobacco may decide to quit for several reasons. Some begin to have health problems, such as asthma, coughing, or respiratory infections. Others find their tobacco habit too expensive or find it difficult to purchase tobacco products if they are under 21. Some teens quit because they do not want to pollute the air with harmful smoke. Some quit when they realize that using tobacco can lead to other risky behaviors, such as the use of alcohol and other drugs. Finally, teens may quit just to break free from the control of nicotine.

Ending the Addiction Cycle

Overcoming nicotine addiction can be difficult, but it is not impossible. Millions of people have done it successfully. It may help to know what to expect when you try to quit. **Nicotine withdrawal** is the process that occurs in the body when nicotine, an addictive drug, is no longer used. Symptoms may include irritability, difficulty concentrating, anxiety, sleep disturbances, and cravings for tobacco. Some people use **nicotine substitutes** to relieve these symptoms. These are products that deliver small amounts of nicotine into the user's system while he or she is trying to give up the tobacco habit. These include gum, patches, nasal sprays, and inhalers. Some are over-the-counter products, while others require a doctor's prescription. It is important not to smoke while also using nicotine substitutes. This can expose the body to dangerous levels of nicotine.

Reading Check

Describe What are the symptoms of nicotine withdrawal?

Getting Help to Quit Tobacco Use

For many people, it takes several tries to quit tobacco use successfully. Joining a **tobacco cessation program**—a course that provides information and help to people who want to stop using tobacco—may improve your chances of quitting on the first try. Many high schools sponsor these programs. Other helpful strategies for quitting are listed below.

- **Prepare for the quit day.** Set a target date and stick to it. Prepare your environment and avoid tobacco triggers.

- **Get support and encouragement.** Tell everyone you know about your plan to quit. Support from family and friends will increase your chance of success.

- **Access professional health services.** Talk to a doctor, join a support group, or enroll in a tobacco cessation program. Other helpful resources include the American Lung Association, the American Cancer Society, the Centers for Disease Control and Prevention (CDC), and local hospitals.

- **Replace tobacco use with healthy behaviors.** Substitute sugarless gum or carrots for tobacco until your cravings pass. Physical activity, stress-management techniques, and avoiding other drugs and alcohol can also help you succeed.

Lesson 2 Review

Facts and Vocabulary

1. What are four reasons that smoking among teens is on a downward trend?

2. List three reasons that you might use to convince a friend to quit using tobacco products.

3. Why might some people use nicotine substitutes when quitting smoking?

Thinking Critically

4. **Evaluate.** How will staying tobacco-free benefit your physical, mental/emotional, and social health?

5. **Synthesize.** Explain how the media influences teens to use and not to use tobacco products.

Applying Health Skills

6. **Refusal Skills.** Write a scenario describing a teen being pressured to use tobacco. Develop three refusal statements that the teen can use to avoid tobacco use.

Writing Critically

7. **Narrative.** Write a short story from the point of view of someone who is trying to quit smoking. Include at least three reasons for quitting and why it might be difficult to quit.

baona/iStock/Getty Images

Promoting a Smoke-Free Environment

BIG IDEA Secondhand smoke is harmful, but there are ways you can reduce your exposure.

REAL LIFE ISSUES

Avoiding Secondhand Smoke. Ken visits his aunt and uncle once a week. Ken's uncle smokes and often lights up a cigarette while Ken is in the room. Ken doesn't like breathing smoke, but he doesn't want to offend his uncle. He is not sure what he can do to persuade his uncle not to smoke. *Write a paragraph about what you would do in this situation if you were Ken.*

After completing the lesson, review and analyze your response to the Real Life Issues question.

Health Risks of Tobacco Smoke

MAIN IDEA Tobacco smoke can harm nonsmokers.

The harmful effects of tobacco smoke aren't limited to smokers. Nonsmokers who breathe air containing tobacco smoke are also at risk for health problems. **Environmental tobacco smoke (ETS),** or secondhand smoke, is air that has been contaminated by tobacco smoke. ETS is composed of **mainstream smoke** and **sidestream smoke**. Mainstream smoke is the smoke exhaled from the lungs of a smoker, and sidestream smoke is the smoke from the burning end of a cigarette, pipe, or cigar. Of the two, sidestream smoke is more dangerous. Because mainstream smoke has already passed through a smoker's lungs, it contains lower concentrations of nicotine, tar, and other harmful chemicals.

Health Risks to Nonsmokers

Inhaling ETS is a serious health risk. ETS from cigarettes, cigars, and pipes contains more than 7,000 chemical compounds. More than 70 of these are carcinogens (cancer-causing substances). Secondhand smoke causes about 3,400 deaths from lung cancer every year. Some studies show that infants and young children who are exposed to ETS are more likely to develop asthma than their peers. ETS also causes eye irritation, headaches, ear infections, and coughing in people of all ages. It worsens asthma and other respiratory problems, and it increases the risk of coronary heart disease.

BEFORE YOU READ

Make an Outline. Use the headings of this lesson to make an outline of what you will learn about the risks of smoking. Use a format like this to help you organize your notes.

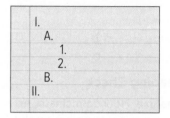

Vocabulary
environmental tobacco smoke (ETS)
mainstream smoke
sidestream smoke

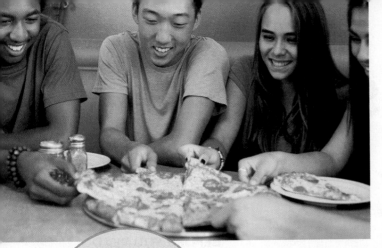

Health Risks to Unborn Children and Infants

Choosing to live tobacco-free is one of the healthiest choices a pregnant female can make for her baby, as well as for herself. Smoking during pregnancy can seriously harm a developing fetus. Nicotine passes through the placenta, constricting the blood vessels of the fetus. Carbon monoxide reduces the oxygen levels in the blood of the mother and fetus. This can reduce fetal growth and increase the risk of miscarriage, prenatal death, premature delivery, low birth weight, deformities, and stillbirths.

The risks of smoking during pregnancy do not end when the baby is born. The infant may also suffer from growth and developmental problems in early childhood. Babies of mothers who smoked during pregnancy or who are exposed to ETS are more likely to die of sudden infant death syndrome (SIDS). In addition, infants exposed to ETS after birth are twice as likely to die of SIDS. They may also have severe asthma attacks, ear infections, or respiratory tract infections.

Smoking is prohibited in many restaurants. **How does this rule protect the health of restaurant customers and employees?**

Reading Check

Analyze How do mainstream smoke and sidestream smoke differ?

Health Risks to Young Children

Young children are particularly sensitive to ETS. Children of smokers are more likely to be in poor health than children of nonsmokers. They tend to have a higher incidence of sore throats, ear infections, and upper respiratory problems. Children who live with smokers also tend to have weaker lungs than children of nonsmokers, as secondhand smoke can also slow lung development.

Another risk of smoking around young children is the example it sets. Children learn by observing. The children of smokers are more than twice as likely to smoke themselves.

Reducing Your Risks

MAIN IDEA You can take action to reduce the effects of ETS.

Since you spend so much time in your home, this is the first place to minimize your exposure to ETS. If a family member smokes, encourage that person to quit. Meanwhile, try to establish smoke-free areas in the house, or make a rule that smokers must go outside. If this is not always possible, air cleaners can help remove some contaminants from the air. Opening windows to admit fresh air will also help.

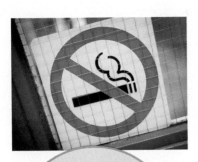

Laws restrict where people may smoke, as well as who can buy tobacco products. **What are the benefits of having smoke-free public places?**

If you have a visitor who smokes, politely ask that person not to smoke inside your home. When you visit the home of a smoker, try to stay outside or in a different room as much as possible. You can also ask to open the windows to let in fresh air. If the smoker is someone other than your friend, you can suggest meeting elsewhere, such as in your home or at a library. In restaurants and other public places, ask to sit in a nonsmoking area. Wherever you can, express your preference for a smoke-free environment.

Creating a Smoke-Free Society

MAIN IDEA Laws help reduce public exposure to ETS.

People who choose to smoke are making a decision that affects the health of others, as well as their own. In the United States, knowledge about the health effects of tobacco use and the costs of tobacco-related illnesses have led to a movement to create a smoke-free society. In fact, one of the goals of *Healthy People 2020* is to reduce tobacco use and the number of tobacco-related deaths.

Medical research shows that any exposure to secondhand smoke can cause health problems. According to the U.S. Surgeon General, the only way to fully protect people from the dangers of ETS is to ban smoking in public places. Many states now prohibit smoking in any workplace. Advertisements aimed at young people encourage them not to smoke. Public service announcements encourage parents not to smoke near their children.

States and local communities are also supporting efforts to create a smoke-free society. Laws now prohibit the sale of tobacco to minors. In addition, some states have successfully sued tobacco companies. The money awarded in these cases may be used to fund anti-smoking campaigns or to offset the medical costs of tobacco use. Finally, community activities that promote a healthy lifestyle give everyone the chance to be a role model for avoiding tobacco use.

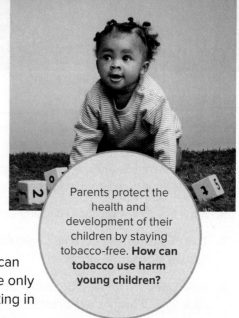

Parents protect the health and development of their children by staying tobacco-free. **How can tobacco use harm young children?**

Character Check

A few of my friends have tried cigarettes. I tell them that I don't agree with their choice, but that we're still friends. I do try to discourage them from smoking and avoid being with them when they use tobacco.

Reading Check

List What are three ways to reduce your exposure to ETS?

Lesson 3 Review

Facts and Vocabulary

1. What is environmental tobacco smoke, and what chemical does it contain?

2. List three ways that ETS affects children.

3. What are two public policies aimed at reducing ETS?

Thinking Critically

4. **Analyze.** How can smoking during pregnancy have long-term effects on the child?

5. **Explain.** Why should you try to avoid ETS, and how can you reduce your exposure to ETS?

Applying Health Skills

6. **Analyzing Influences.** Keep a log of how many tobacco ads you see in one week. Note what type of media was used (print, audio, video), where you saw the ad, and who was targeted. List steps you could take to eliminate these influences in your community.

Writing Critically

7. **Personal.** Describe a situation in which you were exposed to ETS. Include how you felt afterward, physically and mentally. Then write about you could have prevented being exposed to ETS in that situation.

LESSON 1

Vocabulary Review

Correct the sentences below by replacing the italicized term with the correct vocabulary term.

1. A(n) *stimulant* is a cancer-causing substance.

2. Tobacco users can become addicted to the *carbon monoxide* in tobacco.

3. When tobacco burns, it produces a thick, sticky, dark fluid known as *leukoplakia*.

Understanding Key Concepts

After reading the question or statement, select the correct answer.

4. Leukoplakia can develop into which condition?
   a. Emphysema
   b. Oral cancer
   c. Heart disease
   d. Bad breath

5. Which of the following are ways that tobacco harms the cardiovascular system?
   a. Increased heart rate, hardened arteries, chronic bronchitis
   b. Increased heart rate, hardened arteries, increased risk of heart attack
   c. Increased heart rate, chronic bronchitis, emphysema
   d. Chronic bronchitis, emphysema, lung cancer

6. Which of the following is a way that tobacco use immediately affects the body?
   a. Chronic bronchitis
   b. Increased risk of cancer
   c. Leukoplakia
   d. Increased heart rate

Thinking Critically

After reading the question or statement, write a short answer using complete sentences.

7. **Explain.** Is smokeless tobacco less harmful than cigarettes? Why or why not?

8. **Analyze.** If you started smoking today and continued to smoke until you are 30 years old, would you have a higher risk of developing cancer? If so, why?

9. **Explain.** How does nicotine cause an increased risk of stroke?

10. **Discuss.** Kate says that it is her choice to smoke, and that she is the only one who has to worry about her health. How does her decision to smoke affect other people?

11. **Identify.** How can using tobacco impact the social life of a tobacco user?

LESSON 2

Vocabulary Review

Use the correct vocabulary term to complete the following statements.

12. When a tobacco user no longer uses tobacco, the body no longer gets nicotine, and the user experiences _____.

13. A(n) _____ can be used to deliver small amounts of nicotine to the body while a tobacco user is quitting tobacco.

14. A person who wants to successfully quit tobacco could join a(n) _____ that will help the person learn how to quit.

Understanding Key Concepts

After reading the question or statement, select the correct answer.

15. Which is a strategy to keep you from becoming a tobacco user?
   a. Practicing refusal statements
   b. Saving money
   c. Trying a cigarette
   d. Using nicotine gum

16. Which of the following is a reason that a teen tobacco user should quit the habit?
  a. Tobacco use looks sophisticated.
  b. Their friends also smoke.
  c. They can quit as adults.
  d. They will experience health problems.

17. Why do people who are trying to quit tobacco experience physical symptoms such as irritability and anxiety?
  a. They are not committed to quitting.
  b. They are experiencing nicotine withdrawal.
  c. They are upset that other people want them to quit.
  d. They are not engaged in healthier behaviors.

18. Which is *not* a strategy that can help people give up tobacco?
  a. Develop a new daily routine.
  b. Take up a physical activity.
  c. Model adults who smoke.
  d. Join a support group.

19. People gain which health benefit by *not* using tobacco?
  a. Good refusal skills
  b. Friends who do not use tobacco
  c. Lower risk of many diseases
  d. Less money to spend on other interests

Thinking Critically

After reading the question or statement, write a short answer using complete sentences.

20. **Describe.** Why do tobacco users try to quit the habit?

21. **Infer.** Why did tobacco use among teens begin to decrease after 1998?

22. **Identify.** Why do some teens choose to use tobacco and other teens do not?

23. **Predict.** What are two reasons that teen tobacco users find quitting tobacco difficult?

24. **Describe.** What can a person do to quit using tobacco successfully?

Vocabulary Review

Choose the correct term in the sentences below.

25. Environmental tobacco smoke is another name for *secondhand smoke/sidestream smoke.*

26. *Mainstream smoke/Sidestream smoke* comes from a smoker's lungs.

27. Higher concentrations of toxic substances are in *mainstream smoke/sidestream smoke.*

Understanding Key Concepts

After reading the question or statement, select the correct answer.

28. Which is *not* a way that smoking during pregnancy affects the fetus?
  a. Prenatal death
  b. High birth weight
  c. Premature delivery
  d. Developmental problems

29. How can you reduce your risk from ETS?
  a. Become a smoker.
  b. Take vitamins.
  c. Allow visitors to smoke in your house.
  d. Visit places that are smoke-free.

30. Which is a way that the government is reducing ETS exposure?
  a. Banning smoking in public places
  b. Distributing more tobacco licenses
  c. Forming youth antismoking groups
  d. Giving away air cleaners

31. ETS can cause which of these conditions?
  a. Headache
  b. Lung cancer
  c. Sudden infant death syndrome
  d. All of the above

Thinking Critically

After reading the question or statement, write a short answer using complete sentences.

32. Identify. If parents stop smoking, how will that decision help their children's health?

33. Apply. Your friend invites you over for dinner, but you know that your friend's parent smokes. What can you do?

34. Infer. What can you do to promote public policies that support a smoke-free environment?

35. Explain. How does the *Healthy People 2020* program promote health?

36. Analyze. Jim smokes around his friends, who do not smoke. Jim's friends say that they're not worried about the health effects of breathing the ETS created by Jim's tobacco smoke. Are they right *not* to be worried about their health? Explain your answer.

⌐ PROJECT-BASED ASSESSMENT ⌐

Smoking in the Movies

BACKGROUND
Smoking tobacco is discouraged or forbidden in many places. Restaurants, public buildings, schools, offices, airplanes, and even some outdoor parks are smoke-free zones. Yet, many movies continue to show people using tobacco products. In this activity, you will encourage filmmakers to stop showing people smoking in film.

TASK
Create a blog opposing smoking in movies, especially in movies aimed at teens.

AUDIENCE
Students in your school

PURPOSE
Take a public position on the dangers of media that influence teens to smoke tobacco.

PROCEDURE
1. Review your text for information on the health effects of tobacco use.

2. Conduct an Internet search to determine why people start smoking and what influences teens to smoke. Visit government websites and health advocacy organizations to learn their positions on smoking in movies and on television.

3. Search for blogs to study the language, style, and format to use in your own blog.

4. Create a blog making a clear argument opposing smoking in movies.

5. Speak with your principal to see if the blog can be placed on your school's website and updated periodically.

Math Practice

Interpret Graphs. Fred has decided to conduct a survey over the school year to find out what percentage of students in 8th, 10th, and 12th grades at his school reported cigarette use each month. Use the information Fred gathered in the graph to answer Questions 1–3.

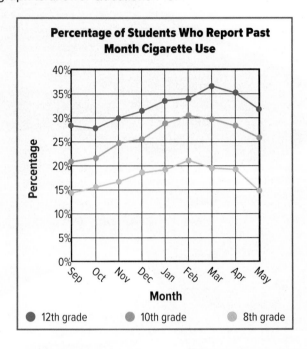

Percentage of Students Who Report Past Month Cigarette Use

● 12th grade   ● 10th grade   ● 8th grade

1. Which grade level had the highest percentage of smokers from September to May?
   a. 8th grade
   b. 10th grade
   c. 12th grade
   d. All grade levels were the same.

2. During which time span was smoking the most common for 8th, 10th, and 12th graders?
   a. Sep.– Oct.
   b. Nov.– Jan.
   c. Jan.– Mar.
   d. Mar.– May

3. In general, what trend is common to all three grade levels from September to May, according to the chart shown here? What influences do you think contributed to this trend?

Reading/Writing Practice

Understand and Apply. Read the passage below, and then answer the questions.

Today you will make a number of decisions. These decisions may or may not have a lasting effect on your life. One decision that will have a lasting effect is the decision not to start smoking. As you know, smoking is dangerous to your health. Smokers have a greater chance than nonsmokers of dying of lung and heart diseases. Cigarette smoke is also dangerous to others: secondhand smoke harms the health of nonsmokers, including the smoker's friends and family. Smoking is also addictive. Tobacco poisons the user, but the nicotine in tobacco smoke makes the user want—and need—more. Many smokers admit that they would like to quit, but they think they can't. Starting is easy; quitting is hard. If you start smoking now, you may be starting a habit that is dangerous to you, your friends, and your family.

1. Which sentence best summarizes the writer's view of smoking?
   a. Many smokers have difficulty quitting.
   b. Smoking is a harmful habit.
   c. Starting is easy, quitting is hard.
   d. Smokers will get lung cancer.

2. How does the writer support the statement that nicotine is addictive?
   a. By explaining that nicotine makes users want more
   b. By stating how easy it is to quit smoking
   c. By telling how easy it is to start smoking
   d. By describing the dangers to nonsmokers

3. Create a podcast to encourage teens not to start smoking.

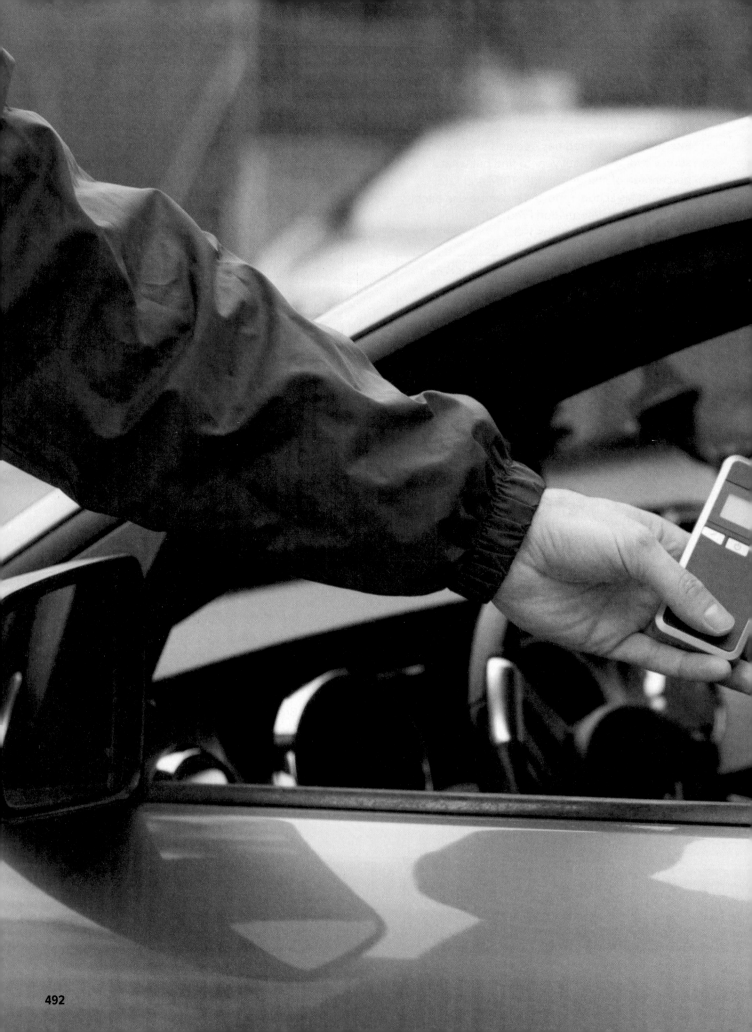

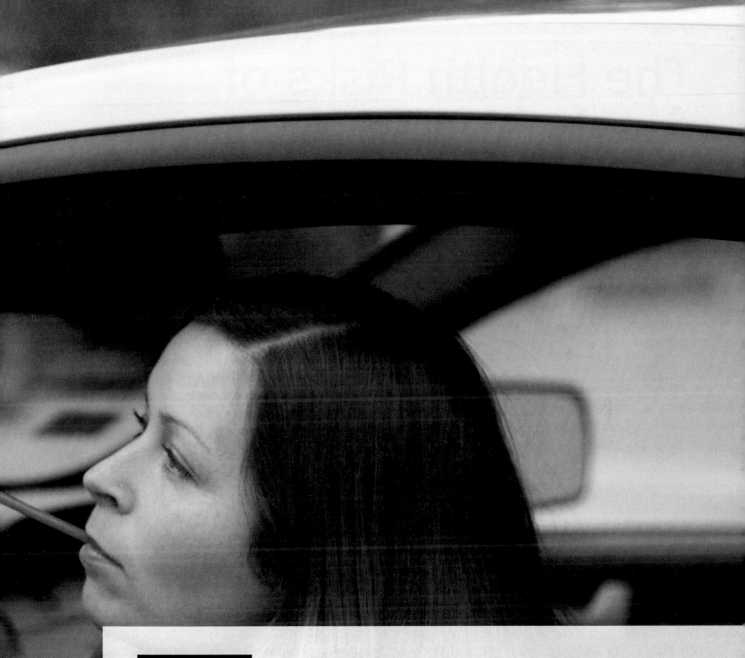

MODULE 21

Alcohol

LESSONS

The Health Risks of Alcohol Use

BEFORE YOU READ

Make an Outline Use the headings of this lesson to make an outline of what you'll learn about the harmful effects of alcohol use. Use a format like this to help you organize your notes.

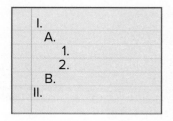

Vocabulary

ethanol
fermentation
depressant
intoxication
binge drinking
alcohol poisoning

BIG IDEA Alcohol use can harm your body and your brain and cause you to make poor decisions.

REAL LIFE ISSUES

Knowing the Risks. Sarah is worried because she has seen her sister, Jamie, experiment with alcohol. Jamie is only in high school, and Sarah feels that her sister does not fully understand the risks of her behavior. Jamie doesn't think there is a problem because she has only had alcohol a few times with her friends. Sarah is concerned that her sister is putting herself at risk, and she knows it's against the law to drink if you are under 21. *Write a dialogue in which Sarah tries to convince Jamie to change her behavior. Sarah should communicate her concern to Jamie.*

After completing the lesson, review and analyze your response to the Real Life Issues question.

Alcohol

MAIN IDEA Alcohol is an addictive drug.

When you look at an advertisement for beer or some other alcoholic drink, what do you see? In most cases, the ad will include images of healthy, happy young people. These images cover up the true story that alcohol—or, more accurately, **ethanol**—is a powerful and addictive drug. It's also physically harmful, especially for teens. Using alcohol during the teen years can affect brain development. Also, in many cases, it can serve as an entry into other types of drug use.

Ethanol is produced naturally during the **fermentation** process, which is the chemical action of yeast on sugars in fruits, vegetables, and grains. It can also be produced synthetically. Alcohol is found in drinks such as beer, wine, and flavored malt-liquor drinks. These drinks contain a combination of ethanol, water, flavoring, and minerals. Spirits, or liquors, such as whiskey and vodka, also contain alcohol.

Short-Term Effects of Alcohol

MAIN IDEA Alcohol impairs the central nervous system.

Alcohol is a **depressant**, or a drug that slows the central nervous system. Using it slows down reaction time, impairs vision, and diminishes judgment.

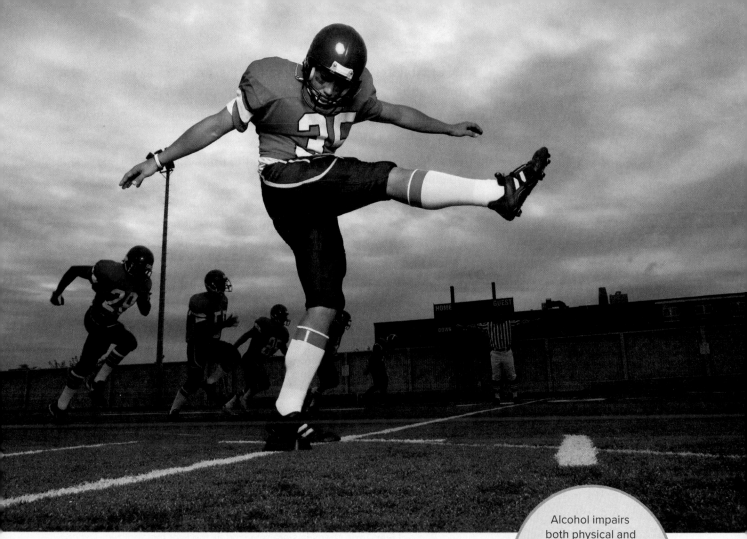

Alcohol impairs both physical and mental abilities. **How can alcohol use decrease your performance in activities that you enjoy?**

Alcohol stays in a person's system until the liver can break it down. If a person drinks alcohol faster than the liver can break it down, he or she will become intoxicated, or "drunk." The amount of alcohol needed to cause **intoxication** will vary from person to person. Intoxication is the state in which the body is poisoned by alcohol or another substance, and the person's physical and mental control is significantly reduced.

Factors That Influence Alcohol's Effects

Alcohol does not affect everyone the same way. Its effects may appear slowly or quickly and may be more or less intense from person to person. Factors that influence alcohol's effects include:

- **Body size.** A smaller person feels the effect of the same amount of alcohol faster than a larger person does.

- **Gender.** Alcohol generally moves into the bloodstream faster in females than in males, mainly because females tend to have smaller bodies.

- **Food.** Having food in the stomach will slow down the passage of alcohol into the bloodstream.

- **Rate of intake.** The faster a person drinks, the more alcohol will stay in the bloodstream because the liver cannot break it down.
- **Amount.** As the amount of alcohol consumed increases, the level of alcohol in the bloodstream rises.
- **Medicine.** Alcohol can interfere with the effects of medicines, and medicine can heighten the effects of alcohol.

Short-Term Effects of Alcohol

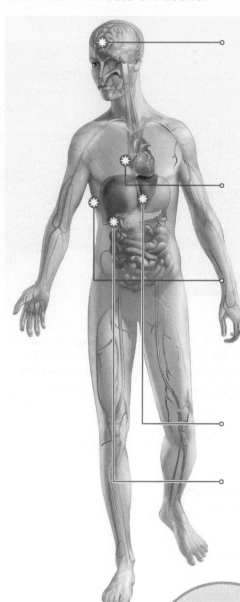

Changes to the Brain

- **Development.** Pathways and connections necessary for learning may be permanently damaged.
- **Memory.** Thought processes are disorganized, and memory and concentration are dulled.
- **Judgment and control.** Judgment is altered and coordination is impaired. Movement, speech, and vision may be affected.
- **Risk of stroke.** Alcohol use may increase risk of stroke in young people.

Cardiovascular Changes

- **Heart.** Small amounts of alcohol can increase the heart rate and blood pressure. High levels of alcohol have the opposite effect, decreasing heart rate and blood pressure. Heart rhythm becomes irregular. Body temperature drops.

Liver and Kidney Problems

- **Liver.** Toxic chemicals are released as the liver metabolizes alcohol. These chemicals cause inflammation and scarring of the liver tissue.
- **Kidneys.** Alcohol causes the kidneys to increase urine output, which can lead to dehydration.

Digestive System Problems

- **Stomach.** Alcohol increases stomach acid production and can cause nausea and vomiting.

Pancreas Problems

- **Pancreas.** Consuming large amounts of alcohol quickly can cause pancreatitis, which is accompanied by acute, severe pain. The pancreas produces enzymes that break down nutrients in foods. Alcohol use can disrupt the absorption of these nutrients.

Physical and mental impairment begin with the first drink of alcohol and increase as more alcohol is consumed.

Alcohol and Drug Interactions

Alcohol can alter the effect of medicines in several ways. It can increase the effectiveness of some medicines and decrease the effectiveness of others. Mixing alcohol with medicine can cause the body to absorb either the drug or the alcohol more slowly. This increases the length of time that the substance stays in the body. Also, when some medications are combined with alcohol, enzymes in the body can change them into chemicals that can damage the liver or other organs. These interactions may lead to illness or even death. Medicines that can interact harmfully with alcohol have warning labels that advise people not to drink while using them.

Long-Term Effects of Alcohol

MAIN IDEA Alcohol use can have negative effects on a person's health.

Alcohol's effects on the body don't end when the liver finishes breaking it down. When used regularly, alcohol can have long-term effects on physical, mental/emotional, and social health. Moreover, the effects of alcohol use are not limited to the drinker. They can also harm others who are close to him or her.

Reading Check

Describe How can alcohol change the way medicine affects your body?

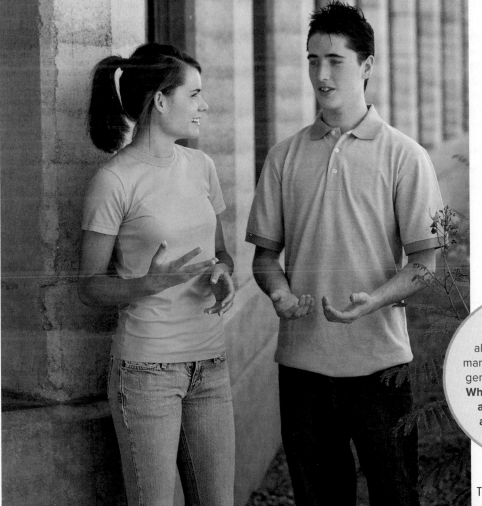

The effects of alcohol depend on many factors, including gender and body size. **Why might women be affected more by alcohol use than men?**

Tim Fuller Photography

Physically, excessive alcohol use over a long period of time can cause damage to nearly every body system. Its effects include:

- damage to brain cells and a reduction in brain size.

- increased blood pressure, which may lead to a heart attack or stroke.

- buildup of fat cells in the liver, which can lead to cell death.

- damage to the lining of the stomach, which can result in ulcers and stomach cancer.

- destruction of the pancreas.

If a person stops using alcohol, some of these physical effects can be reversed over time.

Alcohol use can also have harmful mental/emotional and social effects. Excessive drinking can affect memory and brain function. Alcohol addiction, or alcoholism, is another serious consequence. An addiction to alcohol, like any other addiction, can damage relationships with family, friends, and others.

Reading Check

Explain How does long-term alcohol use affect the liver?

Alcohol has a negative effect on many of the body organs, and excessive long-term alcohol use can cause death.

LONG-TERM EFFECTS OF ALCOHOL			
The Brain	**The Cardiovascular System**	**The Digestive System**	**The Pancreas**
Addiction Physical dependence can lead to the inability to control the frequency and amount of drinking. **Loss of brain functions** Loss of verbal skills, visual and spatial skills, and memory. **Brain damage** Excessive use of alcohol can lead to brain damage and to a reduction of brain size. The learning ability and memory of adolescents who drink even small amounts can be impaired.	**Heart damage** The heart muscles become weakened and the heart becomes enlarged, reducing its ability to pump blood. This damage can lead to heart failure. Reduced blood flow can also damage other body systems. **High blood pressure** Damages the heart and can cause heart attack and stroke.	**Irritation of digestive lining** Can lead to stomach ulcers and cancer of the stomach and esophagus. **Fatty liver** Fats build up in the liver and cannot be broken down, leading to cell death. **Alcoholic hepatitis** Inflammation or infection of the liver. **Cirrhosis of the liver** Liver tissue is replaced with useless scar tissue. Cirrhosis can lead to liver failure and death.	**Swelling of the pancreas lining** The passageway from the pancreas to the small intestine can become blocked, and chemicals needed for digestion cannot pass to the small intestine. The chemicals begin to destroy the pancreas itself, causing pain and vomiting. A severe case of pancreatic swelling can lead to death.

Binge Drinking and Alcohol Poisoning

MAIN IDEA Consuming a large amount of alcohol over a short period of time can be fatal.

One of the riskiest drinking behaviors is drinking large amounts of alcohol in a single session. **Binge drinking**, which is drinking five or more alcoholic drinks at one sitting, is sometimes done on a bet or on a dare. Whatever the reason is, it can have dangerous consequences. Drinking any alcohol can impair a drinker's physical and mental abilities, but binge drinking can seriously harm the drinker's body systems. Alcohol acts as a depressant on body organs. Involuntary actions, such as breathing and the gag reflex that prevents choking, may be suppressed.

A person who drinks too much alcohol may eventually pass out. However, even though the person is unconscious, alcohol that is in the stomach continues to enter the bloodstream. So even though the person has stopped drinking, his or her blood alcohol level will continue to rise. This increases the risk of **alcohol poisoning**, which is a severe and potentially fatal physical reaction to an alcohol overdose. It is dangerous to assume that a person who has passed out after consuming a lot of alcohol will be fine if left to "sleep it off." Some symptoms of alcohol poisoning include:

- mental confusion and stupor.
- coma and an inability to be roused.
- vomiting and seizures.
- slow respiration—ten seconds between breaths or fewer than eight breaths per minute.
- irregular heartbeat.
- hypothermia, or low body temperature, which produces a pale or bluish skin color.

If you suspect that a person has alcohol poisoning, call 911 immediately.

Lesson 1 Review

Facts and Vocabulary

1. What is *intoxication?* What influences how fast a person becomes intoxicated?

2. Explain how alcohol acts as a *depressant* on the central nervous system.

3. What is *binge drinking?* What can happen as a result of binge drinking?

Thinking Critically

4. **Analyze.** Is it safe to take an over-the-counter medicine after drinking alcohol? Explain your reasoning.

5. **Describe.** How can drinking even moderate amounts of alcohol permanently affect teens?

Applying Health Skills

6. **Advocacy.** Write a PSA script that advises other teens of the dangers of binge drinking. Include the health risks and what to do if someone drinks too much alcohol.

Writing Critically

7. **Persuasive.** Write a letter to your city council member asking that police prosecute stores that sell alcohol to anyone who is underage.

Choosing to Live Alcohol-Free

• • • • • • • • • • •

BEFORE YOU READ

Make a Cause-and-Effect Concept Map Draw a box around the phrase "Teen Alcohol Use," as shown here. Write at least three consequences of alcohol use, each in its own box. Connect the consequence boxes to the Teen Alcohol Use box as shown.

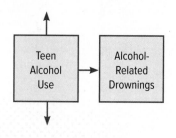

Vocabulary

alcoholism
psychological dependence
physiological dependence
alcohol abuse

• • • • • • • • • • •

BIG IDEA Choosing not to use alcohol protects you from dangerous health consequences.

REAL LIFE ISSUES

Teens and Alcohol Use. The CDC's Youth Risk Behavior Surveillance System survey tracks risk behaviors among teens. In a 2018 survey, 15.5 percent of teens reported using alcohol before the age of 13. *Write a paragraph describing some consequences of teen alcohol use.*

After completing the lesson, review and analyze your response to the Real Life Issues question.

Alcohol Use

MAIN IDEA Several factors influence teen alcohol use.

As you know, it is illegal for teens to use alcohol. Even for those who are old enough to drink legally; however, alcohol use has its risks. One of these risks is **alcoholism**. Alcoholism is a disease in which a person has a physical or psychological dependence on drinks that contain alcohol. Overuse of alcohol can result in **psychological dependence**, a condition in which a person believes that a drug is needed in order to feel good or to function normally. Overuse of alcohol can lead to a **physiological dependence**, a condition in which the user has a chemical need for a drug.

Factors That Influence Alcohol Use

Teens may choose to use alcohol—or to avoid alcohol—for several reasons. Three of the most influential are:

- **Peer pressure.** Teens may be more likely to drink if their friends do. When alcohol is not an accepted activity in a group, by contrast, a teen will not feel pressure to drink.

- **Family.** If a teen's parents discourage and avoid the use of alcohol, the teen is more likely to do the same.

- **Media messages.** The companies that make and sell alcoholic beverages spend billions of dollars each year to link their products with images of youthful, healthy people having a good time. These ads almost never show the negative side of alcohol use.

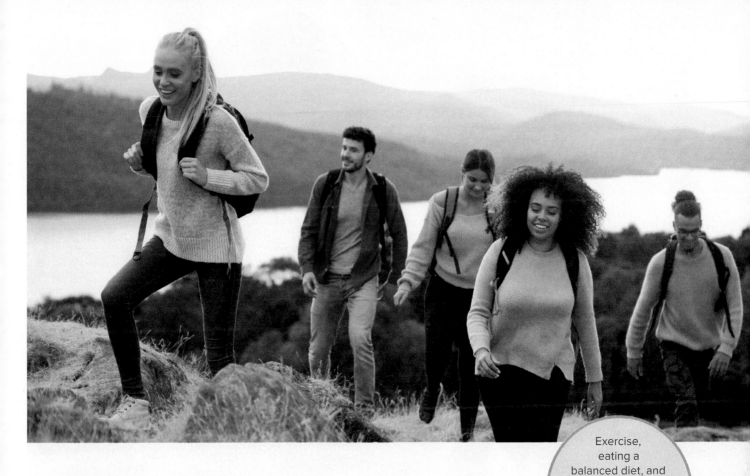

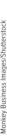

Exercise, eating a balanced diet, and avoiding alcohol can help teens stay healthy. **Why should teens avoid alcohol?**

Advertising Techniques

Advertisers try to make alcohol use seem glamorous and fun. Ads in many places—including billboards, TV and radio, and magazines—may reach children and teens. Alcohol companies also sponsor sporting events, music concerts, art festivals, exhibits, and college events. Alcohol companies may also target teens and young adults by marketing "alcopops." These are beverages that are sweet and look similar to soft drinks. These drinks may look harmless, but they still contain alcohol.

Health Risks of Alcohol Use

MAIN IDEA Alcohol can harm more than just your health.

In the United States, nearly 30 people die each day as a result of alcohol-related traffic accidents. Alcohol use is also linked to deaths from drowning, fire, suicide, and homicide. A nondrinker's risk of being injured increases if that person is with friends who are drinking.

Alcohol and the Law

It is illegal for anyone under the age of 21 to buy, possess, or consume alcohol. Teens who break this law can be arrested and sentenced to a youth detention center. This is a serious consequence, because any arrest and conviction can affect a teen's future. An arrest can limit college and employment options. It can also damage a teen's reputation and cause that teen to lose the trust of friends and family members.

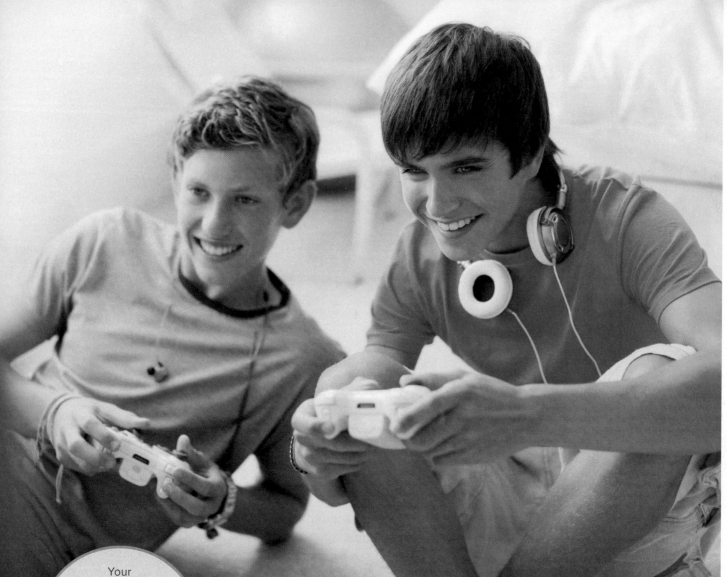

Your decision to avoid alcohol is influenced by the people around you. **How can having friends who do not use alcohol help you to stay alcohol-free?**

Reading Check

Explain How do advertisements try to encourage teens to start drinking?

Alcohol and Violence

Fights are more likely to break out at parties where alcohol is used. Teens who are involved in fights may face disciplinary action from parents, schools, or police. Teens who drink are also more likely to be involved in violent crimes, such as rape, aggravated assault, and robbery. It is estimated that alcohol use is a factor in one-third to two-thirds of sexual assaults and date rapes. Teens can protect their health and safety by avoiding situations where alcohol is present.

Alcohol and Sexual Activity

Alcohol impairs judgment and lowers inhibitions. This may lead people to compromise their values. Teens who use alcohol are more likely to become sexually active at an earlier age and to engage in sexual activity. Approximately 22 percent of sexually active teens use alcohol or drugs before engaging in sexual activity. Teens who drink often are twice as likely to contract an STD as teens who do not drink.

Analyzing the Media

What media images come to mind when you think of advertisements for alcohol? Many ads feature attractive young people whose message seems to be, "You can be like us if you use this product." What are other reasons the people in the ad are enjoying themselves? Conduct an online search using government websites and other trusted sources to examine the guidelines and perceived messages for advertisements for alcohol.

Activity: Technology

Use a critical eye when examining alcohol ads in magazines, television, and billboards. Select three alcohol ads and ask yourself the following questions:

1. What is really being advertised?

2. What is the hidden message?

3. What is the truth?

4. How do the advertisers distort the truth about alcohol?

After analyzing the ads, select one and create a multimedia slide presentation showing how the ad distorts the truth. Use your creativity to show how the ad, or even just elements of the ad, can be misleading.

Alcohol and the Family

An estimated 25 percent of all youth are exposed to excessive alcohol use, or **alcohol abuse**, within their families. Young people who live in a household where a family member abuses alcohol are at a high risk for:

- neglect, abuse, or social **isolation**.
- economic hardship.
- using alcohol themselves.
- physical or mental illness.

Studies show that a person who begins drinking alcohol as a teen is four times more likely to develop a dependence on it than someone who starts drinking in adulthood.

Alcohol and School

Most schools have adopted a zero-tolerance policy for students found using alcohol on school property. Students who use alcohol may be banned from school activities, such as graduation. They may even be expelled from school and put in an alternate education program. Ultimately, these students may find that their options for choosing a college or job are limited.

. . . .

ACADEMIC VOCABULARY

isolation *(noun)*: The act of being withdrawn or separated.

. . . .

Reading Check

List Name three risky behaviors that can be caused by alcohol use.

. . . .

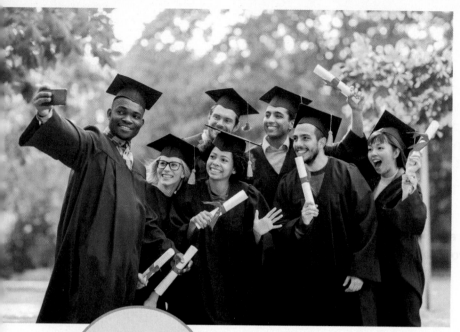

Avoiding Alcohol

MAIN IDEA You will experience many benefits if you choose to live alcohol-free.

There are many adults who choose to live alcohol-free. Others choose to drink alcohol occasionally and responsibly. However, alcohol can be addictive, and once you start drinking, it may be difficult to stop. Teens who start drinking by age 15 are five times more likely to become dependent on alcohol than those who do not start drinking until age 21.

Avoiding alcohol use can help you avoid risky behaviors. **How can teen alcohol use put your future at risk?**

Benefits of Living Alcohol-Free

Many teens today are making the commitment to live alcohol-free. Avoiding alcohol use can improve your life in a variety of ways. Read about each benefit in the list below to learn.

- **Maintaining a healthy body.** You will avoid the damage alcohol can do to the brain and other body organs. You will also decrease your chances of being injured in an accident.

- **Establishing healthy relationships.** You can be open and honest with your family about your activities and habits. Teens who use alcohol may strain their family relationships as they try to keep their drinking a secret.

- **Making healthy decisions.** Drinking alcohol can impair your judgment. By abstaining from alcohol, you can avoid intoxication and make sound decisions that protect your health. You will also reduce the risk of making unhealthy choices, such as drinking and driving or becoming sexually active.

- **Living within the law.** Purchasing or possessing alcohol is against the law for anyone under 21. By remaining alcohol-free, you can avoid arrest and legal problems.

- **Avoiding violence.** Avoiding alcohol reduces your risk of being a victim of or participating in a violent crime.

- **Achieving your goals.** Being alcohol-free allows you to stay focused on your short-term and long-term goals.

Reading Check

Explain How can living alcohol-free help you stay physically and mentally healthy?

Syda Productions/Shutterstock

Refusing Alcohol

One way to avoid alcohol use is to avoid parties or social gatherings where alcohol is served. Instead, plan alcohol-free activities with friends. However, sometimes you may be unable to avoid situations where you may be offered alcohol. Practicing refusal skills will help you build confidence when dealing with peers who use alcohol. Saying no is much easier when you know how you will respond *before* you are faced with the situation. Plan ahead by remembering refusal statements, such as:

- "No thanks, I don't drink."
- "I can't—I need to stay sharp for the game this week."
- "I promised my parents I wouldn't drink."
- "I don't want to risk getting kicked off the team."

If necessary, call your parents or another trusted adult for a ride home.

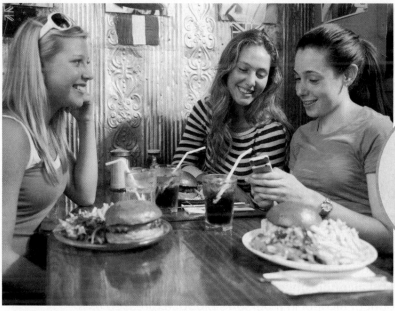

Having a strategy to stay alcohol-free will help you avoid the risks of alcohol use. **What are some ways to avoid using alcohol?**

Lesson 2 Review

Facts and Vocabulary

1. What is *alcohol abuse,* and how are teens likely to be affected if it occurs in their family?

2. How does *alcohol abuse* differ from *alcoholism?*

3. Explain whether teens are at risk of alcohol dependence.

Thinking Critically

4. **Evaluate.** What are four possible consequences of poor decisions made while under the influence of alcohol?

5. **Analyze.** Explain how teens can stay alcohol-free.

Applying Health Skills

6. **Refusal Skills.** You arrive at a party and see that other teens are drinking alcohol. Write a dialogue describing how you use refusal skills effectively to stay alcohol-free.

Writing Critically

7. **Descriptive.** Write a scenario between a teen and a parent. The teen is providing reasons for remaining alcohol-free.

The Impact of Alcohol Abuse

BEFORE YOU READ

Make Note Cards. Label one note card "Alcohol Abuse." Then, make a note card for each vocabulary term in this lesson. On each note card, write what you already know about each term. As you read the lesson, add information to each card about each term.

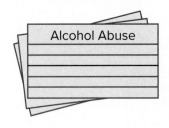

Alcohol Abuse

Vocabulary

blood alcohol concentration (BAC)

alcoholic

recovery

sobriety

. . . .

Reading Check

Explain Why is it dangerous to drive after drinking alcohol?

. . . .

BIG IDEA Problem drinking and alcoholism harm both the drinkers and the people around them.

┌─ **REAL LIFE ISSUES** ─────────────────────────

Living With Alcohol Abuse. Lily's mother drinks alcohol every day, and has several drinks each day. Her mother says that drinking helps her unwind after work. Lily thinks her mother may be an alcoholic. She learned that her mother recently lost her job because she was drinking at work. Lily often finds herself taking care of her mother and is worried about what will happen to her family if her mother cannot stop drinking. *Write a letter to Lily's mother as if you were Lily. In your letter, explain how her mother's drinking is affecting Lily's life.*

After completing the lesson, review and analyze your response to the Real Life Issues question.

└──

Alcohol and Driving

MAIN IDEA Drinking and driving is very dangerous.

Drinking alcohol is always dangerous, but driving after drinking can be disastrous. One-fifth of all teen drivers involved in fatal car accidents have a **blood alcohol concentration (BAC)** of 0.01 percent or more. BAC is the amount of alcohol in a person's blood, expressed as a percentage. Any amount of alcohol in the blood can cause the following effects, all of which can impair a person's driving ability:

- Slow reflexes

- Reduced ability to judge distances and speeds

- Increase in risk-taking behaviors

- Reduced concentration and increased forgetfulness

Driving While Intoxicated

Drunk driving—legally known *as driving while intoxicated (DWI)* or *driving under the influence (DUI)*—is illegal. Adults can be charged with drunk driving if they have a BAC of 0.08 percent. How much alcohol it takes to reach that level will depend not only on how much a person has drunk, but also on the type of drink. The drinker's body size and gender, as well as how fast the alcohol is consumed, can also affect BAC. For people under 21, there is no legal BAC limit, since it's illegal to use alcohol.

COMPARING BEER, WINE, AND SPIRITS		
Drink	Alcohol by Volume	Alcohol Content
Beer *(12 oz.)*	4%	0.5 oz.
Wine *(5 oz.)*	10%	0.5 oz.
Vodka or Whiskey *(1.25 oz.)*	40%	0.5 oz.

Each of these beverages contains the same amount of pure alcohol.

Driving after drinking can have serious, even deadly, results. Possible consequences of DWI or DUI include:

- **Legal consequences.** Drunk drivers face arrest and a court appearance. They may be sentenced to pay a fine or bail, or they may receive jail time. Afterward, they will have a police record.

- **Personal consequences.** After a drunk driving incident, the driver may face severely restricted driving privileges. In some cases, the driver can lose his or her license outright.

- **Financial consequences.** A person charged with drunk driving may have to pay higher insurance rates or may lose his or her insurance entirely.

- **Physical consequences.** Drunk drivers are more likely to be involved in accidents. This puts not only themselves but everyone on the road at risk of injury or death.

Riding in a vehicle with a driver who has been drinking is just as dangerous as if you were the one drinking and driving. If someone you are with has been drinking, find someone else to give you a ride, or call home and ask someone to pick you up.

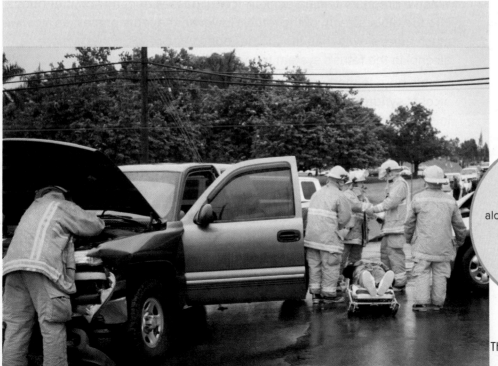

More than 10,500 people died in 2018 in alcohol-related crashes. **What are other consequences of drinking and driving?**

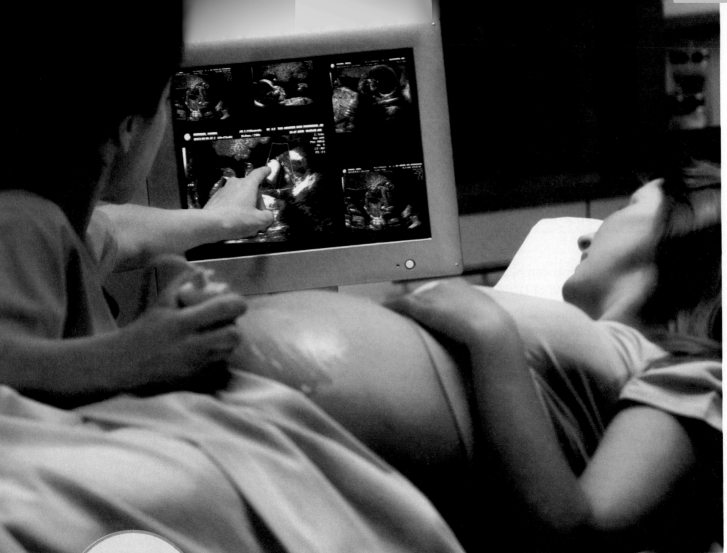

> When a pregnant female drinks, so does her fetus. **What effect can alcohol have on a fetus?**

Alcohol and Pregnancy

MAIN IDEA A female who drinks during pregnancy can harm her fetus.

When a pregnant female drinks, alcohol passes directly from her body into the bloodstream of the fetus. However, the fetus processes alcohol much more slowly than the mother does. As a result, there is more alcohol in the fetus's system for a longer period of time.

Infants born to mothers who drink during pregnancy are at risk for fetal alcohol syndrome (FAS). The effects of FAS are both severe and lasting. Infants born with FAS may have the following problems:

- Small head

- Deformities of face, hands, or feet

- Heart, liver, and kidney defects

- Vision and hearing problems

- Central nervous system problems, developmental difficulties, and poor coordination

- Learning difficulties, hyperactivity, and short attention span

- Anxiety and social withdrawal

Reading Check

Name What are four problems that might affect an infant if the mother drinks alcohol during pregnancy.

FAS is one of the leading preventable causes of mental retardation. To be safe, females who are pregnant, think they might be pregnant, or are trying to become pregnant should not drink *any* alcohol.

Alcoholism

MAIN IDEA Alcoholism is a disease that affects the person who drinks and others around him or her.

Alcoholics are physically or psychologically dependent on alcohol. The behavior of alcoholics varies—some are aggressive and violent, while others may become withdrawn. However, all alcoholics share certain symptoms:

- **Craving.** The person is preoccupied with alcohol and feels a strong need for alcohol to manage tension or stress.

- **Loss of control.** The person is unable to limit his or her alcohol use.

- **Physical dependence.** If alcohol use is stopped, the person has withdrawal symptoms, such as nausea, sweating, shakiness, and anxiety.

- **Tolerance.** The person needs to drink ever-increasing amounts of alcohol in order to feel its effects.

Alcoholism is not limited to any age, race, gender, or ethnic or socioeconomic group. However, growing scientific evidence suggests that alcoholism does run in families. One study shows that children of alcoholics are four times more likely to become alcoholics themselves. Environmental factors can also contribute to alcoholism. These may include friends, culture, peer pressure, availability of alcohol, and stress. One very important factor is the age at which a person starts drinking. People who start in their teens are much more likely to become alcoholics than those who begin drinking as adults.

Alcohol causes serious damage to the liver. Compare the healthy liver (top) with the liver that has been damaged by alcohol abuse. **What effect does alcohol have on the liver?**

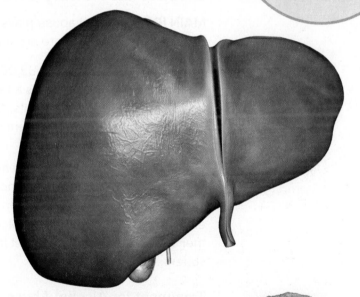

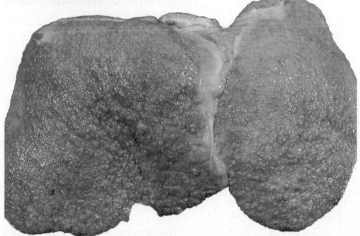

Stages of Alcoholism

Alcoholism develops in three stages: abuse, dependence, and addiction. However, not all alcoholics experience each stage equally. Read about each stage in the list below to learn more.

- **Stage 1—Abuse.** Alcoholism may begin with social drinking. Over time, drinking increases. The person may begin to experience memory loss and blackouts. The person may also begin to lie or make excuses to justify his or her drinking.

- **Stage 2—Dependence.** The person becomes physically dependent on alcohol and is unable to control his or her drinking. The drinker tries to hide the problem, but performance on the job, at school, and at home suffers.

- **Stage 3—Addiction.** In the final stage of alcoholism, the drinker is addicted. By this stage, the liver may be already damaged, and so less alcohol may be required to cause drunkenness. A person who stops drinking at this stage experiences severe withdrawal symptoms.

Reading Check

Describe What are the symptoms of alcoholism?

Effects on Family and Society

MAIN IDEA Alcohol abuse plays a role in crimes and has negative effects on people who are around problem drinkers.

In the United States, about 88,000 people die each year from excessive alcohol use. Alcohol abuse is a factor in the four leading causes of accidental death: car accidents, falls, drowning, and house fires. Alcohol also plays a major role in violent crimes, such as homicide, forcible rape, and robbery.

Often, people who are close to alcoholics develop mentally unhealthy behaviors, such as *codependency*. Codependents ignore their own emotional and physical needs. Instead they focus their energy and emotions on the needs of the alcoholic. In the process, they lose their self-esteem and their trust in others, and their physical health suffers.

Treatment for Alcohol Abuse

Alcoholism cannot be cured, but it can be treated. **Recovery** is the process of learning to live an alcohol-free life. Recovering alcoholics must make a lifelong commitment to **sobriety**, which is living without alcohol. The path to recovery from alcoholism has four stages:

- **Admission.** The person admits to having a drinking problem and asks for help.

- **Detoxification.** The person's body adjusts to functioning without alcohol.

- **Counseling.** The person learns to change behaviors and live alcohol-free.

- **Recovery.** The person takes responsibility for his or her own life.

There are several resources and programs available to help alcoholics and problem drinkers, as well as their families and friends. Groups that help alcoholics include Alcoholics Anonymous and the National Drug and Alcohol Treatment Referral Routing Service, which provides treatment referral and information about treatment facilities. Groups for families include the National Association for Children of Alcoholics and Al-Anon/Alateen, which helps families and friends learn to deal with the effects of living with an alcoholic. Mothers Against Drunk Driving (MADD) and Students Against Destructive Decisions (SADD) focus on education about avoiding alcohol use and other harmful behaviors. Finally, the SAMHSA National Clearinghouse for Alcohol and Drug Information provides general information about alcohol and other drugs.

Reading Check

Explain Describe what an alcoholic must do in order to recover.

Character Check

Demonstrate your commitment to a lifestyle that does not include alcohol use by taking responsibility for your decisions. Write and sign a pledge to stay alcohol free. Share your pledge with your parents and friends. Encourage your friends to sign pledges, too.

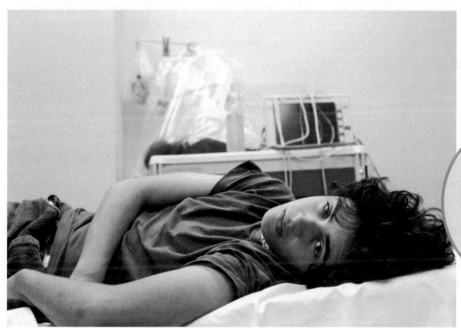

Environmental factors such as peer pressure, stress, cultural surrounds, and friends can contribute to alcoholism.

Lesson 3 Review

Facts and Vocabulary

1. Define the term *blood alcohol concentration (BAC)*. What is the legal BAC for teen drivers?

2. Define the term *fetal alcohol syndrome (FAS)*. What causes it?

3. Explain why an alcoholic experiences detoxification when trying to become sober.

Thinking Critically

4. **Analyze.** How does a moderate amount of alcohol, which otherwise might not be harmful to a female, have the potential to harm her fetus?

5. **Discuss.** What are two possible outcomes of drinking and driving?

Applying Health Skills

6. **Accessing Information.** Use reliable sources to identify community and other resources that help alcoholics and their families. Then, design a webpage that lists these resources.

Writing Critically

7. **Narrative.** Write a one-page story showing how a teen can use refusal skills to avoid getting into a car with a driver who has been drinking.

LESSON 1

Vocabulary Review

Correct the sentences below by replacing the italicized term with the correct vocabulary term.

1. Drinking alcohol can lead to *fermentation*, a state of reduced physical and mental control.

2. *Intoxication* is when a person drinks five or more alcoholic drinks at one sitting.

3. *Binge drinking* is a potentially fatal reaction to an alcohol overdose.

Understanding Key Concepts

After reading the question or statement, select the correct answer.

4. Which is not a short-term effect of alcohol?
   a. Coordination is impaired.
   b. Vision is impaired.
   c. More stomach acid is produced.
   d. Judgment is altered.

5. Which type of person is most likely to be quickly affected by alcohol?
   a. A small female who has not eaten
   b. A large female who just ate dinner
   c. A small male who just ate dinner
   d. A large male who has not eaten

6. Which is a potential consequence of long-term excessive alcohol use?
   a. A heart attack
   b. The need for a liver transplant
   c. Swelling of the brain
   d. An increased ability to control drinking

Thinking Critically

After reading the question or statement, write a short answer using complete sentences.

7. **Describe.** Why are teens who drink more likely to put themselves in risky situations?

8. **Evaluate.** Terry takes a 12-hour allergy medication and then drinks alcohol after waiting an hour. Explain why this is not a safe behavior.

9. **Explain.** How does long-term excessive drinking affect the brain?

10. **Analyze.** Dana drinks only occasionally, but when he drinks he does things that he later regrets. His friends assure him that he is fun when he drinks, and that he should not worry about his actions. Does Dana have a drinking problem? Explain.

11. **Evaluate.** A person passes out after drinking. Explain the dangers of leaving the person alone, and what action should be taken.

LESSON 2

Vocabulary Review

Use the correct vocabulary term to complete the following statements.

12. Teens are likely to experience neglect or abuse if there is _____ in their family.

13. People who have a chemical need for alcohol have a _____.

14. A dependence on drinks with alcohol is called _____.

15. When a person believes that alcohol use is needed to feel good or function normally, that person has a _____.

Understanding Key Concepts

After reading the question or statement, select the correct answer.

16. Which of the following influences teens to stay alcohol-free?
    a. Having peers who drink alcohol
    b. Seeing alcohol ads on TV
    c. Having parents who disapprove of alcohol use
    d. Attending alcohol-sponsored sporting events

17. Which is not a result of the high-risk behaviors associated with alcohol use?
    a. Increased deaths in traffic accidents
    b. Increased frequency of date rape
    c. Suspension from sports teams
    d. Improved job prospects

18. If you stay alcohol-free, which is a likely benefit?
    a. Decreased likelihood of getting a sexually transmitted disease
    b. Increased likelihood of being injured in an accident
    c. Decreased likelihood of making responsible decisions
    d. Increased likelihood of being a victim of violent crime

19. Which is not a strategy to remain alcohol-free?
    a. Planning an alcohol-free party
    b. Practicing refusal statements
    c. Attending parties with people who use alcohol
    d. Calling for a ride home if alcohol is present

Thinking Critically

After reading the question or statement, write a short answer using complete sentences.

20. **Explain.** What are the dangers of adult alcohol use? What are the dangers for teens?

21. **Analyze.** How does sponsoring community events and music concerts help alcohol companies sell their products?

22. **Discuss.** How does teen alcohol use impact the community?

23. **Evaluate.** Why are alcohol-free teens more likely to achieve their long-term goals than teens who use alcohol?

24. **Examine.** Why is avoiding gatherings where alcohol is present the best way to stay alcohol-free?

Vocabulary Review

Choose the correct term in the sentences below.

25. *Blood alcohol concentration (BAC)/Fetal alcohol syndrome (FAS)* is a condition that babies can be born with if a female drinks while pregnant.

26. The amount of alcohol in a person's blood that is expressed as a percentage is *blood alcohol concentration/fetal alcohol syndrome.*

27. An addict who is dependent on alcohol is in/an *sobriety/alcoholic.*

Understanding Key Concepts

After reading the question or statement, select the correct answer.

28. It is illegal for adults to drive when they have what BAC level?
    a. 0.01
    b. 0.02
    c. 0.05
    d. 0.08

29. Which is not likely to occur if a person is caught drinking and driving?
    a. A field sobriety test will be conducted.
    b. The person loses driving privileges.
    c. The person loses insurance coverage.
    d. There will be no penalty.

30. A baby born with FAS may have which of the following?
    a. Anxiety
    b. Facial deformities
    c. Kidney problems
    d. All of the above

31. Which of the following is not part of the stages of alcoholism?
    a. Becoming intoxicated regularly
    b. Going through detoxification
    c. Making excuses for alcohol-related problems
    d. Alcohol taking control of the drinker's life

Thinking Critically

After reading the question or statement, write a short answer using complete sentences.

32. Identify. What effects of alcohol make it risky to drive after drinking?

33. Apply. Jacob's mother is seven months pregnant. She thinks it is alright to start having an occasional glass of wine with dinner because the fetus is mostly developed. What should Jacob tell her?

34. Analyze. What factors increase one's likelihood of becoming an alcoholic?

35. Synthesize. Jesse knows she has a drinking problem and wants help. Explain what she can do to find help.

PROJECT-BASED ASSESSMENT

The Power of Persuasion

BACKGROUND

Companies that sell alcohol often use television advertising to convince people to buy and use their products. Alcohol commercials use powerful combinations of video and audio to sell their product. Anti-alcohol ads may also appear on television. These ads aim to reduce alcohol use among teens.

TASK

Create a webpage about how saying no to alcohol is an attractive and practical option for teens.

AUDIENCE

Students in your class

PURPOSE

Persuade teens to say no to alcohol use.

PROCEDURE

1. Working with a small group, create a list of situations in which teens may be pressured by other teens to use alcohol.

2. Select two possible situations that teens in your school may encounter. Conduct research using reliable sources to learn ways that advertisers might try to persuade teens to use their products.

3. Create a webpage discussing the situations and the possible outcomes, both good and bad. Be sure to include a list of images and possibly videos of commercials for your webpage.

4. Make any necessary revisions to your webpage.

5. Present your final product to your class for input.

Math Practice

Interpreting Graphs. The graph below shows the relationship between blood alcohol level and breath alcohol level. After reviewing the graph, answer the questions that follow.

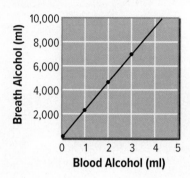

1. Based on the graph, how many milliliters of blood are equivalent to 3150 ml of air?
   a. 1 ml
   b. 1.5 ml
   c. 3 ml
   d. 2100 ml

2. What type of function is shown on the graph?
   a. Exponential
   b. Higher degree
   c. Linear
   d. Quadratic

3. An increase in body temperature of 1.8 degrees F results in an increase of 7 percent in the test results. If a graph similar to the one shown were drawn for a person with a temperature of 97 degrees F, would the slope be greater than or less than the slope of this graph?

Reading/Writing Practice

Understand and Apply. Read the passage below, and then answer the questions.

Having a natural mentor can help teens make positive choices, according to a study by Students Against Destructive Decisions (SADD). Natural mentors can include parents, other family members, teachers, coaches, members of the clergy, and other trusted adults. In the study, 46% of teens who have a natural mentor reported having a higher sense of self. Only 25% of teens who did not have a natural mentor agreed that they have a higher sense of self. More than half of the students surveyed also said that having a natural mentor impacted them in a positive way. Teens are willing to talk to their natural mentors about avoiding alcohol, drugs, and sexual activity.

1. The study's findings show that
   a. a mentor has no influence on teens.
   b. a mentor can help teens make positive choices.
   c. a natural mentor is always a parent.
   d. teens with a natural mentor have a higher sense of self.

2. Based on this article, a natural mentor is
   a. another teen who may be one or two years older.
   b. a parent or other trusted adult.
   c. an adult the teen is paired with through a matching program.
   d. a teacher or school counselor who has had training as a mentor.

3. Write a one-page, persuasive essay describing the importance of having a natural mentor. Describe how mentors can help teens.

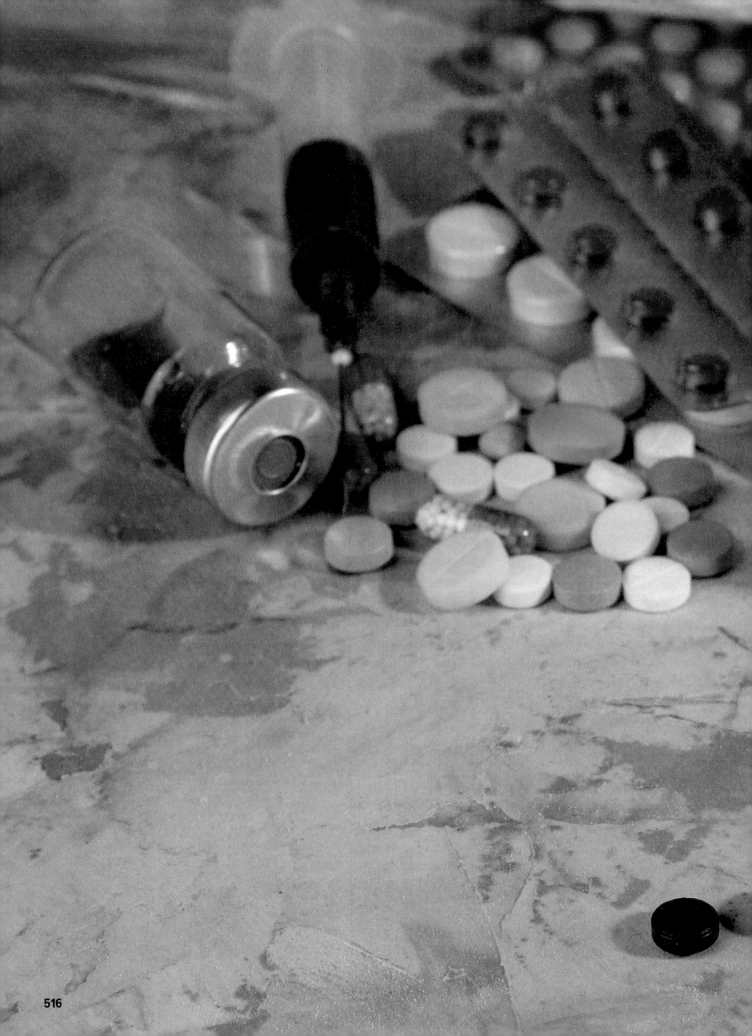

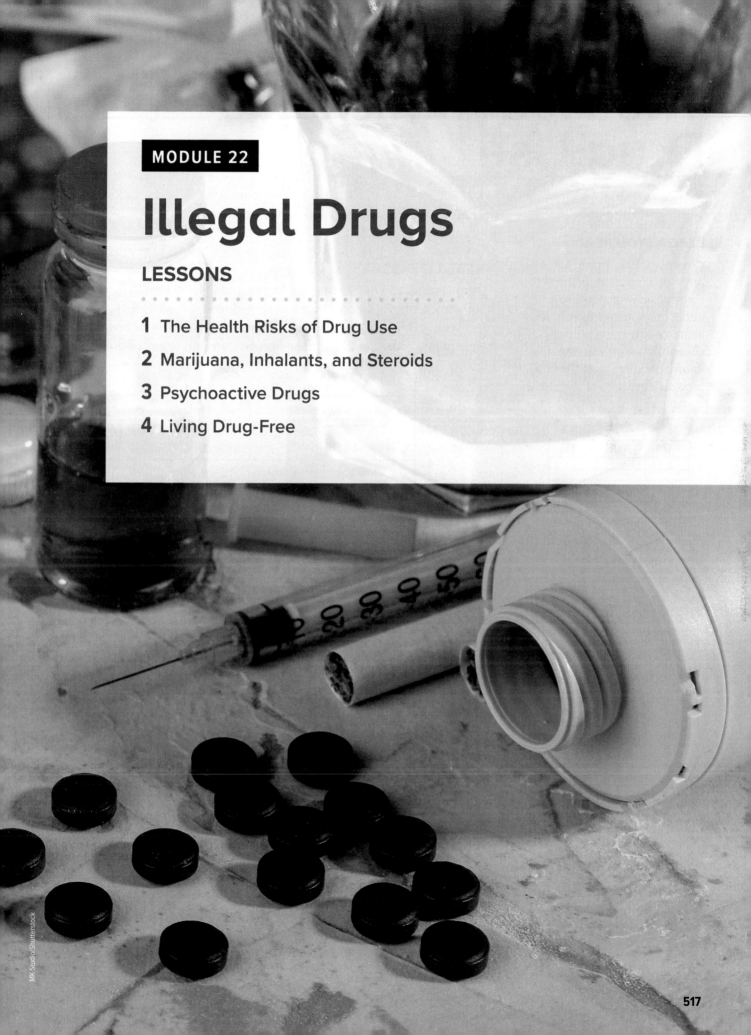

MODULE 22

Illegal Drugs

LESSONS

1 The Health Risks of Drug Use

2 Marijuana, Inhalants, and Steroids

3 Psychoactive Drugs

4 Living Drug-Free

The Health Risks of Drug Use

......

BEFORE YOU READ

Create a K-W-L Chart. Make a three-column chart. In the first column, list what you **k**now about the negative effects of illegal drugs. In the second column, list what you **w**ant to know about this topic. As you read, use the third column to summarize what you **l**earned.

K	W	L

Vocabulary

substance abuse
illegal drugs
illicit drug use
overdose
addiction

......

BIG IDEA Drug misuse and substance abuse are life-threatening behaviors.

REAL LIFE ISSUES

Drug Dangers. The Substance Abuse and Mental Health Services Administration, Drug Abuse Warning Network (SAMHSA) graph shows the number of visits to hospital emergency rooms in 2010 that involved different types of drugs.

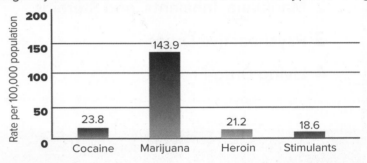

Rate per 100,000 population

Cocaine 23.8 · Marijuana 143.9 · Heroin 21.2 · Stimulants 18.6

Consider what you already know about illicit drug use. Write a paragraph describing some of the potential dangers associated with drug use.

After completing the lesson, review and analyze your response to the Real Life Issues question.

Substance Abuse

MAIN IDEA Substance abuse includes the use of illegal substances, as well as the misuse of legal substances.

You have learned how medicines can be used to cure and prevent disease. Sometimes, people accidentally use medicines in an improper way. In other cases, medicines may be intentionally abused. Deliberately using medicines for non-medical purposes is an example of **substance abuse**. Substance abuse is any unnecessary or improper use of chemical substances for nonmedical purposes. Other forms of substance abuse include the use of **illegal drugs** and the combination of drugs with alcohol. Illegal drugs are chemical substances that people of any age may not lawfully manufacture, possess, buy, or sell. The use of illegal drugs is a crime known as **illicit drug use**. It includes the sale of prescription drugs to people who do not have a doctor's prescription. Although these drugs are legal with a doctor's prescription, it is illegal to take them without a prescription or to give them to others.

Factors That Influence Teens

Illicit drug use is dangerous as well as illegal. So why do some teens do it? There are many factors that can influence teens to try drugs— or to avoid them. These include:

- Peer pressure, or the influence of your friends or social group. For example, teens whose friends avoid drugs are more likely to say no to drugs themselves.

- Family members. Parents and other family members can encourage teens to abstain from drug use.

- Role models such as coaches, athletes, actors, and professionals who speak about the benefits of being drug-free.

- Media messages from TV, radio, websites, movies, and music.

- Perceptions of drug behavior that may lead teens to see drug use as more common than it really is. For example, according to the CDC, more than 70 percent of ninth-graders have never used marijuana.

- Misleading information that makes teens think certain drugs can be beneficial. For instance, some teens believe that steroid use boosts sports performance.

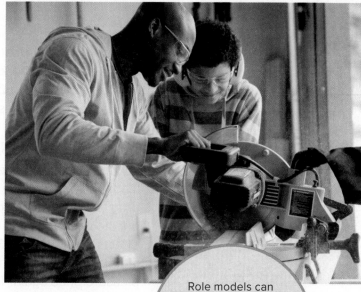

Role models can influence you to avoid drugs. **How would having drug-free role models give you an advantage in resisting drugs?**

Reading Check

Describe How could having a prescription for a legal drug lead to illicit drug use?

How Drugs Affect Your Health

MAIN IDEA Illegal drug use can be deadly.

Unlike medicines, illegal drugs are not tested for quality, purity, or strength. They don't come with labels that list safety guidelines or suggested dosage. Illicit drug use can affect your total health in ways you may not be able to predict.

Effects on Physical Health. Teens who use illegal drugs can experience a variety of harmful physical effects, including some that may be deadly. These reactions can occur with a teen's first drug use. They can also happen to teens who have used a drug in the past and think that they can handle it. The manufacture of illegal drugs is not regulated, so the compounds in each batch of a drug may be different.

One serious danger of drug abuse is the risk of an **overdose**. Also, some illegal drugs are injected with needles. This practice can expose users to diseases such as hepatitis B and HIV. Substance abuse endangers safety, as well. It is a leading cause of crime, suicide, and unintentional injuries.

Effects on Mental Health. Drugs may impair a teen's ability to think and reason. Some drugs, such as Ecstasy, can **alter** the brain's structure and function. Also, teens under the influence of illegal drugs may act in ways that go against their values.

ACADEMIC VOCABULARY

alter *(verb)*: to make different

©Hero/age fotostock

Effects on Social Health. Teens who use drugs may lose friendships with teens who choose to live drug-free. Relationships with family members may also suffer. In addition, some teens may face legal consequences as a result of drug use.

The Cycle of Addiction

Trying a drug just once, or using a drug only a few times, can quickly lead to a serious cycle of **addiction**. In this cycle, the user takes the drug to experience short-term pleasure. As the effects of the drug wear off, the user begins to experience the physical and psychological effects of withdrawal. This leads the user to take the drug again, to relieve these symptoms and to repeat the feelings of short-term pleasure once again. This cycle continues until the addict gets medical help to stop using the drug. Stages in this cycle can include the following:

- **Tolerance.** The body becomes accustomed to the drug, so that the user needs to take more and more of it in order to feel its effects.

- **Psychological dependence.** Over time, the user comes to feel that he or she needs the drug in order to feel good or to function normally.

- **Physiological dependence.** The user's body develops a chemical need for the drug. When the effects of the drug wear off, withdrawal symptoms occur, such as nervousness, insomnia, headaches, vomiting, chills, and cramps. In some cases, these symptoms can be severe enough to cause death.

- **Addiction.** Addiction is a physiological or psychological dependence on a drug. An addict continues to use a drug regularly and compulsively, even while knowing it to be harmful. Because addiction involves both psychological and physiological dependence, addicts have great difficulty ending their drug use on their own. Professional intervention is often necessary to help them stop using illegal drugs.

Reading Check

Explain How does tolerance affect a drug user?

Use of the illegal drug Ecstasy, a stimulant, causes structural and functional changes in the brain. **How can drugs affect your mental health?**

Drugs Take a Heavy Toll

MAIN IDEA In addition to its physical health risks, substance abuse can damage all aspects of your life.

Some people believe that drugs can help them escape from their problems. The reality is that drugs actually create more problems, which affect all aspects of the user's health. On top of that, the dangers of drug use are not limited to the user. Drug abuse can also harm the user's friends and family, as well as society as a whole.

Drug Use and the Brain

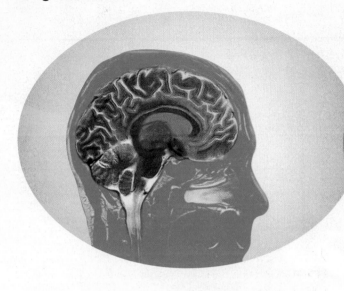

Drug use leads to changes in thinking and the lowering of inhibitions. **What effect could a lowering of inhibitions have on a teen's physical health?**

Consequences for the Individual

Taking drugs lowers inhibitions, which may lead teens to engage in behaviors that put their physical health at risk. For example, they may be more likely to engage in sexual activity. This could put them at risk for unplanned pregnancy or sexually transmitted diseases. They may also behave recklessly in other ways. Teen drug use can lead to increased violence, crime, and accidental death.

Drug use can affect teens' ability to pursue their interests and goals, as well as the goals their parents, teachers, and other adults set for them. Teens who are involved in drug use are more likely to be arrested, and teens who are convicted of a drug offense can be sent to jail. Drug use is also a leading factor in teen depression and suicide.

Consequences for the Family

When a teen abuses drugs, it affects everyone in that teen's life. Teens who use illegal drugs may lose interest in healthy activities. They may stop spending time with friends who value a drug-free lifestyle. Family members will also suffer. They will bear an emotional burden because they feel responsible for the teen and his or her drug use, as well as a financial burden in medical and legal costs.

Consequences for Others

Drug use always harmful, but when the user is a pregnant woman, the unborn child may suffer the most. A developing fetus receives nutrients through the mother's placenta. If a pregnant woman takes drugs, those drugs are passed to the fetus. These drugs have a greater effect on the body of the fetus than they do on the mother. The baby may be born with birth defects, behavioral problems, or a drug addiction. After birth, a nursing mother can still pass traces of drugs to the baby through her breast milk.

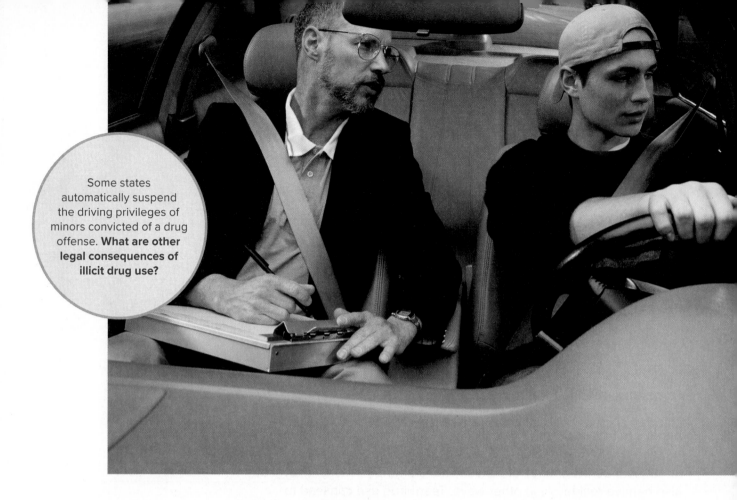

Some states automatically suspend the driving privileges of minors convicted of a drug offense. **What are other legal consequences of illicit drug use?**

Reading Check

Infer How can illicit drug use by one person affect people who do not use drugs?

Character Check

When you resist the pressure to use drugs, you demonstrate that you are responsible and that you have the courage to do the right thing. Join with friends to visit elementary schools. Share with younger students the positive behaviors and actions you use to stay drug free.

Consequences for Society

People who abuse drugs do not just harm themselves and the people who are close to them. They also cause damage to society as a whole. Illegal drug use can lead to drug-related crime and violence. Driving while intoxicated (DWI), also known as driving under the influence (DUI), can result in collisions that cause injuries and deaths.

Drug abuse also affects our nation's economy. Research by the Office of National Drug Control Policy shows that drug abuse costs this country an estimated $180 billion per year. These costs result from:

- lost work hours and productivity due to drug-related illnesses, jail time, accidents, and deaths.

- health care costs and legal fees.

- law enforcement costs and insurance costs due to drug-related damages, injuries, and deaths.

The consequences of drug abuse—mental, emotional, physical, legal, and social—are 100 percent preventable. By choosing a drug-free lifestyle, you avoid these consequences, both for yourself and for others.

Ryan McVay/Getty Images

Trends in Illegal Drug Use

Conduct an online search to determine whether the number of teens who have never used drugs is increasing or decreasing.

A good place to start your search is with the Centers for Disease Control and Prevention's website and searching for the most recent National Youth Risk Behavior Survey. Use websites that end with ".gov" to ensure that they are safe and remember to keep a list of the sources of your research.

Activity: Technology

Once you have found your information, complete the following activity:

1. Write a blog or create a podcast describing the factors that are influencing teens' choices not to use drugs.
2. Include information on the impact of drug use on the individual, family, friends, and the community.
3. Include information on the physical, mental/emotional, social, and legal consequences of drug use.
4. Present your blog or podcast to the class and possibly submit it to the school website.

Lesson 1 Review

Facts and Vocabulary

1. Define the term *overdose*.
2. Describe how an addiction can affect your health.
3. Explain how drug abuse affects society.

Thinking Critically

4. **Infer.** Why might an addiction to a drug become more expensive as the body develops a tolerance to the drug?
5. **Analyze.** Distinguish between *substance abuse* and *illicit drug use*. How are these terms similar? How are they different?

Applying Health Skills

6. **Accessing Information.** Conduct a survey of teens. Ask: What percentage of teens do you think use drugs? Compare your information to statistics from reliable sources. Create a poster presenting your information.

Writing Critically

7. **Persuasive.** Write a dialogue between you and a friend who is thinking about trying an illegal drug. Tell your friend the consequences of drug use.

Marijuana, Inhalants, and Steroids

BEFORE YOU READ

Create a Chart. Create a chart with three columns. Label the columns "Marijuana," "Inhalants," and "Steroids." As you read, list the physical, mental, and legal consequences of each.

Marijuana	Inhalants	Steroids

Vocabulary

marijuana
paranoia
inhalants
anabolic-androgenic steroids

BIG IDEA Three often-abused drugs that can have serious physical and mental side effects are marijuana, inhalants, and anabolic steroids.

REAL LIFE ISSUES

Driving While on Drugs. Studies by the CDC show that 16.5 percent of high school students had ridden with a driver who had been drinking alcohol. Fifteen percent of drivers aged 16–20 involved in fatal motor vehicle crashes had driven under the influence of an illegal substance. After alcohol, marijuana is the drug most often linked to drugged driving. *Write a paragraph that describes what can happen when driving under the influence of illegal drugs.*

After completing the lesson, review and analyze your response to the Real Life Issues question.

Marijuana

MAIN IDEA Using marijuana has serious physical, mental, social, and legal consequences.

Every day, you make choices based on the information that is available to you. Before deciding to see a particular movie, you may read a review. Before deciding what to eat, you might read the list of ingredients. Drugs such as marijuana may be mixed with unknown chemicals and have unexpected effects on your health. Even when you are certain of the source of a drug, using it —or even misusing it—can cause serious harm to your health.

Many states decriminalized the use of **marijuana**, a plant whose leaves, buds, and flowers are usually smoked for their intoxicating effects. In these states, a person will not be charged with a crime if he or she is found carrying less than one ounce of marijuana. Other states have passed laws legalizing the use of marijuana for medical purposes. However, a prescription from a doctor is required to purchase marijuana from an authorized medical marijuana retailer. Despite these changes to laws affecting the use of marijuana, it is still illegal for anyone under the age of 21 to use marijuana or carry any amount of the substance. It is also illegal for anyone to use marijuana in public or to drive while under the intoxicating effects of marijuana.

Health Risks of Marijuana

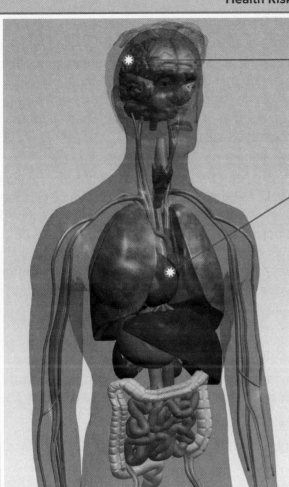

- Hallucinations and paranoia
- Impaired short-term memory, reaction time, concentration, and coordination

- Lung irritation, coughing
- Heart and lung damage
- Increased risk of lung cancer
- Weakened immunity to infection

- Increased appetite
- Increased risk of stillbirth and birth defects
- Changed hormone levels
- In females, risk of infertility
- In males, lowered sperm count and testosterone levels

The effects of marijuana use varies from person to person, and can be influenced by a person's mood and surroundings.

Marijuana is considered a possible *gateway drug*, a drug that may lead the user to try other drugs. All forms of marijuana are mind-altering and can damage the user's health. This is particularly true if marijuana use begins during the teen years. A New Zealand study shows that teens who are heavy users of marijuana lost an average of 8 IQ points between ages 13 and 38.

Physical Consequences of Marijuana Use

Because marijuana is often smoked, users face the same health risks as tobacco smokers. In fact, marijuana smoke contains more cancer-causing chemicals than tobacco smoke.

Medical evidence shows that a compound in marijuana named delta-9-tetrahydrocannabinol, or THC, does reduce the pain and nausea caused by illnesses such as cancer and HIV/AIDS. However, the FDA has approved drugs that deliver THC without the other health risks associated with marijuana use.

Smoking marijuana can also damage the immune system. This makes the user more susceptible to infections. Marijuana poses risks to reproductive health as well. In males, it interferes with sperm production and lowers levels of the male hormone testosterone. In females, by contrast, marijuana raises testosterone levels. This may lead to infertility (the inability to have children).

Mental and Emotional Consequences

Marijuana raises levels of a brain chemical called *dopamine* that produces feelings of pleasure. In some users, marijuana triggers the release of so much dopamine that the user reaches a state of **intense** well-being or elation, known as a "high." When the drug wears off, however, the sensation of pleasure stops, often suddenly. This abrupt letdown is called a "crash."

Marijuana users may experience slowed mental reflexes. Their perception may be distorted, and they may have trouble with thinking and problem solving. Loss of coordination is also common. Users may feel dizzy or have trouble walking. They may also suffer from sudden feelings of anxiety and **paranoia**. Paranoia is an irrational suspiciousness or distrust of others. A few hours after using marijuana, the user can become very sleepy. Also, people using marijuana often have a hard time remembering what has just happened. This short-term memory loss can lead to problems at school and at work.

Mental Effects

- Hallucinations and paranoia
- Impaired short-term memory, reaction time, concentration, and coordination

Heart and Lung Effects

- Lung irritation, coughing
- Heart and lung damage
- Increased risk of lung cancer

Reproductive Effects

- Changed hormone levels
- Increased risk of stillbirth and birth defects
- In females, risk of infertility
- In males, lowered sperm count and testosterone levels

Other Effects

- Increased appetite
- Weakened immunity to infection

Driving and Marijuana Use

Marijuana's mental effects can be deadly if the person gets behind the wheel of a vehicle. The drug interferes with depth perception, increases reaction time, impairs judgment, causes sleepiness, and slows reflexes. The National Highway Traffic Safety Administration (NHTSA) estimates that more than 10 million drivers involved in car crashes were on drugs.

The penalties for driving under the influence of any drug—including marijuana—include suspension of a driver's license, fines, loss of eligibility for federal college loans, and possibly a jail term. If a driver under the influence kills or injures another person, the driver may face still more serious legal penalties, as well as devastating emotional consequences.

Inhalants

MAIN IDEA Inhalants can cause the death of brain cells.

Inhalants are substances whose fumes are sniffed or inhaled to give effect. The category of drugs known as inhalants includes some drugs that are prescribed legally to treat medical conditions such as allergies and asthma. However, the term refers more often to non-medical substances that are inhaled to achieve a high. These substances include solvents, aerosols, glues, paints, varnishes, and gasoline.

Most inhalants suppress the central nervous system. Immediate effects include a glassy stare, slurred speech, impaired judgment, and lack of coordination. Nausea, coughing, nosebleeds, and fatigue are also common. Long-term use can cause liver and kidney damage, blindness, brain damage, paralysis, cardiac arrest, and death.

All inhalants are extremely dangerous, and many are labeled as poisons. Inhalants are harmful even if you are not trying to abuse them. It is possible to inhale the fumes by accident while doing household chores. When using these chemicals, always work in a well-ventilated room. If a project requires long exposure to the fumes, wear a mask.

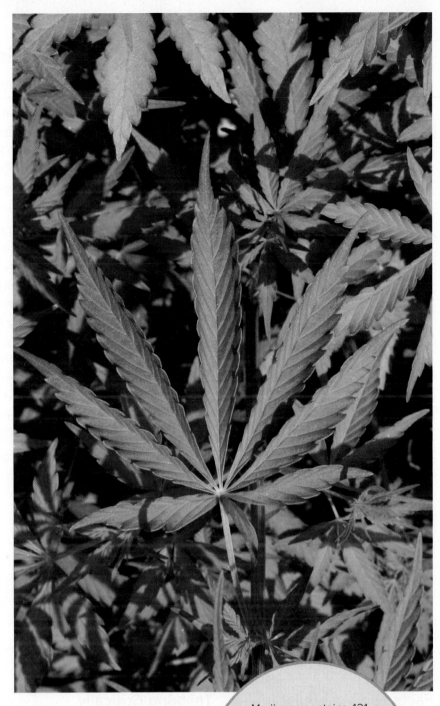

Marijuana contains 421 different chemicals. The main psychoactive ingredient, THC (delta-9-tetrahydrocannabinol), is stored in body fat, and traces of it can be present in the blood for as long as a month. **Why could a marijuana user fail a drug test weeks after using the drug?**

● ● ● ● ● ● ● ● ●

Reading Check

Explain Where does the term *anabolic-androgenic steroids* come from?

● ● ● ● ● ● ● ● ● ● ●

Myths & Reality

Most people understand the dangers of illegal drugs. How much do you know about illegal drugs, like marijuana?

Myth: The effects of marijuana on memory are temporary.

Reality: People normally lose neurons in the hippocampus over time. Chronic marijuana use may speed up that process.

● ● ● ● ● ● ● ● ● ● ●

Consequences of Steroid Use

MAIN IDEA Steroids can cause severe health problems.

Although other types of medicines are called *steroids,* the term is most often used to refer to **anabolic-androgenic steroids**. These are synthetic substances similar to male sex hormones. *Anabolic* refers to muscle building, and *androgenic* refers to increased male characteristics. Steroids may be prescribed for some medical conditions, but using steroids without medical supervision is dangerous.

Steroid use can result in unnatural muscle growth. When combined with physical conditioning, steroids can increase muscle strength. However, the tendons and ligaments do not get stronger, making injuries more likely. Other side effects include weight gain, high blood pressure, and liver and kidney tumors. Steroid users who inject the drug may contract HIV or hepatitis B. These drugs may also cause violent behavior, extreme mood swings, depression, and paranoia. In males, steroids may shrink the testicles, reduce sperm count, cause baldness or development of breasts, and increase the risk for prostate cancer. In females, they may cause baldness, development of facial hair, changes in the menstrual cycle, and a deepened voice.

Any nonmedical use of steroids is illegal. Athletes who use steroids risk being expelled from a team or from an event. They may also face monetary fines, tarnished reputation, and possible jail time.

Lesson 2 Review

Facts and Vocabulary

1. List three of the body systems that are harmed by using marijuana.

2. Define the term *inhalants*.

3. Explain how using steroids to increase muscle strength may result in injury.

Thinking Critically

4. **Infer.** Marijuana users often inhale the smoke very deeply and hold it in their lungs longer than cigarette smokers do. How might this practice make marijuana more dangerous than smoking tobacco?

5. **Compare.** How do the effects of steroids differ in males and females?

Applying Health Skills

6. **Accessing Information.** Research reliable sources to learn more about the dangers of accidentally or purposefully inhaling chemicals. Create a poster showing how inhalants can affect your physical health.

Writing Critically

7. **Persuasive.** Write a public service announcement describing the dangers of driving while under the influence of marijuana.

Psychoactive Drugs

BIG IDEA Psychoactive drugs affect the central nervous system and can be especially damaging to the developing brain and body of a teen.

REAL LIFE ISSUES

Skip This "Trip." Baseball season was finally underway. Alex's team won their first game, so they felt it was time to celebrate. Members of the team are invited to a party by Bob, a guy that Alex just met. Alex has heard that the parties Bob hosts can get a little wild. Bob tells Alex they will have LSD at the party, and encourages him to try some. "It's awesome," says Bob. "No thanks," says Alex. "I'm not into drugs." *Write a paragraph that describes at least three safe activities that can give your body a physical adrenaline rush or stimulate the senses without the use of illegal drugs.*

After completing the lesson, review and analyze your response to the Real Life Issues question.

Effects of Psychoactive Drugs

MAIN IDEA Psychoactive drugs change the functioning of the central nervous system.

The central nervous system (CNS) is amazingly complex. Every human activity, from bending a finger to solving complicated problems, involves the CNS. **Psychoactive drugs** are chemicals that change the way the CNS functions and alter activity in the brain. These drugs fall into four main categories: stimulants, depressants, opiates, and hallucinogens.

Some psychoactive drugs have medicinal value. However, misusing or abusing these drugs can seriously affect the functioning of all the body's systems. The effects on a teen's developing brain and body can be especially damaging. Psychoactive drug use can result in a wide range of health problems, including addiction. Using psychoactive drugs can also impair judgment, leading to risky behavior. This, in turn, may put teens at risk for unintentional injuries, violence, STDs, unintended pregnancy, and suicide. By choosing a drug-free lifestyle, you can protect yourself from all these risks to your health.

BEFORE YOU READ

Make Flash Cards. As you read the lesson, write each vocabulary term on the front of an index card. Write the definition on the back of each card. Use the cards to quiz a partner on the terms and their meanings.

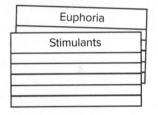

Euphoria
Stimulants

Vocabulary
psychoactive drugs
designer drug
hallucinogens
euphoria
opiates

Health Risks of Psychoactive Drugs

Type of Drug	Consequences to Your Health
Stimulants	
Amphetamines	• Decreased appetite, weight loss, malnutrition • High blood pressure, rapid heartbeat, heart failure, death • Aggressiveness, increased tolerance, addiction
Cocaine	• Nausea, abdominal pain, malnutrition, headache, stroke, seizure, heart attack, death • Exposure to HIV through contaminated needles, addiction
Crack	• Extreme addiction with the same consequences as cocaine • Rapid increase in heart rate and blood pressure, death
Methamphetamine *(Meth)*	• Memory loss, heart and nerve damage • Increased tolerance, addiction
Depressants	
Barbiturates	• Fatigue, confusion, impaired muscle coordination • Reduced heart rate, blood pressure, respiratory function, death
GHB	• Drowsiness, nausea, vomiting, loss of consciousness • Impaired breathing, coma, death
Rohypnol *(roofies)*	• Decreased blood pressure, drowsiness, memory loss, gastrointestinal disturbances
Tranquilizers	• Depression, fever, irritability, loss of judgment, dizziness
Opiates	
Codeine	• Reduced respiratory function, respiratory arrest, death • Exposure to HIV through contaminated needles, addiction
Heroin	• Confusion, sedation, unconsciousness, coma, addiction
Morphine	• Rapid onset of tolerance, addiction
Opium	• Nausea, constipation, addiction
Oxycodone *(OxyContin®)*	• Drowsiness, nausea, constipation, addiction • Reduced respiratory function, respiratory arrest, death
Hallucinogens	
DXM *(tussin)*	• Nausea, dizziness, lack of coordination, rashes • Hallucinations, disorientation, paranoia, panic attacks, seizures
Ecstasy *(MDMA)*	• Confusion, depression, paranoia, muscle breakdown
Ketamine	• Kidney and cardiovascular system failure, death • Memory loss, numbness, impaired motor function
LSD	• Delusions, illusions, hallucinations, flashbacks, numbness, tremors
Mescaline *(peyote)*	• Delusions, illusions, hallucinations, flashbacks, numbness, tremors
PCP	• Loss of appetite, depression, panic, aggression, violent actions
Psilocybin *(mushrooms)*	• Delusions, illusions, hallucinations, paranoia, extreme anxiety, nausea

Club Drugs, Stimulants, and Depressants

MAIN IDEA Club drugs, stimulants, and depressants can cause irreversible health damage.

Some drugs are classified according to their effects. For example, some drugs speed up or slow down the senses, while others affect judgment. Other drugs, such as club drugs, are grouped together based on the settings in which they are used.

Club Drugs

The term *club drugs* refers to various drugs found at concerts and clubs. These drugs can be disguised in foods or slipped into drinks and taken without a person's knowledge. Many club drugs are **designer drugs**, synthetic drugs that are made to imitate the effects of other drugs. Designer drugs can be several hundred times stronger than the drugs they imitate.

Ecstasy (MDMA). Ecstasy, or MDMA, has both stimulant and hallucinogenic effects. **Hallucinogens** are drugs that alter moods, thoughts, and sense perceptions, including vision, hearing, smell, and touch. Ecstasy may cause short-term **euphoria**, a feeling of intense well-being or elation.

Rohypnol. Rohypnol, or "roofies," is a depressant, or sedative. It is also known as the "date-rape drug." Because it is colorless, odorless, and tasteless, it can often be slipped into someone's drink, making that person an easy target for a sexual attack. Victims are at risk for unplanned pregnancy and exposure to STDs, including HIV. Giving anyone a drug without that person's knowledge, or engaging in sexual activity with a person under the influence of a date-rape drug, is a crime.

GHB. GHB, or gamma hydroxybutyric acid, is another CNS depressant. It is **available** as a clear liquid, as a white powder, and in a variety of capsules and tablets. Like Rohypnol, it can be used as a date-rape drug.

Purple Drank or Sizzurp. This drug is another depressant. Prescription cough syrup containing codeine is an ingredient. Users can become addicted and can overdose, possibly leading to death.

Ketamine. Ketamine is an anesthetic used to treat animals. It causes hallucinations and may result in respiratory failure.

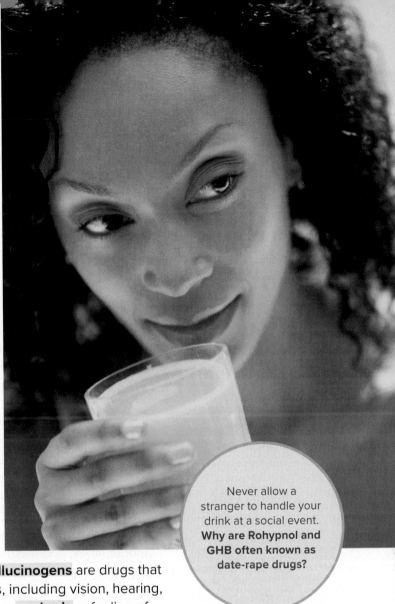

Never allow a stranger to handle your drink at a social event. **Why are Rohypnol and GHB often known as date-rape drugs?**

- - - - - - - - - -

Reading Check

Apply What should you do if you are at a party where people are taking psychoactive drugs?

- - - - - - - - - -

ACADEMIC VOCABULARY

available *(adjective)*: present or ready for immediate use

- - - - - - - - - -

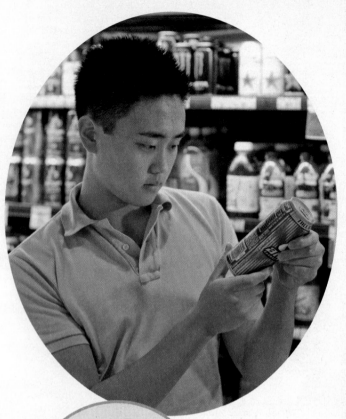

Meth. Methamphetamine, or meth, is a stimulant. Meth is a white, odorless powder that easily dissolves in alcohol or water. Because its nonmedical form is produced in makeshift labs, the drug is readily available but its quality is uncertain. Meth may provide a short-term feeling of euphoria, but often its use also causes depression, paranoia, and delusions. Its use can lead to death.

LSD (Acid). Lysergic acid diethylamide (LSD), or "acid," is a hallucinogen. Users may experience emotions ranging from extreme euphoria to panic, terror, or deep depression. The resulting behaviors may lead to serious injury or death. People who have used LSD may later experience *flashbacks,* in which the emotional effects of the drug reappear long after its actual use.

Other Stimulants

Stimulants speed up the CNS. You may have used some stimulants in the past without even knowing it. The nicotine in tobacco products, for instance, is a powerful stimulant. The caffeine in coffee, tea, cola, and power drinks is also a stimulant. "Energy" or "power" drinks often pack four to ten times the amount of caffeine found in a regular-sized cola. However, other stimulants—such as cocaine, amphetamines, and meth—are illegal and extremely dangerous.

Cocaine. Cocaine is a white powder extracted from the leaves of the coca plant. It is a rapidly acting, powerful, and extremely addictive stimulant. Users may experience a surge of self-confidence and euphoria, followed by an emotional letdown as the drug wears off. Regular cocaine use can lead to depression, fatigue, paranoia, and physiological dependence. Cocaine use can also cause malnutrition and, especially among teens, may result in heart problems. Many cocaine users inject the drug, putting themselves at risk for HIV or hepatitis B from infected needles. An overdose of cocaine can cause death.

Crack. An even more dangerous form of cocaine is crack, also called *rock* or *freebase rock.* Crack reaches the brain in seconds after being smoked or injected. Once in the blood, it causes the heart rate and blood pressure to soar to dangerous levels. Death may result from cardiac or respiratory failure. Mixing crack (or any drug) with alcohol can be fatal. These substances combine in the liver, increasing the risk of death from liver failure.

Amphetamines. Amphetamines are highly addictive stimulants. Some people use them to stay alert, to improve athletic performance, or to lose weight. It is easy to develop a tolerance for these drugs. This can lead the user to take them in ever-increasing amounts. Regular use can result in an irregular heartbeat, paranoia, aggressive behavior, and heart failure.

"Energy drinks" often have so much caffeine that their labels must warn pregnant women and people with high blood pressure not to drink them. **Why is the small serving size of a typical energy drink misleading?**

· · · · · · · · · · · · · ·

Reading Check

Identify Name two legal stimulants that are commonly used.

· · · · · · · · · · · · · ·

Tim Fuller Photography

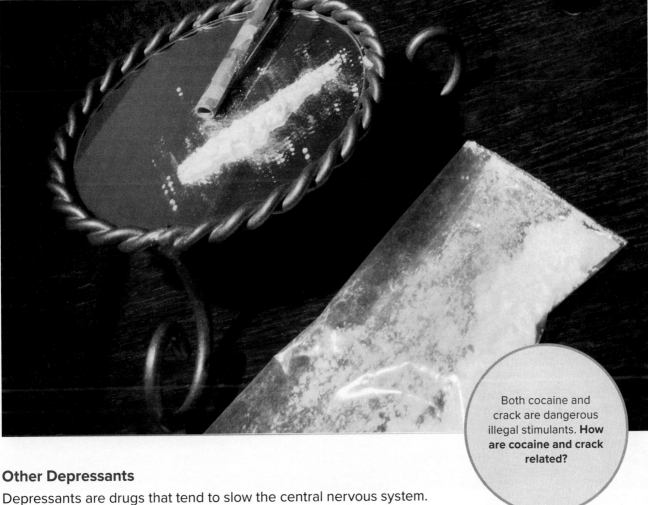

Both cocaine and crack are dangerous illegal stimulants. **How are cocaine and crack related?**

Other Depressants

Depressants are drugs that tend to slow the central nervous system. Alcohol is one commonly used depressant. These drugs are dangerous because they slow heart and breathing rates and lower blood pressure. Combining small amounts of different depressants can cause shallow breathing, weak or rapid pulse, coma, and death.

Barbiturates. Barbiturates are sedatives that are rarely used for medical purposes. Using barbiturates can cause mood changes, excessive sleepiness, and coma. Users may feel intoxicated. Combining these drugs with alcohol can be fatal.

Tranquilizers. Tranquilizers are depressants that relieve anxiety, muscle spasms, and sleeplessness. When they are overused, they can cause physiological and psychological dependence, coma, and death.

Hallucinogens and Opiates

MAIN IDEA Hallucinogens and opiates seriously alter the sensory controls in the brain.

Psychoactive drugs can seriously damage the sections of the brain that interpret input from your senses. Hallucinogens overload the brain's sensory controls. Opiates cause confusion and dull the senses. They are also highly addictive in any form.

Reading Check

Explain Why can combining depressants be dangerous?

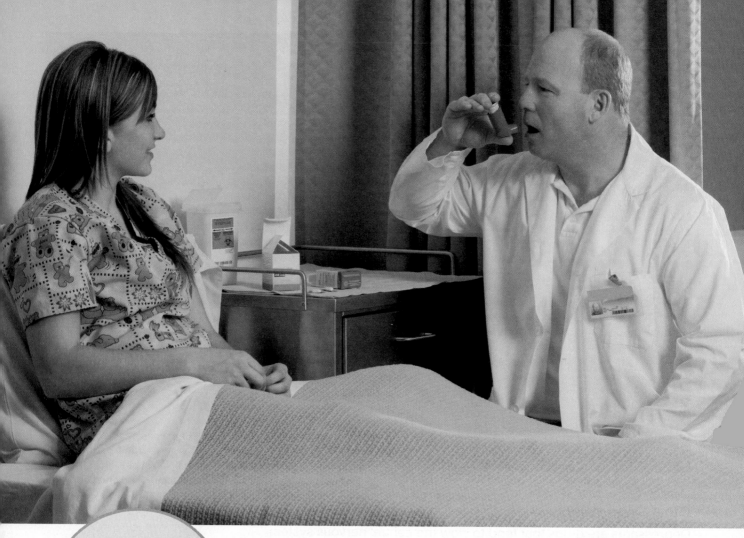

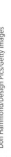

Talk to your doctor or pharmacist about any prescription medications that you are given. **Why is it important for pharmacists to keep records of all sales of opiates?**

· · · · · · · · · · · ·

Reading Check

Apply Why are hallucinogens sometimes fatal?

· · · · · · · · · · · ·

Hallucinogens

Ecstasy, ketamine, acid (LSD), phencyclidine (PCP or angel dust), dextromethorphan (DXM), psilocybin (mushrooms), and mescaline (peyote) are all examples of powerful and dangerous hallucinogens. These drugs overload the sensory controls in the brain, causing confusion, intensified sensations, and hallucinations. This altered mental state can last for several hours or several days. Users may later experience flashbacks, feeling the emotional effects of these drugs long after their actual use.

Hallucinogens can cause serious physical, mental, and emotional harm to users. The effects of these drugs are extremely unpredictable. They alter mood and impair judgment, thoughts, and sense perception, sometimes causing users to behave in ways they normally would not. People using these drugs may believe that they are invincible (immune to harm). Users sometimes harm themselves physically, or behave violently and harm others. Using these drugs can also raise pulse and breathing rates. This can lead to heart or respiratory failure. These drugs may also induce a coma. Most hallucinogens have no medical uses.

PCP. PCP, or angel dust, is one of the most dangerous of all drugs, and its effects vary greatly from user to user. The drug creates a distorted sense of time, increased muscle strength, increased feelings of violence, and the inability to feel pain. Overdoses can cause death, but most PCP-related deaths are caused by the confusion and destructive behavior that the drug produces. For example, PCP users have died in fires because they became disoriented and were unable to feel the pain of burning. Flashbacks can occur at any time, causing pain, confusion, and lack of control.

DXM. DXM, or "tussin," is a cough suppressant sold as an over-the-counter medicine. When used in the recommended dosage, DXM is not dangerous. When misused, it can cause hallucinations, paranoia, panic attacks, nausea, increased heart rate and blood pressure, and addiction.

Mushrooms and Peyote. Psilocybin (mushrooms) and mescaline (peyote cactus) are two hallucinogens found in nature. When eaten, they cause hallucinations, nausea, and flashbacks. Use of these drugs can also lead to poisoning and death when dealers harvest toxic species.

Opiates

Opiates, or narcotics, are drugs such as those derived from the opium plant that are obtainable only by prescription and are used to relieve pain. They include codeine, morphine, oxycodone, and fentanyl. When these drugs are used as prescribed by a health care professional, they are effective pain relievers. In general, these drugs are prescribed to patients who have had surgery. They should be taken for a short time only, and under a doctor's care.

Abusing opiates dulls the senses and can cause drowsiness, constipation, slow and shallow breathing, convulsions, coma, and death. Pharmacists record all sales of opiates because these drugs are addictive.

Codeine. Codeine is a highly addictive ingredient in some prescription painkillers and cough medicines. Even when used exactly as prescribed, the drug can cause drowsiness. For this reason, people taking it should not drive. Codeine use can cause dizziness, labored breathing, low blood pressure, seizures, and respiratory arrest.

Some people may be allergic to codeine. In these individuals, the drug can cause breathing difficulties or mood changes. Codeine has also been linked to death in infants. The CDC has issued a warning against giving any medications containing codeine to infants or small children. If you or someone you know experiences a problem after taking codeine, call 911 immediately.

Morphine. Morphine is a much stronger drug than codeine. It is sometimes prescribed to treat severe pain, but it is generally used only for a short time. Side effects include fast or slow heartbeat, seizures, hallucinations, blurred vision, rashes, and difficulty swallowing.

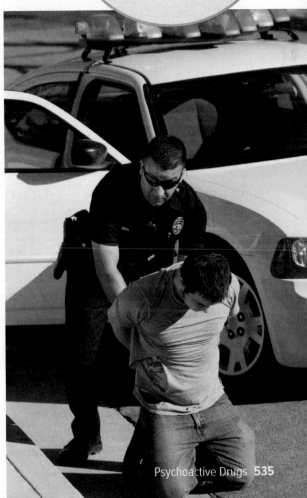

One common effect of meth use is delusions of bugs crawling on the user's skin. As a result, many meth users scratch and pick at their skin until they develop unsightly sores. **What other physical effects can meth use cause?**

Fitness Zone

My "drug" is my favorite sport: running. I don't need to get high on any illegal substance, because when I go for a run, I get all the benefits of a good workout and it makes me feel great. I challenge myself to improve every day, and in the end I have something to be proud of. Keeping my brain and body in top condition for running is the best thing I can do to stay healthy.

• • • • • • • • • • •

Oxycodone. When used properly under the supervision of a doctor, oxycodone is a prescription drug that helps relieve moderate to severe chronic pain. It is often referred to by the brand name OxyContin®. Oxycodone contains a strong opiate. A side effect of this drug is suppression of the respiratory system, which can cause death from respiratory failure.

People can misuse prescription opiates by taking the medicine in a dose other than prescribed, taking someone else's prescription medicine, or taking it to feel its effects even if a person is not experiencing pain. Repeated misuse of prescription opiates can lead to addiction.

Heroin. Heroin is an illegal drug. It is a processed form of morphine that may be injected, snorted, or smoked. Heroin comes in many forms, including a white or brownish powder and a black, sticky tar. Dealers may mix heroin with medicines or household substances to create other forms, such as "cheese heroin."

Heroin slows breathing and pulse rate. It can also cause infection of the heart lining and valves, as well as liver disease. Infected needles used to inject this drug can spread diseases such as HIV and hepatitis B. Large doses can cause coma or death, and fetal death if the user is pregnant. Sometimes, fentanyl is mixed with heroin. Misuse of fentanyl can result in slowed or stopped breathing, unconsciousness, and death.

Several studies have found a link between the misuse of prescription opiates and the use of heroin. The data from a 2011 study showed that about 80 percent of people who used heroin had first misused prescription opiates. Between 1999 and 2018, about 450,000 people in the U.S. died from an overdose involving opiates. Currently, the Centers for Disease Control and Prevention is working with state and local health departments across the U.S. to help respond to and prevent overdoses.

Lesson 3 Review

Facts and Vocabulary

1. Identify the body system that is affected by *psychoactive drugs*.

2. Name the four types of drugs described in this lesson and give an example of each.

3. Define the term *opiates*.

Thinking Critically

4. **Evaluate.** An acquaintance offers you a drug that she says is natural. Does this mean it is safe to take? Why or why not?

5. **Apply.** Why is it important to follow directions from your doctor or pharmacist when taking a prescription drug such as codeine?

Applying Health Skills

6. **Advocacy.** Research the different types of designer drugs, the forms they take, and how they affect health. Use what you have learned to design a website that warns about the dangers of these drugs.

Writing Critically

7. **Narrative.** Write a script convincing a friend not to try drugs. Include data on the harmful effects and health consequences of drug use.

Living Drug-Free

BIG IDEA By deciding not to use drugs, you promote your own health and influence others to do the same.

REAL LIFE ISSUES

A Sister's Advice. When Penny arrives home, her younger sister is sitting outside, crying. "Lisa, what happened?" asks Penny. "A girl at the recreation center offered me drugs," Lisa says. "I didn't know what to do, so I just ran off." Penny gives Lisa a comforting hug. "Sounds like you did the right thing," she assures her. Lisa looks up, her eyes red. "But they're going to make fun of me at school on Monday," she says. "Maybe so," replies Penny, "but would they make fun of you for eating right and working out? I always tell people who offer me drugs that I'm an athlete, and I'm not into that." *Make a list of reasons to say no to drug use.*

After completing the lesson, review and analyze your response to the Real Life Issues question.

Resisting Pressure to Use Drugs

MAIN IDEA Most teens never experiment with illegal drugs.

Peer pressure can be intense during the teen years. When the subject of drug use comes up, you may be told that "everybody's doing it." The fact is, that's not true. Most teens never experiment with illegal drugs. Almost 62 percent of high school students have never tried marijuana, and more than 90 percent have never used cocaine. By deciding to stay drug-free, you protect your health and become a role model to others.

Committing to Be Drug Free

You may feel unsure about saying no to drug use. If your friends put pressure on you to use drugs, however, you may need to ask yourself if they're really your friends. Would a true friend try to make you do something that could hurt you, or something that goes against your values? If you are committed to remaining drug-free, choose friends who share your attitude about drug use, and avoid places where drugs are available. Even a teen who has used drugs in the past can choose to avoid them in the future.

BEFORE YOU READ

Create an Outline. Preview this lesson by scanning the pages. Then, organize the headings and subheadings into an outline. As you read, fill in the outline with important details.

I.	
	A.
	1.
	2.
	B.
II.	

Vocabulary

drug-free school zone
drug watches
rehabilitation

Reading Check

Apply What can you say to someone who pressures you to use drugs by telling you that "everybody's doing it"?

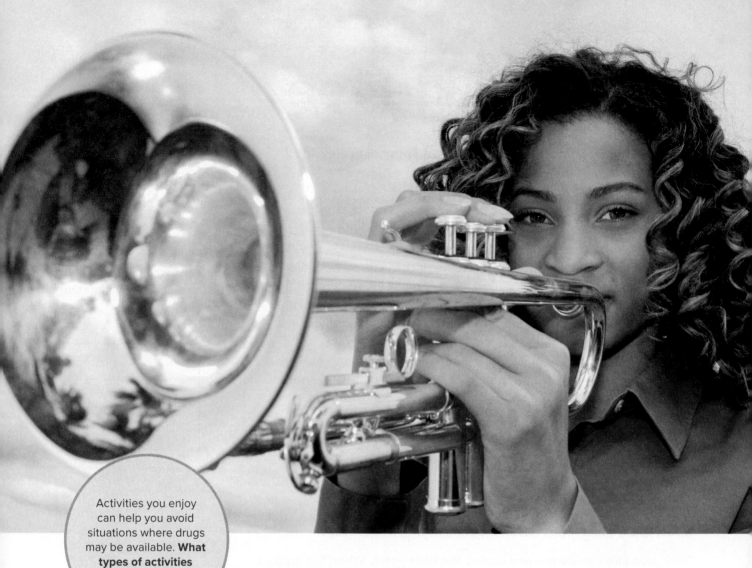

Activities you enjoy can help you avoid situations where drugs may be available. **What types of activities would you choose?**

Refusal skills can help you say no to drugs. You may feel more comfortable if you think of and practice refusal statements ahead of time. Examples of refusal statements include:

- "No thanks, I don't do drugs."

- "I can't. I'm on medication."

- "I'm not interested. That stuff makes me sick."

- "No, I need to be in shape for tomorrow's game."

Healthy Alternatives

Taking part in drug-free activities can help you avoid the dangers of drug use. It can also help build your self-esteem, reinforce your values, and make new friends who can become drug-free role models. Here are a few activities that can provide healthy alternatives to drug use:

- Hobbies, such as photography, cooking, art, or music

- Physical activity, including outdoor recreation, team sports, and individual sports

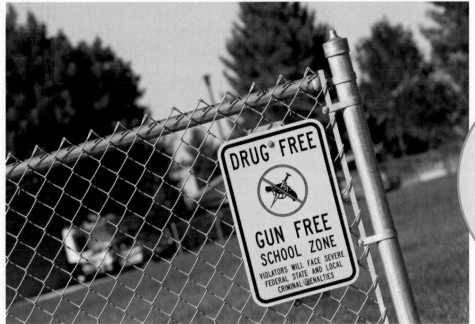

The penalties for using, selling, or possessing drugs in a drug-free school zone are more severe than in other areas. **How far from a school is the border of a typical drug-free school zone?**

- Community activities, such as neighborhood events, political movements, community service, religious activities, and local clubs
- School organizations, including service groups, honor societies, and advocacy groups

Drug Prevention Efforts

MAIN IDEA Schools and communities are working together to support students in their efforts to be drug-free.

Drugs are not just a problem for the people who use them. All of society pays the price for the increased crime, violence, and health care costs that go with drug use. Everyone can help reduce this problem by committing to remain drug-free. In addition, schools and communities are providing ways to help young people avoid drugs.

School Efforts

Near schools, **drug-free school zones** have been established. Within these areas, penalties are often double what they might be for the same drug offense committed elsewhere. Other school efforts to eliminate drug use include drug education classes, zero-tolerance policies, and the expulsion of students found using drugs. Some schools conduct locker searches and maintain police patrols on campus.

Reading Check

Contrast How are some of the penalties for illicit drug use in a drug-free school zone more severe than in other areas?

Community Efforts

Communities across the nation are taking action to prevent drug abuse. One action many communities have taken is to organize **drug watches**. Anti-drug programs in your neighborhood can help protect you, your family and friends, and your entire community from the dangers associated with drug abuse. What if you suspect that someone is abusing drugs at school or in the community? Tell a trusted adult, such as your teacher or your parent or guardian.

Becoming Drug-Free

MAIN IDEA Many types of counseling are available for those who want to become drug-free.

Drug abuse is a treatable condition. However, most drug users need the help of family, friends, or counseling to end their addiction. If a friend or family member shows signs like these, use the list of steps below as a guide to offer help:

- Identify sources of help in your community.

- Talk to the person when he or she is sober. Express your affection and concern, and describe the person's behavior without being judgmental.

- Listen to the person's response. Be prepared for anger and denial.

Warning Signs of Drug Use

The following behaviors may indicate that a person has a drug problem:

- Lies about the drugs he or she is using, constantly talks about drugs

- Stops participating in activities that once were an important part of his or her life

- Changes eating or sleeping habits, shows rapid weight loss

- Takes unnecessary risks, participates in unsafe behaviors

- Gets in trouble with authorities, such as school administrators or police

- Seems withdrawn, depressed, tired, and cares less about appearance

- Has red-rimmed eyes and runny nose not related to colds or allergies

- Has blackouts and forgets what he or she did under the influence

- Has difficulty concentrating

Getting Help

Drug treatment centers offer a safe place to withdraw from drug use and begin **rehabilitation**. Many of these centers provide medications to help with the physical and psychological affects of withdrawal. Types of drug treatment centers include:

- **Outpatient drug-free treatment.** These programs usually do not include medications and often use individual or group counseling.

- **Short-term treatment.** These centers can include residential therapy, medication, and outpatient therapy.

- **Maintenance therapy.** Intended for heroin addicts, this treatment usually includes medication therapy.

- **Therapeutic communities.** These are residences for drug abusers. The centers include highly structured programs that may last from 6 to 12 months.

Drug counselors can also help people **adjust** to a life without drugs. Some counselors use behavioral change strategies to help people become drug-free. These strategies include avoiding people who supply or use the drug, practicing refusal skills, and filling free time with planned, healthy activities.

Former drug users may also attend support groups. These meetings are gatherings of people who share a common problem. These groups provide the long-term support that recovering users need to remain drug-free, in addition to the support of their families.

. . . .

ACADEMIC VOCABULARY

adjust *(verb)*: to bring to a more satisfactory state

. . . .

Lesson 4 Review

Facts and Vocabulary

1. List three healthy alternatives to using drugs.

2. Define the term *drug-free school zone*.

3. Describe *rehabilitation*.

Thinking Critically

4. **Analyze.** Why is it important to commit to being drug-free before drugs are offered to you?

5. **Apply.** Former drug users try to fill their free time with healthy activities. What kinds of healthy activities could a former user try in order to remain drug-free?

Applying Health Skills

6. **Practicing Healthful Behaviors.** List five healthy alternatives to drug use, and share your ideas with the class.

Writing Critically

7. **Narrative.** Write a short story about someone who has stopped using drugs. Describe the types of community resources that provide help.

LESSON 1

Vocabulary Review

Use the correct vocabulary term to complete the following statements.

1. Drug users often find it difficult to stop using drugs without help because _____ involves both psychological and physiological dependence.

2. _____ is any unnecessary or improper use of chemical substances for nonmedical purposes.

3. Taking more than the recommended amount of a prescription drug can lead to serious health problems or even death from a(n) _____.

Understanding Key Concepts

After reading the question or statement, select the correct answer.

4. Which of the following is not usually a factor in deciding to use an illegal drug?
   a. Peer pressure at school
   b. The original source of the drug
   c. How role models live their lives
   d. Messages on television and in movies

5. Which of the following can be a negative consequence of drug use?
   a. Temporary euphoria
   b. Decrease in tolerance
   c. Contraction of an STD
   d. Strengthened refusal skills

Thinking Critically

After reading the question or statement, write a short answer using complete sentences.

6. **Infer.** How might the legal consequences of drug use interfere with a teen's future educational and career goals?

7. **Analyze.** How can illicit drug use affect you if you and your friends do not use drugs?

LESSON 2

Vocabulary Review

Choose the correct term in the sentences below.

8. *Paranoia/Marijuana* is an irrational suspiciousness or distrust of others.

9. Using *anabolic-androgenic steroids/ inhalants* leads to loss of brain cells.

10. *Anabolic-androgenic steroids/Inhalants* can increase muscle strength but not tendon and ligament strength, and causes injuries.

Understanding Key Concepts

After reading the question or statement, select the correct answer.

11. Which consequence of using marijuana can lead to reproductive system problems?
    a. Increased appetite
    b. Feelings of paranoia
    c. Heart and lung damage
    d. Changes in testosterone level

12. Which substance has a legal medical use when used as an inhalant?
    a. Gasoline
    b. Nitrous oxide
    c. Solvent
    d. Varnish

13. Which drugs are not usually taken in through the respiratory system?
    a. Aerosols
    b. Anabolic-androgenic steroids
    c. Marijuana
    d. Nitrous oxide

Thinking Critically

After reading the question or statement, write a short answer using complete sentences.

14. **Analyze.** How could using marijuana harm your social interactions with friends?

15. **Infer.** Why might it be difficult for law enforcement officials to discover and prevent illegal inhalant use?

16. **Extend.** If an athlete chooses to use steroids to increase muscle mass, how does this perceived benefit actually turn out to be a negative consequence?

LESSON 3

Vocabulary Review

Choose the correct word in the sentences below.

17. *Stimulants/Depressants* speed up the central nervous system.

18. Drugs that cause *euphoria/hallucinations* give users a temporary feeling of intense well-being.

19. *Opiates/Hallucinogens* are often obtainable by prescription, but are heavily monitored because they can cause serious addiction.

Understanding Key Concepts

After reading the question or statement, select the correct answer.

20. Which type of psychoactive drug is best known for altering sense perceptions?
    a. Depressants
    b. Hallucinogens
    c. Opiates
    d. Stimulants

21. Which type of psychoactive drug is used medically to block pain messages to the brain?
    a. Depressants
    b. Hallucinogens
    c. Opiates
    d. Stimulants

22. Which hallucinogen is classified as a designer drug?
    a. DXM
    b. LSD
    c. MDMA
    d. PCP

23. Why are Rohypnol and GHB linked to exposure to STDs?
    a. They are highly addictive.
    b. They can be used as date-rape drugs.
    c. They are usually taken intravenously.
    d. They affect the body's immune response.

Thinking Critically

After reading the question or statement, write a short answer using complete sentences.

24. **Infer.** Dangerous drugs are often even more dangerous when mixed together. Why might a drug user take a depressant after taking a stimulant?

25. **Evaluate.** Why could driving under the influence of a psychoactive drug contribute to an accident?

26. **Analyze.** Why is it important for doctors and pharmacists to monitor the legal medical use of opiates?

LESSON 4

Vocabulary Review

Use the correct vocabulary term to complete the following statements.

27. _____ is a way to help drug users fight addiction.

28. A community effort to monitor and report illicit drug use is called a(n) _____.

29. Penalties for drug use are often double what they might be for the same drug offense committed outside of a(n) _____.

Understanding Key Concepts

After reading the question or statement, select the correct answer.

30. Which is *not* a way that communities and schools are helping to prevent drug use?
   a. Organizing drug watches
   b. Providing drug treatment centers
   c. Establishing drug-free school zones
   d. Making it illegal to prescribe addictive medicines

31. Which is *not* a warning sign of drug use?
   a. Allergic reactions
   b. Regular hangovers
   c. Difficulty concentrating
   d. Change in sleeping habits

32. Which type of drug treatment strategy involves a meeting of people who share a common problem?
   a. Support group
   b. Outpatient therapy
   c. Medication therapy
   d. Individual counseling

Thinking Critically

After reading the question or statement, write a short answer using complete sentences.

33. **Connect.** How is peer pressure related to a teen's decision to use or avoid drugs?

34. **Analyze.** Why might it be difficult to determine whether a person has a problem with illegal drugs?

35. **Evaluate.** Why is it important to recognize when someone has an addiction to drugs and to discuss the problem with him or her?

PROJECT-BASED ASSESSMENT

Drugs: Truth and Consequences

BACKGROUND
It is your choice to abstain from illegal drug use. Knowing about the types of illegal drugs and the dangers associated with using them will help reinforce your decision to lead a drug-free life.

TASK
Create a multimedia slide presentation that provides information about drugs and the consequences of drug abuse among teens.

AUDIENCE
Students and adults in your community.

PURPOSE
Educate others about the kinds of illegal drugs that are available. Present information about the effects of illegal drugs and the problems related to teen substance abuse.

PROCEDURE

1. Conduct an online search about the types of illegal drugs and the health consequences of drug use.

2. Use statistics from reliable sources to prove the information you find.

3. Collaborate as a group to create slides for your presentation. Make sure to include any audio or video clips to illustrate your points. Make any necessary revisions.

4. Create the final version of your multimedia presentation.

5. Show your presentation to the class. Ask permission to make the presentation available on your school's website.

Math Practice

Reading Tables. Nonmedical use of substances known as anabolic steroids is considered substance abuse. The consequences of misusing steroids involves more than health risks. There are also legal consequences. The table shows the abuse of anabolic steroids in a past study that involved students from both public and private schools.

Percentage of Teens in Grades 8, 10, and 12 Who Use or Have Used Steroids			
Grade	8th	10th	12th
Ever used	1.9%	2.4%	3.4%
Used in past year	1.1%	1.5%	2.5%
Used in past month	0.5%	0.8%	1.6%

1. If 12,000 of the students studied were tenth graders, how many of them have not used anabolic steroids in the past month?
   a. 96
   b. 180
   c. 11,820
   d. 11,904

2. If 20,000 of the students were eighth graders, how many of them have not ever used anabolic steroids?
   a. 380
   b. 3800
   c. 16,200
   d. 19,620

3. Examine the values in the table. Provide a logical explanation as to why the percentages are higher for older students.

Reading/Writing Practice

Understand and Apply. Read the passage below, and then answer the questions.

It was New Year's Eve, and Carrie was anxious to go to a friend's party. Carrie and her friend, Camille, decided to drive over together. They picked up Camille's new boyfriend, Carl, on the way.

"Hey, let's have some fun tonight," said Carl. "I bought this new drug that everyone's talking about. It'll make the party more fun. What do you say?"

Carrie put her hand up. "I don't want to take drugs. I can have fun without them."

"Aw, come on, everyone's trying it," said Carl. Camille looked at Carrie, then shrugged and looked only slightly apologetic. She really liked this new guy.

"No. It's not for me," Carrie said. "I don't want to use drugs."

1. What is the author's purpose in this piece?
   a. To show how refusal skills work
   b. To illustrate the dangers of drug use
   c. To illustrate the dangers of driving while under the influence of drugs
   d. To tell about the importance of supporting peers through a difficult time

2. What else can Carrie do to avoid drug use?
   a. Describe the physical effects of drug use.
   b. Leave the party and go home.
   c. Tell Camille that Carl's a bad influence.
   d. All of the above

3. Create a pamphlet with pictures or graphics and strong refusal statements showing middle school students how to use refusal skills when offered illegal drugs.

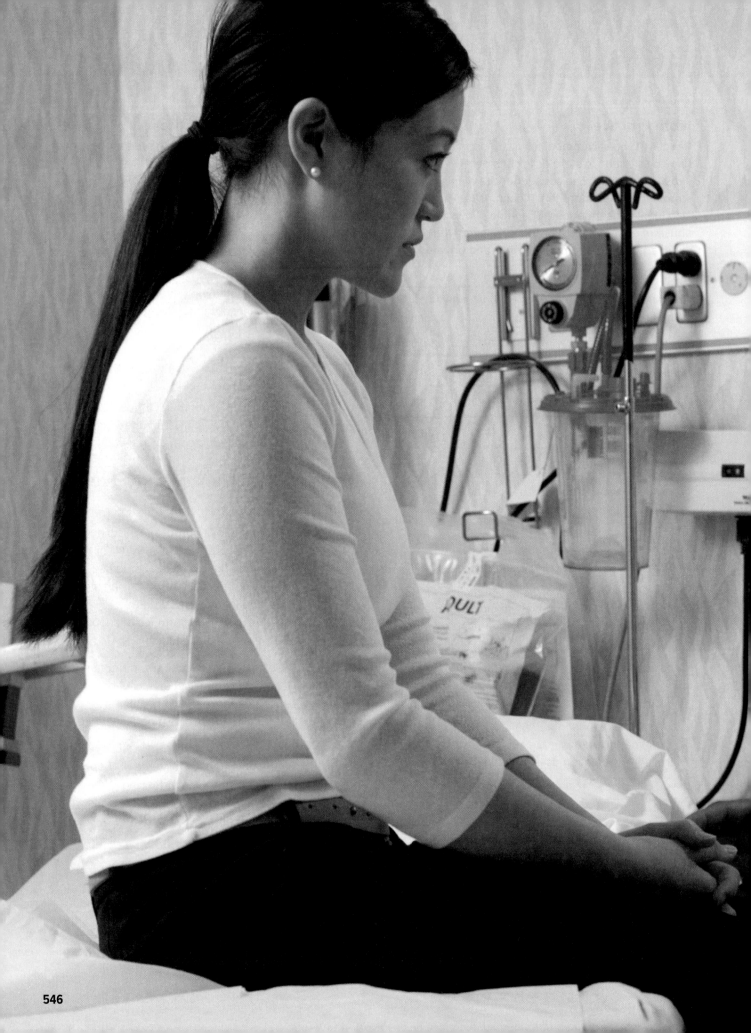

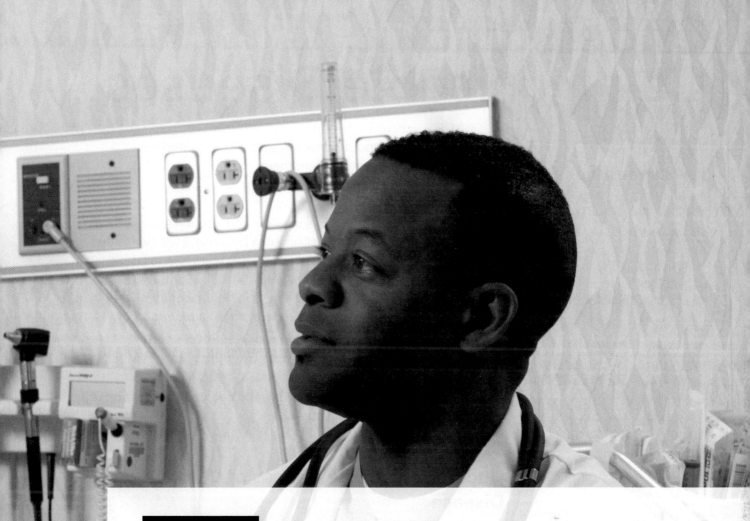

MODULE 23

Communicable Diseases

LESSONS

....

1 Understanding Communicable Diseases

2 Common Communicable Diseases

3 Fighting Communicable Diseases

4 Emerging Diseases and Pandemics

Understanding Communicable Diseases

BEFORE YOU READ

Create a T-Chart. Make a T-chart and label the columns "How communicable diseases are caused" and "How communicable diseases are spread." As you read, fill in the chart with information about both topics.

Causes	Ways Spread

Vocabulary

communicable disease
virus
bacteria
toxin
vector

· · · · · · · · · · · ·

BIG IDEA Learning about communicable diseases and how they spread can help you prevent them.

> ### REAL LIFE ISSUES
>
> **Taking Precautions.** Nolan is very excited about his family's upcoming vacation in Central America because it will be his first time outside the United States. His friends warn him to be careful about drinking unbottled water while in Central America. They say the water might make him sick. Nolan wonders what precautions he can take. *Write a paragraph explaining how Nolan might prepare for the trip. Suggest places where he could find information about potential health risks and how to avoid them.*
>
> After completing the lesson, review and analyze your response to the Real Life Issues question.

Understanding the Causes of Communicable Disease

MAIN IDEA Communicable diseases are caused by several kinds of microorganisms.

Have you ever "caught" a cold or other illness from someone else? If you have, then that illness was a **communicable disease**. A communicable disease is spread from one living organism to another or through the environment. Such illnesses are also described as *contagious* and *infectious*. Communicable diseases occur when pathogens—microorganisms that cause disease—enter your body. If your body does not fight off the invaders fast enough, you can develop an infection. There are several different categories of pathogens, but the most common types are viruses and bacteria.

Viruses

What are the most common diseases that you can think of? Chances are, you thought first of colds and the flu. Both of these common communicable diseases are caused by **viruses**. A virus is a piece of genetic material surrounded by a protein coat. These tiny pathogens invade the cells of living organisms in order to reproduce. Once a virus has penetrated a cell, it begins to multiply. The new viruses burst out of the cell and start taking over other cells.

As the virus multiplies and spreads, disease sets in and the body's immune system jumps into action. Usually, the virus runs its course and is killed by the immune system. Antibiotics do not work against viruses, although they can sometimes treat the symptoms of a virus.

Bacteria

Bacteria are single-celled microorganisms that are everywhere. They can be found nearly everywhere on earth, as well as on and in your own body. Fortunately, most bacteria are harmless. Some are even helpful, like the ones that help you digest food. Some bacteria, however, can cause diseases. In some cases, disease-causing bacteria may produce **toxins,** or substances that kill cells or interfere with their functions.

Unlike diseases caused by viruses, a bacterial disease can often be treated with antibiotics. However, the overuse of antibiotics has caused some bacteria to evolve in ways that make them resistant to these drugs. Infections caused by these antibiotic-resistant strains are much harder to treat.

Antibiotic resistance. In a given population of bacteria, a few individual bacteria may be naturally resistant to an antibiotic. These individuals survive and multiply. They can pass the genes that make them resistant to other bacteria. Soon there is an entire population of bacteria that are resistant to antibiotics. Species of bacteria that cause pneumonia, tuberculosis, and staph infections are among those that have developed antibiotic resistance. Some species of fungi that cause disease, including those that cause yeast infections, have also developed antibiotic resistance. If you are prescribed antibiotics, always take them according to the doctor's instructions.

• • • • • • • • • • • •

Reading Check

Describe How does a virus affect the body?

• • • • • • • • • • • •

Every common communicable disease can be traced to a particular type of pathogen. **Which of the diseases listed here have you experienced?**

DISEASES BY TYPE OF PATHOGEN				
Viruses	**Bacteria**	**Fungi**	**Protozoa**	**Rickettsias**
• common cold	• bacterial foodborne illness	• athlete's foot	• malaria	• typhus
• influenza (flu)	• strep throat	• ringworm	• amoebic dysentery	• Rocky Mountain spotted fever
• viral pneumonia	• tuberculosis	• vaginal yeast infection	• sleeping sickness	
• viral hepatitis	• diphtheria			
• polio	• gonorrhea			
• mononucleosis	• Lyme disease			
• measles	• bacterial pinkeye			
• AIDS	• bacterial pneumonia			
• viral meningitis	• bacterial meningitis			
• chicken pox				
• herpes				
• rabies				
• smallpox				
• West Nile virus				

Other Pathogens

Several other types of microorganisms can also cause disease. These include:

- **Fungi.** These plantlike organisms can infect the lungs, the mucous membranes, and the skin. Athlete's foot is a common fungal disease.

- **Protozoa.** These single-celled organisms are larger and more complex than bacteria. Malaria is an example of a disease caused by protozoa.

- **Rickettsias.** This is a type of microorganism which resembles bacteria. They often enter the body through insect bites. Typhus is caused by rickettsias.

How Diseases Spread

MAIN IDEA Diseases can be transmitted in a variety of ways.

Pathogens infect humans and other living things in a variety of ways. Some spread directly from person to person, while others are passed on through objects or through the air. Knowing how diseases are transmitted is your first line of defense against them.

Direct Contact

Many pathogens spread from one person to another through direct contact. This can include touching, biting, kissing, or sexual contact. Other methods of transmission include:

- **Puncture wounds.** A person may get tetanus from stepping on a rusty nail.

- **Childbirth.** A pregnant woman may transmit an infection to her unborn child through the placenta.

- **Contact with infected animals.** Animal bites and scratches can sometimes transmit disease.

Indirect Contact

You don't have to be in direct **contact** with a person to become infected. Sometimes, indirect contact can be just as dangerous.

Contaminated Objects. If you touch an object (for example, a doorknob) that an infected person has touched, you could pick up pathogens on your hands. These pathogens can then enter your body if you rub your eyes. To protect yourself, keep your hands away from your mouth, nose, and eyes, and wash your hands regularly.

Vectors. Pathogens are often spread by **vectors**. Vectors are organisms that carry and transmit pathogens to humans or other animals, such as flies, mosquitoes, and ticks. Diseases that spread this way are called *vector-borne diseases*. Some examples include malaria, West Nile virus, and Lyme disease.

Contaminated Food and Water. When food is improperly handled or stored, harmful bacteria can develop. This can happen not only with meat and fish, but with fruits and vegetables as well. Water supplies that become contaminated with human or animal feces can also spread illnesses, such as hepatitis A.

Airborne Transmission

When an infected person sneezes or coughs, pathogens are released into the air as tiny droplets that can travel as far as ten feet. Even when the droplets evaporate, the pathogens may float on dust particles until they are inhaled. Other pathogens, such as fungal spores, are also small enough to spread this way. Diseases that can spread through the air include chicken pox, tuberculosis, influenza, and inhalation anthrax.

Taking Precautions

MAIN IDEA You can take steps to prevent infection.

There is no guaranteed way to avoid communicable diseases completely. However, a few simple precautions can dramatically reduce your risk.

Wash Your Hands

The single most effective way to protect yourself from catching or spreading diseases is to wash your hands regularly. Make sure to clean both hands thoroughly with soap and warm water. Always wash your hands:

- Before you eat.

- After you use the bathroom.

- After handling pets.

- Before and after inserting contact lenses or applying makeup.

- After touching anything that an infected person has handled.

Reading Check

Identify List three ways communicable diseases can be spread.

Japan is known for being a very polite society. People who have colds or the flu often wear masks when they go outdoors. **Why do you think people in some cultures wear masks when they are ill?**

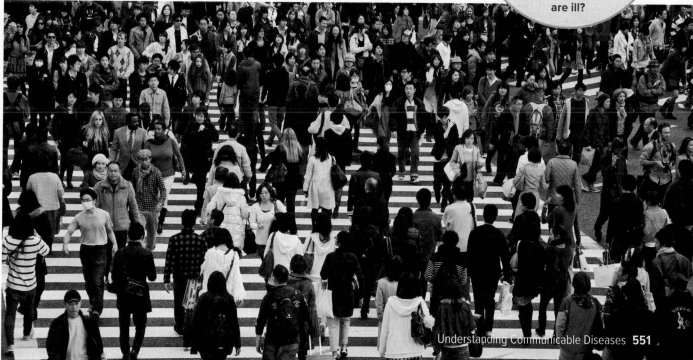

Thomas La Mela/Shutterstock

Reading Check

Explain How do a healthful diet and regular physical activity help you avoid communicable diseases?

Character Check

One simple action can demonstrate your respect for your own health and the health of others. Every time you wash your hands properly you reduce the risk of spreading potential pathogens, especially when you prepare food or when you touch objects that others may put in their mouths. What other safe food handling habits can you practice?

Protect Yourself from Vectors

Some vector-borne diseases, such as West Nile virus and bird flu, are on the rise. To protect yourself, limit the time you spend outside at dawn and dusk, when mosquitoes are most active. When you do go outside, wear pants and long-sleeved shirts to avoid insect bites, and use insect repellant. Also, avoid all contact with dead birds.

Other Prevention Strategies

Several additional strategies can also help reduce your chance of getting or spreading communicable diseases:

- Cover your mouth when you cough or sneeze, and wash your hands after using a tissue.

- Avoid sharing personal items, such as eating utensils.

- Handle food properly.

- Eat well and exercise. Getting the right nutrients and staying fit will help your body fight infection.

- Avoid tobacco, alcohol, and other drugs.

- Abstain from sexual contact.

Lesson 1 Review

Facts and Vocabulary

1. Define the word *communicable*.

2. List three ways that communicable diseases are spread through indirect contact.

3. Describe how a virus is different from bacteria.

Thinking Critically

4. **Analyze.** The fungus that causes athlete's foot lives in warm, moist places. What can you do to reduce your risk of infection when you are in gym locker rooms or other public places?

5. **Synthesize.** If you had a cold, what actions would you take to prevent spreading the illness to other people?

Applying Health Skills

6. **Practicing Healthful Behaviors.** Create an e-mail announcement that your school could send to parents at the beginning of the school year. In your e-mail, give strategies for avoiding communicable diseases such as the flu or the common cold.

Writing Critically

7. **Narrative.** Write a short story from the point of view of bacteria or a virus. Describe how the bacteria or virus finds its way into someone's body, and what happens when it gets there.

Common Communicable Diseases

BIG IDEA You can lower your chances of catching a communicable disease by learning about the causes and symptoms of these diseases, and how to avoid them.

REAL LIFE ISSUES

Passing It On. The Centers for Disease Control and Prevention keeps track of seasonal flu information for schools and childcare providers. Their records show that students miss nearly 22 million school days each year due to the common cold. The flu, a more serious illness, sends more than 200,000 people in the U.S. to the hospital each year. *Write a paragraph explaining how you can protect yourself and others from the spread of illnesses.*

After completing the lesson, review and analyze your response to the Real Life Issues question.

BEFORE YOU READ

Create a K-W-L Chart. Make a three-column chart. In the left column, write what you **k**now about common communicable diseases. In the middle column, write what you **w**ant to know about these diseases. As you read, use the third column to summarize what you **l**earned.

K	W	L

Vocabulary

respiratory tract
mucous membrane
pneumonia
jaundice
cirrhosis

Respiratory Infections

MAIN IDEA Many diseases begin as respiratory infections.

Many communicable diseases occur in the **respiratory tract**, which is a passageway that connects the nose, throat, and lungs. This passageway connects the outside world to the inside of your body. The most common respiratory infections are colds, influenza, pneumonia, strep throat, and tuberculosis.

Common Cold

The common cold is a viral infection that causes inflammation of the **mucous membranes**. This is the lining of various body cavities, including the nose, ears, and mouth. Sneezing, a sore throat, and a runny nose are the most common symptoms. Cold germs can spread through direct contact with an infected person, indirect contact with contaminated objects, or airborne transmission.

Because colds are caused by viruses, they have no cure. All you can do is wait for your body to fight off the infection. The best treatment is to get plenty of rest and drink lots of liquids.

Influenza

Influenza, or the flu, is a viral infection of the respiratory tract. Symptoms include high fever, fatigue, headache, muscle aches, and coughing. Like the common cold, the flu can spread through the air or through direct or indirect contact.

•••••••••••••

Reading Check

Identify Name at least three respiratory infections.

•••••••••••••

Because the flu is a viral infection, antibiotics can't cure it. Antiviral drugs may be effective in treating flu symptoms if taken early enough. In most cases, though, people treat the flu with proper nutrition, lots of liquids, and plenty of rest.

Many people choose to get a flu vaccination once a year. This shot protects you from one type of flu virus that may be common that year. Getting a yearly flu vaccine is especially important for older adults and people with chronic health problems.

Pneumonia

In severe cases, the flu can lead to **pneumonia**. This is an infection of the lungs in which the air sacs fill with pus and other liquids. The symptoms of this illness are similar to those of the flu, which means that sometimes people can have pneumonia without realizing it. People who are vulnerable to pneumonia include older adults and those who already have the flu.

Pneumonia can be caused by a virus or by bacteria. Viral pneumonia is sometimes treated with antiviral drugs. Bacterial pneumonia, if diagnosed early enough, can be treated with antibiotics. Pneumonia can be fatal, especially when it strikes older adults and people with lung or heart problems.

Strep Throat

Strep throat is a bacterial infection spread by direct contact with an infected person or through airborne transmission. Symptoms include sore throat, fever, and enlarged lymph nodes in the neck. Left untreated, strep throat can lead to serious problems, including heart damage. Strep throat can be treated with antibiotics.

Tuberculosis

In the mid-19th Century, tuberculosis, or TB, killed one of seven people in the United States. In the early 1990s, the rates of TB in the U.S. began to rise again. Statistics from 2012 indicate that TB is again decreasing in the U.S. with 9,945 cases reported that year.

There are many methods of spreading communicable diseases. **What can you do every day to reduce your risk of infection?**

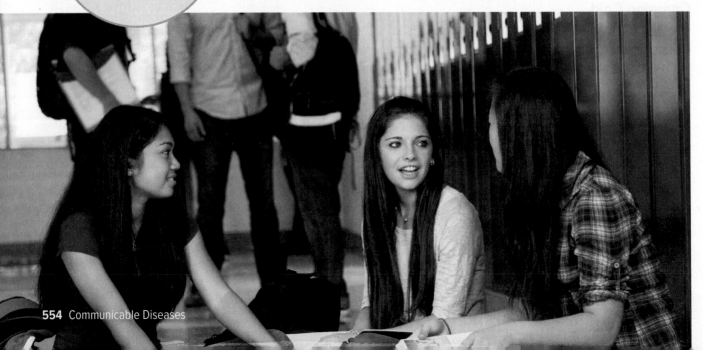

Jon Feingersh/Blend Images LLC

TB is a bacterial disease that usually attacks the lungs. It spreads through the air. TB is not spread by shaking another person's hand, sharing food or drink, touching bed linens or toilet seats, sharing toothbrushes, or kissing. Symptoms of TB include fatigue, coughing, fever, weight loss, and night sweats. The disease affects people with weakened immune systems due to other diseases.

Most people who are infected with TB bacteria never develop the disease because the immune system prevents the bacteria from multiplying and spreading. This condition is called latent TB infection, meaning that the bacteria live inside the body without making a person ill. For those people with TB disease, antibiotics are prescribed. In some cases, the disease has become resistant to some antibiotics. In these cases, a doctor must prescribe several antibiotics at one time to treat the disease.

Avoiding Respiratory Infections

Some respiratory infections are mild, while others are very serious. However, the same few habits can help protect you from all of them:

- Avoid close contact with sick people. If you're ill, stay home to protect others.

- Wash your hands often.

- Avoid touching your mouth, eyes, and nose.

- Strengthen your immune system with a healthful diet and physical activity.

- Abstain from smoking.

Hepatitis

MAIN IDEA There are three common types of hepatitis.

Hepatitis is a viral infection that causes inflammation of the liver. There are at least five different kinds of hepatitis, but the most common are types A, B, and C. Vaccines are available for hepatitis A and B, but because the disease comes from a virus, there is no cure.

- Hepatitis A usually attacks the digestive system through contact with the feces of an infected person. Common symptoms include fever, vomiting, fatigue, abdominal pain, and **jaundice**, which is a yellowing of the skin and eyes. The best ways to avoid hepatitis A are to stay away from people who are infected and to wash your hands thoroughly after using any public restroom.

- Hepatitis B has symptoms similar to those of hepatitis A, but it can also cause liver failure and a scarring of the liver called **cirrhosis**. This virus can be spread through sexual contact or through contact with an infected person's blood. To protect yourself from hepatitis B, abstain from sexual activity and the use of illegal drugs. Also, avoid getting tattoos or body piercings, and do not share personal items such as razors and toothbrushes.

- Hepatitis C is the most common blood-borne infection in the United States. Its symptoms include jaundice, dark urine, fatigue, abdominal

Reading Check

Identify Which of the body's organs is affected by hepatitis?

pain, and loss of appetite. Hepatitis C can lead to chronic liver disease, liver cancer, and liver failure. The disease is most often spread by direct contact with needles that are contaminated with infected blood. You can lower your chances of infection by abstaining from illegal drug use and sexual activity and by not sharing personal care items.

Other Communicable Diseases

MAIN IDEA Staying informed about communicable diseases can protect your health.

Respiratory infections and hepatitis are the most common communicable diseases in this country. However, there are many others. The more you know about these diseases and how they are transmitted, the better your chances of avoiding them.

COMMON COMMUNICABLE DISEASES					
	Mononucleosis	**Measles**	**Whooping Cough**	**Meningitis**	**Chicken pox**
Type/ Transmission	Virus; spread by direct contact, including sharing eating utensils and kissing	Virus; spread by coughs, sneezes, or a person talking	Bacteria; spread by coughs and sneezes, or spending time in close contact	Virus or bacteria; spread by direct or indirect contact	Virus; spread through air or contact with fluid from blisters
Symptoms	Chills, fever, sore throat, fatigue, swollen lymph nodes	High fever, red eyes, runny nose, cough, bumpy red rash	Cough, followed by a high-pitched "whoop" sound; fever; vomiting; exhaustion	Fever, severe headache, nausea, vomiting, sensitivity to light, stiff neck	Rash, itching, fever, fatigue
Treatment/ Prevention	Rest if tired	No definite treatment; vaccine for prevention	Antibiotics; vaccine for prevention	Viral meningitis: antiviral medicine if severe; bacterial meningitis: antibiotics; vaccine available	Rest, stay home so others aren't infected; vaccine available

Lesson 2 Review

Facts and Vocabulary

1. Describe how the common cold is different from the flu.

2. List three ways to prevent a respiratory tract infection.

3. Describe whether hepatitis can be treated successfully with antibiotics.

Thinking Critically

4. **Explain.** Why do you think the respiratory tract is where most infections from communicable diseases occur?

5. **Cause and Effect.** How does hepatitis spread from one illegal drug user to another?

Applying Health Skills

6. **Accessing Information.** Research the website for your state's Health Department. Write a brief summary of the information you find about communicable diseases in your state.

Writing Critically

7. **Persuasive.** Create a handout for elementary school students about the importance of washing your hands regularly. The handout should convince young people that hand washing is one of the best ways to avoid catching communicable diseases.

Fighting Communicable Diseases

BIG IDEA By learning about and practicing prevention strategies, you can help your body stay healthy.

REAL LIFE ISSUES

Too Busy to Stay Healthy. Ashley's friend Sang called from home to say she has a cold and will not be in school today. Sang says she feels tired all the time because her schedule is so busy. In addition to school, Sang has a part-time job and also volunteers at a local animal shelter. Ashley has also noticed that Sang often skips lunch. ***Write a dialogue between Sang and Ashley in which they discuss how Sang's behavior may be contributing to her colds. The girls should come up with ideas for Sang that will help her avoid catching colds so often.***

After completing the lesson, review and analyze your response to the Real Life Issues question.

BEFORE YOU READ

Create Vocabulary Cards. Write each new vocabulary term on a separate note card. For each term, write a definition based on your current knowledge. As you read, fill in additional information related to each term.

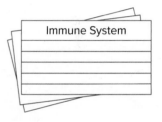
Immune System

Vocabulary
immune system
inflammatory response
phagocyte
antigens
lymphocyte
immunity

Physical and Chemical Barriers

MAIN IDEA Physical and chemical barriers make up your body's first line of defense against pathogens.

You wear a coat or sweater to stay warm, a hat to keep the sun off your head and face, and a helmet for head protection when you ride a bike. All of these are barriers that protect your body. In the same way, your body has its own built-in barriers to deal with invasion from microscopic pathogens. There are two kinds of barriers that protect you: physical and chemical. Physical barriers, such as the skin, block pathogens from entering your body. Chemical barriers, such as the enzymes in tears, destroy these tiny invaders.

The Immune System

MAIN IDEA Your body's immune system is your best ally in the fight against communicable diseases.

Although your body's physical and chemical barriers stop many pathogens before they can cause infection or disease, pathogens can—and do—sneak past these defenses. That's when your **immune system** goes to work. The immune system is a network of cells, tissues, organs, and chemicals that fights off pathogens.

The immune system fights pathogens using two major strategies: the inflammatory response and specific defenses.

The Inflammatory Response

Have you ever gotten a splinter or a cut? If so, you probably remember that the affected area became red and swollen. These are symptoms of the **inflammatory response**, which is a reaction to tissue damage caused by injury or infection. Your immune system knows a foreign object such as a splinter might have pathogens on it. It also knows that a cut could allow pathogens to get into your body. It triggers the inflammatory response to stop the invading pathogens, as well as to prevent further injury to the tissue. The inflammatory response works against all types of pathogens. It includes the following actions:

1. In response to tissue damage and invading microorganisms, blood vessels near the area of injury expand. This allows more blood to flow to the area and begin fighting the invading pathogens.

2. Fluid and cells from the bloodstream put pressure on the nerve endings, causing pressure and pain.

3. White blood cells, called **phagocytes**, surround the pathogens and destroy them with special chemicals. Pus, which is a mass of dead white blood cells and damaged tissue, may build up at the site of inflammation if bacteria are present.

4. With the pathogens killed and tissue damage under control, the body begins to repair the tissue.

> Your body uses physical and chemical barriers to fight pathogens. **Which barriers are physical? Which are chemical?**

Physical and Chemical Barriers

Tears and saliva contain enzymes that disable and even destroy pathogens.

Mucous membranes form a protective lining for your mouth, nose, and many other parts of your body. These membranes produce mucus, a sticky substance that traps pathogens before they can cause infection, then carries the trapped pathogens to other parts of the body for disposal.

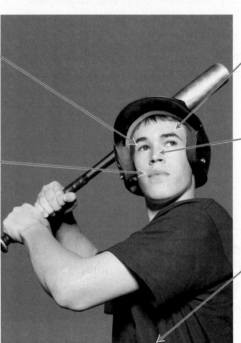

Skin is like a personal coat of armor, stopping most pathogens in their tracks as they try to enter the body.

Cilia are small hairs that line parts of your respiratory system. Cilia sweep mucus and pathogens to the throat, where they can be swallowed or coughed out.

Gastric juice in the stomach destroys many pathogens that enter your body through the nose or mouth.

Specific Defenses

Some pathogens may survive the inflammatory response. This **enables** the body to trigger specific defenses in reaction to certain pathogens. This process is called the *immune response.*

The immune system can recognize particular pathogens because of substances called **antigens,** found on their surfaces. (Toxins also contain antigens and can trigger the immune response.) Certain types of white blood cells use antigens to detect pathogens and destroy them. If your body ever detects the same antigens again, it will remember them and activate specific defenses to block the infection.

Lymphocytes

Lymphocytes are specialized white blood cells that coordinate and perform many functions of the immune response. There are two types of lymphocytes: T cells and B cells.

T Cells. There are several types of T cells, each with its own function:

- Helper T cells trigger the production of B cells and killer T cells.

- Killer T cells attack and destroy infected body cells. These cells don't attack the pathogens, only the infected cells.

- Suppressor T cells coordinate the actions of other T cells. They suppress, or "turn off," helper T cells when the infection has been cleared.

B Cells. These lymphocytes have just one job: producing antibodies. Each B cell is programmed to make one type of antibody that is specific to a certain pathogen. Antibodies perform a variety of different jobs, including:

- attaching to antigens to mark them for destruction.

- destroying invading pathogens.

- blocking viruses from entering body cells.

The Immune Response
1. Pathogens invade the body.

1. Pathogens invade the body.

2. Macrophages engulf the pathogen.

3. Macrophages digest the pathogen, and T cells recognize antigens of the pathogen as invaders.

4. T cells bind to the antigens.

5. B cells bind to antigens and helper T cells.

6. B cells divide to produce plasma cells.

7. Plasma cells release antibodies into the bloodstream.

8. Antibodies bind to antigens to help other cells identify and destroy the pathogens.

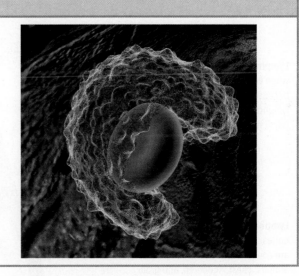

Purestock/SuperStock

Immune System Memory

Your immune system can "remember" the antigens it has dealt with in the past. When antigens activate certain T cells and B cells, the cells become "memory lymphocytes." These special memory cells circulate in your bloodstream and through the lymphatic system. When memory cells recognize a former invader, the immune system sends antibodies and killer T cells to stop it. This gives you **immunity** to future attacks from this pathogen. Immunity is the state of being protected against a particular disease. There are two types of immunity: active and passive.

Active Immunity. This type of immunity develops from natural or artificial processes. Your body develops naturally acquired active immunity when it is exposed to antigens from invading pathogens. For example, if you've had measles or been vaccinated against it, your immune system remembers and will attack the antigens for the measles virus.

Artificially acquired active immunity results from a vaccine. A vaccine is a preparation of dead or weakened pathogens that are introduced into the body to stimulate an immune response. Vaccines cause your immune system to produce disease-fighting antibodies without causing the disease itself. Today, more than 20 serious human diseases can be prevented by vaccination. For some diseases, you need to be vaccinated only once in your life. For other diseases, such as measles, tetanus, and influenza, you may need to be vaccinated at regular intervals.

Passive Immunity. You acquire passive immunity when your body receives antibodies from another person or an animal. This type of immunity is temporary, usually lasting only a few weeks or a couple of months.

The lymphatic system circulates antibodies to give you protection against many diseases. This protection can last throughout your life. **What role do lymphocytes play in fighting disease?**

Immunity and the Lymphatic System

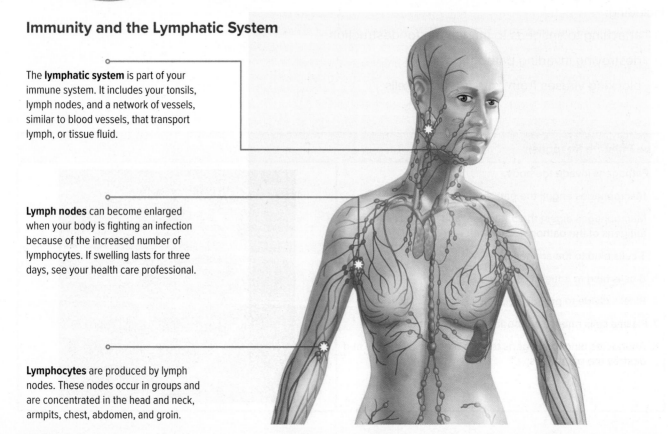

The **lymphatic system** is part of your immune system. It includes your tonsils, lymph nodes, and a network of vessels, similar to blood vessels, that transport lymph, or tissue fluid.

Lymph nodes can become enlarged when your body is fighting an infection because of the increased number of lymphocytes. If swelling lasts for three days, see your health care professional.

Lymphocytes are produced by lymph nodes. These nodes occur in groups and are concentrated in the head and neck, armpits, chest, abdomen, and groin.

Like active immunity, passive immunity can be either natural or artificial. Natural passive immunity occurs when antibodies pass from mother to child during pregnancy or while nursing. Artificial passive immunity happens when you receive an injection prepared with antibodies that are produced by an animal or a human immune to the disease.

Prevention Strategies

MAIN IDEA Strategies for preventing the spread of disease include practicing healthful behaviors, tracking diseases, and getting vaccinations.

The immune system is a powerful fighter against infection. You can keep it tuned up and in good working order by eating a nutritious, well-balanced diet and getting regular physical activity. In addition, you can take preventive measures to avoid disease and stay healthy. These include frequent hand washing, handling food properly, avoiding insect bites, and abstaining from sexual contact.

Tracking Reportable Diseases

Community, national, and global efforts also play a crucial role in fighting communicable disease. Agencies such as the Centers for Disease Control and Prevention (CDC) and the World Health Organization (WHO) keep a constant watch on the spread of diseases around the world. By tracking infections such as hepatitis, influenza, cholera, and yellow fever, they can often predict where the diseases might strike next. This information helps countries prepare and develop their own prevention strategies.

Vaccinations

In the past, smallpox killed hundreds of millions of people. Today, thanks to the smallpox vaccine, the disease has been essentially wiped out. Scientists and health care workers are always trying to stay one step ahead of communicable diseases and develop new vaccines. Vaccines fall into four categories. Read about each one to learn more.

- **Live-virus vaccines.** These specially weakened pathogens can be grown in laboratories. Although most of their disease-causing characteristics are gone, they can still stimulate the immune system to produce antibodies. The vaccine for measles, mumps, and rubella (MMR) and the vaccine for chicken pox are produced this way.

- **Killed-virus vaccines.** These vaccines use dead pathogens. Even though the pathogens are no longer active, they can still trigger an immune system response. Flu shots, the Salk vaccine for polio, and the vaccines for hepatitis A, rabies, cholera, and plague are all killed-virus vaccines.

- **Toxoids.** These are inactivated toxins from pathogens. They are used to stimulate the production of antibodies. Tetanus and diphtheria immunizations use toxoids.

- **Other types.** New and second-generation viruses are on the cutting edge of disease-fighting technology. One example is the vaccine for hepatitis B, which is made from genetically altered yeast cells.

Reading Check

Identify Name three ways that your immune system helps protect you against pathogens.

Reading Check

Explain Why is it important to track communicable diseases?

Myths and Reality

Have you ever had the flu before? What about a flu shot?

Myth: The side effects of a flu shot are worse than getting the flu.

Reality: For the vast majority of people, the worst side effect of a flu shot is a sore arm. The nasal mist flu vaccine can cause nasal congestion, a sore throat, and a cough in some people.

Immunization for All. When you receive a vaccine, you are not only keeping yourself healthy, but also helping to protect everyone around you. A small number of people cannot get vaccines because they are allergic to one or more of the ingredients. For some people, a vaccine will not confer immunity. That means that these people have an increased risk of infection. However, if people around them have received a vaccine, it reduces the transmission of the disease. Reducing the transmission of the disease helps protect people that cannot receive vaccines . Overall, vaccination reduces the number of people who are at risk for a communicable disease. That's why it's important to keep your immunizations up-to-date. To find out which immunizations you need, ask your family physician or local health department. Maintaining a record of your vaccinations will help you keep track of when you need "booster" shots.

Data show that vaccinations help keep the number of infections to a minimum. For example, by 1974 almost 80 percent of children in Japan were vaccinated against whooping cough. Only 393 cases of whooping cough were reported that year, with no deaths. Two years later, in 1976, only 10 percent of infants were receiving whooping cough vaccines. In 1979, more than 13,000 cases of whooping cough were reported, with 41 deaths. In subsequent years as the percentage of infants being vaccinated increased, the number of cases decreased.

Most schools and preschools require students to show proof of current immunizations before admission. Each state also has its own laws about immunization and school attendance. Make sure you know and follow the public health policies and government regulations in your community. Remember, everyone can play an active role in preventing the spread of communicable diseases.

Lesson 3 Review

Facts and Vocabulary

1. Describe the purpose of the inflammatory response.

2. Describe the difference between *active immunity* and *passive immunity*.

3. Define the term *phagocyte*.

Thinking Critically

4. **Analyze.** Discuss the meaning of *memory* as it applies to the immune system. How is it similar to your brain's memory?

5. **Synthesize.** You could say that your good health is the result of a successful partnership between you and your body. Support this statement using facts from the lesson.

Applying Health Skills

6. **Analyzing Influences.** A healthy immune system depends on a healthful diet and regular physical activity. Consider the influences that might affect your ability to practice these habits. In what ways do these influences make it easier for you to stay healthy? In what ways do they make it more difficult?

Writing Critically

7. **Expository.** Write a paragraph explaining why keeping your own vaccinations up to date is a duty not only to yourself but also to the people around you.

Emerging Diseases and Pandemics

BIG IDEA Today, infectious diseases have the potential to spread quickly throughout the world.

REAL LIFE ISSUES

Bacteria in Your Food. The Centers for Disease Control and Prevention (CDC) reports that in 2019, more than 1.35 million cases of Salmonella were reported in the United States. About 400 people die each year from severe cases of Salmonella contamination. *Think about foods that you or your family have purchased or prepared. Write a paragraph describing how bacteria can be found in foods, which can lead to a foodborne illness.*

After completing the lesson, review and analyze your response to the Real Life Issues question.

Emerging Infections

MAIN IDEA Some diseases are becoming more dangerous and widespread.

Vaccines and modern technology have saved millions of lives, but communicable diseases are still the top cause of deaths worldwide. Health experts label some communicable diseases as **emerging infections**. These are communicable diseases whose occurrence in humans has increased within the past two decades, or threatens to increase in the near future. Scientists now believe that some diseases once thought to be noncommunicable may, in fact, be caused by pathogens. Such diseases include Alzheimer's, diabetes, and coronary artery disease.

COVID-19

COVID-19 is a respiratory illness caused by a new coronavirus. Coronaviruses cause respiratory infections in humans and other animals that range from the common cold to SARS and COVID-19. Symptoms of COVID-19 include fever, dry cough, fatigue, and difficulty breathing. Some people experience a loss of taste or smell, headache, vomiting, and diarrhea. In March 2020, the World Health Organization (WHO) declared COVID-19 a **pandemic**. A pandemic is a global outbreak of an infectious disease.

BEFORE YOU READ

Organize Information. Make a table and label the columns "Disease," "How It's Spread," and "Prevention Strategies." As you read, fill in the chart with information about the emerging infections discussed in this lesson.

Disease	How It's Spread	Prevention Strategies

Vocabulary

emerging infection
pandemic
giardia
epidemic

Zika Virus

Zika virus is transmitted primarily by mosquitoes and causes symptoms that include fever, rash, fatigue, headache, and muscle and joint pain. Zika virus can also be transmitted through sexual contact and blood transfusions. If infection occurs during pregnancy, Zika virus can cause birth defects. It can also result in preterm birth, stillbirth, and other complications. Although there were prior outbreaks, it was not until an outbreak in 2015 that an association between Zika virus and birth defects was discovered. As of 2020, 86 countries and territories have reported cases of Zika virus.

Ebola Virus Disease (EVD)

Ebola virus disease is caused by several viruses that are closely related. Symptoms of EVD include fever, fatigue, headache, and hemorrhaging. EVD is transmitted by direct contact with blood or body fluids of an infected person or a person who has died from EVD. Contact with items, such as bedding and medical equipment contaminated with body fluids of someone who is infected or has died from EVD can also result in transmission. Treatment involves treating symptoms. Since EVD was first recognized in 1976, there are have been multiple outbreaks, mostly in countries in Africa.

H1N1 Virus

The H1N1 virus is a respiratory virus normally found in pigs. It is a combination of human, pig, and avian flu viruses, and it can spread from human to human. Symptoms include fever, sore throat, runny nose, body aches, and fatigue. More than 70 countries, including the United States, have reported cases of the H1N1 virus. In late 2013, the H1N1 virus again emerged in the U.S., primarily causing illness among young and middle-aged adults.

Emerging infections spread in several ways. **Why is Lyme disease increasing today?**

FACTORS BEHIND EMERGING INFECTIONS		
The Factor	**How It Happens**	**Examples**
Transport across borders	Infected people and animals carry pathogens from one area to another; sometimes spread by insect carriers such as mosquitoes.	Dengue fever, found mostly in South and Central America and Asia, has now appeared in the southwestern United States. West Nile encephalitis has spread from Asia and Africa to Europe and the Americas. Both diseases are carried by mosquitoes.
Population movement	As residential areas expand, people move closer to wooded areas.	Lyme disease in the United States
Resistance to antibiotics	Widespread use of antibiotics gives rise to drug resistant pathogens.	The pathogens that cause tuberculosis, gonorrhea, and a type of pneumonia are resistant to one or more antibiotics.
Changes in food technology	Mass production and distribution of food mean that a small amount of pathogens can infect a great number of people.	*E. coli* and *Salmonella* have been responsible for widespread outbreaks of illness.
Agents of bioterrorism	Some pathogens are deadly even in tiny amounts, and they can be dispersed over a large area.	In 2001, envelopes containing anthrax spores were sent to government and media figures in the United States.

Avian Influenza

Avian influenza, or bird flu, is caused by a virus that occurs naturally among birds. Wild birds carry the virus in their intestines and usually do not get sick from it.

However, the virus has spread to domesticated birds, such as chickens, ducks, and turkeys, through contact with water, feed cages, or dirt contaminated by wild birds. Avian influenza can pass to humans who have direct contact with infected birds or contaminated surfaces. In rare cases, mostly in Asia, people have died from bird flu. Because there is no vaccine and no cure, health authorities are watching this disease very carefully.

Reading Check

Explain Why are health organizations so worried about avian influenza?

Salmonella and E. coli

Salmonella and *E. coli* are bacteria that sometimes live in animals' intestinal tracts. If people come in contact with these bacteria by eating contaminated food produced by these animals, they may become ill. Illnesses can spread quickly to large areas if contamination occurs in central agricultural or food-processing facilities and contaminated food products are distributed to cities and towns all over the world. Storing foods carefully and cooking meat to proper temperature will kill *Salmonella* and *E. coli* bacteria.

Recreational Water Illnesses

Swimming is fun and a good source of physical activity. However, if the water is not regularly treated with disinfectants, chlorine, or other chemicals, it can also spread *recreational water illness,* or RWI. RWIs can occur when water is contaminated by harmful strains of bacteria such as *E. coli* or by **giardia**, a microorganism that infects the digestive system.

RWIs are most commonly spread through swallowing or having contact with water contaminated with untreated sewage or feces from humans or animals. RWIs are on the rise throughout the world, particularly in areas where raw sewage is dumped in untreated waterways. To help prevent RWIs, don't swim when you have diarrhea. Try not to let water in your mouth, and definitely try not to swallow it. Also, remember to practice good hygiene: take a shower before swimming, and wash your hands after using the bathroom.

Swimming is a fun way to stay fit, but it can pose a risk of getting an RWI. **What actions can you take to avoid RWIs?**

Other Emerging Infections

Other emerging infections that pose serious health threats include HIV/AIDS, Lyme disease, West Nile virus, SARS, and mad cow disease. Many factors are involved in the development and spread of emerging diseases. As with other highly communicable diseases, awareness is the first step toward prevention.

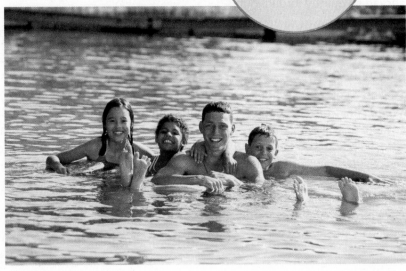

Tom Stewart/CORBIS

- **HIV/AIDS.** HIV is the virus that causes AIDS. This disease is not new, but it is spreading and has become a global health threat.

- **Lyme Disease.** This disease is transmitted to humans through tick bites. Lyme disease is on the rise because, as suburban **communities** grow, people build their homes ever closer to heavily wooded areas, where ticks thrive. To protect yourself, avoid bushy areas with high grass. When you go hiking, wear insect repellant and cover your skin.

- **West Nile Virus.** Mosquitoes sometimes feed on birds carrying the West Nile virus, a pathogen commonly found in Africa, the Middle East, and West Asia. When infected mosquitoes bite humans, they often transfer the virus. About 20 percent of those bitten by an infected mosquito will develop West Nile fever, a potentially severe illness.

- **SARS.** Severe Acute Respiratory Syndrome, or SARS, is a viral illness first reported in Asia in 2003. The illness spread to more than two dozen countries, killing almost 800 people. Health and government agencies were able to contain the virus and stop the spread of illness.

- **Mad Cow Disease.** This disease, which affects the brain functions of cattle, is also known as bovine spongiform encephalopathy, or BSE. Scientists are worried that BSE could spread to humans. It reached **epidemic** proportions in Great Britain. An epidemic is a disease outbreak that affects many people in the same place and at the same time.

Reemerging Infections. A reemerging infection is a disease that was once under control but is now threatening to become widespread again. One example is cholera, an infection of the small intestine that causes severe diarrhea. Cholera spreads through contaminated water and tends to occur in places with poor sanitation or overcrowding. A major cholera outbreak occurred in Haiti in 2010.

How Diseases Affect the World

MAIN IDEA Diseases can spread with amazing speed.

The world's countries are connected through trade and travel. These connections make it easy for infectious diseases to spread. For example, an American tourist can pick up an infection in another country, return home, and spread it to his family, friends, and coworkers.

If a disease spreads rapidly enough, it can become a pandemic. An outbreak of avian flu or *E. coli* in a small area of the globe can quickly spread and threaten the health of entire countries, even continents. Some pandemics are actually diseases that have been around for a while and have previously been treated with antibiotics. Because these drugs are so widely used, however, some pathogens have mutated into new forms that are resistant to antibiotics. This happens through a three-stage process:

1. Pathogens invade the body and cause illness.

2. Antibiotics attack the pathogens.

3. The pathogens that survive the antibiotics reproduce, creating a new generation of drug-resistant pathogens.

Reading Check

Explain Why can pandemics spread so quickly throughout the world?

Character Check

Having a cold feels awful. When I have a cold, I don't want to pass it onto anyone else. If I have to go to school, I make sure that I sneeze into my elbow. I also try to prevent the spread of the cold by washing my hands several times during the day.

Keeping pandemics under control requires constant research to find the causes and the cures for emerging diseases. Health agencies plan for pandemics and develop rapid-response strategies to combat them. They also work to control future pandemics through education. For instance, the U.S. government has launched programs that will educate the public about flu pandemics.

Mutation of Pathogens

The increased development of antibiotics has saved countless lives. However, because antibiotics are so widely used, some pathogens have mutated into new forms that are resistant to antibiotics. Pathogens become drug-resistant in a three-step process:

- Pathogens invade the body and cause illness.

- Antibiotics attack the pathogens.

- The pathogens that survive the antibiotics reproduce, creating a new generation of drug-resistant pathogens.

Travel is exciting, but it can also pose health risks. **How does air travel contribute to the spread of infection?**

Lesson 4 Review

Facts and Vocabulary

1. Define the term *emerging infection*.

2. Describe how recreational water illnesses are most commonly spread.

3. Explain how a *pandemic* is different from an *epidemic*.

Thinking Critically

4. **Evaluate.** If a friend told you that you don't need to worry about infectious diseases because you can always take antibiotics, what would you say?

5. **Analyze.** In a Colorado meatpacking plant, a vat of hamburger meat has been infected with *E. coli* bacteria. Weeks later, people in a dozen American states get sick. How might the contamination have occurred over such a large area?

Applying Health Skills

6. **Accessing Information.** Choose one emerging disease from this lesson that you want to know more about. Research how the disease spreads, and find as many tips for avoiding the disease as you can.

Writing Critically

7. **Expository.** You have been asked to write a column for an airline magazine that explains emerging diseases to travelers. Think about what air travelers in particular need to know about how diseases spread, and what they can do to stop a disease from becoming a pandemic.

LESSON 1

Vocabulary Review

Correct the sentences below by replacing the italicized term with the correct vocabulary term.

1. A(n) *infection* is an organism that causes disease.

2. A substance that kills cells or interferes with their functions is called a(n) *vector*.

3. When pathogens in the body multiply and damage body cells, a(n) *virus* results.

Understanding Key Concepts

After reading the question or statement, select the correct answer.

4. The common cold and influenza are caused by
   a. overeating.
   b. viruses.
   c. bacterial infection.
   d. exposure to toxins.

5. Malaria, West Nile virus, and Lyme disease are examples of diseases that are spread by
   a. vectors.
   b. contaminated utensils.
   c. sexual contact.
   d. contaminated water.

Thinking Critically

After reading the question or statement, write a short answer using complete sentences.

6. **Explain.** If the body's immune system cannot fight off an infection, what happens?

7. **Identify.** Name the process by which bacteria multiply themselves.

8. **Synthesize.** Describe at least three strategies for reducing your risk of getting or spreading communicable diseases.

9. **Evaluate.** Consider your role in preventing disease. How do your behaviors affect the health of your community as well as your own health?

LESSON 2

Vocabulary Review

Use the correct vocabulary term to complete the following statements.

10. The lining of body cavities (such as the mouth) is made of _____.

11. The passageway that makes breathing possible is the _____.

12. Influenza can lead to _____, a potentially fatal infection of the lungs.

Understanding Key Concepts

After reading the question or statement, select the correct answer.

13. Which of the following habits probably will not help you avoid respiratory tract infections?
    a. Rinsing with mouthwash
    b. Frequent hand washing
    c. Avoiding close contact with ill people
    d. Abstaining from smoking

14. Some strains of tuberculosis have become resistant to which form of treatment?
    a. Bed rest
    b. Surgery
    c. Dietary changes
    d. Antibiotics

15. What is the most common blood-borne infection in the United States?
    a. Hepatitis A
    b. Hepatitis B
    c. Hepatitis C
    d. None of the above

Thinking Critically

After reading the question or statement, write a short answer using complete sentences.

16. **Evaluate.** What is the best treatment for the common cold?

17. **Identify.** Receiving a flu vaccine once a year is especially important for which groups of people?

18. **Explain.** Why do doctors sometimes have to prescribe several antibiotics for a person in order to treat one disease?

19. **Synthesize.** Explain how peer pressure might contribute to the spread of hepatitis B.

LESSON 3

Vocabulary Review

Choose the correct word in the sentences below.

20. *Antigens/Lymphocytes* are substances that are capable of triggering an immune response.

21. *Inflammation/Immunity* is the state of being protected against a particular disease.

22. A preparation of dead or weakened pathogens used to stimulate an immune response is called a(n) *vaccine/antibody.*

Understanding Key Concepts

After reading the question or statement, select the correct answer.

23. What is the role of phagocytes in the inflammatory response?
    a. They prevent pus from building up.
    b. They surround and destroy pathogens.
    c. They trigger the production of T cells.
    d. They cause blood vessels to expand.

24. If you receive antibodies from another person or an animal instead of producing them in your own body, it is called
    a. communicable disease.
    b. specific defense.
    c. active immunity.
    d. passive immunity.

25. Live-virus, killed-virus, toxoid, and second-generation virus are all categories of
    a. vaccines.
    b. antigens.
    c. preventive strategies.
    d. antibiotics.

26. To remain effective, some vaccinations
    a. must have passive immunity.
    b. contain amateur pathogens.
    c. must be repeated at regular intervals.
    d. are most successful if given when a person is young.

Thinking Critically

After reading the question or statement, write a short answer using complete sentences.

27. **Identify.** What two major strategies does the immune system use to fight pathogens?

28. **Explain.** Why do health agencies like the CDC and WHO track and monitor the spread of diseases?

29. **Synthesize.** If you do not receive up-to-date immunizations, how might your future be affected?

LESSON 4

Vocabulary Review

Correct the sentences below by replacing the italicized term with the correct vocabulary term.

30. West Nile encephalitis is an example of a(n) *acute infection.*

31. A global outbreak of an infectious disease is called a(n) *mutation.*

32. *Antibody* is a microorganism that infects the digestive system.

Understanding Key Concepts

After reading the question or statement, select the correct answer.

33. The incidence of emerging infections is
    a. decreasing.
    b. increasing.
    c. holding steady.
    d. virtually nonexistent, thanks to modern medicine.

34. The most effective way to prevent infection from *Salmonella* and *E. coli* is to
   a. visually inspect food before eating.
   b. avoid eating salmon.
   c. cook meat thoroughly.
   d. wash your hands after you eat.

35. Which of the following is *not* a strategy for preventing the spread of RWI?
   a. Relying on chlorine treatments
   b. Staying out of the water when you have diarrhea
   c. Keeping water from entering your mouth when you are swimming
   d. Taking a shower before swimming

Thinking Critically

After reading the question or statement, write a short answer using complete sentences.

36. **Explain.** How do emerging infections happen?

37. **Describe.** What are the three steps of pathogen mutation?

38. **Evaluate.** What is the impact of travel on the spread of diseases?

PROJECT-BASED ASSESSMENT

Victory for Vaccines

BACKGROUND
Polio is a communicable disease caused by a virus. The disease can affect the brain and spinal cord and cause paralysis. In the early 1950s, a polio epidemic in the United States killed many people, mostly children. By 1975 the disease was almost completely eliminated in the United States.

TASK
Conduct research on Dr. Jonas Salk and Dr. Albert Sabin, including their role in the near eradication of polio. Present your findings to the class by developing a website or video.

AUDIENCE
Students in your class

PURPOSE
Make people aware of the importance of vaccinations in controlling disease.

PROCEDURE

1. Use online resources to find articles about polio.
2. Learn how the vaccines for polio were discovered.
3. Tell how the two vaccines differ from each other.
4. Explain why there are still some cases of polio in the United States.
5. Describe the efforts that are being made to eliminate polio in the rest of the world. What health groups are involved in the effort?
6. Prepare your website or video based on your research and present to your class.

Math Practice

Solve Problems. Use the passage below to answer Questions 1–3.

If you have ever had a bacterial infection, you have seen how quickly bacteria can multiply in your body. Bacteria reproduce by dividing in two in a process known as binary fission. *Under ideal conditions, binary fission takes about 15 minutes. However, this time can vary from 10 minutes to 24 hours.*

Starting with a single bacterium, how can you find out how many bacteria exist after a certain length of time? After one reproductive cycle, you have two bacteria, or 2¹. After two cycles, you have four, or 2². You can summarize this pattern with the formula $B = 2n$, *where B is the number of bacteria, and n is the number of reproductive cycles.*

1. One bacterium has a reproductive cycle of 30 minutes. How many bacteria will there be at the end of four hours?
   a. 16
   b. 120
   c. 256
   d. 512

2. How many bacteria exist after seven reproductive cycles?
   a. 14
   b. 64
   c. 128
   d. It depends on the length of the reproductive cycle.

3. What would be the shape of a graph on which time is plotted on the *x*-axis and number of bacteria is plotted on the *y*-axis? Where is the slope of the line the steepest?

Reading/Writing Practice

Understand and Apply. Read the passage below, and then answer the questions.

I can't wait to go camping again with my family this summer. We always have a great time. Last year my best friend, Randy, came with us. I'm hoping he wants to go again, even after the argument we had last time.

It was late in the afternoon at the campsite, and we were walking along the river. I knew the mosquitoes would be coming out soon, so I took a bottle of insect repellent out of my backpack and sprayed it on my exposed skin. I told Randy he should do the same, but he just laughed. "You worry too much," he said. I told him mosquitoes carry diseases that can spread to people, and that it's important to prevent insect bites. He put on the insect repellent, but he was annoyed. Things were tense between us for a while, but we got over it. Still, I wonder if it will happen again this year.

1. When did the author decide it was time to apply insect repellent?
   a. Noon
   b. Late afternoon
   c. Sunset
   d. Before going to bed

2. What reason did the author give Randy as to why it's important to put on insect repellent?
   a. Insect bites can be painful.
   b. Mosquitoes are annoying.
   c. Mosquitoes carry diseases that can spread to people.
   d. Insect bites are the leading cause of infection among teens.

3. How do you think the author felt during this encounter? Do you think he handled the situation appropriately? Explain.

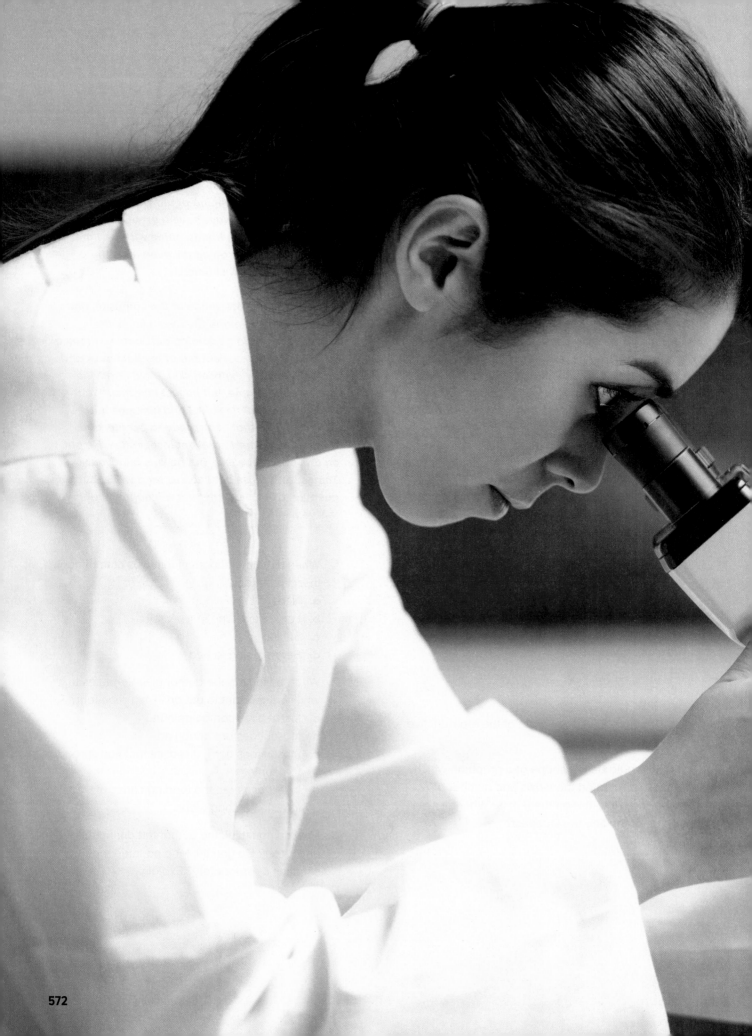

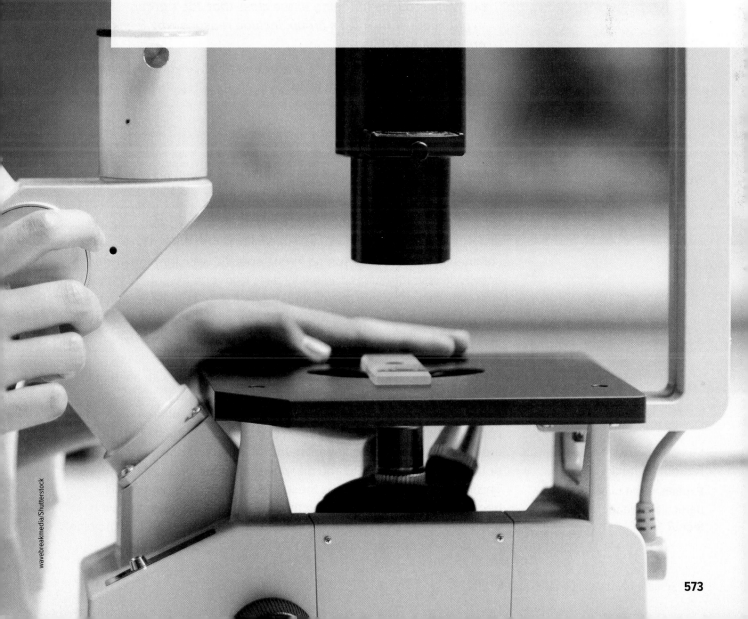

MODULE 24

Sexually Transmitted Diseases and HIV/AIDS

LESSONS

Sexually Transmitted Diseases

BEFORE YOU READ

Create a Cluster Chart. Draw a circle and label it "STDs." Use surrounding circles to identify common STDs. As you read, continue filling the chart with more details about each type of infection.

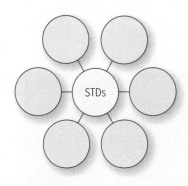

Vocabulary

asymptomatic

. . . .

Reading Check

Explain What makes STDs particularly dangerous for teens?

. . . .

BIG IDEA Sexually transmitted diseases (STDs) are highly communicable infections that are contracted through sexual contact.

REAL LIFE ISSUES

Developing Awareness. Today is the third session of the juniors' human sexuality class, and the topic is diseases and infections that are spread through sexual contact. Tricia and her friends do not want to go to class. They say they've heard it all before, and besides, it's embarrassing to talk about. Joe and his friends think they should attend because the more they know, the safer they'll be. ***Write reasons for going to the class that Joe's group might suggest to Tricia's group. Include reasons why teens are at risk for STDs.***

After completing the lesson, review and analyze your response to the Real Life Issues question.

What Are STDs?

MAIN IDEA Any person who has sexual contact with another person risks contracting a sexually transmitted disease.

AIDS, herpes, and gonorrhea are all examples of sexually transmitted diseases, also known as sexually transmitted infections. These communicable diseases spread in one specific way: through sexual activity. These infections can easily pass from one person to another. However, they can only do so when there is direct genital contact or the exchange of semen or other body fluids. Any person who has sexual contact with another person risks contracting an STD. This risk increases as the number of sexual partners a person has rises.

Some STDs are caused by bacteria and can be cured with antibiotics. Others are caused by viruses and have no cure, though their symptoms can often be controlled. Early diagnosis and treatment are crucial to controlling or curing an STD. However, some of the most common STDs are often **asymptomatic**, meaning that individuals show no symptoms, or the symptoms are mild and disappear after the onset of the infection. This lack of symptoms makes these STDs particularly dangerous because people may not realize that they are infected. People with undiagnosed STDs may not seek treatment. They may also unknowingly pass the infection on to future sexual partners.

STDs IN THE UNITED STATES		
STD	Estimated Number of New Cases Each Year	Reported Cases (2018)
Chlamydia	2.86 million	1,800,000
Genital Herpes	776,000	300,000
Gonorrhea	820,000	583,000
Trichomoniasis	1 million	3,700,000
Syphilis	55,400	35,000

This chart shows the discrepancy between the estimated number of new STD cases in the United States and the number of reported cases. **Why do you think such a large percentage of STDs are undiagnosed and unreported?**

Common STDs

MAIN IDEA There are approximately 25 different STDs, six of which are considered the most common.

There are approximately 25 known STDs worldwide. The six considered the most common are genital HPV infection, chlamydia, genital herpes, gonorrhea, trichomoniasis, and syphilis. The table summarizes the symptoms and possible long-term effects of these six STDs. In general, the effects are more serious in females than in males, and females are also more likely to suffer complications. However, all infected people can experience significant effects from STDs—both physical and psychological.

Genital HPV Infections

Genital HPV infections are caused by the human papillomavirus (HPV), a group of more than 100 kinds of viruses. More than 40 of these viruses are **transmitted** through sexual contact. HPV infections can cause genital warts, which appear as bumps or growths on or near the genitals. Over 20 million people in the United States are infected with HPV each year.

ACADEMIC VOCABULARY

transmit (verb): to send from one person or place to another

Most genital HPV infections do not have symptoms and will disappear without medical treatment. However, some HPV infections, if not diagnosed and treated, may cause abnormal Pap tests or, more seriously, may result in certain types of cervical cancer. A vaccine is now available for protection against HPV. It is not a cure, but it is recommended to reduce the number of cases of cervical cancer.

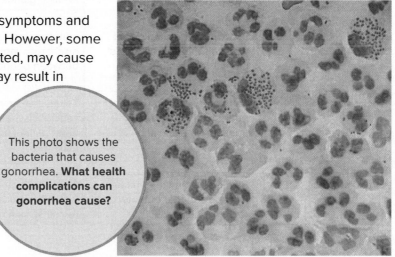

This photo shows the bacteria that causes gonorrhea. **What health complications can gonorrhea cause?**

Image courtesy of the Centers for Disease Control and Prevention/Joe Miller.

Chlamydia

Chlamydia is a bacterial infection that affects the reproductive organs of both males and females. In 2018 almost 1.8 million new cases of chlamydia were reported. The disease is three times more likely to affect females than males. However, less than half of all cases are reported because, like genital HPV, chlamydia often produces no symptoms. Thus, sexually active teens may not know they are infected, do not seek testing, and go untreated. Chlamydia is the most common STD among teens.

If left untreated, chlamydia can cause serious complications. Females can develop pelvic inflammatory disease (PID) and suffer chronic pelvic pain or infertility. Untreated chlamydia can also lead to infertility in males. Pregnant females with chlamydia can deliver prematurely, and the infants born to infected mothers may develop eye disease or pneumonia, as well as fatal complications. Also, females with chlamydia are up to five times more likely to become infected with HIV if they are exposed to the virus.

This chart shows the symptoms and possible long-term effects of common STDs. **Why is delayed treatment for STDs never a healthy choice?**

STD SYMPTOMS			
STD	**Symptoms in Males**	**Symptoms in Females**	**Possible Long-Term Effects**
Genital HPV Infection	Genital warts on the penis, scrotum, groin, anus, or thigh	Genital warts in or around the vagina, vulva, cervix, or anus	Development of cervical cancer in females
Chlamydia	Penis discharge; burning during urination; itching or burning sensations around penis	Lower abdominal or back pain; nausea; fever; bleeding between periods; pain during intercourse; muscle ache; headache; abnormal vaginal discharge; burning sensation when urinating	In males, inflammation of urethra; In females, inflammation of cervix, damage to fallopian tubes, chronic pelvic pain, infertility
Genital Herpes	Blisters on or around genitals or rectum; sores that can take weeks to heal; flu-like symptoms, including fever and swollen glands	Blisters on or near vagina or rectum; sores that can take weeks to heal; flu-like symptoms, including fever and swollen glands	Psychological distress; can cause life-threatening infection in baby born to mother with the disease
Gonorrhea	Burning sensation when urinating; green, yellow, or white discharge from penis; painful, swollen testicles	Pain or burning when urinating; increased vaginal discharge; vaginal bleeding between periods	In males, painful condition of testicles leading to infertility if untreated (epididymitis); In females, chronic pelvic pain and infertility
Trichomoniasis	Temporary irritation inside penis; mild burning after urination or ejaculation	Thick, gray or yellowish green vaginal discharge with strong odor; painful urination; vaginal itching	Discomfort; higher susceptibility to other STDs; premature or low-birth-weight babies born to infected pregnant females
Syphilis	Single sore on the genitals (sores disappear but infection remains); skin rash	Single sore on the vagina (sores disappear but infection remains); skin rash	Serious damage to internal organs, including brain, heart, and nerves

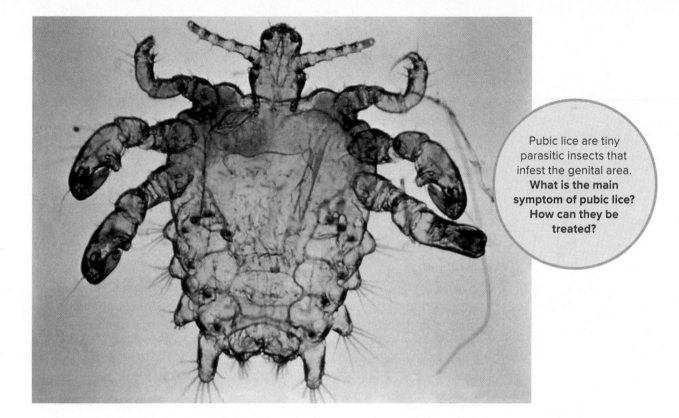

Pubic lice are tiny parasitic insects that infest the genital area. **What is the main symptom of pubic lice? How can they be treated?**

Genital Herpes

Genital herpes is caused by the herpes simplex virus (HSV). There are two different strains of this virus. HSV-1 usually causes cold sores in or near the mouth, while HSV-2 typically causes genital sores. However, either type can infect both the mouth and the genitals. In the United States, it is estimated that one of every six people has genital herpes.

Many people infected with genital herpes are asymptomatic and do not know they have the infection. If symptoms do occur, the first outbreak will usually appear as blisters on the genitals or rectum within two weeks of the virus being transmitted. The blisters break, leaving sores that can take several weeks to heal. Usually the first sores are followed by shorter, less severe outbreaks that can occur on and off for years. Antiviral treatments can lessen the frequency of these outbreaks, but the disease has no cure.

Gonorrhea

Gonorrhea is a bacterial STD that usually affects the mucous membranes. It is the second most commonly reported infectious disease in the United States. The CDC estimates that more than 700,000 Americans are infected with gonorrhea each year, but only half of these infections are reported.

Many males with gonorrhea are asymptomatic, and infected females may show only mild symptoms. Left untreated, gonorrhea can lead to severe health problems, such as infertility. The bacteria can also spread to the bloodstream and cause permanent damage to the body's joints. Females can pass the infection to their babies during childbirth. These babies may contract eye infections that cause blindness.

Trichomoniasis

Trichomoniasis is caused by a microscopic protozoan that infects the vagina, urethra, and bladder. About 3.7 million people in the U.S. have the disease. However, only 30 percent of these people develop symptoms. Some males have a temporary irritation inside the penis, mild discharge, or slight burning during and after urination or ejaculation. Infected females often experience *vaginitis,* an inflammation of the vagina that causes discharge, irritation, and itching. Females with trichomoniasis are also more likely to contract HIV if they are exposed to it. Babies born to infected females are often premature and have low birth weights.

Syphilis

Syphilis, an infection caused by small bacteria called spirochetes, attacks many parts of the body. The infection passes through three stages. In the first stage, a sore appears on the external genitals or the vagina. The disease can be passed to another person through direct contact with this sore during sexual activity. At this stage, the disease can be easily treated.

If the infection goes untreated, the sore heals after a couple of weeks, but the infection remains. In the second stage, the infection produces a skin rash. As in the first stage, the untreated rash will disappear, but the infection remains and progresses to the third stage. During this stage, syphilis can damage internal organs, cause brain dementia, and may cause death.

The STD Epidemic

MAIN IDEA Accurate health information and responsible behavior will help fight the STD epidemic.

The United States currently faces an STD epidemic. The Centers for Disease Control and Prevention (CDC) estimates that medical costs connected to STDs are now more than $15.9 billion a year. Each year, approximately 20 million people are infected with an STD, and almost half of them are under the age of 24. However, as the chart shows, many of these cases will not be diagnosed, treated, or reported, creating a serious health crisis. STD cases may go undiagnosed or untreated due to:

- **embarrassment or fear.** Some people are too ashamed or afraid to seek medical help.

- **lack of symptoms.** Many people infected with STDs are asymptomatic and do not know they have a disease. Infected individuals may unknowingly transmit the disease to others.

Reading Check

Explain Why is it important for STDs to be diagnosed as soon as possible?

- **misinformation.** If STD symptoms disappear without treatment, the infected person may mistakenly believe the disease has been cured. People may not have all the facts and may receive wrong information from friends.
- **notification policies.** State laws require health care providers to report some, but not all, STDs. People who have contracted HPV or genital herpes are not required to report their infections or to inform any partners of their condition.

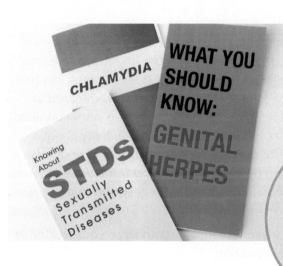

The CDC provides important updated information about STDs at their website. **Where else might you find reliable information about STDs?**

Lesson 1 Review

Facts and Vocabulary

1. Define the term *sexually transmitted disease*.
2. Name four common STDs.
3. In the United States, approximately how many people are infected with an STD each year?

Thinking Critically

4. **Synthesize.** How can you communicate the danger of STDs to other teens?
5. **Analyze.** Why is it important to learn about the reasons STDs go undiagnosed and untreated?

Applying Health Skills

6. **Accessing Information.** Create a directory identifying resources in your community where teens can find accurate information about the diagnosis and treatment of STDs.

Writing Critically

7. **Expository.** Describe the cause-and-effect relationship between the reasons many STDs go unreported and undiagnosed and the current STD epidemic in the United States.

Ken Karp/McGraw-Hill Education

Preventing and Treating STDs

BEFORE YOU READ

Create an Outline. Preview this lesson by scanning the pages. Then organize the headings and subheadings into an outline. As you read, fill in your outline with important details.

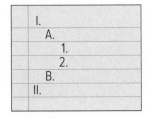

I.		
	A.	
		1.
		2.
	B.	
II.		

Vocabulary

antibiotics

ACADEMIC VOCABULARY

guideline (*noun*): an outline of conduct

BIG IDEA All STDs are preventable and most can be treated, but some are incurable.

REAL LIFE ISSUES

Making Personal Decisions. Jake and Maria have been dating for six months. Lately, Maria has been more and more insistent that they take their relationship "to the next level." Jake has had two previous sexual relationships, but he has now decided to practice abstinence. He made his decision based partly on what he learned about STDs. He now thinks sexual activity is not worth all the risks. *Write a dialogue between Maria and Jake. Include an explanation of the risks that you think Jake is talking about, and show how Jake might respond in a healthful way.*

After completing the lesson, review and analyze your response to the Real Life Issues question.

Prevention Through Abstinence

MAIN IDEA The most successful method to prevent the spread of STDs is abstinence.

About 9 million American teens contract STDs each year. Some of these are bacterial infections, such as chlamydia or gonorrhea, which can be treated and cured with **antibiotics**. Antibiotics are a class of chemical agents that destroy disease-causing microorganisms while leaving the patient unharmed. Others, such as genital herpes and HPV, are incurable viral infections. Any STDs that are not diagnosed and treated early can result in serious long-term or permanent health problems. In some cases, an untreated STD can result in death.

The only method that is 100 percent successful in preventing STDs is abstinence from sexual activity. The following **guidelines** can help you protect your health and stay committed to abstinence:

- Set personal limits on physical affection. Be clear about your decision and discuss it with those who are close to you.

- Avoid dating someone who is sexually active or who pressures you to go beyond your limits.

- Avoid attending parties or situations where you may feel pressured to engage in sexual activity.

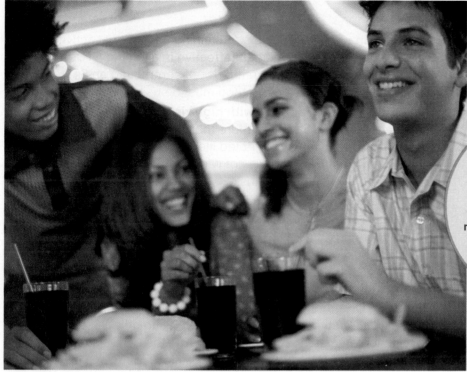

Group outings are one way to enjoy the company of friends and avoid pressure to engage in sexual activity. **Why might you want to discuss your commitment to abstinence with your friends?**

- Avoid people who make fun of your decisions or encourage high-risk behaviors, such as the use of alcohol or drugs.

- Choose group outings where you can enjoy the company of friends and avoid pressure to engage in sexual activity.

- Practice refusal skills. Use words and body language to resist the pressure to engage in sexual activity.

Understanding the Risks

Each month about 1.5 million teens are diagnosed with an STD. Teens are at high risk partly because many teens are unaware of a partner's past behavior. It is impossible to look at someone and tell if that person has an STD. Even asking the other person if he or she has an STD cannot completely prevent STDs from being passed from one person to another. Some people may not be aware that they have an STD if the person is asymptomatic. To remain safe, abstinence is the only 100 percent sure method of preventing STDs.

Avoiding High-Risk Behaviors

About half of all new STDs infections each year occur in people aged 15 to 24 years old. Because many STDs go undiagnosed, it is not enough for a partner simply tell you that he or she is uninfected. Avoiding high risk behaviors is the best prevention. These behaviors include:

- **being sexually active with more than one person.** This includes having a series of sexual relationships with one person at a time. Being sexually active with even one partner puts a person at risk, but the risk increases with the number of partners.

Reading Check

Explain How can the use of alcohol and other drugs increase a person's risk of contracting an STD?

- **engaging in unprotected sex.** Abstaining from sexual activity is the only method that is 100 percent effective in avoiding STDs. However, barrier protection can reduce the risk of contracting an STD. In order to be effective, the barrier method must be used correctly.
- **engaging in sexual activity with high-risk partners.** Such partners include those who have had more than one sexual partner in the past and those who have injected illegal drugs. Taking a person's word about past behaviors is not wise. Sexual activity with just one infected person puts you at risk.
- **using alcohol and other drugs.** Alcohol can lower inhibitions and cause teens to engage in sexual activity when they might otherwise choose not to. To safeguard your health, it's important to be in control of your decisions.

HPV Vaccine

The Food and Drug Administration (FDA) has approved the HPV vaccine to protect against four types of HPV infections. Health officials recommend the vaccine for females 11–26 years old. In 2011, the CDC also recommended that males between the ages of 11–26 receive the vaccine.

DIAGNOSIS METHODS AND TREATMENTS FOR STDs		
STD	**Diagnosis Method**	**Treatment/Cure**
Genital HPV Infection	Pap test in females; genital warts diagnosed by a physical examination	No cure; warts may clear up without medication or by using medications applied by patient; or may clear up with treatments performed by a health care provider
Chlamydia	Urine tests; tests on specimen collected from the infected site	Treated and cured with antibiotics
Genital Herpes	Visual inspection by a health care professional; testing of infected sore; blood tests	No cure; antiviral medication can shorten and prevent outbreaks
Gonorrhea	Laboratory test (Gram's stain); urine test	Treated and cured with antibiotics; successful treatment becoming difficult due to increase of drug-resistant strains; medication stops infection but cannot repair damage done by disease
Trichomoniasis	Physical examination and laboratory test	Prescription drug, metronidazole, given by mouth in a single dose; both partners should receive treatment at same time
Syphilis	Physical examination; blood test	Curable with penicillin or other antibiotics; treatment will not repair damage already done

Diagnosis methods and successful treatments for common STDs vary.

Diagnosing and Treating STDs

MAIN IDEA Only a health care professional can accurately diagnose and treat an STD.

If STDs are not diagnosed and treated early, they can have serious long-term consequences. Teens who believe they might be infected with an STD should talk to a health care professional as soon as possible. Many public health clinics provide information and treatment free of charge. Keep in mind that not all genital infections are STDs. Some are simply localized skin infections or rashes. Only a trained professional can determine which test will most effectively screen for a particular STD.

When an STD has been diagnosed, a health care professional will prescribe the most effective medication and monitor the patient's treatment. STDs cannot be cured using common household products, homemade remedies, or over-the-counter treatments. A health professional, such as a school nurse, can provide facts about STDs and how they are treated. Also, remember that taking medicines prescribed to others is not only risky, it is also illegal.

Antibiotics can effectively treat bacterial STDs, but viral STDs are incurable. However, medications can lessen the discomfort from sores and skin irritations caused by viral STDs. The table summarizes methods of diagnosing and treating common STDs.

Act Responsibly

Everyone is responsible for helping to prevent the spread of STDs. One way to control this epidemic is to practice abstinence. Another is to report any known infections. Public health clinics can sometimes help locate past partners to make sure they get medical treatment. Ultimately, however, it is the responsibility of any person infected with an STD to notify everyone with whom he or she has had sexual contact in the past. Informing someone else about a possible STD could save a life.

Reading Check

Explain Which types of STDs can be treated and possibly cured? Which cannot?

Myths & Reality

A person you know at school says that STDs cannot be transmitted the first time you become sexually active. You're not sure you agree.

Myth: STDs cannot be transmitted the first time you become sexually active.

Reality: STDs can be transmitted any time you are sexually active. Also, sexually active means any type of sexual activity. An STD is a virus or infection, and cannot determine whether it's your first time.

Lesson 2 Review

Facts and Vocabulary

1. Name the only method that is 100 percent effective in preventing the spread of STDs.

2. Identify two high-risk behaviors that can lead to contracting an STD.

3. Define the term *HPV vaccine*.

Thinking Critically

4. **Synthesize.** Predict situations that could lead to pressure to engage in sexual activity, and identify ways to avoid these situations.

5. **Analyze.** Explain the causes and consequences of teen health risk behaviors that could result in STD infection, and describe prevention strategies.

Applying Health Skills

6. **Refusal Skills.** Write a scenario in which one teen is pressuring another to engage in behavior that puts both at high risk for contracting an STD. The second teen should use refusal skills to respond to the pressure.

Writing Critically

7. **Persuasive.** Write a public service announcement urging teens to get medical help for all health problems, including suspected STDs. Include local resources for medical care.

HIV/AIDS

BEFORE YOU READ

Create a K-W-L Chart. Make a three-column chart. In the first column, list what you **k**now about HIV/AIDS. In the second column, list what you **w**ant to know about this topic. As you read, use the third column to summarize what you **l**earned.

K	W	L

Vocabulary

acquired immune deficiency syndrome (AIDS)
human immunodeficiency virus (HIV)

. . . .

BIG IDEA HIV is the virus that causes AIDS, a disease that weakens the body's immune system and may have fatal consequences.

REAL LIFE ISSUES

Finding Out the Facts. Cal and Mia heard a rumor at school that a senior tested positive for HIV. "I'm not going to soccer with the seniors," declares Mia. "I don't want to come into contact with their sweat." Cal laughs. "Get real. You can't get HIV from sweat!" Mia shoots back. "Well, sweat's a bodily fluid, isn't it?" *Write a list of true/false questions about HIV/AIDS that Mia and her friends might have about how HIV is transmitted.*

After completing the lesson, review and analyze your response to the Real Life Issues question.

What is HIV/AIDS?

MAIN IDEA HIV/AIDS weakens the body's immune system.

Acquired immune deficiency syndrome (AIDS) is a disease in which the immune system is weakened. It has become one of the deadliest diseases in human history. More than 32 million people around the world have died from AIDS, including more than 675,000 Americans. AIDS is caused by the **human immunodeficiency virus (HIV)**, which is a virus that attacks the immune system. When this virus enters the body, it finds and destroys the white blood cells that fight disease. In the final stages of an HIV infection, the immune system is destroyed, and AIDS develops.

HIV infection is a worldwide concern. Health care officials estimate that 37.9 million people around the world currently have HIV/AIDS. Approximately 21 percent of newly reported HIV/AIDS infections in 2018 were reported among people aged 13 to 24. Every year, about 8,000 young people become infected worldwide.

Health care officials view HIV/AIDS as a *pandemic,* a global outbreak of infectious disease. The seriousness of this pandemic is greatly increased because many of the people who are infected do not know it. Many experts and scientists consider HIV/AIDS to be the most serious public health problem facing the world.

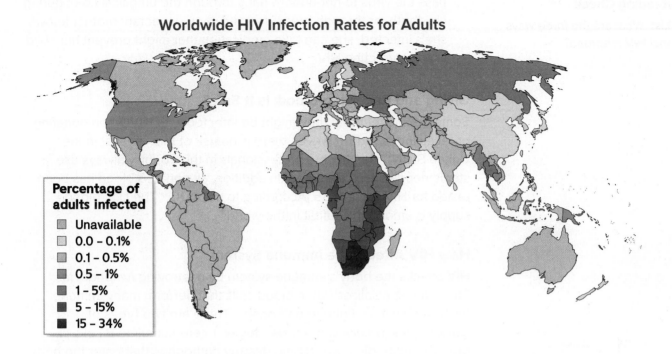

Worldwide HIV Infection Rates for Adults

Percentage of adults infected
- ☐ Unavailable
- ☐ 0.0 – 0.1%
- ☐ 0.1 – 0.5%
- ☐ 0.5 – 1%
- ☐ 1 – 5%
- ☐ 5 – 15%
- ■ 15 – 34%

Understanding HIV/AIDS

MAIN IDEA HIV/AIDS is transmitted in a variety of ways.

HIV is a fragile virus and cannot live outside the human body. Exposure to air at room temperature kills the virus, so HIV cannot be spread through airborne transmission. It also cannot spread through casual contact (such as shaking hands) or through insect bites. Although the virus has been found in the sweat, tears, and saliva of infected persons, the amount is too small to be considered dangerous.

HIV is transmitted among humans only when one person's infected blood, semen, or vaginal secretions come in contact with another person's broken skin or mucous membranes. Mucous membranes can be found in the mouth, eyes, nose, rectum, and genitals. HIV spreads in three ways:

- **During sexual intercourse.** HIV can enter the bloodstream through microscopic openings in tissues of the vagina, the anus, the mouth, or the opening in the penis. People with STDs are more vulnerable to HIV infection because STDs cause changes in the body's membranes that make it easier for HIV to penetrate them.

- **By sharing needles.** Needles that are used by someone with the HIV infection will become contaminated with HIV. Using a needle that someone with the virus has used can transmit the virus directly into the bloodstream. Needles used for body piercings and tattoos can pose a risk because they may come into contact with contaminated blood. If the needles are not properly cleaned or sterilized, they can pass the infection to other customers.

Reading Check

Explain How are HIV and AIDS related?

- **From mother to baby.** A pregnant female infected with HIV can pass the virus to her unborn baby through the umbilical cord, during childbirth, or through breast-feeding. If an expectant mother knows she's infected, she can take medication that might prevent her child from contracting HIV.

Giving and Receiving Blood: Is It Safe?

Some people fear that they might be infected with HIV when donating or receiving blood. However, there is no risk of this, at least in the United States. Health care professionals in this country always use sterile needles to draw blood. In addition, all donated blood has been tested for HIV since 1985. According to the CDC, "The U.S. blood supply is among the safest in the world."

How HIV Affects the Immune System

HIV attacks the body's immune system by destroying *lymphocytes*. These are specialized white blood cells that perform many immune functions, such as fighting pathogens. There are two types of lymphocytes: B cells and T cells. Helper T cells stimulate B cells to produce antibodies, which help destroy pathogens that enter the body. AIDS attacks the body's killer T cells.

Once inside the cell, HIV is safe from attack by the immune system's antibodies. **How does this make HIV particularly dangerous?**

How HIV Attacks Cells

1. HIV attaches to cell surface.
2. Virus core enters cell and goes to nucleus.
3. Virus makes a copy of its genetic material.
4. New virus assembles at cell surface.
5. New virus breaks away from host cell.

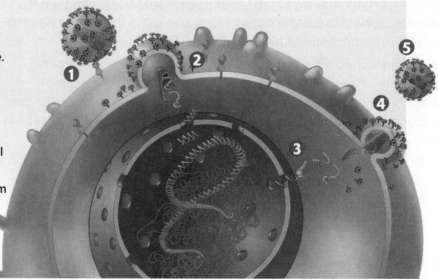

Once HIV is **confined** within a cell, it is safe from attack by antibodies. The virus reproduces itself inside the T cells and eventually destroys them. As more cells are destroyed, the immune system becomes weaker and weaker. In time, the body becomes vulnerable to *AIDS-opportunistic infections*. These are infections that the body would be able to fight off if the immune system were healthy. HIV infection moves through identifiable stages before progressing to AIDS:

- **Acute Infection Stage**. This stage begins within two to four weeks of infection. A person may become sick with a severe flu-like illness. Some of the symptoms experienced can include fever, swollen glands, sore throat, rash, muscle and joint aches, fatigue, and headache. During this stage, the virus is reproducing rapidly in the body. During the acute infection stage, the levels of HIV in the bloodstream are very high. The virus takes over helper T cells and destroys them. During this stage, the person with HIV can easily transmit the virus to others through sexual activity or drug use, as well as other methods of transmission.

- **Clinical Latency Stage.** During this stage, the HIV virus continues to reproduce in the body. This stage is sometimes referred to as the asymptomatic stage because the person may not feel ill. The clinical latency stage can last for decades if a person is being treated for HIV. For those not being treated, this stage can last for up to an average of 10 years.

- **AIDS.** When the helper T-cells drop to less than 200, or one of several AIDS-opportunistic infections are present, the disease has progressed to the AIDS stage.

While the three stages are identifiable, no timetable exists to determine how long each individual will remain in a stage, or how healthy a person with HIV will remain. Several factors determine each individual's health status. These include how healthy the person was when infected, and whether the person maintains good nutrition, exercises regularly, and avoids tobacco use after infection.

Lesson 3 Review

Facts and Vocabulary

1. Explain how HIV affects the human immune system.

2. Describe two ways you can protect yourself from contracting HIV/AIDS.

3. Explain why the body's antibodies fail to protect people from HIV.

Thinking Critically

4. **Analyze.** Why has the CDC implemented mandatory testing for all donated blood?

5. **Synthesize.** How does the immune system respond to the presence of HIV in the body?

Applying Health Skills

6. **Advocacy.** Create a poster or public service announcement that warns teens about the risks of contracting HIV/AIDS.

Writing Critically

7. **Expository.** Write an essay that explains the relationship between HIV and AIDS. Discuss why the infection is considered one of the world's deadliest diseases.

Preventing and Treating HIV/AIDS

BEFORE YOU READ

Organize Information. Make a three-column chart. Label the columns "Prevention," "Diagnosis," and "Treatment." As you read, fill in the chart with information about how HIV/AIDS can be prevented, diagnosed, and treated.

Prevention	Diagnosis	Treatment

Vocabulary

antibody
rapid test
antibody screening test

ACADEMIC VOCABULARY

estimate *(verb)*: to determine roughly the size or extent of

BIG IDEA HIV/AIDS is preventable and treatable, but it is incurable.

REAL LIFE ISSUES

Worried About HIV. Tony is concerned about his older sister, Kari. She confided that she enjoys college life, but she and her friends are under a lot of pressure to have sex and to experiment with alcohol and other drugs. Kari is committed to abstinence, so she's chosen to hang out with people who respect her decision. Yesterday, however, one of her closest friends told her that he tested positive for HIV. Kari was shocked and upset by the news that someone she cares about deeply is infected with HIV. *Write a dialogue between Tony and Kari. How might Tony express his concern and support for his sister?*

After completing the lesson, review and analyze your response to the Real Life Issues question.

Preventing HIV/AIDS

MAIN IDEA There are many actions you can take to avoid contracting HIV/AIDS.

The CDC estimates that more than one million Americans live with HIV, and 50,000 are infected each year. About 8,300 of them are between the ages of 13 and 24. Teens who are sexually active or who use intravenous drugs are at the highest risk. The graph shows the number of HIV/AIDS cases reported among teens between 1999 and 2011.

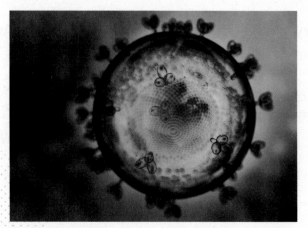

There is no way to tell just by looking whether a person is HIV-positive. The CDC **estimates** that 20 percent of the people in the United States who are infected with HIV do not know they are infected. Because of this, they may unknowingly spread the virus to others.

MedicalRF.com

HIV/AIDS Among Teens

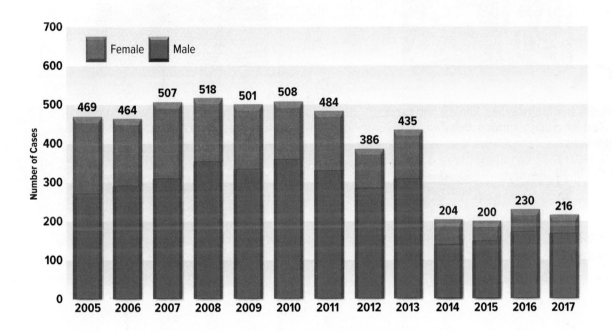

Protecting Yourself From HIV

Fortunately, there are steps you can take to protect yourself from HIV/AIDS. The two most important are to practice abstinence and to avoid sharing needles. Avoiding situations where drug or alcohol use might compromise your judgment will help you maintain your decision to remain abstinent. The diagram illustrates additional strategies you can use to avoid infection.

Notice that the listed behaviors for avoiding HIV all involve relationships. For example, sharing a needle always involves another person. The other people in your life play nearly as big a role in determining your HIV/AIDS risk as you do. Ask yourself:

- What do I know about the people in my life and their behaviors?
- Will they put me at risk for getting HIV/AIDS?
- How can I be sure another person is not HIV-positive?

Knowing as much as you can about the people around you and their behaviors can help you make responsible and informed decisions. It also helps to practice your refusal skills so that you will be prepared if you are pressured to take part in any high-risk behaviors.

Ways to Prevent HIV and AIDS

Practice abstinence. HIV is spread through semen and vaginal secretions. Wait to be sexually active until you are ready for a monogamous, lifelong relationship.

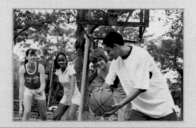

Avoid sharing needles or syringes used to inject drugs, including steroids.

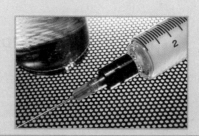

Avoid sharing needles, knives, and razors used for cutting, tattoos, body art, or body piercing.

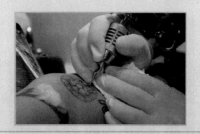

Avoid situations and events where you might feel pressured to engage in sexual activity or drug and alcohol use.

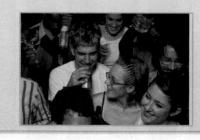

Diagnosing HIV/AIDS

MAIN IDEA Several tests are used to diagnose HIV/AIDS.

Because 1 in 5 people with HIV are unaware that they have the infection, the CDC recommends that everyone aged 13 to 64 be tested at least once. People in high-risk groups should be tested more frequently.

Typically, a blood sample or an oral specimen from between the inside of the cheek and the gum is collected and sent to a laboratory for analysis. Results are usually available within two weeks. At most testing sites, qualified personnel are available to answer questions, make referrals, and explain results.

Types of Laboratory HIV Tests

After collecting samples and sending them to a laboratory, technicians screen the sample for the presence of the HIV **antibody**. An antibody is a protein that acts against a specific antigen. These antibodies do not occur naturally in a person's body; they are produced only in the presence of an infection. The most common laboratory tests used for HIV screening are the nucleic acid test (NAT), antigen/antibody screening tests, and rapid antibody screening tests. A **rapid test** is an HIV test that produces results in only 20 minutes. Three types of rapid tests can be used. They are the rapid antibody screening test, the oral fluid antibody self-test, and the home collection kit.

Reading Check

Identify What are successful methods to avoid contracting HIV/AIDS?

A NAT test looks for the presence of the virus in the blood. This test is expensive and is generally used only when a person has recently been in a high-risk situation, or if the person is displaying early signs of HIV infection. When the NAT test is used, an antigen/antibody test is usually done at the same time.

Antigen/antibody screening test. An antigen/antibody screening test, also known as an EIA test, looks for the presence of HIV antigens and antibodies in the blood. Antigens are foreign substances in the blood. They cause the immune system to become active. If the results are positive, that means HIV antibodies are present.

One of three types of rapid tests may be used in situations where the infected person might not come back to learn the results of an HIV test. With the rapid antibody screening test, a small sample of blood or oral fluid is used. A home collection kit is similar. A small sample of blood is collected at home and then sent to a laboratory where it is tested. Another test is the oral fluid antibody self-test. This test produces results in 20 minutes, and may be used at home, at a community testing center, or in a clinic.

Follow-up Tests. If a test for HIV is returned showing a positive result, an additional test is done to confirm the first test. Further testing is also done to distinguish the type of HIV antibodies, and to look directly at the virus.

Cost of Testing. HIV testing is fully covered by health insurance. To help prevent the spread of HIV, public health departments will offer the test free-of-charge. The local public health department can provide information on free testing, and may offer locations for free tests on the agency's website.

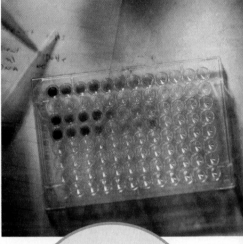

In a positive EIA test, HIV antibodies bind to the HIV antigens on a plastic bead coated with HIV proteins. **Under what circumstances would HIV antibodies appear in a tissue or blood sample?**

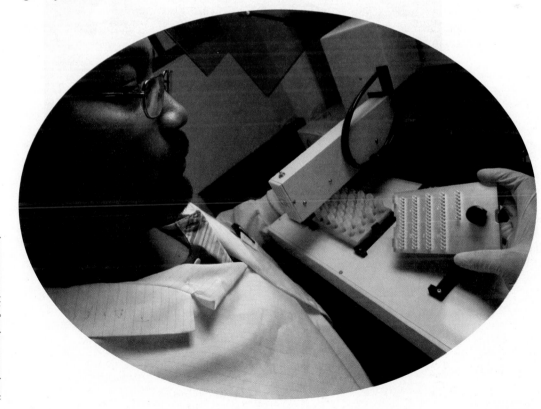

Reading Check

Explain Why is testing necessary for those who suspect they have contracted HIV/AIDS?

Character Check

Each individual can play a role in curbing the spread of HIV by staying informed and spreading the word about this disease. Take the time to read articles about HIV/AIDS. Share information with family and friends about recent developments in treatment and research to find a cure.

Benefits of Early Diagnosis

There are several benefits to early testing and diagnosis of HIV/AIDS. Early detection allows a person to:

- Begin proper medical care early to slow the progress of HIV.

- Avoid behaviors that could spread the virus to others.

- Gain peace of mind when the results are negative.

Treating HIV/AIDS

MAIN IDEA Medications can slow the progress of HIV/AIDS, but there is no cure.

No drug yet exists to cure HIV/AIDS. However, since the early 1980s, drugs have been developed that slow the progress of HIV and treat some of its symptoms. To slow the growth of the virus, people take a combination of drugs, a treatment known as antiretroviral therapy (ART). In 2006, the FDA approved a once-daily, single-pill treatment for HIV/AIDs.

Many of the HIV drugs available are also used to treat the opportunistic infections that can attack a weakened immune system. AIDS-opportunistic illnesses include pneumonia and some types of cancers that can ultimately cause death.

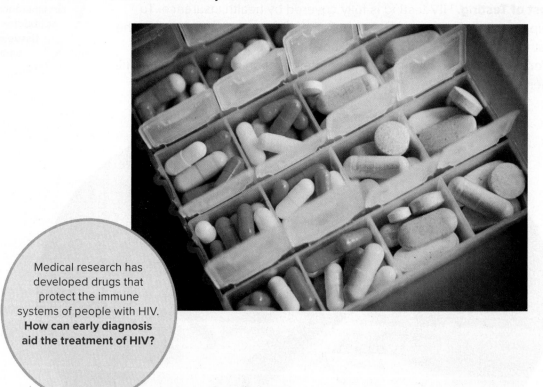

Medical research has developed drugs that protect the immune systems of people with HIV. **How can early diagnosis aid the treatment of HIV?**

AIDS Awareness Campaign

HIV/AIDS affects everyone. Conduct an Internet search to find the number of people, along with age ranges, who have been diagnosed with AIDS over the last decade. The CDC and the National Institutes of Health (NIH) are good websites to begin your search for this information.

Activity: Technology

Work in groups to create a campaign to raise awareness of HIV/AIDS prevention. Use the information that was gathered from the Internet search. Each member of your team will be responsible for completing one item for the campaign. Campaign materials can include the following:

- A blog, website, or wiki.

- Public service announcement script for a podcast.

- Opinion article for an e-newsletter or the school's website.

The materials should encourage teens to avoid behaviors that can put them at risk for HIV/AIDS.

Lesson 4 Review

Facts and Vocabulary

1. Name the tests used to detect HIV.

2. Name the test used to confirm a diagnosis of HIV once antibodies are detected.

3. Explain what you can do to check the accuracy of HIV/AIDS home testing kits.

Thinking Critically

4. **Synthesize.** What are the benefits of getting tested for HIV when an infection is suspected?

5. **Analyze.** When and for what reasons are blood or tissue samples tested more than once for HIV?

Applying Health Skills

6. **Advocacy.** Working in small groups, plan a classroom, school, or community project to help support AIDS research.

Writing Critically

7. **Expository.** Write an essay discussing how a teen's health and social life might be affected if the teen tested positive for HIV.

LESSON 1

Vocabulary Review

Use the correct vocabulary term to complete the following statements.

1. People infected with STDs often do not realize they have an infection because many STDs can be _____.

2. Health experts say that the United States currently faces an STD _____.

Understanding Key Concepts

After reading the question or statement, select the correct answer.

3. STDs can be passed from person to person through
   a. casual contact such as shaking hands.
   b. the air by coughing or sneezing.
   c. sexual contact.
   d. all of the above.

4. If left untreated, all STDs
   a. can lead to serious health problems.
   b. will eventually cure themselves.
   c. will become asymptomatic.
   d. lead to infection by HIV/AIDS.

Thinking Critically

After reading the question or statement, write a short answer using complete sentences.

5. **Describe.** Give one reason why STDs go undiagnosed and untreated.

6. **Compare and Contrast.** What are the differences in the ways that STDs affect males and females?

LESSON 2

Vocabulary Review

Correct the sentences below by replacing the italicized term with the correct vocabulary term.

7. Many STDs can be treated and some cured with medications called *HPV vaccines*.

8. A *refusal skill* is the deliberate decision to avoid sexual activity.

Understanding Key Concepts

After reading the question or statement, select the correct answer.

9. Which is not a high-risk behavior?
   a. Engaging in sexual activity with multiple partners
   b. Engaging in unprotected sexual activity
   c. Using alcohol and other drugs
   d. Abstaining from sexual activity

10. Getting a diagnosis and treatment is
    a. acting responsibly.
    b. crucial for those infected with STDs.
    c. a healthful behavior.
    d. all of the above.

11. Treatment of an STD
    a. does not prevent reinfection.
    b. isn't always necessary.
    c. can be postponed.
    d. always cures the infection.

Thinking Critically

After reading the question or statement, write a short answer using complete sentences.

12. **Compare and Contrast.** Identify the differences and similarities between viral and bacterial STDs.

13. **Discuss.** Which STD can be prevented by a vaccine? What are its limitations? Who is eligible to receive this vaccination?

14. **Evaluate.** Why is preventing STD transmission more effective than treating STDs?

15. **Explain.** What are antibiotics? How are they used to treat STDs?

Vocabulary Review

Choose the correct term in the sentences below.

16. *HIV/Mucous membrane* is transmitted through the bloodstream.

17. *Lymphocyte/AIDS* is the final stage of HIV infection.

18. Health care officials consider AIDS to be a(n) *antibody/pandemic*.

Understanding Key Concepts

After reading the question or statement, select the correct answer.

19. During the course of HIV/AIDS, the infected person
    a. gets stronger.
    b. should not hug anyone or shake hands.
    c. needs less and less medication.
    d. becomes vulnerable to opportunistic illnesses.

20. Which of the following is not a way that HIV attacks cells?
    a. The virus attaches itself to the cell's surface.
    b. The virus makes a copy of its genetic material.
    c. The virus shrinks cells.
    d. The new virus assembles at cell surface.

21. It is difficult for antibodies to fight AIDS because
    a. HIV weakens antibodies.
    b. HIV destroys white blood cells.
    c. HIV is protected once it enters cells.
    d. HIV mutates rapidly.

Thinking Critically

After reading the question or statement, write a short answer using complete sentences.

22. **Explain.** Describe how HIV infection progresses in the body.

23. **Identify.** Name three ways HIV is transmitted.

24. **Evaluate.** What misinformation causes some people to stay away from those infected with HIV? Why is this information wrong?

Vocabulary Review

Use the correct vocabulary term to complete the following statements.

25. The _____ test is the first test that technicians use to screen for HIV.

26. If the initial test produces positive results twice, a(n) _____ test is run.

27. The _____ allows samples to be tested on site rather than sending them to labs.

Understanding Key Concepts

After reading the question or statement, select the correct answer.

28. A person who thinks he or she is infected with HIV/AIDS should
    a. use a home testing kit.
    b. hide the condition from others.
    c. get a medical diagnosis right away.
    d. hope that symptoms do not appear.

29. About one-fourth of the people infected with HIV/AIDS

    a. are males.

    b. are females.

    c. don't know they are infected.

    d. will never develop symptoms.

30. People who are infected with HIV/AIDS, but don't know it,

    a. won't become as ill as those who know they have the virus.

    b. don't need to change their high-risk behaviors.

    c. don't need to practice abstinence.

    d. can unknowingly spread the virus to others.

Thinking Critically

After reading the question or statement, write a short answer using complete sentences.

31. **Explain.** The number of HIV/AIDS infections is much higher in developing nations than in developed countries. Why might this number be higher in some countries?

32. **Identify.** What are some benefits of early diagnosis of HIV/AIDS?

PROJECT-BASED ASSESSMENT

Knowledge is Power

BACKGROUND

Access to accurate information can prevent the spread of STDs. How much do the teens in your school know about STDs?

TASK

Use a free online survey tool to create a survey to determine areas in which students in your school are uninformed or misinformed about STDs. Create a webpage that provides students with accurate information about STDs, including the fact that abstinence is the only 100 percent effective way to prevent infection.

AUDIENCE

Teens in your school

PURPOSE

Educate students about STDs by providing accurate information.

PROCEDURE

1. Collaborate as a group to use the information in the module to make up the questions for the online survey.

2. Select 20 or more students in your school and ask them to answer the questions.

3. Analyze the answers to determine areas in which students are uninformed or misinformed.

4. Create a webpage that provides the needed information.

5. Present your group's webpage to your class.

Math Practice

Interpret Graphs. The bar graph below shows the number of new cases of different STDs reported in the United States. Study the bar graph, and then answer the questions.

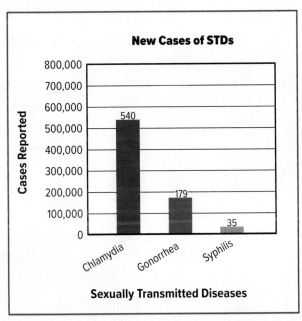

New Cases of STDs

Cases Reported

- Chlamydia: 540
- Gonorrhea: 179
- Syphilis: 35

Sexually Transmitted Diseases

Source: Centers for Disease Control and Prevention, 2018

1. If the population of the United States is about 328 million, what is the ratio of infection for chlamydia this year?
   a. 1 in 60
   b. 1 in 600
   c. 1 in 6,000
   d. 1 in 60,000

2. How much more common is chlamydia infection than gonorrhea?
   a. Twice as common
   b. Three times more common
   c. Four times more common
   d. Six times more common

3. Using the bar graph, explain how you would predict the rates of STD infection for people in your state.

Reading/Writing Practice

Understand and Apply. Read the passage below, and then answer the questions.

During the late 1980s, Ryan White was the face of AIDS for many Americans. Ryan contracted AIDS through a blood transfusion. Many members of his community mistakenly believed that AIDS could spread through casual contact. They pressured the school board to ban Ryan from attending school. Ryan's family took his case to court, and he was eventually allowed to return to school. Ryan became an AIDS educator. He spoke of the need for everyone to learn about AIDS and to treat affected people with compassion and dignity. Ryan lived for six years following his AIDS diagnosis. He died in 1990 at age 18. Later that year, Congress passed the Ryan White Comprehensive AIDS Resources Emergency (CARE) Act. Today, the act provides about $1.5 billion annually to care for people living with HIV/AIDS.

1. What is the purpose of this passage?
   a. To describe an early case of AIDS
   b. To describe the fear of HIV/AIDS
   c. To show how Ryan fought AIDS
   d. To blame public officials

2. What was the result of the publicity surrounding Ryan's case?
   a. It helped Ryan live longer.
   b. It allowed Ryan to return to school.
   c. It provided the public with factual information about HIV/AIDS.
   d. It increased the hostility against Ryan.

3. Write a paragraph explaining how HIV can and cannot be spread. Explain why the virus can be spread only in certain ways.

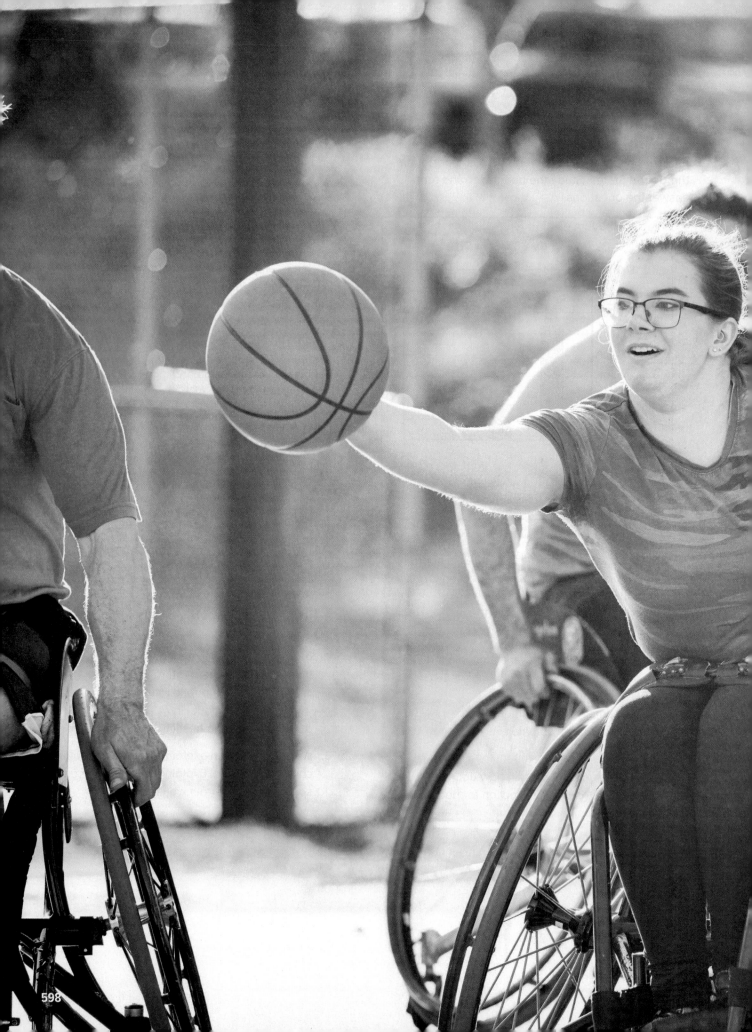

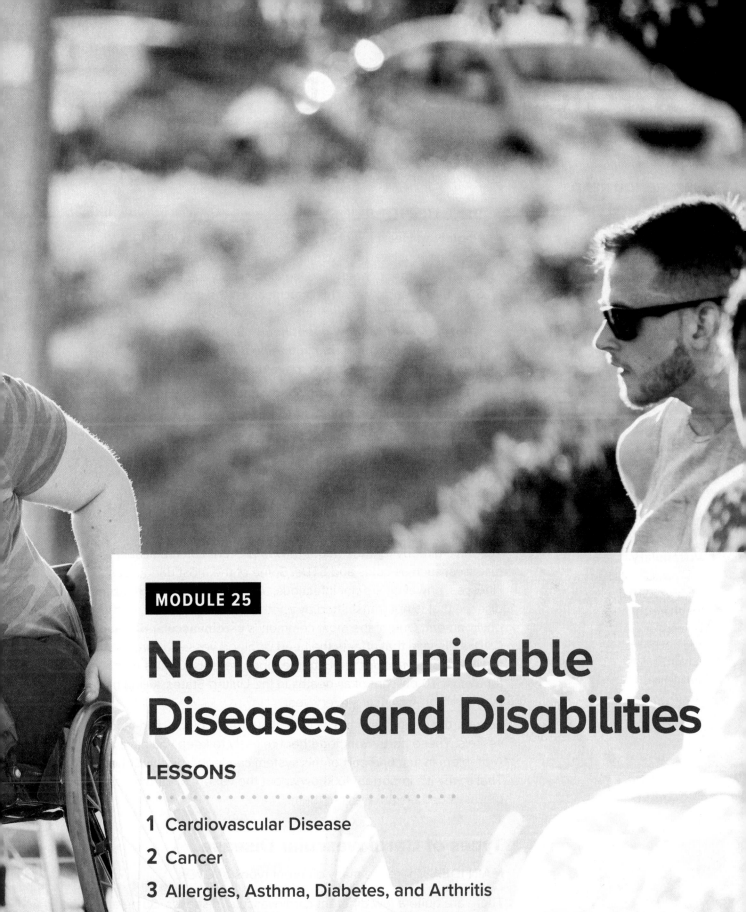

Noncommunicable Diseases and Disabilities

LESSONS

1 Cardiovascular Disease

2 Cancer

3 Allergies, Asthma, Diabetes, and Arthritis

4 Physical and Mental Challenges

Cardiovascular Disease

BEFORE YOU READ

Create a Cluster Chart.
Draw a circle and label it "Cardiovascular Disease," or CVD. Use surrounding circles to identify factors that contribute to this disease. As you read, continue filling in the chart with more details.

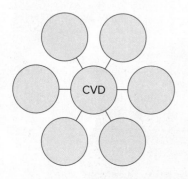

Vocabulary

noncommunicable disease
cardiovascular disease
hypertension
atherosclerosis
arteriosclerosis
angina pectoris
arrhythmias
stroke

BIG IDEA Preventive behaviors can reduce your risk for cardiovascular disease and stroke.

REAL LIFE ISSUES

Neglected Hearts. According to the CDC, about 600,000 people die of heart disease in the U.S. every year—that's 1 in 4 deaths. Coronary heart disease alone costs the U.S. more than $108 billion each year. This total includes the cost of health care services, medications, and lost productivity. *Think about what you already know about heart disease. Write a paragraph explaining why you think it is important to fight heart disease before it even develops.*

After completing the lesson, review and analyze your response to the Real Life Issues question.

Cardiovascular Disease

MAIN IDEA The heart, blood, and blood vessels are at risk for a number of potentially serious diseases.

You have already learned about how to prevent communicable diseases, such as colds and STDs. Some of the most dangerous illnesses, however, are not infectious. A **noncommunicable disease** is a disease that is not transmitted by another person, a vector, or the environment. One of the most common is **cardiovascular disease**, or CVD, a disease that affects the heart or blood vessels. *Cardio* refers to the heart, and *vascular* refers to the blood vessels. CVD is responsible for almost 40 percent of all deaths in the United States, killing more than a million Americans every year.

Your cardiovascular system includes your heart, blood, and blood vessels. These parts work together tirelessly to keep you alive and well. A problem in just one part of this system can jeopardize your health. That's why it's important to know about the variety of cardiovascular diseases and how to prevent them.

Types of Cardiovascular Disease

MAIN IDEA There are many different types of CVDs.

There are quite a few different cardiovascular diseases. Some affect the heart, others affect the blood, and some affect the system as a whole. As you read about these diseases, think about how each one is caused and what you can do to reduce your risk.

Hypertension

High blood pressure can damage the heart, blood vessels, and other body organs if it continues over a period of time. It is also a major risk factor for other types of CVDs. Because **hypertension**, or high blood pressure, often has no symptoms in its early stages, it is sometimes called a "silent killer."

High blood pressure can occur at any age, but it is more common among people over the age of 35. It is estimated that about one-third of American adults have hypertension. People can often treat this condition just by managing their weight, eating a healthful diet, and staying physically active. However, medication is also available.

Atherosclerosis

When you were born, the lining of your blood vessels were smooth and elastic. What is the condition of your blood vessels today? If you smoke, have high blood pressure, or have high cholesterol levels, a fatty substance called plaque can build up on your artery walls. This condition is known as **atherosclerosis**, a disease characterized by the accumulation of plaque on artery walls. People with atherosclerosis have a condition called **arteriosclerosis**, hardened arteries with reduced elasticity.

The main cause of atherosclerosis is making unhealthful food choices—specifically, foods that have large amounts of saturated fat and cholesterol. Sometimes a blood clot forms near plaque buildup and blocks the artery. If this artery supplies blood to the heart or the brain, a heart attack or stroke may result.

Diseases of the Heart

Every day, your heart pumps about 100,000 times, moving blood to all parts of your body. Like every other part of your body, it needs oxygen from the blood in order to function. When the blood supply to the heart is reduced or blocked, the heart does not get the oxygen it needs. The result may be chest pain (angina pectoris) or heart muscle damage (heart attack). Other common diseases of the heart include arrhythmias and congestive heart failure. Doctors use a variety of techniques to diagnose and treat heart disease.

Reading Check

Identify What are some healthful behaviors that can prevent atherosclerosis?

The artery on the far left is healthy, while the other arteries show evidence of atherosclerosis. **What lifestyle choices can increase your risk for atherosclerosis?**

Healthy and Unhealthy Arteries

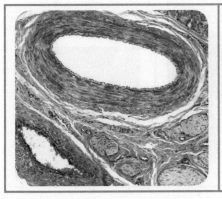 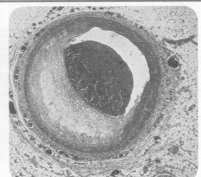 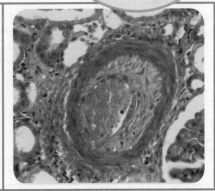

As medical technology advances, more diagnostic tools and treatment options become available. **Which treatment option uses a small balloon to clear a blocked artery?**

Angina Pectoris. Chest pain that results when the heart does not get enough oxygen is called **angina pectoris**. Angina pectoris is usually caused by atherosclerosis. The pain of angina usually lasts from a few seconds to a few minutes. This pain should be taken seriously, since it is a warning sign that the heart is not getting enough blood. It can sometimes be treated with medication.

Arrhythmias. Irregular heartbeats, or **arrhythmias**, happen when the heart skips a beat or beats very fast or very slowly. Arrhythmias are quite common and usually don't cause problems. However, some types are serious and should always be checked by a doctor. In one type, called *ventricular fibrillation,* the electrical impulses that **regulate** heart rhythm become rapid or irregular. This is the most common cause of *cardiac arrest,* in which the heart stops beating regularly. Cardiac arrest can lead to sudden death. It can be treated with cardiopulmonary resuscitation (CPR) or the use of an automated external defibrillator.

DIAGNOSING AND TREATING HEART DISEASE

Diagnostic Tools

Electrocardiogram (EKG)	Magnetic Resonance Imaging (MRI)	Angiography	CT Scan
Produces graph of heart's electrical activity. Shows heart function. 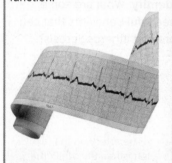	Uses powerful magnets to produce images. Shows heart damage and defects. 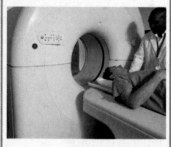	Thin, flexible tube guided through blood vessels to the heart. Dye is injected, and motion X-rays taken to look for heart obstructions. 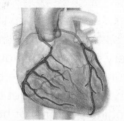	The patient lies on a table inside a doughnut-shaped machine. Scans create multiple images of the heart. Scans show calcium blockages in arteries and vessels. Scans show heart function.

Treatment Options

Coronary Bypass	Angioplasty	Pacemaker	Laser Intervention
Healthy vein removed from another area to create a detour around blocked artery. 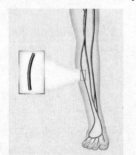	Tube with balloon inserted into blocked artery. Balloon inflated against artery walls, then deflated and removed. Metal structure may remain to keep artery open.	Implanted in chest. Sends electrical impulses to heart to make it beat regularly. 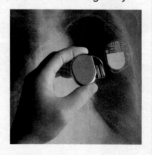	Laser fiber inserted into blocked artery. Laser vaporizes the blockage and restores the flow of blood. 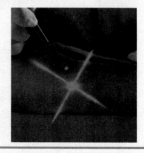

Heart Attack. Heart attack is not the same thing as cardiac arrest, which occurs due to an electrical problem with the heart. A heart attack occurs when a restricted blood supply damages the heart muscle. Many heart attacks cause intense chest pain, but about 25 percent produce no symptoms or less common symptoms, such as shortness of breath. Nausea and fatigue are more common in women. Anyone who experiences the following warning signs of heart attack should call 911 immediately:

- Pressure, fullness, squeezing, or aching in the chest area

- Pain spreading to arms, neck, jaw, abdomen, or back

- Chest discomfort with shortness of breath, dizziness, sweating, nausea, or vomiting

Congestive Heart Failure. This occurs when the heart gradually weakens and can no longer pump blood at its usual rate and force. Congestive heart failure cannot be cured, but it can improve through ongoing treatment, such as medication and healthful behaviors. In other cases, a heart transplant may be needed. Transplant centers consider each case individually based on factors such as age, other health concerns, and willingness to make lifestyle changes. Hearts and other organs for transplant are collected from people who have signed up to become donors through their state's donor registry. The government website www.organdonor.gov provides information about how to become an organ donor.

In many cases sudden cardiac arrest can be reversed if CPR or electric shock using a defibrillator is applied. **Why is it important to have defibrillators available in many different public places?**

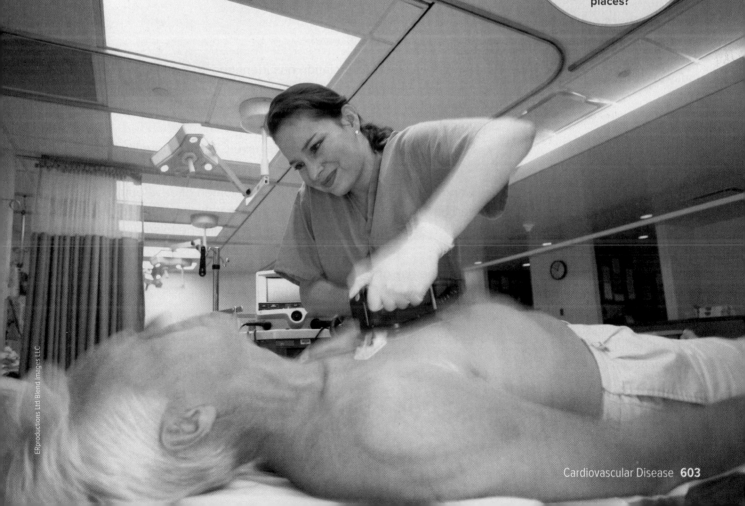

ERproductions Ltd/Blend Images LLC

Stroke

Cardiovascular disease (CVD) can affect the brain as well as the heart. Sometimes an artery supplying blood to the brain becomes blocked or bursts, resulting in a **stroke**—an acute injury in which blood flow to the brain is interrupted. A stroke that occurs because of a burst blood vessel is called a cerebral hemorrhage. Stroke can cause problems such as paralysis. The damage depends on the size of the stroke and what part of the brain is affected.

Warning signs of stroke include severe headache, numbness on one side of the body, confusion, trouble walking, dizziness, and trouble seeing out of one or both eyes. Today, treatments exist that can stop a stroke as it is occurring. Drugs known as clot busters can break up a clot and restore the normal flow of blood to the brain.

What Teens Need to Know

MAIN IDEA CVD can begin during the teen years.

Did you know that CVD can start to develop during adolescence or even childhood? Autopsy results on teens who died from causes other than CVD found that one in six already showed signs of CVD. Those with known risk factors, such as smoking or diabetes, were more likely to have blood vessel damage. A teen with damaged blood vessels may not experience any symptoms until later in adulthood, but the danger is already there.

Reading Check

Identify What are three decisions you could make today to reduce your risk of CVD?

Myths & Reality

Diseases are very complex. Do you think you understand everything about cardiovascular disease?

Myth: Most people with cardiovascular disease die suddenly.

Reality: Cardiovascular disease usually causes people to become progressively ill and debilitated, especially if it is not managed properly.

Risk Factors

The American Heart Association has identified several factors that increase the risk of heart attack and stroke. There are some factors that you can control. Unfortunately, there are also some that are unavoidable:

- **Heredity.** Children whose parents have CVD are more likely to develop CVD themselves.

- **Gender.** Men have a greater risk than women of developing CVD and having heart attacks. However, research shows that older women are less likely than men of the same age to survive a heart attack.

- **Age.** The risk of CVD increases with age. Approximately 80 percent of people who die of CVD are 65 or older.

Knowing about these risk factors can help you make healthful decisions to reduce your risk. For example, if CVD runs in your family, you can make a strong commitment to control your weight, exercise regularly, avoid tobacco use, and eat foods low in fat and cholesterol.

CVD RISK FACTORS YOU CAN CONTROL		
Risk Factor	**Preventive Measure**	**Why It's Important**
Tobacco Use	Avoid using tobacco.	About 20 percent of deaths from CVDs are smoking related. For teens, tobacco use is the biggest risk factor.
	Avoid secondhand smoke.	About 46,000 nonsmokers who are exposed to secondhand smoke die from CVDs each year.
High Blood Pressure	Have your blood pressure checked regularly.	High blood pressure strains your cardiovascular system.
	Eat healthfully, exercise regularly, and manage your weight.	
High Cholesterol	Eat fewer high-fat and high-cholesterol foods, and get regular physical activity.	High cholesterol can cause plaque to form in your arteries.
Physical Inactivity	Be sure you get at least 30 to 60 minutes of physical activity every day.	Physical activity strengthens your heart and helps you maintain a healthy weight.
Excess Weight	Maintain a healthy weight.	Excess weight puts a strain on the heart and raises blood pressure and blood cholesterol levels. It also increases your risk for type 2 diabetes (a risk factor for heart disease).
Stress	Use stress-management techniques.	Constant stress raises blood pressure.
Alcohol and Drug Use	Abstain from alcohol and other drugs.	Too much alcohol raises blood pressure and can cause irregular heartbeat or heart failure. Some illegal drugs increase heart rate and blood pressure and can result in heart failure.

An Exercise Campaign

Moderate exercise helps keep people healthy. Exercise burns calories, builds muscle, and helps the heart stay strong. Some people feel that exercise must be done for at least an hour and must be strenuous. Conduct an Internet search for examples of forms of exercise that are not strenuous and time-consuming.

Activity: Technology

Exercise can be as simple as a brisk walk, and most of the benefits are gained in the first half hour. More people should know that moderate exercise for just 30 minutes per day is an effective way to maintain or improve cardiovascular health.

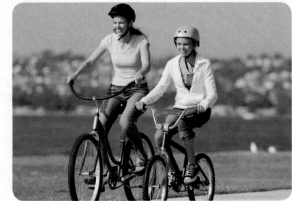

Based on your Internet research, create a campaign to encourage teens to exercise for 30 minutes per day. The campaign should help teens understand why exercise is important, what kinds of exercises help their cardiovascular systems, and how much exercise people need. Create a webpage for the school's website that will inspire teens to begin a moderate exercise program.

Lesson 1 Review

Facts and Vocabulary

1. Define the term *cardiovascular disease*.

2. Describe what can happen if hypertension is not treated.

3. Define the term *stroke*.

Thinking Critically

4. **Compare and Contrast.** How is stroke similar to heart attack? How is it different?

5. **Synthesize.** How can practicing healthy lifestyle behaviors today help lower your risk for cardiovascular disease in the future?

Applying Health Skills

6. **Practicing Healthful Behaviors.** Evaluate your daily habits. What decisions can you make today to replace unhealthful choices with healthful ones?

Writing Critically

7. **Persuasive.** Imagine you have a friend who says you don't need to worry about CVD until you are older. Write a letter convincing this friend that it's important to start taking preventive measures now.

Cancer

BIG IDEA Cancer takes many different forms and can affect people of all ages.

REAL LIFE ISSUES

Making a Healthful Choice. Amy is worried about her granddad. He is a longtime smoker, and Amy has learned in school that smoking can lead to health problems, such as heart disease and cancer. Amy and her mom both want her granddad to quit smoking. They have decided to write letters telling him how they feel when they see him smoking. They want him to know how important he is to them and why they want him to stay healthy. *What should Amy write to encourage her granddad to stop smoking? How can she use the letter to express her concern and support? Summarize your thoughts in a paragraph.*

After completing the lesson, review and analyze your response to the Real Life Issues question.

BEFORE YOU READ

Create a K-W-L Chart. Make a three-column chart. In the first column, write what you know about the behaviors or lifestyle choices that can lead to cancer. In the second column, write what you want to know about cancer risk factors. As you read, use the third column to summarize what you learned.

K	W	L

Vocabulary

cancer
tumor
malignant
metastasis
benign
biopsy
remission

What Is Cancer?

MAIN IDEA Cancer has a variety of forms and affects different areas of the body.

Cells are the building blocks of your body. Approximately 100 trillion of these tiny cells are constantly growing, dividing, dying, and replacing themselves inside you. Although most new cells are normal, some are not. **Cancer** occurs when abnormal cells reproduce rapidly and uncontrollably.

How Cancer Harms the Body

When abnormal cells build up inside otherwise normal tissue, they can form a **tumor**. This is an abnormal mass of tissue that has no natural role in the body. Many people assume that a tumor means cancer, but that is not always the case. In fact, there are two kinds of tumors: malignant and benign. A **malignant**, or cancerous, tumor does not stay in one place. It spreads to neighboring tissue and enters the blood or lymph to travel to other parts of the body. This process is called **metastasis**. As cancer cells spread throughout the body, they divide and form new tumors.

A **benign**, or noncancerous, tumor, by contrast, grows slowly. It is surrounded by membranes that prevent it from spreading. Does this mean that it is harmless? No, not always. A benign tumor can still put pressure on your organs and tissues and interfere with normal body functions. It can also block arteries, veins, and other passages. For example, a benign tumor in the brain could block the brain's blood supply.

TYPES OF CANCER			
Organ Affected (new cases/year)	**Some Risk Factors**	**Symptoms**	**Screening and Early Detection Methods**
Skin (96,480) Most common type of cancer in the United States	Exposure to ultra-violet (UV) radiation from the sun, tanning beds, sunlamps, and other sources	Change on the skin, especially a new growth, a mole or freckle that changes, or a sore that won't heal	Physical exam, biopsies
Breast (271,270) Second leading cause of cancer death for women	Genetic factors, obesity, alcohol use, physical inactivity	Unusual lump; nipple that thickens, changes shape, dimples, or has discharge	Self-exam, mammogram
Prostate (174,650) Found mostly in men over 55	Possible hereditary link, possible link to high-fat diet	Frequent or painful urination; inability to urinate; weak or interrupted flow of urine; blood in urine or semen; pain in lower back, hips, or upper thighs	Blood test
Lung (228,150) Leading cause of cancer deaths in the United States	Exposure to cigarette smoke, radon, or asbestos	No initial symptoms; later symptoms include cough, shortness of breath, wheezing, coughing up blood, hoarseness	Chest X-ray
Colon/Rectum (145,600) Second leading cause of cancer deaths in the United States	Risk increases with age	Often no initial symptoms; later, blood in feces; frequent pain, aches, or cramps in stomach; change in bowel habits; weight loss	Test for blood in the stool, rectal exam, colonoscopy
Mouth (14,310) Occurs mostly in people over 40	Use of tobacco, chewing tobacco, or alcohol	Sore or lump on mouth that doesn't heal; unusual bleeding; pain or numbness on lip, mouth, tongue, or throat; feeling that something is caught in the throat; pain with chewing or swallowing; change in voice	Dental/oral exam
Cervix (13,170)	History of infection with human papillomavirus (HPV)	Usually no symptoms in early stages; later, abnormal vaginal bleeding, increased vaginal discharge	Pap test
Testicle (9,560) Most common cancer in men ages 15 to 34	Undescended testicle; family history of testicular cancer	Small, hard, painless lump on testicle; sudden accumulation of fluid in scrotum; pain in region between scrotum and anus	Self-exam

NIH, National Cancer Institute 2019; American Cancer Society, Cancer Facts & Figures, 2019.

Types of Cancer

Cancers can develop in almost any part of the body. Cancers are classified according to the tissues they affect:

- **Lymphomas.** These are cancers of the immune system.

- **Leukemias.** These are cancers of the blood-forming organs.

- **Carcinomas.** These are cancers of the glands and body linings, including the skin and the linings of the digestive tract and lungs.

- **Sarcomas.** These are cancers of the connective tissue, bones, ligaments, and muscles.

Risk Factors for Cancer

MAIN IDEA Risk factors for cancer include lifestyle behaviors.

Every day, your body produces countless healthy, normal cells—but it also produces some abnormal ones. Your immune system usually kills these abnormal cells before they become cancerous. However, when the immune system is weak or when the abnormal cells multiply faster than the immune system can destroy them, cancer may develop.

Carcinogens

Many cancers develop because of exposure to a carcinogen. Tobacco and UV light are two of the most common carcinogens.

Tobacco Use. The number one cause of cancer deaths in the United States is tobacco use. About 70 different carcinogens have been linked to tobacco and tobacco smoke. About 90 percent of lung cancers are caused by smoking. About 40 percent of all cancers are **linked** to tobacco use. On average, smokers live 1 year fewer than nonsmokers.

This risk factor is not limited to smokers. Smokeless tobacco is a major risk factor for oral cancer, which affects the lips, mouth, and throat. Nonsmokers who are exposed to secondhand smoke are also at risk because they breathe in nicotine and other toxic chemicals.

Radiation. Another common carcinogen is ultraviolet (UV) radiation. The glow of a suntan may look attractive, but it is actually your skin's reaction to damage from the sun. UV rays from the sun are the main cause of skin cancer. Tanning beds and sunlamps also emit UV radiation, which is just as damaging as the sun's rays.

Reading Check

Explain Are benign tumors harmless? Why or why not?

ACADEMIC VOCABULARY

link *(verb)*: to connect

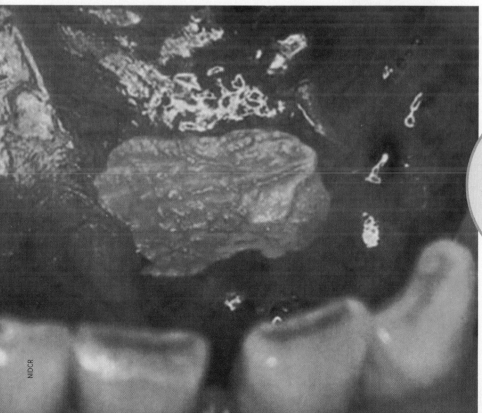

NIDCR

This person's cancer may have been caused by using smokeless tobacco. **Smokeless tobacco is a major risk factor for what kind of cancer?**

Sexually Transmitted Diseases

Some sexually transmitted diseases can lead to cancer. For example, certain forms of human papillomavirus, or HPV, can cause cervical cancer. The hepatitis B virus, another STD, can cause cancer of the liver.

Dietary Factors

Being obese increases a person's risk for cancer. A diet that is high in fat and low in fiber is linked to cancers of the colon, breast, and prostate. Here's why:

- Fats make colon cells more vulnerable to carcinogens. Colon cells divide faster if the diet is high in fat, increasing the risk that abnormal cells will form.

- Dietary fiber speeds the movement of waste through the intestines and out of the body. If a person's diet is low in fiber, the waste moves more slowly, giving carcinogens in the waste more time to act on the body's cells.

Reducing Your Risk

Sometimes cancer seems to strike people at random. That is one of the most frightening aspects of the disease. Although some factors may be beyond your control, you can dramatically lower your cancer risk by practicing healthful behaviors.

Reading Check

Explain Why is it important to eat high-fiber foods?

How You Can Reduce Your Cancer Risk

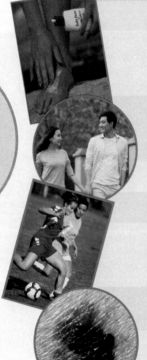

There are many healthful behaviors you can practice to reduce your risk for cancer. **How many of these behaviors do you already practice?**

Protect your skin from UV radiation.

Avoid tobacco and alcohol. Tobacco is the single major cause of cancer death in the United States. Excess alcohol increases the risk of several types of cancer, including mouth and throat cancer.

Practice abstinence from sexual activity to reduce the risk of sexually transmitted diseases. Hepatitis B can cause liver cancer, and HPV can cause cancers of the reproductive organs.

Be physically active.

Maintain a healthy weight.

Eat nutritious foods. Include 2–4 servings of fruits and 3–5 servings of vegetables every day. These foods are good sources of fiber, and some contain compounds that act against carcinogens.

Follow an eating plan that is low in saturated fat and high in fiber.

Recognize the warning signs of cancer. Do regular self-exams to detect cancer early.

Detecting Cancer

MAIN IDEA Early detection is the key to successful cancer treatment.

The survival rate for people with cancer depends on two main factors: the type of cancer and how early it is found. Early detection is the key to successful cancer treatment. Catching cancers early, in turn, depends on both self-examination and medical examination.

- Self-examination involves checking your own body for possible signs of cancer. Many types of cancer, including those of the breasts, testicles, and skin, are discovered early through self-examination.

- Medical examination, or medical screening, involves testing by a doctor for early signs of cancer. As medical technology continues to advance, doctors are able to detect cancers earlier than in the past. About half of all new cancer cases each year are detected during a routine medical screening.

If a doctor thinks cancer is a possibility, a **biopsy** may be ordered. A biopsy is the removal of a small piece of tissue for examination. This procedure is usually needed to determine whether cancer is present. Doctors also use X-rays and other imaging techniques to help determine a tumor's location and size.

Reading Check

Identify What are three actions you could take to reduce your risk for cancer?

WARNING SIGNS OF CANCER	
The warning signs listed below do not necessarily indicate cancer, as there may be other causes. However, all are serious enough to bring to a doctor's attention right away.	
Fever, fatigue, pain, and discoloration of the skin. These general signs can sometimes indicate cancer.	**Thickening or lump in breast or other body part.** Many cancers can be felt through the skin.
Change in bowel habits or bladder function. This may suggest colon, bladder, or prostate cancer.	**Indigestion or trouble swallowing.** Though usually harmless, these symptoms can sometimes indicate cancer of the stomach, esophagus, or throat.
Sores that will not heal. Persistent sores on skin, mouth, or genitalia should be examined promptly.	**Change in wart or mole.** Change in color or size might indicate skin cancer.
Unusual bleeding or discharge. This could be present in phlegm, stool, urine, or discharge from vagina or nipples.	**Nagging cough or hoarseness.** This could indicate cancer of the lungs, larynx, or thyroid.

A person with any of these warning signs should see a doctor as soon as possible. **What is a warning sign of skin cancer?**

Treating Cancer

MAIN IDEA There are many options for treating cancer.

Treatment options for cancer have expanded greatly in recent years. The methods used to treat cancer depend on several factors, such as the type of cancer and whether a tumor has spread from its original location. Treatment may include one or more of the methods listed below:

- Surgery removes some or all of the cancerous masses from the body.
- Radiation therapy uses radioactive substances to kill cancer cells and shrink cancerous masses.
- Chemotherapy uses chemicals to destroy cancer cells.
- Immunotherapy activates a person's immune system to recognize specific cancers and destroy them.
- Hormone therapy uses medicines to interfere with the production of certain hormones, such as estrogen, that help cancer cells grow. These treatments kill cancer cells or slow their growth.

If treatment succeeds in removing the cancer or getting it under control, the cancer is said to be in **remission**. This is a period of time when symptoms disappear. Today, more and more cancer survivors are able to lead full, active lives.

Reading Check

Identify Which cancer treatment option uses chemicals to destroy cancer cells?

Fitness Zone

When I told my doctor that some of my older relatives have gotten cancer, she told me that eating a healthy diet and making healthy lifestyle choices can reduce my risks. Making healthier choices could mean 375,000 fewer cancer diagnoses in the U.S. every year. That convinced me to make better choices to protect my health.

Lesson 2 Review

Facts and Vocabulary

1. Define the term *metastasis*.

2. Name two methods to use for early cancer detection.

3. Identify three cancer treatment options.

Thinking Critically

4. **Synthesize.** Based on what you know about your own lifestyle and what you now know about the risk factors for cancer, do you need to change any of your behaviors? Explain.

5. **Evaluate.** How does technology help in detecting and treating cancer?

Applying Health Skills

6. **Refusal Skills.** Based on what you have learned in this lesson, explain what you might say to someone who is trying to pressure you into using tobacco.

Writing Critically

7. **Expository.** Research the procedures used for early detection of cancer. Then write a short essay analyzing the benefits of health screenings, checkups, and early detection. Include information from your research to support your analysis.

Allergies, Asthma, Diabetes, and Arthritis

BEFORE YOU READ

Create Vocabulary Cards. Write each new vocabulary term on a separate index card. For each term, write a definition based on your current knowledge. As you read, fill in additional information related to each term.

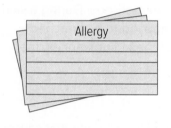

Vocabulary

allergy
histamines
diabetes
arthritis
rheumatoid arthritis

• • • • • • • • • • • •

BIG IDEA Practicing self-management strategies can help reduce the severity of allergies, asthma, diabetes, and arthritis.

REAL LIFE ISSUES

Using Good Judgment. Eliza feels good about volunteering at the local animal shelter on weekends. She loves taking care of the animals, but she always ends up leaving with a runny nose, an itchy throat, irritated eyes, and sneezing attacks. Eliza thinks she may have allergies, but she has not seen a doctor. She is worried that she won't be able to continue working with animals if she can't find a way to control her allergy symptoms. *Write a letter offering advice on how you think Eliza should handle her allergy symptoms.*

After completing the lesson, review and analyze your response to the Real Life Issues question.

Allergies

MAIN IDEA Allergies are caused by a variety of substances.

If you are sneezing and have a runny nose, you might have a cold—or it might be an **allergy**. An allergy is a specific reaction of the immune system to a foreign and frequently harmless substance. Have you ever noticed how many advertisements for allergy medicines are on TV and in magazines? That's because allergies are a very common noncommunicable illness.

The substances that cause allergies are called *allergens.* They include pollen, certain foods, dust, mold spores, chemicals, insect venom, animal dander, and certain medicines. When these substances make their way from the environment into your body, they can trigger an *allergic reaction.* Suppose, for example, that you have an allergy to pollen. If you come into contact with pollen, your body reacts this way:

1. The pollen enters your body, which treats it as a foreign invader.
2. Antigens on the surface of the pollen attach to special immune cells in the linings of the nasal passage.
3. These immune cells release **histamines**, which are chemicals that can stimulate mucus and fluid production.
4. Histamines cause sneezing, itchy eyes, runny nose, and other allergy symptoms.

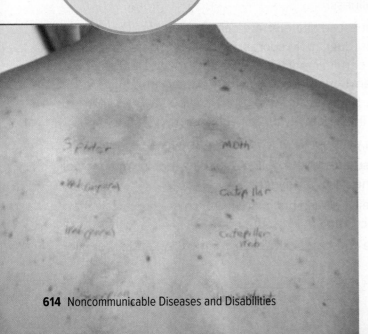

Reading Check

Describe How does the production of histamines affect the body?

Allergy Symptoms

There are many kinds of allergic reactions, ranging from mild to life-threatening. Some allergies, like Eliza's, produce sneezing, itchy eyes, and a scratchy throat. Others cause a rash or itchy, raised bumps on the skin, known as hives. More dangerous symptoms include:

- Severe hives
- Itching or swelling of an area stung by an insect
- Difficulty breathing or swallowing
- Swelling of the tongue, mouth, or eyes
- Sharp drop in blood pressure, which can cause dizziness

If someone you know experiences a severe allergic reaction, call 911 immediately.

Diagnosing Allergies

Sometimes you can diagnose an allergy yourself. For example, you may notice that you break out in a rash after eating certain foods. In many cases, though, tests are needed to identify the source of an allergic reaction. Blood tests and skin tests are common methods. During a skin test, small amounts of possible allergens are applied to a scratched area of the skin. If a person is allergic to any of these substances, the skin in that area will swell and turn red.

Treating Allergies

The simplest way to deal with an allergy is to avoid the allergen that causes it. Many people avoid peanuts, milk, or foods made with these ingredients because of allergies. However, some allergens cannot always be avoided. In such cases, people with allergies can take antihistamines, which help control their symptoms. Some antihistamines can cause side effects or worsen other medical conditions, such as heart or lung problems. Your doctor or pharmacist can tell you which medication will work best for you. If your allergies are severe, your doctor may prescribe a single, injectable dose of medicine that you carry with you at all times. This fact-acting medicine could save your life during a severe allergy attack.

Skin tests can determine which substances cause an individual to have allergic reactions. **Why are several different substances used when doing skin patch tests?**

Asthma

MAIN IDEA Asthma has no cure, but it can be managed.

More than 18 million adults and 7 million children in the United States have asthma. This disease can develop at any age, but about one-third of asthma sufferers are under the age of 18. Asthma can be life threatening, so those who have it must take the condition seriously and learn to manage it.

Dr. Frank Perlman, M.A. Parson/CDC

If you have asthma, your bronchial tubes are highly sensitive to certain substances, called *triggers*. Common asthma triggers include air pollution, pet dander, tobacco smoke, microscopic mold, pollen, and dust mites. Exercise may also trigger an asthma attack. During an attack, the muscles of the bronchial walls tighten and produce extra mucus. Symptoms may range from minor wheezing to severe difficulty in breathing.

Managing Asthma

People with asthma are usually under a doctor's care and take prescribed medications. They can also help themselves with these self-management strategies:

- **Monitor the condition.** Learn to recognize the warning signs of an attack: shortness of breath, chest tightness or pain, coughing, or sneezing. Responding quickly can help prevent attacks or keep them from getting worse.

- **Manage your environment.** Avoid exposure to tobacco smoke, wash bedding frequently, and be aware of the air quality in your area.

- **Manage stress.** Stress can trigger an asthma attack. Learn relaxation and stress-management techniques to reduce your risk.

- **Take medication properly.** Medications help relieve symptoms, prevent flare-ups, and make air passages less sensitive to triggers. Many people with asthma use *bronchodilators,* or inhalers. These devices deliver medicine that relaxes and widens the respiratory passages.

Reading Check

Identify Name three triggers that can cause an asthma attack.

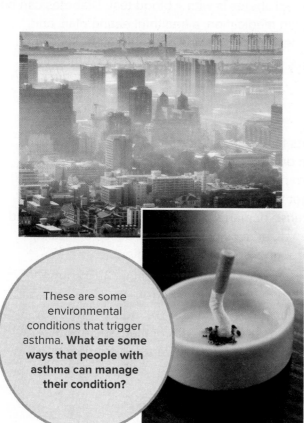

These are some environmental conditions that trigger asthma. **What are some ways that people with asthma can manage their condition?**

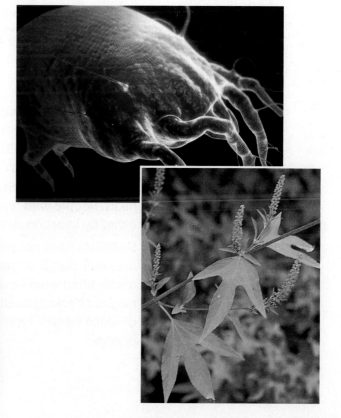

(tl)Don Bayley/E+/Getty Images, (tr)MedicalRF.com, (b)Adam Gault/age fotostock, (br)Steven P. Lynch

Diabetes

MAIN IDEA Type 2 diabetes is on the rise.

It's likely you know someone with **diabetes**. This is a chronic disease that affects the way body cells convert sugar into energy. It is one of the fastest-growing diseases in the United States, with almost 1.5 million new cases diagnosed in 2018. Young people are especially at risk today.

In some people with diabetes *(or diabetics),* the pancreas does not produce enough *insulin,* a hormone that helps glucose from food enter body cells and provide them with energy. Other diabetics do produce enough insulin, but the cells don't **respond** normally to it. As a result, glucose builds up in the blood instead of being delivered to cells. Symptoms of diabetes include:

- Frequent urination
- Excessive thirst
- Unexplained weight loss
- Sudden changes in vision
- Tingling in hands or feet
- Frequent fatigue
- Sores that are slow to heal
- More infections than usual

The only way to diagnose diabetes is with a blood test. Diabetes can be successfully managed with medication, a healthful eating plan, and regular moderate exercise. If the disease is not treated, the long-term effects include blindness, kidney failure, limb amputations, heart disease, and stroke.

Type 1 Diabetes

Type 1 diabetes accounts for 5 percent of all diabetes cases in young people. This form of the disease appears suddenly and progresses quickly. The body fails to produce insulin, glucose builds up in the blood, and cells don't get the energy they need. Over time, the high blood sugar level can cause damage to the eyes, kidneys, nerves, and heart. People with type 1 diabetes must take daily doses of insulin, either by injection or through a specially attached pump.

Scientists have not yet been able to determine what causes type 1 diabetes. Some suspect an environmental trigger—for example, an unidentified virus—that stimulates an immune response. The body begins attacking itself and destroys the cells of the pancreas that produce insulin. Type 1 diabetes is thus known as an autoimmune disease.

Type 2 Diabetes

In this form of diabetes, the body is unable to make enough insulin or to use insulin properly. Type 2 diabetes accounts for 90 to 95 percent of all cases of diabetes. It typically appears after age 40, but growing numbers of younger people—even children and teens—are developing this disease. This increase is directly linked to the increase in childhood obesity. Some scientists fear that type 2 diabetes will become an epidemic for two reasons: there are more older people in the population, and there are more obese and inactive young people.

There are two healthful behaviors that can help prevent type 2 diabetes:

- **Choose low-fat, low-calorie foods.** People whose eating plans are high in fat, calories, and cholesterol have an increased risk of diabetes.

- **Engage in regular physical activity.** Being active helps control weight and lowers blood cholesterol levels.

People with diabetes can live full, normal lives if they manage their condition. This includes monitoring their blood sugar levels, making healthful eating decisions, getting plenty of physical activity, and taking prescribed medications.

Reading Check

Explain What is one reason that type 2 diabetes is increasing among young people?

Arthritis

MAIN IDEA Arthritis is a major cause of disability.

Arthritis is a group of more than 100 different diseases that cause pain and loss of movement in the joints. It is more common in older adults, but it can affect people of all ages. The two main forms of arthritis are osteoarthritis and rheumatoid arthritis. Both can be debilitating, limiting movement in the affected joints. There is currently no cure for either type, but self-management techniques can reduce pain and improve movement.

Osteoarthritis

Half of all arthritis cases involve osteoarthritis. This condition causes cartilage—the strong, flexible tissue that cushions your joints—to become pitted and frayed. In time, it may wear away completely, causing the bones to rub painfully against each other. Osteoarthritis mainly affects the large, weight-bearing joints, such as the knees and hips. However, the fingers, feet, lower back, and lower joints are also at risk. People with osteoarthritis experience aches and soreness, especially when moving.

Several strategies can help reduce your risk of developing osteoarthritis:

- **Control your weight.** Maintaining a healthy weight reduces stress on your joints.

- **Stay active.** Physical activity strengthens your joints.

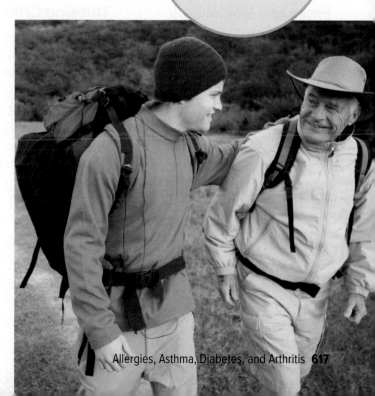

Staying active will help keep your joints strong. **What other healthful behaviors can help prevent arthritis?**

Corbis

Allergies, Asthma, Diabetes, and Arthritis **617**

Myths & Reality

Do you think you've got diabetes all figured out? Consider this fact.

Myth: I don't have a family history of diabetes, so I will not get it.

Reality: While some people inherit a great risk of developing diabetes, many people without a family history of diabetes are diagnosed with it. Weight and physical activity are other factors that can determine whether you will develop diabetes.

• • • • • • • • • • • •

- **Prevent sports injuries.** Warm up before exercising, participate in strength training, and use protective equipment to avoid joint injuries.

- **Protect against Lyme disease.** If left untreated, Lyme disease can result in a rare form of osteoarthritis. When walking in wooded areas, use insect repellant and wear long-sleeved shirts and pants.

Rheumatoid Arthritis

Rheumatoid arthritis is a disease characterized by the debilitating destruction of the joints due to inflammation. It is an autoimmune disorder. It is three times more common in women than in men. Symptoms usually first appear between the ages of 20 and 50, but the disease can also affect young children. Some of the symptoms and side effects include:

- joint pain, inflammation, swelling, and stiffness.

- deformed joints that can't function properly.

- possible fever, fatigue, and swollen lymph nodes.

Rheumatoid arthritis affects mainly the joints in the hand, foot, elbow, shoulder, knee, hip, and ankle. The effects are usually symmetrical, meaning that both sides of the body develop the same symptoms at the same time. Treatments focus on relieving pain, reducing inflammation, and keeping the joints flexible. Treatment methods include medication, exercise, rest, joint protection, and physical and occupational therapy.

Lesson 3 Review

Facts and Vocabulary

1. Define the term *histamines*. What role do they play in an allergic reaction?

2. Name three strategies for managing asthma.

3. Name the two main forms of arthritis.

Thinking Critically

4. **Synthesize.** If someone has allergies, is it safer to stay indoors or to get as much fresh air as possible? Explain.

5. **Evaluate.** Many people have diabetes but are not aware of it. What makes this lack of awareness dangerous?

Applying Health Skills

6. **Practicing Healthful Behaviors.** Make a three-column chart. In the first column, list the four diseases described in this lesson. In the second column, identify risk factors for each disease. In the third column, write down actions you can take to reduce your risk for each disease.

Writing Critically

7. **Narrative.** Write a story about a teen who has one of the diseases covered in this lesson. Describe how the condition affects the teen's daily life and how he or she manages the disease.

Physical and Mental Challenges

BIG IDEA People with physical and mental challenges deserve to be treated with dignity and respect.

REAL LIFE ISSUES

Dealing with a Disability. Peter was born with a physical disability that affects the way he walks. He doesn't need a wheelchair or a cane, but when he walks, he looks very different from most people. It also takes him longer to get from one place to another. Because he moves more slowly, Peter is always the last one picked for team sports. He sometimes hears people laughing at him. ***What would you say to someone who laughs at Peter? In a paragraph, explain why this behavior is wrong.***

After completing the lesson, review and analyze your response to the Real Life Issues question.

Physical Challenges

MAIN IDEA Most physical challenges affect sight, hearing, and motor ability.

About 37 to 56 million American adults have some kind of **disability**. A disability is any physical or mental impairment that limits normal activities, including seeing, hearing, walking, or speaking. The range of physical challenges is quite broad. However, most of them fall into one of three categories: sight impairment, hearing impairment, or motor impairment.

Sight Impairment

More than 3 million Americans are either blind or have low vision. In the United States, about 1.3 million people are legally blind, and at least 5 million have some degree of sight impairment that cannot be corrected with glasses or contact lenses. Sight impairment is more common among older adults, but it can affect people of all ages.

Blindness can also result from an injury, but disease is a much more common cause. The most common causes of blindness are:

- **Complications from diabetes,** in which high blood sugar levels cause damage to the retina. This is the leading cause of blindness.

- **Macular degeneration,** a condition in which the retina wastes away. This is the main cause of blindness in people over 55.

BEFORE YOU READ

Create a T-Chart. Make a two-column chart. Label one column "Physical Challenges" and the other "Mental Challenges." As you read, fill in the columns with examples and descriptions of each.

Physical Challenges	Mental Challenges

Vocabulary

disability
profound deafness
intellectual disability
Americans with Disabilities Act (ADA)

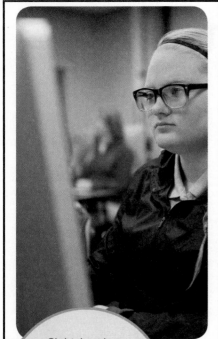
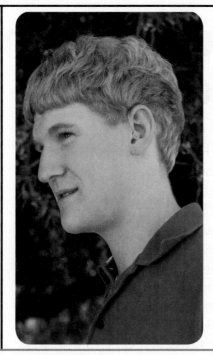
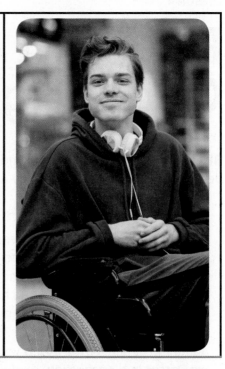

Sight, hearing, and motor impairment are examples of physical disabilities. **How has technology affected people with disabilities?**

· · · · · · · · · · · ·

Reading Check

Identify What is the number one cause of blindness?

· · · · · · · · · · · ·

- **Glaucoma,** a disease that damages the eye's optic nerve.
- **Cataracts,** a condition in which the eye's lens becomes clouded.

Regular eye exams can catch many eye conditions early. This can help prevent blindness or slow its progress.

Hearing Impairment

Almost 30 million Americans have disabilities that affect their ability to hear. Hearing problems range from mild difficulty to **profound deafness,** which is hearing loss so severe that a person affected cannot benefit from mechanical amplification, such as a hearing aid. A variety of factors can cause hearing impairments, including:

- **Heredity.** If one or both parents have hearing impairment, their child is more likely to develop it as well.
- **Injury.** An injury to the ears or head, such as a skull fracture, can cause hearing loss.
- **Disease.** Ear infections, brain tumors, measles, and other conditions can lead to hearing loss.
- **Obstruction.** Hearing loss is sometimes caused by a buildup of wax or a bone blockage in the ear.
- **Nerve damage.** Nerve damage often occurs with age, but it can also be the result of repeated exposure to loud noises, such as stereos, video games, and concerts.

We live in a noisy world, and some experts think the increase in environmental noise is why hearing loss may be occurring earlier in people's lives than it did a few decades ago. Fortunately, it is easy to protect yourself. Wear earplugs if you're exposed to loud noise, and turn down the **volume** if you're listening to music through earphones. Anyone who works around loud machinery, airplanes, or other sources of loud noise should wear earplugs to protect hearing.

Hearing loss can be a gradual process. If you ever notice any changes in your hearing, it may be time to visit an *audiologist,* a specialist in hearing problems.

ACADEMIC VOCABULARY

volume *(noun):* the degree of loudness

Motor Impairment

Tasks that are simple for most people—tying a shoe, climbing the stairs, opening a jar, lifting a glass—can be a challenge for people with a motor impairment. Motor impairments result when the body's range of motion and coordination are affected by a brain injury or a nervous system disorder.

People with motor impairments may cope with physical challenges in different ways, depending on their situation. There are several treatments and devices that have helped many people with motor impairment adapt to their situation:

- **Physical therapy** helps people keep their joints flexible and their muscles stretched, improving their ability to move around.

- **Occupational therapy** helps people learn how to perform everyday tasks so that they can lead independent lives.

- **Assistive devices** help people perform everyday tasks. Examples include motorized wheelchairs and special computers, as well as artificial limbs for people with missing limbs. People who cannot use their hands and arms can also use mouth sticks or head sticks to operate a wheelchair or send instructions to a computer.

Mental Challenges

MAIN IDEA Mental disabilities have been linked to several different causes.

One challenge that affects a person's ability to live independently is **intellectual disability**. This is a below-average intellectual ability present from birth or early childhood and associated with difficulties in learning and social adaptation. Several factors can cause intellectual disability, including injury, disease, and brain abnormality. Additional factors include the following (click on each to learn more):

- **Genetic disorders.** Disorders such as Down syndrome, phenylketonuria (PKU), Tay-Sachs, and Fragile X syndrome can cause intellectual disability in infancy.

- **Behaviors during pregnancy.** Expectant mothers who use alcohol or other drugs greatly increase the risk of giving birth to babies with intellectual disability, low birth weight, or fetal alcohol syndrome.

- **Rubella infection during pregnancy.** Immunization against rubella, either during childhood or in the first three months of pregnancy, reduces the risk of infection.

- **Restricted oxygen supply.** Restricted oxygen supply during birth can cause intellectual disability in infants. Head injury, stroke, and certain infections such as meningitis can also limit oxygen supply, causing intellectual disability in older individuals.

Reading Check

List What are three factors that may cause intellectual disability?

Accommodating Differences

MAIN IDEA It is important to provide equal treatment and opportunities for people with physical and mental challenges.

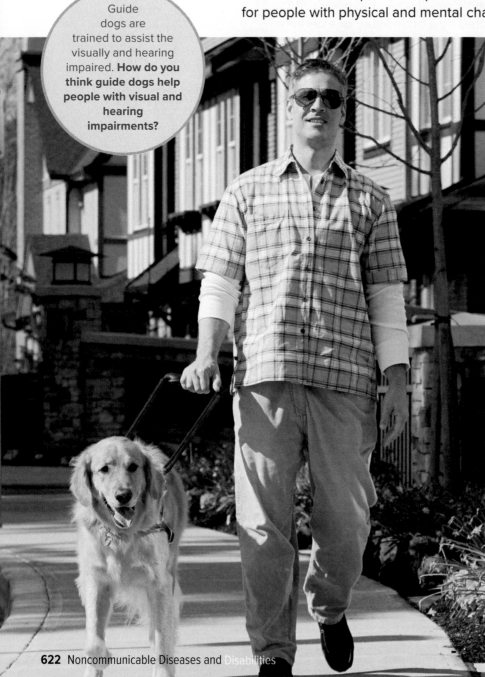

Guide dogs are trained to assist the visually and hearing impaired. **How do you think guide dogs help people with visual and hearing impairments?**

In recent decades, the federal government has begun to address the difficulties of living with disabilities in our society. Advocacy efforts have resulted in laws and policies that address discrimination. These policies are based on the principle that people with disabilities should have the same opportunities as everyone else. For example, policies now require that public transportation vehicles and building entrances must be wheelchair accessible. This helps people with motor impairments to participate freely in business and social activities.

Image Source/Getty Images

One specific law relating to physical and mental disabilities is the **Americans with Disabilities Act (ADA)**. The ADA is a law prohibiting discrimination against people with physical or mental disabilities in the workplace, transportation, public accommodations, and telecommunications. The law was passed in 1990 and revised in 2010. The ADA includes the following provisions:

- Employers with 15 or more employees must give qualified individuals with disabilities an equal opportunity to benefit from employment-related opportunities.

- State and local governments must make their buildings and other facilities accessible. They must also communicate effectively with people who have vision, hearing, or speech disabilities.

- Telephone companies must set up telecommunications relay services (TRS) that allow callers with hearing and speech challenges to communicate with assistance.

In 1998, the government passed another law, the Workforce Investment Act. This law ensures that any information posted to a website by a government agency must be accessible to those who are disabled.

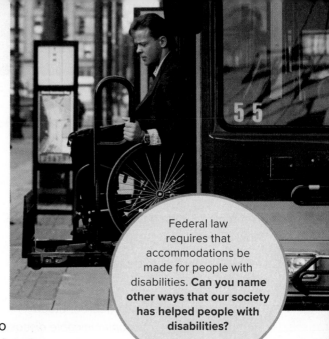

Federal law requires that accommodations be made for people with disabilities. **Can you name other ways that our society has helped people with disabilities?**

Character Check

Learning sign language can give you the ability to communicate with people who are deaf. It is also a way of showing that you care about the needs of others. Do some research to find organizations in your area that offer classes in sign language. Learn some simple signs so that you can communicate with people who are deaf.

Lesson 4 Review

Facts and Vocabulary

1. Name three common causes of blindness.

2. Define the term *assistive device*.

3. Explain whether intellectual disabilities are preventable.

Thinking Critically

4. **Analyze.** What are some challenges that someone with a sight or hearing impairment might have commuting to work each day?

5. **Evaluate.** Why is it important to make buildings and services accessible to people with physical and mental challenges?

Applying Health Skills

6. **Advocacy.** Create a flyer that promotes better understanding of physical and mental challenges and empathy for people with these disabilities. Include appropriate information and statistics.

Writing Critically

7. **Expository.** Write about the accommodations your school has made to assist people with physical or mental challenges. Describe these accommodations and explain whether your school needs to make any additional accommodations.

Physical and Mental Challenges **623**

LESSON 1

Vocabulary Review

Correct the sentences below by replacing the italicized term with the correct vocabulary term.

1. *Heart attack* is an acute injury in which blood flow to the brain is interrupted.

2. High blood pressure is also known as *atherosclerosis.*

3. A disease that affects the heart or blood vessels is called a *noncommunicable disease.*

Understanding Key Concepts

After reading the question or statement, select the correct answer.

4. Which of the following statements is true about stroke?
   a. A stroke can cause paralysis.
   b. A stroke is an acute injury that affects the liver.
   c. During a stroke, blood flow to the brain increases.
   d. During a stroke, the brain gets too much oxygen.

5. Which of the following statements is *not* true about tobacco use?
   a. About 20 percent of deaths from cardiovascular disease are smoking related.
   b. People who smoke less than a pack a day are generally safe from cardiovascular disease.
   c. Cardiovascular disease can be caused by exposure to secondhand smoke.
   d. For teens, tobacco use is the number one risk factor for cardiovascular disease.

Thinking Critically

After reading the question or statement, write a short answer using complete sentences.

6. **Explain.** What is the difference between a communicable disease and a noncommunicable disease?

7. **Describe.** How can a high cholesterol level cause atherosclerosis?

8. **Analyze.** What happens during congestive heart failure?

9. **Explain.** Why is it important to learn about cardiovascular disease as a teen, rather than waiting until you are older?

LESSON 2

Vocabulary Review

Use the correct vocabulary term to complete the following statements.

10. A(n) _____ is an abnormal mass of tissue that has no natural role in the body.

11. Cancer-causing substances are called _____.

12. During a(n) _____, a doctor removes a small piece of tissue for examination.

Understanding Key Concepts

After reading the question or statement, select the correct answer.

13. Which of the following is true about malignant tumors?
    a. They are inconvenient but harmless.
    b. They stay in their original location.
    c. They travel to other parts of the body via the blood or lymph.
    d. They occur only in older adults.

14. Which of the following statements is true about cancer?
    a. Smoking is the leading cause of cancer deaths in the United States.
    b. Cancer is a hereditary disease.
    c. People who live in moderate or cool climates have a low risk for cancer.
    d. Metastasis can be stopped with a healthful diet.

15. What percentage of all cancer deaths are caused by dietary risk factors?
- **a.** 10
- **b.** 20
- **c.** 30
- **d.** 40

Thinking Critically

After reading the question or statement, write a short answer using complete sentences.

16. Describe. What happens during metastasis?

17. Explain. Why is it important to pay attention to the moles on your skin?

18. Identify. What are three cancers that can be detected through self examination?

19. Evaluate. What is the connection between abstaining from sexual activity and reducing cancer risk?

LESSON 3

Vocabulary Review

Correct the sentences below by replacing the italicized term with the correct vocabulary term.

20. Chemicals that can stimulate mucus and fluid production are called *allergens*.

21. *Arthritis* affects the way body cells convert sugar into energy.

22. *Allergy* is a condition in which the airways in the lungs become narrowed.

Understanding Key Concepts

After reading the question or statement, select the correct answer.

23. Severe hives and difficulty swallowing are symptoms of a serious
- **a.** asthma attack.
- **b.** diabetic seizure.
- **c.** allergic reaction.
- **d.** arthritic condition.

24. The only way to diagnose diabetes is by
- **a.** watching for the key symptoms.
- **b.** undergoing a biopsy procedure.
- **c.** receiving an eye exam.
- **d.** getting a blood test.

25. The main areas affected by osteoarthritis are
- **a.** internal organs, such as the liver.
- **b.** weight-bearing joints, such as the knees.
- **c.** the neck and shoulders.
- **d.** the sinuses.

Thinking Critically

After reading the question or statement, write a short answer using complete sentences.

26. Identify. What are four strategies for managing asthma?

27. Explain. Why are some scientists concerned that type 2 diabetes will become an epidemic?

28. Synthesize. How can your family reduce asthma triggers in your home?

LESSON 4

Vocabulary Review

Use the correct vocabulary term to complete the following statements.

29. _____ is hearing loss so severe that hearing aids have no effect.

30. The _____ is a law that prohibits discrimination against people with disabilities.

Understanding Key Concepts

After reading the question or statement, select the correct answer.

31. Glaucoma and diabetes complications are two common causes of
- **a.** deafness.
- **b.** mental illness.
- **c.** blindness.
- **d.** paralysis.

32. What percentage of Americans have some type of disability?
a. 5
b. 10
c. 20
d. 40

33. Advocates for people with physical and mental challenges believe that
a. people are defined by their disabilities.
b. people with disabilities should have different opportunities.
c. everyone must learn to read braille.
d. buses and building entrances should be wheelchair accessible.

Thinking Critically

After reading the question or statement, write a short answer using complete sentences.

34. Identify. What are the three main categories of physical challenges?

35. Analyze. What is the role of heredity in hearing impairment?

36. Explain. What are three ways that assistive devices help people with motor impairments?

37. Evaluate. Discuss the impact of the Americans with Disabilities Act. How does it affect the lives of people with physical and mental challenges?

PROJECT-BASED ASSESSMENT

Reducing Risk

BACKGROUND

Scientists have identified behaviors and treatments that decrease the risk of noncommunicable diseases. While some risk factors for these diseases are related to heredity, gender, and age, many other factors can be modified to reduce disease risk.

TASK

Choose one of the diseases discussed in the module, research it, and develop a multimedia presentation illustrating the nature of the disease.

AUDIENCE

Students in your class and adults in the community

PURPOSE

Inform people about the nature, risk factors, and treatment of a particular noncommunicable disease.

PROCEDURE

1. Choose a noncommunicable disease discussed in the module.

2. Conduct an Internet search to learn more about the disease.

3. Find illustrations and video clips showing the effect of the disease.

4. Include information on positive, preventive measures that lower risks related to the disease. Be sure to also include recent medical advances in the diagnosis and treatment of the disease.

5. Collaborate as a group to create a multimedia presentation incorporating all these aspects.

6. Present your presentation to your class.

Math Practice

Interpret Graphs. Frequent sunburns can lead to melanoma, a deadly type of skin cancer. The bar graph below shows the percentage of high school students who reported getting sunburned. Use the graph to answer the questions that follow.

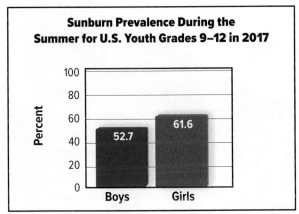

Sunburn Prevalence During the Summer for U.S. Youth Grades 9–12 in 2017

Adapted from Centers for Disease Control and Prevention Statistics, 2017.

1. Which group makes up the greatest percentage of all youth surveyed?
   a. Girls who got a sunburn that summer
   b. Girls who did not get a sunburn that summer
   c. Boys who got a sunburn that summer
   d. Boys who did not get a sunburn that summer

2. What percentage of boys did *not* get a sunburn that summer?
   a. 28.5%
   b. 47.3%
   c. 66.3%
   d. 71.5%

3. If you examined a representative sample that consisted of 500 boys, how many would have gotten a sunburn that summer?

Reading/Writing Practice

Understand and Apply. Read the passage below and then answer the questions.

It's the last home game of the season, and Lincoln High School's basketball team is headed for another victory. The team has compiled its best-ever record this season. Some people attribute this success to Shawn, the assistant manager. Shawn is intellectually disabled. His impairment prevents him from being a regular player, but he loves helping manage the team and practicing with the players. He's so devoted to the team that players say he inspires them to play harder. As the clock runs down, cheers fill the gymnasium. Lincoln wins! At the team's annual banquet, the coach presents Shawn with a special Most Valuable Player award for his contribution to the team.

1. How would you best describe Shawn's role on the basketball team?
   a. He helps organize the equipment.
   b. He is the team's point guard.
   c. His enthusiasm inspires the players to give their best effort on the court.
   d. He practices but doesn't play.

2. What message does Shawn's MVP award send to other students and faculty?
   a. intellectual disability is a barrier to athletic achievement.
   b. Teens with mental disabilities can make valuable contributions.
   c. It is important to treat Shawn differently.
   d. Other teams should ask Shawn to be their assistant manager.

3. Describe the effect that Shawn's success might have on other students with physical or mental challenges.

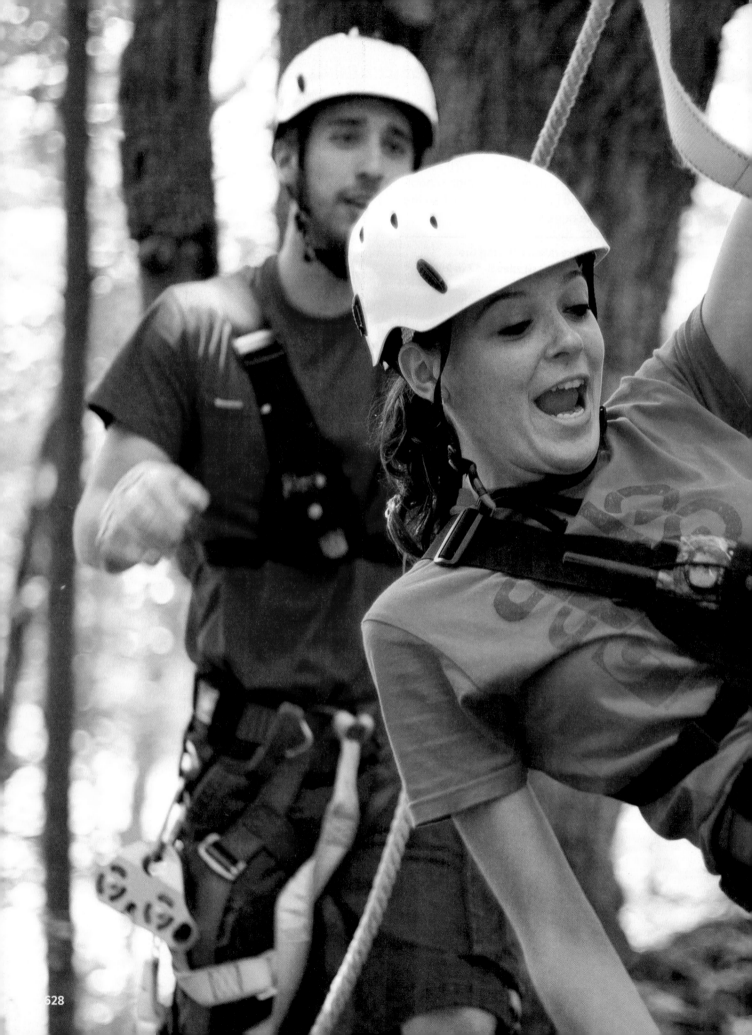

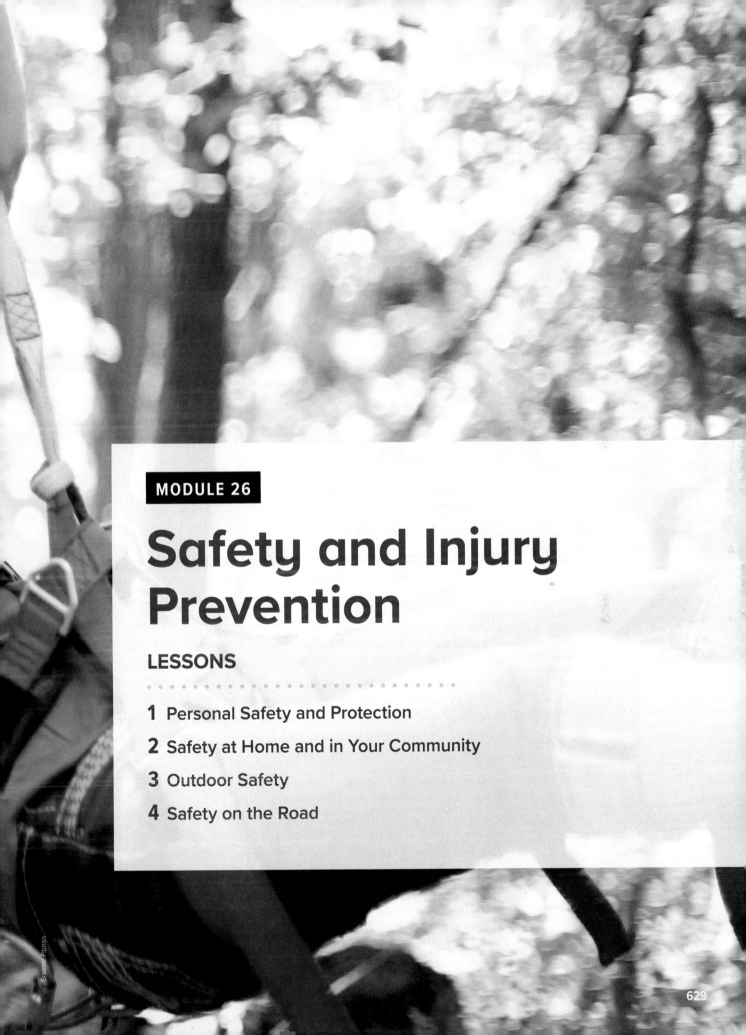

Safety and Injury Prevention

LESSONS

1 Personal Safety and Protection

2 Safety at Home and in Your Community

3 Outdoor Safety

4 Safety on the Road

Personal Safety and Protection

• • • • • • • • • • • •

BEFORE YOU READ

Create a T-Chart. Make a chart with two columns labeled "Personal Safety" and "Internet Safety." As you read, fill in each column with information about types of risks and how to avoid them.

Personal Safety	Internet Safety

Vocabulary

personal safety
self-defense
cyberbullying

• • • • • • • • • • • •

BIG IDEA Learning basic safety precautions can help you avoid threatening or harmful situations.

REAL LIFE ISSUES

Safety First. As many as 35 percent of teens, or 1 in 3 young people, say they have been victims of electronic aggression or cyberbullying. Ten percent of teens found pictures of themselves online that were posted without their permission. Ten percent learned that cyberbullies pretended to be them while communicating with others. *Write a paragraph describing safety strategies that could reduce your chances of becoming a victim of a crime.*

After completing the lesson, review and analyze your response to the Real Life Issues question.

Safety Strategies

MAIN IDEA The key to personal safety is learning how to recognize and avoid dangerous situations.

Did you know that teens are the victims of more violent crimes than any other age group? Teens are more likely than younger children to go out at night, but they are less likely than adults to watch out for **personal safety**. Personal safety is the steps you take to prevent yourself from becoming the victim of crime. People living in urban areas report the highest rates of violent crime. However, crime can occur in any neighborhood and among any ethnic or socioeconomic group. About half of all violent crime occurs within one mile of a victim's home, and many victims know their attackers.

One way that you can protect yourself from crime is to avoid the places where it is more likely to occur. For example, you can avoid walking alone at night and stick to brightly lit, well-traveled streets, rather than isolated areas such as alleys or parks. However, sometimes crime finds you. For instance, someone might follow you home from school, or you might see someone carrying a gun or other weapon in school. If you cannot avoid a dangerous situation, you can do the next best thing: know how to protect yourself. To reduce your risk of becoming a victim of crime, remain aware of your surroundings and take precautions to protect your belongings.

Learning to Protect Yourself

Self-defense includes any strategy for protecting yourself from harm. One of the best self-defense strategies is to be aware of what's happening around you, even when you are in familiar places. Projecting a strong, confident image also helps. Criminals are more likely to attack those who look vulnerable, confused, or inattentive to their surroundings. You can show confidence by holding your head high and walking with a deliberate stride.

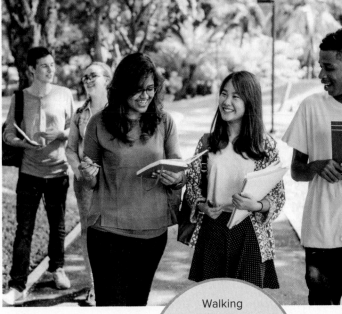

Walking with groups can help protect you from being a victim of crime. **Why does being in a group offer protection?**

If you think you are being followed in a public place, there are several things you can do. Let the stalker know that you are aware of his or her presence. Try changing directions or crossing the street. If necessary, seek help from someone nearby or enter a business that's open. If you are attacked or about to be attacked, do whatever is necessary to escape, such as running, yelling, or kicking. Shout "fire" instead of "help"—it's more likely to get a response. Here are some additional tips to help you avoid attack:

- If you carry a cell phone, make sure it's easy to get to. Remember that dialing 911 will connect you with emergency services anywhere in the United States.

- Wear comfortable shoes so that you can move quickly.

- Carry your wallet or purse in a place that makes it difficult to grab. Avoid displaying expensive jewelry, electronics, or anything that would attract a thief.

- If you drive, park your car in a well-lit area and keep it locked. Check before getting in to make sure that no one is inside, and lock the doors as soon as you get in.

- Never hitchhike or give a ride to anyone you do not know well. Keep in mind that even someone you've met before could be dangerous.

- Get on and off public transportation in busy, well-lit areas. Sit near the driver or with a group of people.

- Know the locations of public places where you can seek help if you need it.

- When you go out, let your family know where you're going and when you'll be back. Call home if your plans change.

Self-Defense Classes. Self-defense classes can teach you additional strategies for protecting yourself. When you hear "self-defense," you may think of martial-arts style fighting, and some classes do teach these skills. However, self-defense classes can also teach you how to size up a situation, figure out what to do, and catch an attacker off-guard. Most importantly, these classes can give you the confidence you need to defeat an attacker.

Reading Check

Cause and Effect Give two examples of behaviors that can help you avoid a dangerous situation.

Rawpixel.com/Shutterstock

Staying Safe Online

MAIN IDEA Teens need to protect themselves online.

Today's teens know that the Internet can be incredibly useful. More and more teens and young adults have personal webpages and use the Internet for a variety of purposes. Unfortunately, the Internet can also be a dangerous place. The hazards you can **encounter** range from upsetting situations—like being insulted in an instant message, blog, or text message—to physical threats, such as Internet predators.

This doesn't mean that being online isn't worth the risks. It just means that you need to know how to protect yourself. Here are a few precautions to take when you're online:

- **Keep your identity private.** Avoid posting personal information in any public space. This includes your full name, address, phone number, financial information, passwords, and anything else a stranger could use to track you down in the real world.

- **Be cautious about taking online relationships offline.** Agreeing to meet in person with someone you've met online could be risky. You have no way of knowing who the person really is. If you decide to go, arrange to meet in a public place and bring a parent or other trusted adult.

- **Don't respond to inappropriate messages.** If anyone sends you a message that makes you feel uncomfortable for any reason, tell a parent or other trusted adult.

- **Let your parents or guardians know what you're doing online.** Tell them about the people you meet online, just the same way you'd talk to them about the friends you see in the real world.

ACADEMIC VOCABULARY

encounter *(verb)*: to experience

Reading Check

List What are three types of information you should keep private while online?

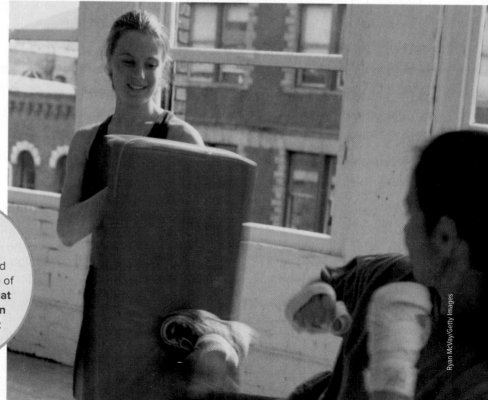

Self-defense classes can boost your confidence and help you take charge of your own safety. **What other strategies can you use to protect yourself?**

Ryan McVay/Getty Images

How Technology is Used to Bully

MAIN IDEA Cyberbullies can spread hurtful messages quickly.

Cyberbullying is cruel or hurtful contact using technology. Cyberbullies use electronic technology to harass people, threaten them, or spread rumors. Cyberbullying allows one person to bully another without ever seeing the victim in person. It's likely that the victim is unable to identify the cyberbully.

Cyberbullies use technology to bully others. A cyberbully may forward a private photo via text or email using a phone, tablet, or computer that embarrasses another person. The cyberbully may post an unflattering photo or send a humiliating message to a social media site. They might also send a message to groups of students and others. Cyberbullying can also occur in online forums, chat rooms, and gaming communities. The technology and social media sites are not the cause of cyberbullying, but they are the tools used by bullies. As more adolescents and teens use technology, the incidence of cyberbullying has increased. The School Crime Supplement from the National Center for Education Statistics and Bureau of Justice Statistics reported that 15 percent of students in grades 6–12 have been bullied online or via text.

Whether bullying is done in person or through technology, it has negative effects on a person's physical, mental/emotional, and social health. Teens who are cyberbullied are more likely to:

- use alcohol and drugs.
- skip school.
- experience in-person bullying.
- be unwilling to attend school.
- receive poor grades.
- have lower self-esteem.
- have more health problems.

Coping With Electronic Aggression

About 16 percent of teens say they have experienced cyberbullying, also known as *electronic aggression.* Such contact can come from people you know or from strangers you've had no contact with offline. It can range from immature and annoying to threatening and scary.

To avoid becoming a target of electronic aggression, one important rule is to keep an eye on your own communication style, both online and in text messages. When you use a website, learn its rules for postings, and stick to them. Also, be careful how you word your messages. What you think is just a joke may come across as an attack or an insult to someone else. Avoid getting into "flame wars," trading insults back and forth over the Internet. The other person may have started it, but you don't have to respond.

Reading Check

List What are three effects of cyberbullying?

If you receive a hurtful message online, the best way to cope is usually to ignore it. Cyberbullies are often looking for attention. If you don't react, they'll find someone who will. If the bullying continues, however, seek help from a trusted adult. Take screenshots or save the messages as evidence and contact your Internet service provider (ISP) or wireless phone company. It may be possible to block all future communications from the cyberbully. If any actual crime has been committed, such as making violent threats, contact the police.

Reading Check

List What are three strategies to use social media safely, respectfully, and legally?

Preventing Cyberbullying

MAIN IDEA Cyberbullies use several types of technology to attack another person.

The best way to avoid becoming the victim of a cyberbully is to do what you can to prevent it from occurring. Each teen who uses social media can help to prevent the spread of cyberbullying. Avoid including personal information about yourself in text messages, email, or social networks.

Another important rule to remember is that any photo that you post online will remain online forever. Even if you delete a photo, a person with good computer skills can retrieve the image. This includes photos that are sent via email, posted to a social network site, or sent via text. When cyberbullying occurs, write down and report the behavior. Other steps you can take to stop cyberbullies include:

- Do not respond to cyberbullying messages.

- Do not forward cyberbullying messages.

- Block the person who is cyberbullying.

- Visit social media safety centers to learn how to block users.

- Keep evidence of cyberbullying. Write down the dates, times, and descriptions of incidents. Save and print screenshots, e-mails, text messages, etc.

The Internet can be a useful tool for keeping in touch with your friends. **What precautions should you take to protect your safety online?**

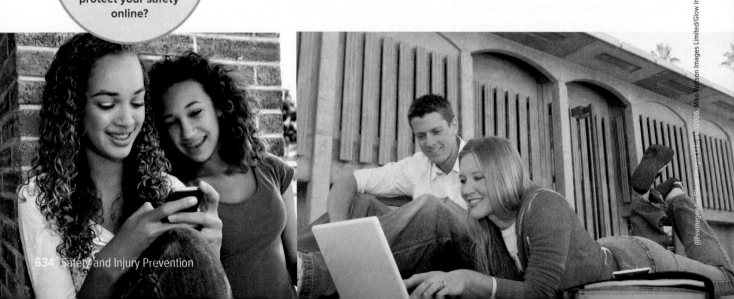

- Report cyberbullying to your social media site so it can take action against users abusing its terms of service. Use your evidence.

- Report cyberbullying to Internet and cell phone service providers so they can take action against users abusing their terms of service. Use your evidence.

- Report cyberbullying to law enforcement. Cyberbullying can be considered a crime. Some state laws also cover off-campus bullying that creates a hostile school environment. Use your evidence.

- Report cyberbullying to your school. Cyberbullying can create a disruptive environment at school and is often related to in-person bullying. The school can use your evidence to help stop the behavior and develop its anti-bullying policy.

Avoiding Internet Predators

Cyberbullies try to hurt their victims. They attempt to make these victims feel threatened and helpless. Internet predators, on the other hand, use online contact to build up trust so that they can lure victims into a face-to-face meeting. To avoid falling victim to Internet predators, follow the general guidelines for online safety. Keep your identity, personal information, and passwords private. Be cautious about meeting in person with someone you've met online. If you do decide to meet in person, tell a trusted adult what you are doing, where you are going, and when you plan to be back. If you're ever in an online conversation that makes you feel uncomfortable or threatened—for any reason—close the application or chat window, leave the site, and let a trusted adult know about the incident.

Fitness Zone

I'm really careful to avoid exercising outside after dark. When I go for a walk with my mom in the evenings, we wear reflective clothing so other people can see us, and we use flashlights so we can see where we're going. We also walk against traffic so we can see what's coming toward us.

Lesson 1 Review

Facts and Vocabulary

1. What steps can you take to protect yourself from an attack when entering or leaving a car?

2. Name two threats you may encounter on the Internet.

3. Describe precautions you can take to avoid becoming the target of a cyberbully.

Thinking Critically

4. **Evaluate.** Why is it important to avoid dangerous situations, even if you know how to defend yourself?

5. **Synthesize.** Gina is walking home from school when she notices someone is following her. What could she do to protect herself?

Applying Health Skills

6. **Communication Skills.** Suppose you have been posting on a message board about current events. The group is debating a political issue that you have strong opinions about. Write a message you could post that expresses your opinions in a way that is respectful toward those who disagree with you.

Writing Critically

7. **Creative.** Write lyrics for a pop song or rap about personal safety. Choose a topic in this lesson as the basis for your lyrics.

Safety at Home and in Your Community

BEFORE YOU READ

Organize Information.
Use a T-chart to organize the information in this lesson. On one side, list causes of accidental injuries. On the other side, list safety precautions that can prevent them.

Causes	Safety Precautions

Vocabulary

unintentional injury
accident chain
fire extinguisher
smoke alarm
Occupational Safety and Health Administration (OSHA)

BIG IDEA Reducing the potential for accidents can help you stay safe at home and at work.

REAL LIFE ISSUES

Fire Safety. Lucius and his family are moving into a new house. As he's examining his new bedroom on the second floor, his dad comes in and looks out the window. "We'll need to find a place to store a ladder," he says. "This window's your emergency exit in case of fire. Come to think of it, we need to develop a fire safety plan for the whole house." *What do you think is involved in developing a fire safety plan? Why is it important to have such a plan?*

After completing the lesson, review and analyze your response to the Real Life Issues question.

The Accident Chain

MAIN IDEA Many accidental injuries are preventable.

Not all accidents pose a threat to your health. For example, accidentally leaving your English report at home doesn't hurt anything except your grade. The kind of accidents that pose a real danger are the ones that result in **unintentional injuries**. These are injuries resulting from an unexpected event. Every year, more than 20 million children and teens suffer unintentional injuries that require medical attention or restrict their activities.

Fortunately, many of these injuries are preventable. You can often avoid them by breaking the **accident chain**, a sequence of events that leads to an unintentional injury. Breaking just one "link" in this chain—that is, stopping just one of the events—can prevent an injury.

Keeping Your Home Safe

MAIN IDEA Safety precautions can prevent injuries at home.

Accidents in the home are one of the top causes of injury and death in the United States. Common types of household accidents include fires, falls, and poisonings. You can reduce the risk of such accidents by following some basic safety precautions.

The Accident Chain

Breaking any of the links in this chain can prevent the accident and the resulting injury.	
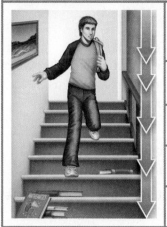	**An Unsafe Situation** Mark's alarm clock didn't go off this morning. As a result, he overslept and has to rush to get ready for school.
	An Unsafe Habit Mark often leaves his books on the stairs.
	An Unsafe Action Mark hurries down the stairs without watching where he's going.
	The Accident Mark trips over his books and falls down the stairs.
	The Consequences Mark lands on his wrist and sprains it. He's also late for school.

Preventing Fires

Common causes of household fires include burning candles and incense, smoking, kitchen fires, and faulty electrical wiring. To prevent fires in your home, follow these precautions:

- Keep matches, lighters, and candles away from children. Don't leave burning candles unattended.

- Make sure that smokers extinguish cigarettes completely, and that no one smokes in bed.

- Don't leave cooking food unattended. Clean stoves and ovens to prevent grease build-up, which can catch fire.

- Follow the operating instructions for using space heaters and other heat sources.

If a fire does occur, two life-saving devices can help you escape without harm. The first is a **fire extinguisher**. These are portable devices that help in putting out small fires. Keep an all-purpose fire extinguisher in your kitchen—one that is approved for flammable materials, flammable liquids, and electrical fires. Make sure that everyone in the house knows how to use it. The second important safety device is a **smoke alarm**. It produces a loud warning noise in the presence of smoke. Having working smoke alarms in your home more than doubles your chances of surviving a fire. Every home should have a smoke alarm on each floor, near the kitchen and bedrooms.

Test your smoke alarms once a month, and change the batteries twice a year. **How do smoke alarms protect your safety?**

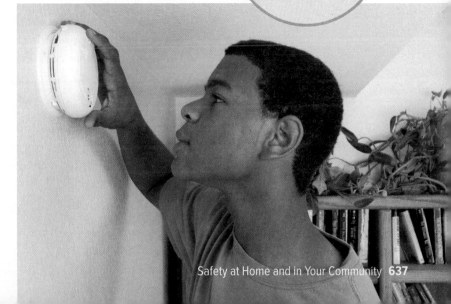

Tim Fuller Photography

Of course, a smoke alarm can only warn you of a fire; it can't get you to safety. Identify an escape path from every room of your home and a designated spot to meet up with your family after you get out. If you have to escape from a fire, stay close to the ground so that you can crawl under the smoke. If your clothes catch fire, stop, drop, and roll to put out the flames.

Staying Safe With Electricity

Because wiring problems are a common source of house fires, knowing about electrical safety can help prevent electrical fires as well as electric shocks. Here are some safety tips to follow:

- Avoid overloading your electrical system.

- Inspect electrical cords regularly. If you find any worn or exposed wiring, unplug the appliance *immediately* and avoid using it again.

- Make sure extension cords are properly rated for their intended use and have polarized (three-prong) plugs.

- Avoid running electric cords under rugs or behind baseboards. Prevent furniture from sitting on the cords, and avoid attaching cords to the walls with nails or staples.

- Avoid using an electrical appliance near water, and never reach into water to retrieve a dropped appliance without unplugging it first.

- In homes with small children, cover unused outlets with safety caps.

Preventing Falls

Falls are responsible for about half of all accidental deaths in the home. To reduce the risk of injury from falls, take precautions in these areas of the home:

- **Stairs.** Keep stairways well lit, in good repair, and free of clutter. Staircases should have sturdy handrails, and all stair coverings should be securely fastened down. Never put small rugs at the foot of a staircase.

- **Bathrooms.** Put nonskid mats or strips in the tub or shower. Keep a night-light in the bathroom so people don't trip in the darkness.

- **Windows.** If there are small children in the home, install window guards on the upper floors. However, make sure the windows can be opened in case of a fire.

- **Kitchens.** Keep the floor clean, and mop up spills promptly. Use a sturdy step stool to get things down from high places.

- **Living areas.** Keep the floor clear of clutter. Use nonskid rugs or place nonskid mats under rugs. Keep phone and electrical cords out of the flow of traffic.

Preventing Poisonings

Many of the items you keep around the house—cleaning supplies, bug sprays, medicines, and even cosmetics—can be harmful or even fatal if swallowed. The two most important steps for preventing poisonings in your home are:

- **Store products safely.** Store all medications and other hazardous substances in childproof containers, and keep them out of the reach of children. Put locks or safety latches on cabinets where dangerous chemicals are stored. Discard medicines that are past their expiration date. Remember to protect pets as well as children: Avoid storing household chemicals near pet food or water dishes, and clean up spills promptly.

- **Pay attention to labels.** Unless directed by a doctor, never take more of a drug than the label recommends. Consult with your doctor if you are taking two or more drugs to make sure it is safe to combine them. Also, follow instructions for using household chemicals, such as cleaning fluids. Mixing chemicals can result in dangerous fumes, explosions, home fires, and burns. Lastly, make sure that fuel-burning appliances, such as grills or kerosene lamps, are properly vented to prevent carbon monoxide poisoning.

Common Household Poisons

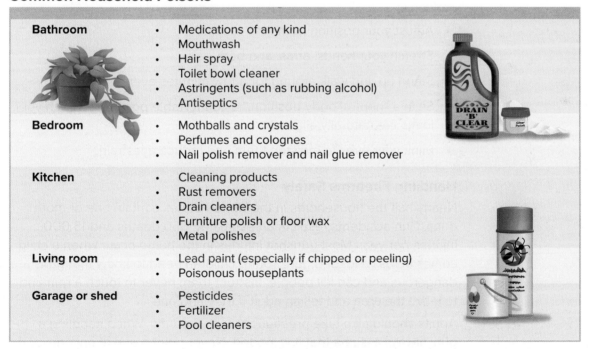

Bathroom	• Medications of any kind • Mouthwash • Hair spray • Toilet bowl cleaner • Astringents (such as rubbing alcohol) • Antiseptics
Bedroom	• Mothballs and crystals • Perfumes and colognes • Nail polish remover and nail glue remover
Kitchen	• Cleaning products • Rust removers • Drain cleaners • Furniture polish or floor wax • Metal polishes
Living room	• Lead paint (especially if chipped or peeling) • Poisonous houseplants
Garage or shed	• Pesticides • Fertilizer • Pool cleaners

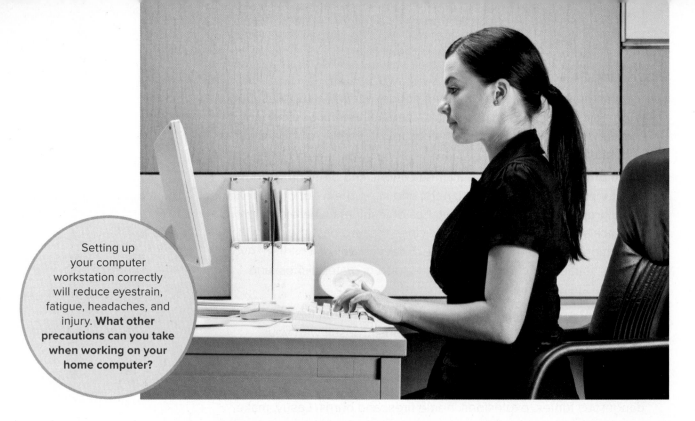

Setting up your computer workstation correctly will reduce eyestrain, fatigue, headaches, and injury. **What other precautions can you take when working on your home computer?**

Using Computers Safely

When you use a computer at home, you may need to sit in one place for a long time, staring at the screen and making the same movements over and over. This can lead to eyestrain and sore muscles. It can also cause injuries of the wrists, hands, or arms. Here are a few ways to reduce these problems:

- Adjust your position from time to time.

- Stretch your hands, arms, and body.

- Stand up and walk around for a few minutes every hour or so.

- Sit in a "neutral body position," a comfortable posture in which your joints are naturally aligned.

- Blink your eyes to moisten them and reduce eyestrain.

Handling Firearms Safely

Nearly half the households in the United States contain one or more guns. Gun accidents result in an estimated 650 deaths and 15,000 injuries per year. Most gunshot injuries in the home occur when a child comes across a loaded gun. Young children need to know that guns are dangerous and can kill people. Instruct them never to touch a gun and to leave the area and tell an adult if they find one.

Adults should also take precautions with firearms. When handling a gun, always assume that it is loaded. Never point a gun at anyone, and keep your finger off the trigger except when firing. Add a trigger lock to the gun and store it unloaded in a locked cabinet. Lock ammunition away separately, and keep the keys where children can't get to them.

Guarding Against Intruders

Accidents aren't the only threat to the safety of your home. There is also the risk that an intruder could break in and steal things, or even commit a violent attack. To keep intruders out, follow these guidelines:

- Keep your doors and windows locked. Deadbolt locks are the most secure kind. If doors or windows are damaged, repair them promptly. Avoid hiding a spare key outside the house; instead, give a key to a neighbor you trust.

- Use a peephole to identify people who come to the door. Never open the door to a stranger, and never tell people that you're home alone.

Reading Check

Describe What are three ways that you can stay safe at home?

REAL WORLD CONNECTION

Accidents and Unintentional Injuries

The graph below compares the top five causes of nonfatal unintentional injuries to Americans between the ages of 15 and 19. Study the graph, then answer the questions that follow.

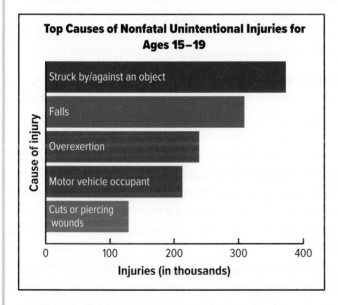

Top Causes of Nonfatal Unintentional Injuries for Ages 15–19

Cause of injury (top to bottom): Struck by/against an object; Falls; Overexertion; Motor vehicle occupant; Cuts or piercing wounds

Injuries (in thousands): 0, 100, 200, 300, 400

Activity: Mathematics

Assume the total number of nonfatal unintentional injuries for this age group was 2 million.

1. What percentage of these injuries resulted from falls?

2. What percentage of all injuries do the five causes listed here account for?

3. Identify at least three steps you could take to reduce your risk of accidents and unintentional injuries.

CONCEPT Numbers and Operations: Percents

A percent can be used to express the relationship between two numbers (A and B). To calculate what percent of B is represented by A, use this formula: $(A \div B) \times 100$. For example, $(2 \div 8) \times 100 = 25$. Therefore, 2 is 25 percent of 8.

- Make sure your answering machine message does not tell callers that you're away from home.

- If you come home and see something suspicious, such as an unknown car parked in your driveway or a window that's been forced open, don't go inside. Instead, call the police from a neighbor's house.

Keeping Your Community Safe

MAIN IDEA You can work with others to protect your safety at school, at work, and in your community.

You've learned about some ways to make your home a safer place, but your life isn't limited to your home. You have a right to be safe everywhere you go—at school, at work, and in your community. Many communities are taking the following steps to make neighborhoods safer.

- **Increased police presence.** Putting more police officers on the streets can reduce crime by as much as 15 percent.

- **Neighborhood Watch programs.** Through these programs, citizens watch for suspicious activity and report it to the police.

- **After-school programs.** These programs give students a place to go during after-school hours, when many crimes are committed. Keeping students in a safe place makes them less likely to commit crimes and less likely to become victims.

- **Improved lighting in public areas.** Better lighting can discourage crime by making it harder to commit crimes under cover of darkness.

Safety at School

Violence in schools can include fights between students, bullying, gang activity, and the presence of weapons. Other problems that can make school an unsafe environment include vandalism and alcohol and drug use. Eliminating these problems takes a joint effort. Click on each item in the list below to learn what school staff, students, and parents can do to make schools safer.

- **School Staff.** School staff can develop security procedures. These may include hiring security guards, working cooperatively with the police, or using metal detectors to keep weapons out. Schools can also put disciplinary policies in place to deal with offenders. Some schools have adopted "zero-tolerance" policies, which means that a student can be expelled or **suspended** for a single offense.

- **Students.** Students can develop peer mediation programs to help settle conflicts. They can report crimes or other suspicious activities to school staff. They can also help make their school a healthier, safer environment by cleaning up graffiti, leading anti-violence groups, and getting others involved in community service.

- **Parents.** Parents can play a role by being aware of the conditions in their children's schools. They can become involved in school affairs by joining parent-teacher groups, chaperoning field trips and other school events, and helping out in the classroom.

Reading Check

Cause and Effect List three problems that can make schools less safe. Identify three strategies for dealing with these problems.

Safety on the Job

Millions of teens in the United States hold full-time or part-time jobs. Part-time or summer jobs offer a way to earn extra cash, build responsibility, and learn useful skills. However, work also has its risks. Each year, about 52,600 teen workers suffer injuries or illnesses serious enough to send them to a hospital emergency room.

The federal government has enacted laws to protect the health of young workers. First, all employers must meet standards set by the **Occupational Safety and Health Administration (OSHA)**. OSHA is the agency within the federal government that is responsible for promoting safe and healthful conditions in the workplace. Other laws place limits on the kinds of jobs that teens can do. For example, workers under 18 years old are not allowed to drive forklifts, work as miners or loggers, operate certain types of power-driven equipment, or work with explosives or radioactive materials.

Teen employees and their employers can also take steps to prevent work-related injuries. Young workers can know the risks of their jobs, follow safe work practices, and refuse to work in unsafe conditions. Employers can provide adequate training and supervision.

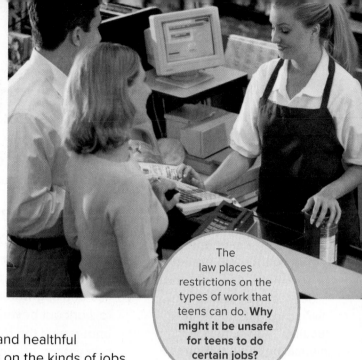

The law places restrictions on the types of work that teens can do. **Why might it be unsafe for teens to do certain jobs?**

Character Check

Teens who obey laws and respect authority demonstrate good citizenship. Good citizenship also involves doing your part to make your community safer. What are some ways you can demonstrate good citizenship to reduce crime in your community?

Lesson 2 Review

Facts and Vocabulary

1. Define the term *unintentional injuries*.

2. Identify two important pieces of fire safety equipment.

3. List two steps you can take to prevent poisonings in your home.

Thinking Critically

4. **Synthesize.** Seventeen-year-old Claude finds his father's shotgun on the kitchen table. It looks like his dad was interrupted in the middle of cleaning it. What should Claude do?

5. **Analyze.** What factors may make teens especially vulnerable to being injured on the job?

Applying Health Skills

6. **Practicing Healthful Behaviors.** Think of a specific job that a teen might have. Develop a list of strategies for preventing injuries on the job.

Writing Critically

7. **Narrative.** Write a short story about an accident involving a teen. Your story should clearly show each of the steps in the accident chain and how all of them work together to result in the accident.

Safety at Home and in Your Community **643**

Outdoor Safety

BEFORE YOU READ

Create a Cluster Chart. In the center of a sheet of paper, write "Outdoor Activities" and circle it. Surround it with circles labeled "Camping and Hiking," "Winter Sports," "Swimming and Diving," and "Boating." As you read, add information about staying safe during each type of activity.

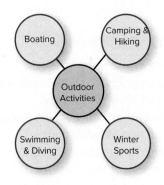

Vocabulary

personal flotation device

. . . .

BIG IDEA Common sense and caution can minimize the risk of accidental injuries during outdoor activities.

REAL LIFE ISSUES

Playing It Safe. Outdoor activities can be fun, but they can also pose a risk of injury. Using the right safety equipment for your sport can reduce the risk of injury. So can taking precautions like drinking water to stay hydrated and avoiding the desire to work out beyond your current capabilities. To help you understand the risk, the DHHS provides information on the percentage of accidents caused by various sports. *Write a paragraph describing the safety equipment that is needed to participate in various outdoor activities.*

After completing the lesson, review and analyze your response to the Real Life Issues question.

Outdoor Recreation

MAIN IDEA Planning ahead can protect you from injury during outdoor activities such as camping, hiking, and winter sports.

Imagine this: you've just come back to your campsite after a day of hiking in the woods with your friends. Now you're relaxing around the campfire, toasting marshmallows and swapping stories. This cheerful scene is possible because you thought ahead of time about where to go, what to do, and what to bring. This is the most important general rule for all kinds of outdoor activities: *plan ahead.* Here are some specific ways to do just that:

- **Know your limits.** Stick with tasks that match your level of ability. Brush up on necessary skills ahead of time.

- **Bring supplies.** Take plenty of safe drinking water. Never drink the water from lakes, rivers, or streams; it may contain harmful pathogens. Plan simple meals and store the food safely. Don't forget first-aid supplies and any medications you normally take.

- **Plan for the weather.** Check the local weather forecast and plan for the expected conditions.

- **Wear appropriate clothing.** Choose clothes that are right for the weather and will protect you from poisonous plants and insects. Dress in layers to adjust to changing temperatures.

- **Tell people your plans.** Let your family know where you're going and when you'll be back. If possible, carry a cell phone for emergencies. A sports whistle can also be useful as a way to signal for help.

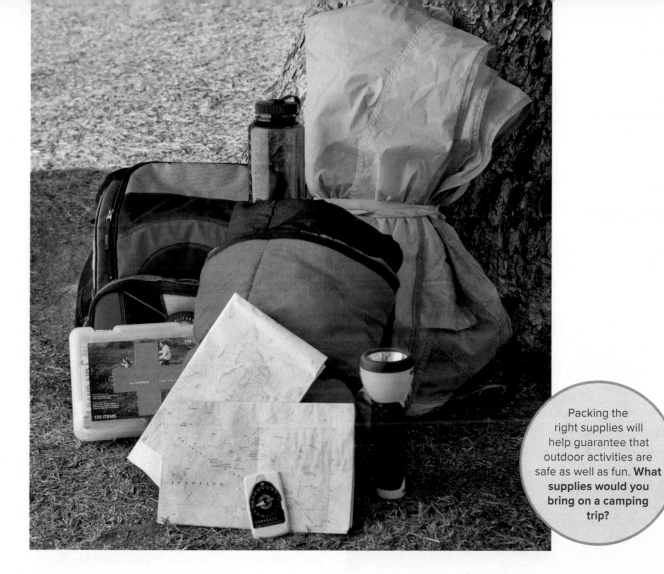

Packing the right supplies will help guarantee that outdoor activities are safe as well as fun. **What supplies would you bring on a camping trip?**

Camping and Hiking

There's nothing like a day out on the trails or a night sleeping under the stars. You just need to steer clear of bears, poison ivy, and sprained ankles! The guidelines below offer more information about how to enjoy your stay in the woods and reduce your risk of injury.

- **Camp with a group.** Having at least one other person with you means there's always one person to go get help if the other is sick or injured.

- **Stick to well-marked trails.** In case you do get lost, bring a map and a compass, and know how to use them.

- **Be cautious around wildlife.** Don't feed wild animals. Avoid keeping food in or near sleeping areas, where wild animals may come looking for it.

- **Take care with fires.** Before starting a campfire, make sure it's **legal**. Keep fires at least ten feet away from your tent, and put them out completely before going to bed.

- **Respect the environment.** If there aren't any trash bins at your campsite, pack your waste with you when you go.

• • • • • • • • • •

ACADEMIC VOCABULARY

legal (*adjective*): permitted by law

• • • • • • • • • • •

Winter Sports

When you take part in cold-weather activities, wear warm, layered clothing to protect you from frostbite (skin and tissue damage) and hypothermia (dangerously low body temperature). To avoid sunburn, you should also apply sunscreen to all exposed skin. Choose a sunscreen with an SPF of at least 15. Also, as with all other outdoor activities, make sure you have a buddy with you to help out in an emergency.

- **Sledding.** Make sure your equipment is in good condition. Choose safe spots to sled in: gently sloped hills with plenty of space and a level area to come to a stop at the bottom. Avoid sledding on or near frozen lakes, because the ice may not be solid.

- **Ice skating.** The most important rule is to skate only in designated areas. Never skate anywhere you don't know the thickness of the ice. Wear skates that fit comfortably and support your ankles.

- **Skiing, snowboarding, and snowmobiling.** These sports can result in serious injuries, including broken bones and head injuries. To protect yourself, wear an approved, well-fitting ski helmet. Also, make sure that your other equipment, such as boots and bindings, fits well and is in good condition. Stick to marked trails that are appropriate for your level of ability. Remember to look both ways and uphill before crossing or merging onto a trail. When heading downhill, give the people ahead of you the right of way, since they may not be able to see you coming from behind. If you need to stop, get to the side of the trail, out of the path of others.

Water Safety

MAIN IDEA Following safety precautions can prevent drowning and other water-related injuries.

Swimming, boating, and other water sports are great ways to find relief from the summer heat. However, it's important not to lose sight of water safety. Every year, nearly 3,500 people die from drowning. Although most drowning incidents involve young children, people of all age groups need to pay attention to water safety guidelines.

Proper clothing and equipment are two of the keys to outdoor winter safety. **What kind of clothing should you choose for cold-weather activities?**

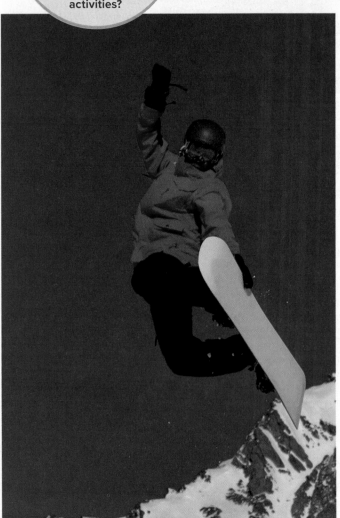

Swimming and Diving

The most important rule for safety in the water, of course, is to know how to swim. Know your limits as a swimmer. If you're just learning, don't try to keep up with skilled swimmers. Instead, stick to shallow areas where you can touch the bottom. If you are a strong swimmer, keep an eye on friends who aren't as skilled as you are. Finally, no matter how good a swimmer you are, never go in alone. Even experienced swimmers could suffer a muscle cramp or other medical emergency. Here are a few more rules for safe swimming and diving:

- Only swim in designated areas where there's a lifeguard present. Obey "No Swimming" and "No Diving" signs—they're there for a reason.

- Dive only into water that you know is deep enough. Diving into shallow water could result in permanent spinal cord damage or death.

- When swimming, always enter the water feet first. Check for hidden rocks and other hazards.

- Avoid swimming near piers and reefs. These areas are often subject to rip currents that can drag swimmers out into open water.

- If you get caught in a current, avoid trying to fight it. Swim with the current until it releases you, then return to the shore.

- Pay attention to the weather. When it's hot, drink plenty of fluids and reapply sunscreen frequently. If you start to shiver, get out of the water.

- Be prepared for emergencies. Knowing first aid can help you save a life.

Boating

Every year, more people die in boating accidents than in airplane crashes or train wrecks. Following a few common-sense guidelines can help you stay safe while boating.

- Make sure the person handling the boat is experienced. Never ride in a boat with an operator who has been using alcohol or other drugs.

- Always wear a **Personal flotation device (PFD)**, also known as a life jacket. PFDs come in a wide variety of types and styles for boaters of different ages and levels of swimming ability. Inflatable toys or "water wings" are *not* a substitute for an approved PFD.

- Plan ahead and check weather reports. If a storm is predicted, avoid going out onto the water. If you are already on the boat, head back to shore immediately.

- Make sure someone on land knows where you are and when you expect to be back.

Preventing Drowning

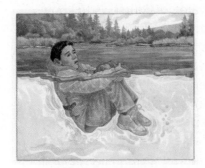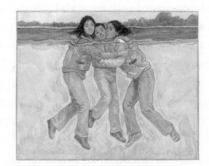

Reading Check

Classify List two safety tips you should follow when swimming and two tips for safe boating.

Myths & Reality

Do you like to swim? Maybe you've never considered the risk of drowning before.

Myth: Drowning takes a long time to occur.

Reality: Children are most at risk for drowning, and a child can lose consciousness under water in 20 seconds.

When canoeing or kayaking, you should be prepared to end up in the water at some point. Because the water is likely to be cold, dress in layers and choose synthetic fabrics that will wick moisture away from your body. Know your limits when canoeing or kayaking, and don't attempt rivers or rapids that are beyond your abilities. Make sure you know how to handle a boat properly and recognize river hazards before heading out on the water.

The same safety rules that apply to boating also apply to personal watercraft. According to the U.S. Coast Guard, 60 percent of all accidents involving personal watercraft occur because of lack of experience or speeding. Some states have laws governing the use of personal watercraft devices. For example, there may be age limits for operating one, or a test you have to pass before you can use them.

Lesson 3 Review

Facts and Vocabulary

1. Identify three strategies for preventing accidental injuries while hiking or camping.

2. List three general safety guidelines for participating in winter sports.

3. Describe the leading safety rule when diving.

Thinking Critically

4. **Analyze.** You and your friend Jake are skiing. Jake suggests trying the advanced slope, even though you're both beginners. What are the possible consequences of going along with this idea?

5. **Synthesize.** You and your family are taking a boat out on the lake for the afternoon. What supplies and safety equipment should you bring with you?

Applying Health Skills

6. **Decision Making.** Some friends invite you to go on a canoe ride. You've never canoed before and don't know how to handle the boat. On a sheet of paper, outline a response to this situation, using the six steps of the decision-making process.

Writing Critically

7. **Personal.** Write a journal entry in your notebook about a day spent doing some kind of outdoor activity. You may describe an activity you have actually done, or a fictitious one. Discuss the steps you took to protect your health and safety while outdoors.

Safety on the Road

BIG IDEA Drivers, pedestrians, and others on the road need to follow rules to stay safe.

REAL LIFE ISSUES

Limits on Driving. Shang was excited when he passed his driver's test. The first thing he did was to ask his dad if he could borrow the car that night to take a friend to the movies. He was surprised and disappointed when his dad said, "I don't think that's a good idea. You just got your license, and driving at night is a lot trickier. You need practice driving at night." *Write a dialogue in which Shang and his dad use good communication and conflict resolution skills to reach an acceptable solution.*

After completing the lesson, review and analyze your response to the Real Life Issues question.

Auto Safety

MAIN IDEA Paying attention and following the rules of the road are the keys to safe driving.

Did you know that motor vehicle crashes are the leading cause of death for people between the ages of 15 and 20? Young drivers are more than twice as likely to be involved in a crash as the rest of the population. This is why **vehicular safety**—obeying the rules of the road and exercising common sense and good judgment while driving— is such an important issue for teens.

The most important rule of driving safety is: pay attention to what you're doing. According to the National Highway Traffic Safety Administration at least 80 percent of car crashes occur as a result of **distracted driving**. The driver may be talking on a cell phone, drowsy, or lost in thought. To reduce driver distractions, some states have passed laws requiring that drivers use only hands-free cell phones and never send text messages while driving. You can do your part to reduce distractions when you're driving. Position the seat and mirrors and buckle your safety belt before you start the car. Adjust the radio and temperature controls before you start moving.

Below are some examples of things you need to pay attention to when you're in the driver's seat.

- **Other drivers.** Be aware of the cars around you and how they're moving. Make sure other drivers can see you by switching on your headlights at night and in bad weather.

- **Road conditions.** Reduce your speed if the road is icy or wet, if the heavy snow or rain is limiting your vision, if a lane narrows, if there are sharp curves ahead, or if there is construction or heavy traffic.

BEFORE YOU READ

Organize Information. Draw a chart with three columns. In the first column, list facts you already know about traffic safety. In the second, list questions about this topic you would like to have answered. As you read, fill in the third column with the answers.

Facts	Questions	Answers

Vocabulary

vehicular safety
distracted driving
graduated licensing
road rage
defensive driving

Reading Check

Analyze Pick one source of distracted driving and analyze how it may lead to an auto accident.

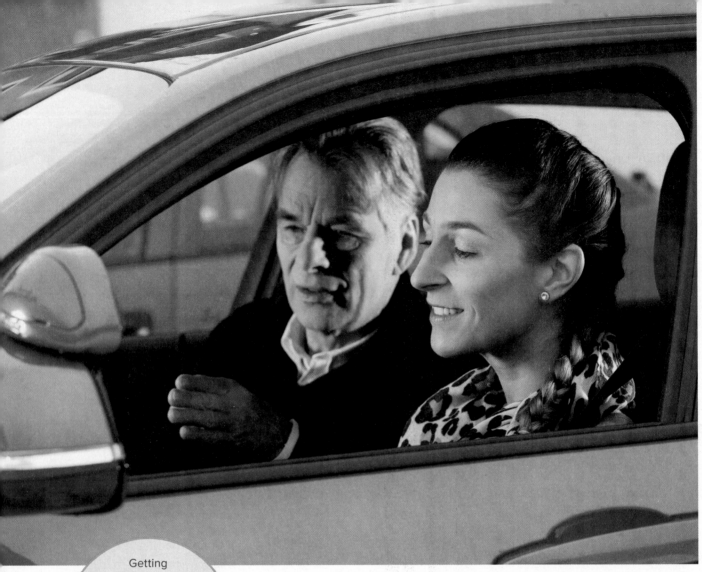

Getting lessons from an experienced driver will help you improve your driving skills. **Why might young or inexperienced drivers be more likely to get into accidents?**

- **Your physical state.** Drowsiness can impair your reaction time and your judgment. If you feel tired, try to wake yourself up by stopping for a snack or a bit of exercise. If you're still drowsy, pull over at the nearest safe, well-lit area and call home.

- **Your emotional state.** Being angry or upset can affect your driving. If you find yourself getting worked up behind the wheel, ask someone else to drive, or if you're alone, pull over to a safe spot until you calm down.

Teen Drivers

Young drivers may be more likely to get into accidents because they lack the experience and skills needed to drive safely. They are more likely than older drivers to underestimate the hazards of the road. They are also more likely to take risks such as running red lights or driving after using alcohol or drugs.

Driving Do's and Don'ts

Do:	Don't:
• Maintain a safe speed—not too fast, not too slow.	• Drive after using alcohol or any other depressant.
• Maintain a safe distance from other cars. Follow the three-second rule; when the car in front of you passes an object, you should pass it at least three seconds later.	• Drive while drowsy.
	• Use a cell phone while driving.
	• Be distracted by adjusting the radio or other controls.
• Signal all turns.	• Eat food while driving.
• Obey traffic signals.	• Drive with someone who has been drinking alcohol or using illegal drugs.
• Let other drivers merge safely.	
• Wear your safety belt, and make sure your passengers wear theirs.	• Use your horn inappropriately. It's meant to be a warning signal; save it for that.

To protect inexperienced drivers and others on the road, many states have **graduated licensing** programs. Graduated licensing is a system that slowly increases driving privileges over time. Many programs have three stages: learner, provisional, and full driver's license. Each stage has a different set of driving restrictions. Some states have also prohibited teen drivers from using cell phones while driving.

Avoiding Road Rage

Suppose you're driving along, minding your own business, when another driver suddenly swerves into your lane without signaling, forcing you to slam on your brakes. Some drivers respond to this type of situation with **road rage**. This means responding to a driving incident with violence. Road rage behaviors can include:

- honking, shouting, gesturing, or flashing lights.
- chasing or tailgating another vehicle.
- cutting off another car or forcing it off the road.
- deliberately hitting or bumping another car.
- threatening or physically attacking another driver.

If you witness these kinds of behaviors, stay a safe distance away. If you're threatened, lock your doors and head for the nearest police station. Never try to retaliate, or the conflict could turn deadly.

Being a Responsible Driver

Unfortunately, you can't always trust other drivers to drive safely. To protect yourself, you need to practice **defensive driving**. This means being aware of potential hazards on the road and taking action to avoid them. When you drive defensively, you not only take responsibility for your own behavior but also keep an eye out for others. A car that is weaving, crossing the center line, making wide turns, or braking without warning may have an impaired driver. If you spot such a vehicle, keep your distance, or pull over and notify the police.

Passengers can help reduce the risk of accidents as well. The most important way to do this is to avoid distracting the driver from the road. You can also take responsibility for your own safety. Always wear your seat belt, and never get into a vehicle with an impaired driver. Ask the person for the keys, and if he or she refuses, call a parent or other trusted adult for help.

• • • • • • • • • • • •

Reading Check

Identify Problems and Solutions Name two actions you can take to stay safe while driving.

• • • • • • • • • • • •

Sharing the Road

MAIN IDEA Everyone on the road shares a responsibility to follow traffic laws.

Everybody on the road has a responsibility to watch out for everybody else. When you're driving, you need to keep an eye out for cyclists and pedestrians. By the same token, when you're on foot, on a bike, or skating, you need to be aware of vehicles and follow the rules of the road.

Pedestrian Safety

Obviously, the safest place to walk is on the sidewalk. If there isn't a sidewalk, walk on the left side of the road, facing oncoming traffic. This will make it easier for cars to see you. It also makes it easier for you to see them and get out of their way if a driver comes too close. Cross streets only at marked crosswalks or, if there are no crosswalks, at a corner. Before you cross a street, look left, then right, then left again. Make sure the cars have seen you and stopped before stepping into the street.

Bicycle Safety

Riding a bike is a great way to get around and get some exercise at the same time. Here are some tips for safe cycling:

- Always wear a safety-approved helmet that fits properly.

- Obey traffic laws.

- Signal turns about half a block before reaching the intersection. Extend your left arm straight out to the side to signal a left turn. Bend your left arm upward at the elbow to signal a right turn.

- Ride single file, and keep to the far right side of the road. Watch out for obstacles such as opening car doors, sewer gratings, soft shoulders, and cars pulling into traffic.

- Avoid tailgating motor vehicles or riding closely behind a moving vehicle.

- Look left, right, and left again before riding into the stream of traffic.

- Dress to be seen. Wear bright colors in the daytime and reflective clothing at night. Make sure your bike has reflectors on the front and rear, on both wheels, and on both pedals.

• • • • • • • • • • •

Reading Check

Classify Identify two safety rules that apply to pedestrians, cyclists, and skaters.

• • • • • • • • • • •

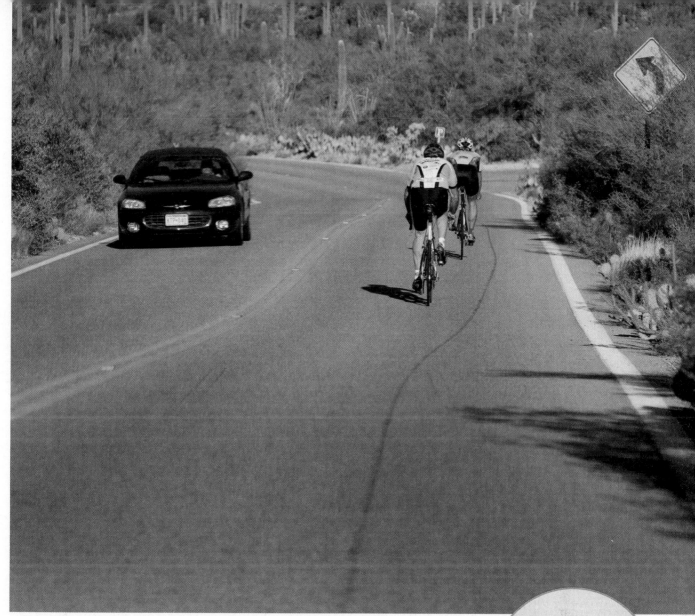

Skating Safety

To protect yourself while skating, wear the proper equipment: helmet, pads, wrist guards, and gloves. If you're a beginner, avoid skating in high traffic areas. Watch out for pedestrians, cyclists, and others on the sidewalks. Avoid skating in the street, and cross streets safely when you come to them. If you start to lose your balance, crouch down so that you won't have as far to fall. Try to keep your body loose, and try to roll if you fall down. Trying to absorb the force of the fall with your arms could lead to wrist injuries.

Small Motor Vehicle Safety

Small motor vehicles include motorcycles, mopeds, and all-terrain vehicles (ATVs). Motorcycles and mopeds are motor vehicles, just like cars, and are subject to the same traffic laws. Motorcyclists must have a special motorcycle license in addition to their driver's license.

Cyclists ride with the flow of traffic and obey the same traffic signs and signals as cars. **What are some safety measures you can take when riding a bike?**

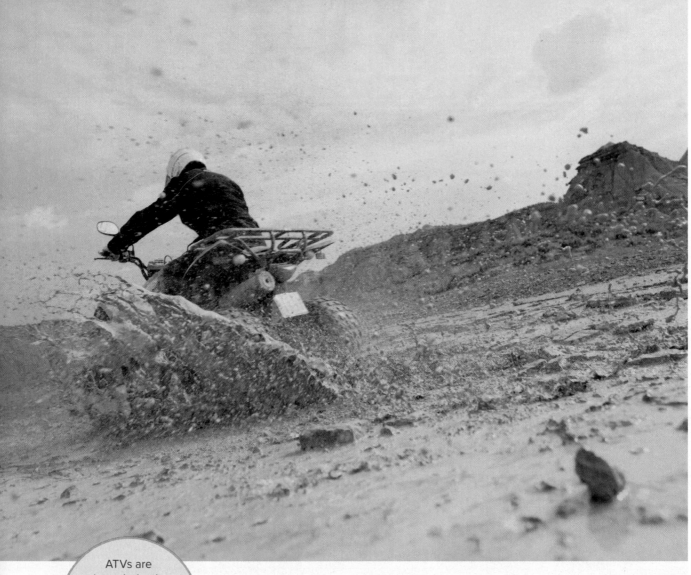

ATVs are intended only for off-road use. **Why might it be hazardous to take an ATV out on paved roads?**

According to the NHTSA, motorcyclists and their passengers are 35 times more likely to die in a crash than people in cars. Head injuries cause the most deaths in motorcycle accidents. In 20 states, all motorcyclists and passengers must wear protective helmets. In another 27 states, motorcyclists and passengers under the age of 18 are required to wear helmets. Helmets should meet the standards set by the U.S. Department of Transportation (DOT). Wearing sturdy clothing that covers the arms and legs also provides some protection. Just as with cars, passengers should avoid riding on a motorcycle if the driver is impaired by drug or alcohol use.

All-Terrain Vehicles (ATVs). Another type of small vehicle is the ATV. ATVs have four wheels. These off-road vehicles are used for recreation, as well as for work on many farms and ranches. However, an ATV is not a toy, and it's important to take safety precautions when using one. About 46 percent of all victims of ATV accidents are under 16 years old.

In 2008, the Consumer Product Safety Commission (CPSC) banned ATVs with three wheels. The CPSC is also proposing other rules for safe ATV use. These include licensing ATV users, restricting people under age 16 from using ATVs, and requiring all ATV users to complete safety classes. To operate ATVs safely, follow these guidelines:

- Only one person should ride on an ATV at a time.
- Avoid using attachments that will reduce the stability and braking of the ATV.
- Wear appropriate gear when riding an ATV. In addition to a DOT-approved helmet, you should wear eye protection, a long-sleeved shirt, long pants, gloves, and boots that cover your ankles.
- Avoid taking an ATV out on paved roads.
- Avoid ATV drivers who have been using alcohol or drugs.

Myths & Reality

Next time you think you're "too cool" for a seat belt, consider this fact about safety belts in cars.

Myth: By not fastening the safety belt, a passenger has a good chance of surviving an accident by being thrown clear of the car.

Reality: By not wearing a safety belt, a passenger might be thrown from the car in an accident. That would normally not be helpful, though. There is a 25 percent greater chance of being killed in an accident if you are thrown from the car.

Lesson 4 Review

Facts and Vocabulary

1. Identify the most important rule of driving safety.
2. Identify three behaviors associated with road rage.
3. Name one safety equipment item that is recommended for both cycling and in-line skating.

Thinking Critically

4. **Evaluate.** According to an old saying, "It's better to be alive than right." How could this saying be applied to vehicular safety?
5. **Evaluate.** What are some of the risks associated with operating motorcycles, mopeds, and ATVs?

Applying Health Skills

6. **Advocacy.** Work with a small group to produce a safety guide that educates teens and others on how to stay safe while operating a motorcycle, moped, or ATV. Produce your guide as a video, public service announcement, brochure, or comic book.

Writing Critically

7. **Expository.** List three risks you might face while driving, skating, or riding a bicycle. Then write a paragraph explaining how your behavior can increase or reduce these risks.

LESSON 1

Vocabulary Review

Correct the sentences below by replacing the italicized term with the correct vocabulary term.

1. Recognizing and avoiding dangerous situations is a part of *everyday precautions*.

2. Learning how to size up a situation, figure out what to do, and catch your attacker off-guard are examples of *martial arts*.

3. Cruel or hurtful online contact is called *harassment*.

Understanding Key Concepts

After reading the question or statement, select the correct answer.

4. If you think you are being followed in a public place, you should
   a. pretend you aren't aware of the stalker.
   b. go into a business that's open.
   c. challenge your attacker.
   d. avoid making a scene.

Thinking Critically

After reading the question or statement, write a short answer using complete sentences.

5. **Analyze.** How does letting your family know your plans protect your personal safety when you go out?

6. **Make Inferences.** Why might a person trying to escape from an attacker be more likely to get a response by shouting "fire" instead of "help"?

7. **Compare and Contrast.** How do the tactics used by cyberbullies differ from those used by Internet predators?

LESSON 2

Vocabulary Review

Use the correct vocabulary term to complete the following statements.

8. The kinds of accidents that pose a real danger are the ones that result in a(n) _____.

9. The _____ is a sequence of events that leads to an unintentional injury.

10. A(n) _____ is a portable device for putting out small fires.

11. A(n) _____ is a device that produces a loud warning noise in the presence of smoke.

12. The agency within the federal government that is responsible for promoting safe and healthful conditions in the workplace is called _____.

Understanding Key Concepts

After reading the question or statement, select the correct answer.

13. How often should smoke alarms be tested to make sure they are working?
    a. Every week
    b. Every month
    c. Twice a year
    d. Once a year

14. What is responsible for approximately half of all accidental deaths in the home?
    a. Poisonings
    b. Fire
    c. Electrical shock
    d. Falls

15. Which of the following steps can students take to improve the safety of their schools?
    a. Hire security guards.
    b. Put metal detectors at school entrances.
    c. Adopt zero-tolerance policies for offenses.
    d. Develop peer mediation programs.

Thinking Critically

After reading the question or statement, write a short answer using complete sentences.

16. Identify. What are the five steps in the accident chain?

17. Explain. How does following rules for electrical safety help prevent home fires?

18. Analyze. Why is it dangerous to mix household chemicals, such as cleaning fluids?

LESSON 3

Vocabulary Review

Use the correct vocabulary term to complete the following statement.

19. Wearing warm, layered clothing will protect you from _____, or a dangerously low body temperature.

20. Another name for a(n) _____ is a life jacket.

21. Damage to the skin and tissue caused by the cold is _____.

Understanding Key Concepts

After reading the question or statement, select the correct answer.

22. When skiing, snowboarding, or snowmobiling, you should give the right of way to
  a. the people ahead of you.
  b. the people coming from behind you.
  c. the people to your left.
  d. the people to your right.

23. The only safe place to swim is
  a. in a swimming pool.
  b. in a lake or river.
  c. in a designated area with a lifeguard present.
  d. near piers and reefs.

24. Which of the following water safety rules applies *only* to boating?
  a. Know how to swim.
  b. Don't go out alone.
  c. Pay attention to the weather.
  d. Always wear a life jacket.

Thinking Critically

After reading the question or statement, write a short answer using complete sentences.

25. Explain. Why should you avoid keeping food in or near sleeping areas while camping?

26. Evaluate. What is the advantage of having a buddy with you for all types of outdoor activity?

27. Apply. What should you do if you get caught in a current while swimming?

LESSON 4

Vocabulary Review

Correct the sentences below by replacing the italicized term with the correct vocabulary term.

28. *Traffic law* is a system that gradually increases driving privileges over time.

29. Responding to a driving incident with violence is called *highway anger*.

30. *Responsiveness* means being aware of potential hazards on the road and taking action to avoid them.

Understanding Key Concepts

After reading the question or statement, select the correct answer.

31. The National Highway Traffic Safety Administration (NHTSA) estimates that at least 25 percent of car crashes happen when a driver
    a. is not paying attention.
    b. is not wearing a safety belt.
    c. is angry or upset.
    d. is on wet or icy roads.

32. The proper place to ride a bicycle is
    a. on the left side of the road, facing oncoming traffic.
    b. on the far right side of the road.
    c. as close to the middle of the road as possible.
    d. on the sidewalk.

33. All-terrain vehicles (ATVs) should be ridden only
    a. on paved roads.
    b. by licensed drivers.
    c. for recreation.
    d. by one person at a time.

Thinking Critically

After reading the question or statement, write a short answer using complete sentences.

34. **Analyze.** What factors make teen drivers more likely to be involved in accidents?

35. **Evaluate.** What are the advantages of graduated licensing?

36. **Apply.** What should you do if you start to lose your balance while on a skateboard?

⌐ PROJECT-BASED ASSESSMENT

Preventing Poisonings

BACKGROUND

Households contain a surprising number of toxic substances. Cleaners, paints, medicines, and even some houseplants can be poisonous. Many home poisonings involve small children. A tiny amount of a toxic substance can be deadly. Treatment often depends on the type of poison. The good news is that most poisonings can be prevented.

TASK

Create a public service announcement (PSA) that can be played over the school intercom.

AUDIENCE

Families in your community

PURPOSE

Provide families with information to prevent household poisonings.

PROCEDURE

1. Review the poison prevention information presented in this module.

2. Conduct an Internet search to find additional information on poison prevention.

3. Collaborate as a group to compile a list of steps people can take to prevent household poisonings. Add emergency measures that can be taken if someone is poisoned.

4. Find the 24-hour toll-free number for the Centers for Disease Control and Prevention's poison control hotline.

5. Present the PSA to your class. Get permission from your principal to play the PSA over the school intercom.

Math Practice

Interpret Graphs. The bar graph below shows the percentage of total hospitalized injuries based on a sample size of 650,000 people. Use the graph to answer Questions 1–3.

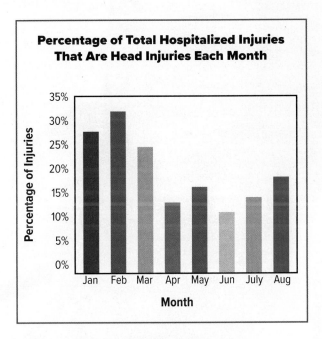

Percentage of Total Hospitalized Injuries That Are Head Injuries Each Month

1. If 32% of the sample size were injured in February, how many people were injured?
   a. 175,000
   b. 208,000
   c. 324,000
   d. 475,000

2. Which month had the fewest number of injuries?
   a. January
   b. April
   c. June
   d. August

3. Approximately how many injuries occurred during the month with the fewest injuries?
   a. 117,000
   b. 91,000
   c. 71,500
   d. 65,000

Reading/Writing Practice

Understand and Apply. Read the passage below, and then answer the questions.

A fire broke out Thursday night in the home of the Levin family in Deep Valley. Mr. and Mrs. Levin and their two children, Sam and Jamie, escaped unhurt. "Our smoke detector saved our lives," reported Debbie Levin. "It woke us all up out of a sound sleep. Dave and I went to check on the kids, but they were already on their way out—crawling under the smoke just the way we taught them." "It's really worth the effort to make a fire safety plan and have drills with your kids," added Dave Levin. The Levins escaped to the home of their neighbors, the Johnsons, and called the fire department. Firefighters were able to extinguish the blaze before it caused significant damage.

1. Which of the following sentences would best complete the third paragraph?
   a. The fire was caused by bad wiring.
   b. We have a fire extinguisher on hand.
   c. The Johnsons let us use their phone to call the fire department.
   d. Our kids knew exactly what to do in this situation.

2. What is the purpose of this passage?
   a. To urge people to buy fire extinguishers
   b. To report a neighborhood fire
   c. To explain how smoke detectors work
   d. To generate sympathy for the Levins

3. Write a conclusion for this article that describes how the fire in the Levin home started. Include advice on how readers can protect themselves from fires in their own homes.

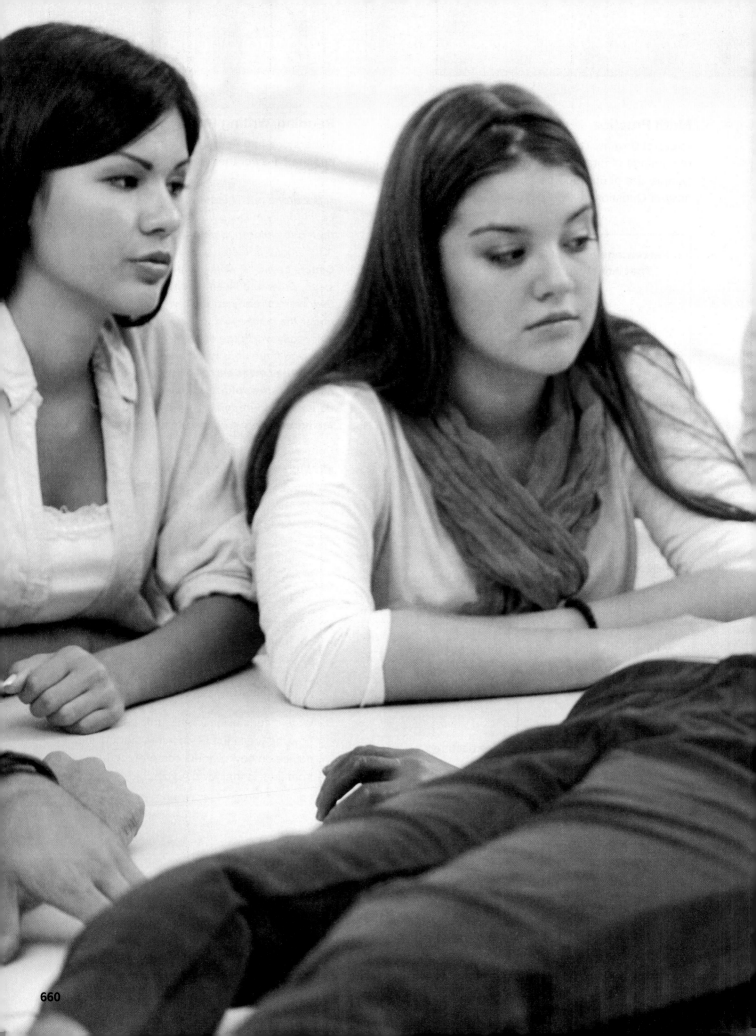

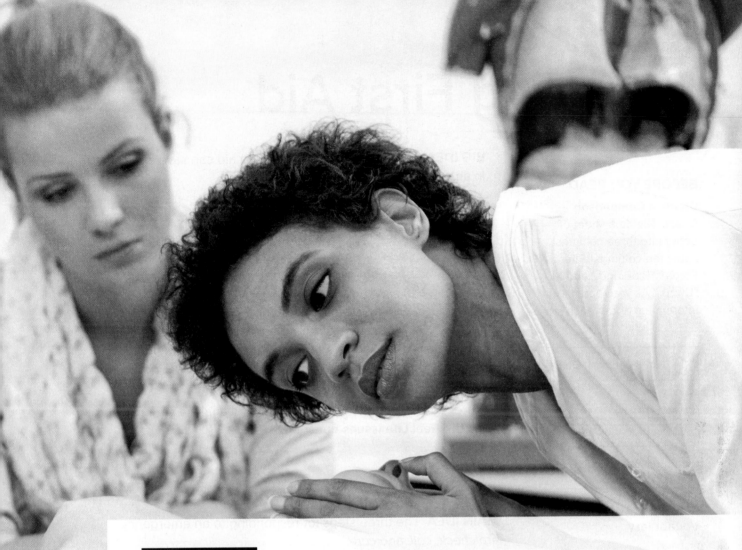

MODULE 27

First Aid and Emergencies

LESSONS

1 Providing First Aid

2 CPR and First Aid for Shock and Choking

3 Responding to Other Common Emergencies

4 Emergency Preparedness

Providing First Aid

. . . .

BEFORE YOU READ

Create a Comparison Chart. Divide a sheet of paper into three columns. Label the columns "First Steps," "Bleeding," and "Burns." As you read, fill in information about each topic.

First Steps	Bleeding	Burns

Vocabulary

first aid
Good Samaritan laws
universal precautions

. . . .

BIG IDEA Knowing how to perform first aid can save a life in an emergency.

REAL LIFE ISSUES

Helping Out a Stranger. Eva was driving in her neighborhood when she saw someone lying by the side of the road. She pulled over and got out of her car. The person was a woman wearing a bicycle helmet. An overturned bike was lying nearby. Cautiously, Eva touched her shoulder. "Hey, are you okay?" she asked. "Can you move?" The woman responded with a muffled groan. *Write a conclusion to this story that shows how Eva responded to this emergency and what effect her actions had on herself and on the stranger she helped.*

After completing the lesson, review and analyze your response to the Real Life Issues question.

First Steps in an Emergency

MAIN IDEA The three steps for responding to an emergency are *check, call,* and *care.*

If you ever find yourself facing an emergency—a car crash, a hurricane, or even a terrorist attack—will you know what to do? In a situation like this, knowing **first aid** could save someone's life. First aid is the immediate, temporary care given to an ill or injured person until professional medical care can be provided. In the seconds and minutes right after an emergency strikes, first aid can mean the difference between life and death. By learning and using proper first-aid procedures, you can help prevent further injuries and reduce the number of victims who die.

Recognizing an emergency is the first step in responding to it. The next step is to check the scene to make sure it's safe for you to respond. Look out for such hazards as downed electrical lines or oncoming traffic that might put you at risk if you approach. Remember, you can't help the other person if you become injured yourself. Once you've determined that the scene is safe, you can take steps to help.

The Three Cs

The "three Cs" of emergency care are *check, call,* and *care.* Here's how to put them into practice:

- **Check the victim.** A victim who is unconscious or has a life-threatening condition (for example, someone who is not breathing) needs immediate care. If anyone else is around, call out to that person to help you with the victim. Only move the victim if he or she is in direct physical danger or if you must move the victim in order to provide lifesaving care.

- **Call 911 or your local emergency number.** If the victim is in need of immediate care, get someone else at the scene to call 911 while you provide first aid. If no one else is present, make the call yourself. Emergency operators may be able to talk you through the steps of helping the victim. Stay on the line until help arrives.

- **Care for the victim.** If possible, get the victim's permission before giving first aid. If the victim refuses help, respect his or her decision. However, if the victim can't speak to give permission, don't hesitate to provide care. Most states have **Good Samaritan laws** that will protect you. These are statutes that protect rescuers from being sued for giving emergency care.

Reading Check

Identify What are the three Cs of emergency care?

Providing proper first-aid procedures at the scene of an accident can help prevent further injuries and help save lives.

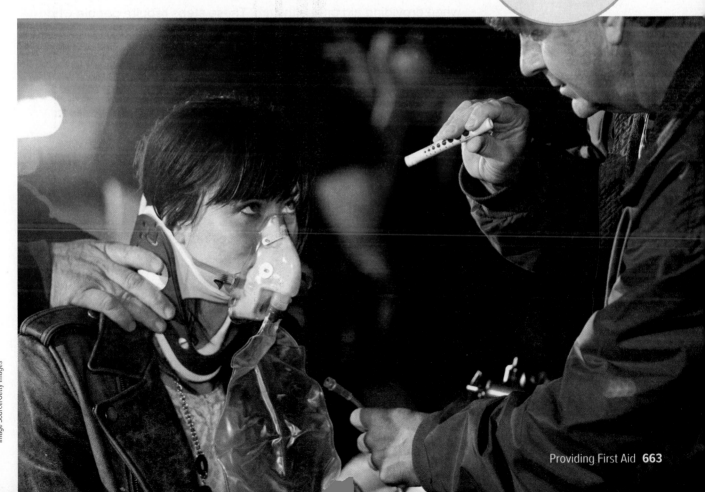

Image Source/Getty Images

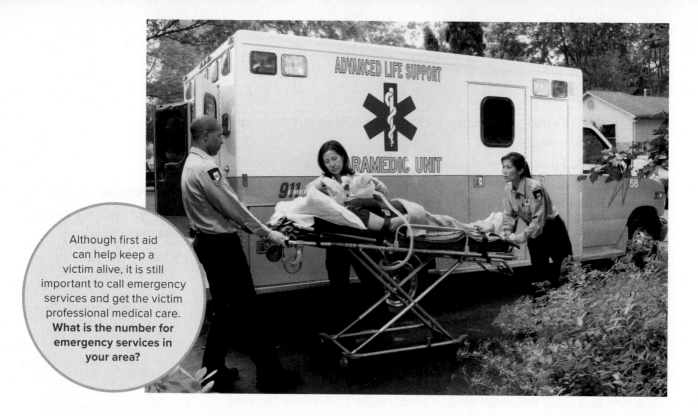

Although first aid can help keep a victim alive, it is still important to call emergency services and get the victim professional medical care. **What is the number for emergency services in your area?**

Universal Precautions

One risk of giving first aid is that blood and other body fluids can carry pathogens, including the viruses that cause AIDS and hepatitis B. To protect yourself, follow **universal precautions**, which are steps taken to prevent the spread of disease through blood and other body fluids when providing aid or health care. These steps require people who provide first aid or medical care to treat all body fluids as if they could carry disease. Universal precautions include:

- wearing sterile gloves whenever you could come into contact with someone's blood or body fluids.

- washing hands immediately after providing first aid.

- using a mouthpiece, if one is available, when providing rescue breathing.

First Aid for Bleeding

MAIN IDEA The steps for treating bleeding depend on the type of injury and how severe it is.

If you slip on an icy sidewalk and scrape your hand, the wound may bleed, but it won't be a medical emergency. **Minor** injuries that cause bleeding, such as small cuts and scrapes, can usually be treated at home. Severe bleeding, however, can be a life-threatening emergency. The appropriate first aid for bleeding depends on what type of wound you are dealing with and how severe the bleeding is.

Paul Burns/Getty Images

Types of Open Wounds

Open wounds are injuries in which the skin is broken. Types of open wounds include the following:

- **Abrasions.** Also known as scrapes, these occur when the skin is scraped against a hard surface, bursting the tiny blood vessels in the outer layer of skin. The chief danger with this type of wound is that dirt and bacteria can penetrate the skin. It's important to clean the wound well to prevent infection and speed healing.

- **Lacerations.** These are cuts caused by a sharp object slicing through the layers of skin. Minor lacerations can be treated at home, but medical care is needed for deep cuts, cuts that won't stop bleeding, and cuts on the face and neck. These wounds may require stitches. A tetanus booster may also be needed.

- **Punctures.** A puncture wound is a small but deep hole caused by a sharp and narrow object (such as a nail) that pierces the skin. Puncture wounds do not usually cause heavy bleeding, but they do carry a high risk of infection, including tetanus infection. If a puncture wound is deep, dirty, or in the foot, see a doctor. The victim may need a tetanus shot or booster.

- **Avulsions.** An avulsion occurs when skin or tissue is partly or completely torn away from the body. Such wounds usually require stitches. If a body part, such as a finger, is partly or completely separated from the body, seek emergency medical care right away. If possible, wrap the severed body part in a cold, moist towel to preserve the tissue; doctors may be able to reattach it.

Controlling Bleeding

When treating an open wound on someone other than yourself, wear clean protective gloves. If medical help is needed, call 911 before taking any other steps. Next, wash the wound thoroughly with mild soap and running water to remove dirt and debris. Then follow these steps to control the bleeding:

- If possible, raise the wounded body part above the level of the heart.

- Cover the wound with sterile gauze or a clean cloth.

- Press the palm of your hand firmly against the gauze. Apply steady pressure to the wound for five minutes or until help arrives. Do not stop to check the wound; you may interrupt the clotting of the blood.

Myths & Reality

Have you ever had a bad burn? Maybe someone told you to put butter on it. Do you think that was helpful in healing?

Myth: Putting butter on a burn will help it heal.

Reality: Butter may actually seal in the heat and make a burn feel worse. Butter can also trap germs in the burned skin, increasing the likelihood of infection.

Reading Check

Classify Which kind of burn always requires professional medical care?

- If blood soaks through the gauze, add another gauze pad on top of the first and continue to apply pressure.

- Once the bleeding slows or stops, **secure** the pad firmly in place with a bandage or strips of gauze or other material. The pad should be snug, but not so tight that you can't feel the victim's pulse.

- If you can't stop the bleeding after five minutes, or if the wound starts bleeding again, call for medical help (if you have not done so already). Continue to apply pressure to the wound until help arrives.

Certain types of injuries can cause internal bleeding—blood spilling from a damaged blood vessel into one of the body's cavities. Internal bleeding is difficult to detect. However, bleeding from the eyes, nose, mouth, or ears may be a sign that internal bleeding is occurring. Internal bleeding requires emergency care, so call for help right away. While waiting for help to arrive, you can take steps to prevent the victim from going into shock.

First Aid for Burns

MAIN IDEA Treatment for burns depends on the severity of the burn.

Burns can occur in a variety of ways. Burns caused by heat are the most common type. They may occur as a result of exposure to flame, touching a hot object such as a stove, scalding with hot water or steam, or overexposure to the sun (sunburn). Burns can also result from exposure to electricity or to certain chemicals, such as bleach. Chemical and electrical burns require special first-aid procedures.

First-degree burns and small second-degree burns are considered minor and can be treated with these steps:

1. Cool the burned area by holding it under cold, running water for at least five minutes. If this isn't possible, immerse the burned area in cool water or wrap it in cold, wet cloths. Do not use ice, which may cause frostbite and further damage the skin.

2. Cover the burn loosely with a sterile gauze bandage.

3. The victim may take an over-the-counter pain reliever. Make sure the victim isn't allergic to the medication.

4. Minor burns usually heal without further treatment, although the skin may be discolored. If signs of infection develop—including increased pain, redness, fever, swelling, or oozing—seek medical help.

Some second-degree burns and all third-degree burns require immediate medical care. Call 911 and provide first aid until help arrives. Cover the burned area with a clean, moist cloth, but do not remove burned clothing unless it is still smoldering. Do not immerse a large burned area in cold water; the burn victim could go into shock. Be prepared to give first aid for shock or loss of circulation.

Types of burns

First-degree burns involve only the outer layer of skin. This outermost layer is called the epidermis. In a first-degree burn, the skin becomes red, and the burned area may become swollen and painful. First-degree burns are considered minor burns unless they involve a major joint or cover large areas of the hands, feet, face, groin, or buttocks.

Second-degree burns involve the epidermis and the underlying layers of skin (the dermis). The skin becomes very red and develops blisters. There is severe pain and swelling. A second-degree burn no larger than 2 to 3 inches in diameter can be treated as a minor burn. Larger burns, or burns that affect the hands, feet, face, groin, buttocks, or a major joint, require professional medical care.

Third-degree burns, the most serious kind, involve all layers of the skin and may penetrate the underlying tissues. The skin may be charred black or may appear white and dry. It may also be possible to see muscle and even bone. These burns can destroy nerve endings, so victims may not experience pain. Third-degree burns require immediate medical attention.

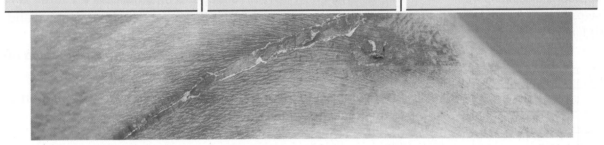

Lesson 1 Review

Facts and Vocabulary

1. List the three first steps for responding to an emergency.

2. Identify the four types of open wounds.

3. Describe the procedure for treating a minor burn.

Thinking Critically

4. **Synthesize.** Suppose that you are looking after your seven-year-old neighbor. The boy steps on a tack and gets a puncture wound in his foot. How would you respond?

5. **Evaluate.** Which types of open wounds are most likely to require professional medical care? Why?

Applying Health Skills

6. **Advocacy.** Write a persuasive flyer designed to encourage other teens to learn first aid. Your flyer should explain the value of knowing first aid and the situations in which it can be useful.

Writing Critically

7. **Narrative.** Write a short story in which a teen responds to a medical emergency and provides appropriate first aid.

CPR and First Aid for Shock and Choking

BEFORE YOU READ

Organize Information. Make a three-column chart. Label the columns "CPR," "First Aid for Shock," and "First Aid for Choking." As you read, fill in the appropriate columns with the steps in each first-aid procedure.

CPR	Shock	Choking

Vocabulary

chain of survival
cardiopulmonary resuscitation (CPR)
defibrillator
rescue breathing
shock

. . . .

BIG IDEA Medical emergencies that are life threatening include loss of breathing, shock, and choking.

REAL LIFE ISSUES

Learning CPR. Lauren babysits her nephew on Tuesday nights while her sister attends class. Her sister wants Lauren to take CPR and child safety classes at a local community college so that she will know how to respond to an emergency. Lauren isn't sure that she wants to spend her weekend learning first aid and CPR, since she may never have to use these life-saving techniques. *Write a letter to Lauren, explaining why it could be important for Lauren to learn CPR and first aid.*

After completing the lesson, review and analyze your response to the Real Life Issues question.

The Chain of Survival

MAIN IDEA In a medical emergency, a victim's life depends on a specific series of actions called the *chain of survival*.

The most urgent medical emergencies are often those in which the victim is unresponsive—unable to speak or react to his or her surroundings. This condition can result from a heart attack, a stroke, or cardiac arrest. In this type of emergency you need to act quickly, because the first few minutes are usually the most critical. The key is to know what to do, remain calm, and take action.

An unresponsive victim is in immediate danger. Her or his best hope for survival lies in the **chain of survival**. This is a sequence of actions that maximize the victim's chances of survival. It includes the following links:

- **A call to emergency medical services.** This first step is important for all victims. The 911 operator will ask you questions about the victim's condition and instruct you about what to do next. If the victim's heart has stopped, you will be instructed to move on to the next link in the chain of survival.

- **CPR, or cardiopulmonary resuscitation.** CPR is a first-aid procedure that combines rescue breathing and chest compressions to supply oxygen to the body until normal body functions can resume. It provides the victim with a chance to survive until medical help arrives.

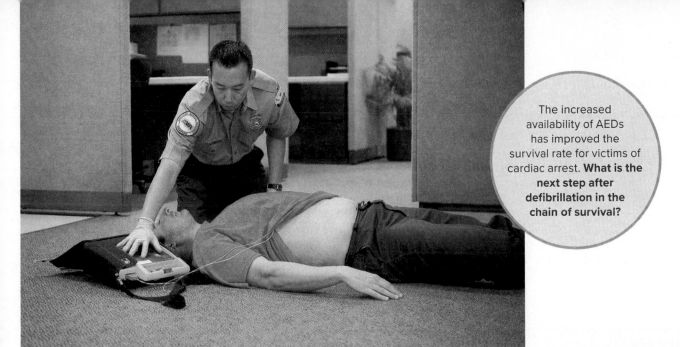

The increased availability of AEDs has improved the survival rate for victims of cardiac arrest. **What is the next step after defibrillation in the chain of survival?**

- **Use of a defibrillator.** A defibrillator is a device that delivers an electric shock to the heart to restore its normal rhythm. An increasing number of public places now provide automated external defibrillators (AEDs).

- **Advanced care.** Paramedics and other trained medical personnel can provide the care needed to keep the victim alive on the way to the hospital.

Reading Check

Make Inferences What is the purpose of the chain of survival?

CPR

MAIN IDEA CPR can save the life of a person whose heartbeat or breathing has stopped.

The second link in the chain of survival is to perform cardiopulmonary resuscitation, or CPR on the victim. Currently, two forms of CPR are recommended for use. An emergency medical specialist or trained individual will perform CPR that combines chest compressions with **rescue breathing**. This is breathing for a person who is not breathing on his or her own. A person using this form of CPR should be trained in the technique.

A person who is untrained in giving CPR can perform an updated form of the procedure called *Hands-Only™ CPR*. Hands-Only™ CPR eliminates the need for rescue breathing and focuses on chest compressions. If no trained person is present, an untrained person should begin Hands-Only™ CPR before paramedics arrive. In some parts of the country, 911 dispatchers are taught how to talk an untrained person through the steps of CPR.

McGraw-Hill Education

Hands-Only™ CPR for Adults

The first thing to do when you encounter an injured person is call 9-1-1. Before performing CPR on an adult, check to see whether the person is conscious. Tap the victim on the shoulder while shouting, "Are you okay?" If the victim doesn't respond, look at the victim's chest to determine if he or she is breathing. Performing chest compressions on a victim who is not in cardiac arrest can cause injury.

If you are confident that the victim is not breathing, begin Hands-Only™ CPR. The first diagram shows how to position your hands over the victim's chest and begin chest compressions. Aim to complete 100 chest compressions each minute, continuing until the victim responds or until paramedics arrive.

ADULT CPR
The basic process of Hands-Only™ CPR for adults focuses on chest compressions.

Check to see if the victim is breathing. Look, listen, and feel for normal breathing for five to ten seconds. Signs of normal breathing include

- seeing the person's chest rise and fall.
- hearing breathing sounds, including wheezing, gurgling, or snoring.
- feeling air moving out of the person's mouth or nose.

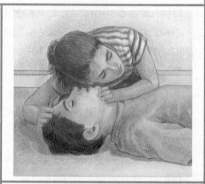

Begin chest compressions. To position your hands correctly, follow these steps:

1. Use your fingers to find the end of the victim's sternum (breastbone), where the ribs come together.

2. Place two fingers over the end of the sternum.

3. Place the heel of your other hand against the sternum, directly above your fingers (on the side closest to the victim's face).

4. Place your other hand on top of the one you just put in position. Interlock the fingers of your hands and raise your fingers so they do not touch the person's chest.

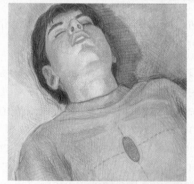

Perform chest compressions using the following procedure:

1. Straighten your arms, lock your elbows, and line your shoulders up so they are directly above your hands.

2. Press downward on the person's chest, forcing the breastbone down by 1.5 to 2 inches (3.8 to 5 cm).

3. Begin compressions at a steady pace. You can maintain a rhythm by counting, "One and two and three and . . ." Press down each time you say a number.

4. Try to perform 100 chest compressions per minute.

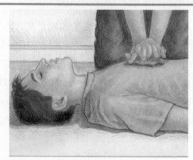

Because the Hands-Only™ CPR procedure is both easy to remember and effective, experts consider people more likely to perform it than conventional CPR. The American Heart Association considers any attempt at CPR to be better than no attempt at all to provide help.

The AHA still recommends taking a course in conventional CPR, which includes training in both rescue breathing and giving high-quality chest compressions. Experts say that conventional CPR may still be better than Hands-Only™ CPR for certain victims, including:

- Infants and young children

- An adult who has collapsed, but no one saw it happen

- Drowning victims or people suffering life-threatening breathing problems

CPR for Infants and Children

The second diagram illustrates how to position your hands when performing CPR on an infant or young child. The cycle of CPR for children under the age of 8 includes 30 chest compressions alternating with 2 rescue breaths. The procedure for infants and young children also differs in several other ways:

- When performing CPR on a newborn baby, open the airway and give two breaths *before* beginning chest compressions.

- When performing chest compressions on an infant, using the heel of your hand can be too forceful and may cause injury. Instead, use three fingers, positioned on the baby's sternum at the center of the chest. Press the sternum down about one-third to one-half the depth of the baby's chest.

Reading Check

Compare and Contrast List three ways in which CPR for infants differs from CPR for adults.

INFANT AND CHILD CPR

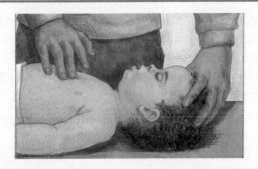

- This image shows how to position your fingers to perform chest compressions on an infant.

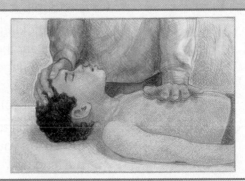

- This image shows how to position your hands for chest compressions on a child between one and eight years old.

- To perform chest compressions on a child between one and eight years old, you can either use the heel of one hand or use both hands as in adult CPR. Position your hands about two finger widths above the end of the sternum and press the sternum down about one-third to one-half the depth of the child's chest.

- When performing rescue breathing on a baby, place your mouth over the baby's nose and mouth at the same time—not the mouth only, as for an adult.

- Do not use a breathing mask designed for adult CPR when performing CPR on an infant.

Other Emergencies

MAIN IDEA Choking and shock are life-threatening medical emergencies that require immediate attention.

The chain of **survival** does not apply to every medical emergency. If a person is choking, rescue breathing will not help because the airway is blocked. Knowing the specific first-aid procedures for choking and shock can save lives in a medical emergency.

First Aid for Choking

Choking occurs when an object, such as a piece of food, becomes stuck in a person's windpipe, cutting off the flow of air. Clutching the throat is the universal sign for choking. Other signs of choking include inability to speak, difficulty breathing, an inability to cough forcefully, turning blue in the face or lips, and loss of consciousness.

If you see these signs in an adult, help the person immediately by performing abdominal thrusts. If someone else is nearby, ask that person to call 911 while you help the victim. For a choking infant, perform back blows and chest thrusts to dislodge the object.

If the choking victim is unconscious, lower the person to the floor and try to clear the airway. Reach into the mouth and sweep the object out with one finger. Be careful not to push the obstruction deeper into the throat. If the obstruction cannot be dislodged, begin performing CPR. The chest compressions may dislodge the object.

If you begin to choke when you're alone, you can perform abdominal thrusts on yourself by covering your fist with the other hand and pushing upward and inward. Another method is to bend over a rigid structure, such as a countertop or the back of a chair. Press against it to thrust your abdomen upward and inward.

ACADEMIC VOCABULARY

survival *(noun)*: the continuation of life or existence

Reading Check

Explain How can you help a choking adult?

TREATMENT FOR CHOKING

If an adult is choking:

1. Stand behind the victim and wrap your arms around his or her waist. (For a pregnant or obese victim, wrap your arms around the rib cage.)

2. Make a fist with one hand and grasp it with your other hand.

3. Pull your hands into the abdomen with a quick, upward thrust.

4. Repeat the abdominal thrusts until the object is dislodged.

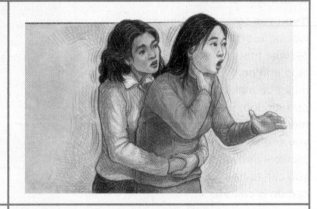

If an infant is choking:

1. Sit down and hold the baby facedown over your forearm, which should be resting on your thigh.

2. With the heel of your hand, give the infant five gentle but firm blows between the shoulder blades.

3. If this doesn't dislodge the object, turn the infant face-up, with the head lower than the body. Perform five chest compressions as you would when performing infant CPR.

4. If the baby still isn't breathing, have someone call emergency services immediately while you repeat the back blows and chest thrusts. If breathing doesn't resume, begin infant CPR.

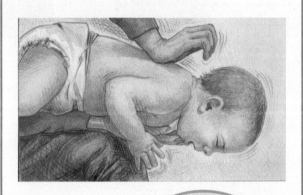

First Aid for Shock

Shock is a life-threatening condition in which the heart is not delivering an adequate supply of blood to the body. Symptoms of shock include:

- cold, clammy skin, which may appear pale or grayish.

- weak, rapid pulse and altered breathing.

- dull, staring eyes, which may have dilated pupils.

- faintness, weakness, confusion, or loss of consciousness.

Use abdominal thrusts on a choking adult. For an infant, alternate back blows with chest thrusts. **Why do you think different methods are used for adults and infants?**

If someone displays these symptoms, call 911 right away. If the victim is conscious and doesn't have an injury to the head, neck, legs, or spine, get him or her to lie down and raise his or her legs about 12 inches. If the victim has any wounds or other injuries, give first aid for these while you wait for help to arrive. Some shock victims become anxious or agitated, so try to keep the person calm. Monitor the victim's breathing, and be prepared to start CPR immediately if breathing stops. Loosen the victim's clothing and try to keep him or her warm and comfortable. Do not give the victim anything to eat or drink. If the victim vomits, drools, or starts bleeding from the mouth, roll him or her into the recovery position.

If you see someone who has just suffered an injury, don't assume that someone else will stop and help. Everyone else might be making that same assumption. Be a responsible member of your community. If you see someone who needs medical assistance, do what you can to help, even if all you can do is call 911.

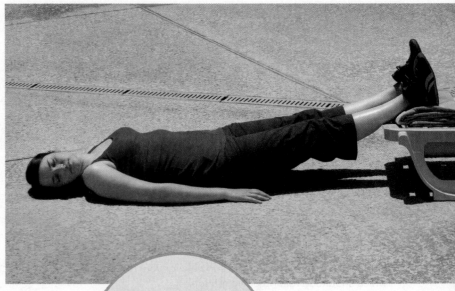

A person suffering from shock should lie down with the legs elevated, unless the person has an injury to the head, neck, legs, or spine. **What purpose might raising the victim's legs serve?**

Lesson 2 Review

Facts and Vocabulary

1. Identify the steps in the chain of survival.

2. Describe the basic cycle of CPR.

3. Describe the universal sign for choking.

Thinking Critically

4. **Evaluate.** Why is calling emergency services the first step in the chain of survival?

5. **Analyze.** Explain how the strategy for responding to choking differs, depending on whether the victim is an adult or an infant.

Applying Health Skills

6. **Accessing Information.** Use community or Internet resources to find out where and when CPR classes are offered in your area. If possible, arrange to take one of these classes.

Writing Critically

7. **Creative.** Write a jingle that uses rhyme and rhythm to help people remember the steps for a first-aid procedure discussed in this lesson.

Tim Fuller Photography

Responding to Other Common Emergencies

BIG IDEA You can use first aid to deal with common emergencies such as muscle and bone injuries, impaired consciousness, animal bites, nosebleeds, and poisoning.

REAL LIFE ISSUES

Feeling Faint. Kim has been looking forward to the school dance all month. On the day of the dance, she's so excited that she forgets to eat lunch. At the dance, she is having a great time out on the hot, crowded dance floor. Then she starts to feel dizzy, and the next thing she knows, she's lying outside on the ground. Looking up, she sees a teacher and a couple of her friends. "You fainted," the teacher explains. "You need to lie still for a while." Kim is embarrassed. She wants to reassure the teacher that she's fine and go back to the dance. *Write a dialogue between Kim and the teacher. Show how the two of them deal with Kim's situation in a way that protects her health.*

After completing the lesson, review and analyze your response to the Real Life Issues question.

BEFORE YOU READ

Create a T-Chart. On one side of the chart, list common medical emergencies. On the other side, list strategies to deal with each type of emergency.

Emergencies	Strategies

Vocabulary

unconsciousness
concussion
poison
poison control center
venom

Muscle, Joint, and Bone Injuries

MAIN IDEA Muscle and joint injuries can be minor or severe, but bone injuries are always medical emergencies.

As you have learned, sports and other physical activities can result in injuries to your muscles, joints, and bones. These kinds of injuries can occur in other situations as well. For example, you could sprain your ankle by tripping over a branch, break your arm in a car crash, or dislocate your shoulder falling from a ladder. Safety precautions can help prevent injuries like these, but accidents can still happen. That's why you should know the proper first-aid procedures for treating injuries such as strains, sprains, fractures, and dislocations.

Muscle and Joint Injuries

Two common and fairly minor injuries are strains and sprains. A strain is a tear in a muscle, while a sprain is an injury to the ligaments around a joint. These injuries produce similar symptoms, including pain, stiffness, swelling, difficulty moving the affected body part, and discoloration or bruising of the surrounding skin. Strains and sprains vary in severity.

Severe strains and sprains will require medical care. Call 911 for emergency medical help if:

- the victim is unable to move the affected muscle or joint.
- the pain is severe.
- the injury is bleeding.
- the joint appears deformed.
- you hear a popping sound coming from the joint.

The P.R.I.C.E. Procedure You can treat minor strains and sprains with the P.R.I.C.E. procedure. The steps in this procedure are:

- **Protect** the affected area by wrapping it in a bandage or splint.
- **Rest** the injured body part for at least a day,
- **Ice** the area to reduce swelling and pain. Wrap ice cubes in a cloth or towel and hold it against the affected area for 10 to 15 minutes at a time, three times a day.
- **Compress** the affected area by wrapping it firmly, but not too tightly, in a bandage.
- **Elevate** the injured body part above the level of the heart, if possible.

You can gradually begin to use the affected body part again as the pain and swelling subside. If the swelling lasts more than two days, see a doctor.

Fractures and Dislocations

Injuries to bones include fractures and dislocations. A fracture is a break in a bone. A dislocation is a separation of a bone from its normal position in a joint. Symptoms for both injuries include severe pain, swelling, bruising, and inability to move the affected body part. The limb or joint may be visibly misshapen, discolored, or out of place.

Fractures and dislocations are emergencies that require immediate medical care. The first-aid procedures for both conditions are the same:

1. Call 911 or your local emergency medical service.
2. Do your best to keep the victim still and calm.
3. If the skin is broken, rinse it carefully to prevent infection, taking care not to disturb the bone. Cover the wound with a sterile dressing, if available.
4. If necessary, apply a splint. A splint will immobilize the injured body part to prevent further injury. Attach any kind of rigid support—such as a board or stick—to the injured body part with strips of cloth, immobilizing the area extending above and below the injured bone.
5. Apply an ice pack to reduce pain and swelling.
6. If the injury does not affect the head, neck, legs, or spine, have the victim lie down with the legs raised about 12 inches to prevent shock.

Reading Check

Compare and Contrast Name one way in which fractures and dislocations are similar and one way in which they differ.

Unconsciousness

MAIN IDEA A victim who loses consciousness for any amount of time requires medical care.

Nearly any major injury or illness can cause **unconsciousness**. This is the condition of not being alert or aware of your surroundings. Alcohol and drug abuse can also cause a person to lose consciousness. Victims who are unconscious are not able to respond to simple commands. They also cannot cough or clear their throats, putting them at risk of choking.

If you encounter someone who has lost consciousness, call 911, check the victim's breathing, and be prepared to perform CPR if necessary. If the victim is breathing and does not seem to have an injury to the spine, lay the victim down on his or her side. Bend the top leg so that the hip and knee joints form right angles, and gently tilt the victim's head back to open the airway. This position, known as the *recovery position,* will help the victim breathe. Keep the victim warm until help arrives.

Fainting

Fainting is a temporary loss of consciousness that occurs when not enough blood is flowing to the brain. If you see someone faint, try to catch the person to stop him or her from falling. Lay the victim on the floor and elevate the legs. Loosen any tight clothing around the victim's neck. If the person vomits, quickly roll him or her into the recovery position. If the victim does not regain consciousness within a couple of minutes, call 911. Otherwise, just keep the victim lying still for 10 to 15 minutes.

A single episode of fainting may not be serious. However, it is a warning that your body needs medical attention. Victims of fainting should see a doctor as soon as possible if they have never fainted before or they are fainting frequently.

The recovery position is the safest position for an unconscious person because the airway is protected. **Why is it important to keep the airway open?**

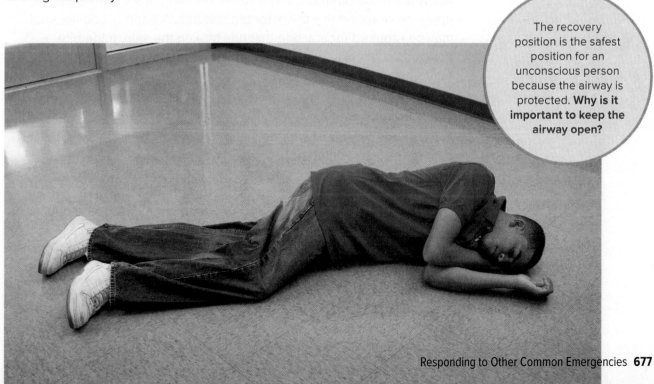

Tim Fuller Photography

. . . .

Reading Check

Explain What can you do to help someone who is unconscious, has fainted, or has a concussion?

. . . .

Concussion

A **concussion** is a jarring injury to the brain that can cause unconsciousness. Anyone who loses consciousness or experiences memory loss or confusion because of a head injury might have a concussion. Call 911 for all cases of suspected concussion. If the victim is conscious, have him or her lie down. Use first aid to treat any bleeding while you wait for help to arrive. If the victim is unconscious, avoid moving him or her if there is reason to suspect a head or neck injury. Otherwise, you can place the victim in the recovery position.

Other Common Emergencies

MAIN IDEA It's important to learn first-aid procedures for emergencies such as animal bites, nosebleeds, and poisoning.

Other common medical emergencies include animal bites, nosebleeds, and poisoning. Learning proper first-aid procedures will help you stay calm and respond appropriately in the event of an emergency.

Animal Bites

Animal bites can transmit serious diseases. One such disease is rabies, a viral infection that can be deadly if not treated immediately. Once a person develops symptoms of rabies, the disease cannot be cured. However, a vaccine can prevent the disease if it is given within two days of exposure to the virus. Anyone who is bitten by an unknown or wild animal should **seek** emergency medical care immediately.

In general, animal bites should be treated like any other open wound. If you're providing first aid to a bite victim, wash your hands thoroughly and put on protective gloves. Then, wash the bite area thoroughly with mild soap and water. Apply pressure as needed to stop any bleeding. Apply antibiotic ointment and a sterile dressing. If the wound swells, apply ice wrapped in a towel for ten minutes. A tetanus booster shot may be required for any bite that has broken the skin. If the bite develops signs of infection (such as redness, pain, or swelling), seek emergency medical care.

Nosebleeds

Nosebleeds can occur after an injury to the nose or when very dry air causes the lining of the nose to become irritated. An occasional nosebleed isn't a cause for concern. If your nose starts bleeding, sit down and squeeze the soft part of the nose between your thumb and finger, holding the nostrils closed, for five to ten minutes. Breathe through your mouth and lean forward to avoid swallowing the blood. An ice pack or cold compress applied to the bridge of the nose may also help. If the bleeding doesn't stop after 20 minutes, seek emergency medical help.

Poisoning

A **poison** is any substance that causes injury, illness, or death when it enters the body. A poison can be a solid, liquid, or gas. Almost 2.5 million cases of poisoning occur in the United States each year, resulting in nearly 1,000 deaths.

The first step in any suspected case of poisoning is to contact a **poison control center**. This is a round-the-clock service that provides emergency medical advice on how to treat victims of poisoning. You can reach the American Association of Poison Control Centers at www.poisonhelp.org or at 1-800-222-1222. Keep this information in your phone and dial it at once in any case of suspected poisoning. Even if you aren't sure the victim has been poisoned, call right away, rather than wait for symptoms to develop. Some poisons require quick action to minimize damage to the victim or prevent death. When you contact a center, be prepared to provide:

- your name, location, and telephone number.
- the victim's condition, age, and weight.
- the name of the poison, when it was taken, and the amount of poison that was involved. If you do not have this information, tell as much as you know.

The poison control expert will provide you with step-by-step instructions on how to treat the victim. Do not give the victim any medication unless the expert tells you to do so.

Insect and Spider Bites or Stings. The stings of insects such as bees, hornets, and wasps, as well as the bites of certain spiders, are painful but usually not dangerous. If someone is allergic to the poisonous secretions, called **venom,** of these insects or spiders, and has been stung, call 911. For other cases, follow these steps:

- Remove the stinger by scraping it off with a firm, straight-edged object such as a credit card. Do not use tweezers, since they may squeeze the stinger and release more venom.
- Wash the site thoroughly with mild soap and water to help prevent infection.

Pinching the nostrils closed will stop almost all nosebleeds. **What factors can trigger a nosebleed?**

FORMS OF POISONING		
How Poison Enters the Body	**Examples**	**What Action to Take**
Swallowing	Household cleaners, medicines	Call poison control and follow instructions. You may be instructed to give the victim a small amount of milk or water or to induce vomiting. Do not take these actions unless instructed to do so.
Inhalation	Carbon monoxide from heating fixtures, fumes from certain solvents, fumes produced by mixing cleaning products together	Get the victim to fresh air right away. Then call poison control. Be prepared to perform rescue breathing if necessary.
Through the eyes	Any strong chemical that enters the eye	Flush the eye with fresh water for 15 to 20 minutes. Call poison control.
Through the skin	Caustic chemicals such as drain cleaner or rust remover; certain pesticides	Remove clothing the poison has touched. Rinse skin with running water for 15 to 20 minutes. Call poison control.

- Apply ice (wrapped in a cloth) to the site for ten minutes to reduce pain and swelling. Alternate ten minutes on, ten minutes off.

- Antihistamines and anti-itch creams may help reduce itching.

- If the victim shows signs of a severe reaction, such as weakness, difficulty breathing, or swelling of the face, call 911 immediately.

Poisonous Plants. Most people are allergic to poison ivy, poison oak, and poison sumac. Exposure to these plants will cause itching, swelling, redness, burning, and blisters at the site of the contact. If you brush up against one of these plants, avoid rubbing your skin. Doing so will spread the plant oils that cause an allergic reaction. Washing the area immediately with soap and water may prevent a reaction. Take care to wash any clothing or other objects that have touched the plant as well. If an allergic reaction develops, an over-the-counter cream or an oral antihistamine may ease the itching.

Exposure to poison ivy, poison oak, and poison sumac can cause itching, swelling, and blisters. **What should you do if you accidentally brush against one of these plants?**

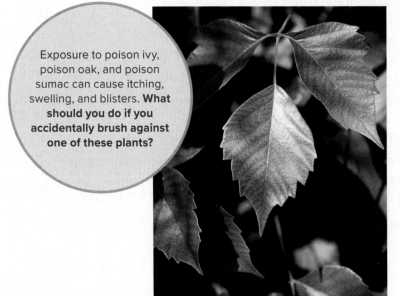

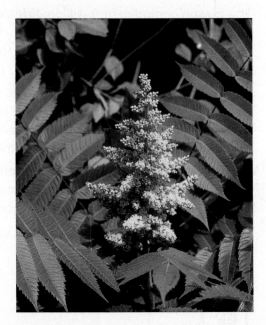

Snakebites. Certain types of snakes can inject venom into the victim's body. In the United States, varieties of poisonous snakes include rattlesnakes, copperheads, water moccasins (also known as cottonmouths), coral snakes, and cobras. You should treat any snakebite seriously unless you are absolutely sure of the species. Follow these steps:

- Call 911 for medical help and follow the dispatcher's instructions.

- Try to keep the victim from moving. Keep the affected body part below chest level to reduce the flow of venom to the heart.

- Remove rings and other constricting items, since the affected area may swell up.

- Try using a snakebite suction kit, if one is available in your first-aid kit.

- Do *not* apply a tourniquet, use cold compresses, cut into the bitten area with a blade, suck the venom out by mouth, or give the victim any medications without being advised to do so by a doctor or 911 dispatcher.

Reading Check

Identify List one thing you can do in the event of a snakebite.

Fitness Zone

A lot of people like the saying "No pain, no gain," but my coach says that feeling pain during exercise means something is wrong. Coach says that if you feel pain, you should stop exercising right away. Listen to your body. It knows the difference between real pain and the discomfort of a muscle working.

Lesson 3 Review

Facts and Vocabulary

1. List the symptoms of a fracture or dislocation.

2. Explain why the recovery position is the safest position for an unconscious person.

3. List the first step in any case of suspected poisoning.

Thinking Critically

4. **Evaluate.** Why should you always seek professional medical care for fractures and dislocations?

5. **Analyze.** List the items you would need to treat a bee sting in a victim who is not allergic to the venom.

Applying Health Skills

6. **Practicing Healthful Behaviors.** Make a poster illustrating the steps of the P.R.I.C.E. procedure.

Writing Critically

7. **Narrative.** Write a newspaper-style article about a child or teen who is bitten by a wild animal. The article should describe the steps the victim and his or her parents take to treat the wound and prevent rabies and other diseases.

Emergency Preparedness

BEFORE YOU READ

Organize Information. Write "Weather Emergencies & Natural Disasters" in a circle. Surround this circle with the following terms: "Thunderstorms," "Hurricanes," "Tornadoes," "Blizzards," "Floods," "Earthquakes," and "Wildfires." As you read, add information about each type of emergency.

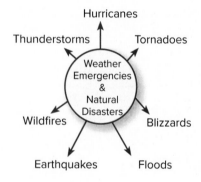

Vocabulary

hurricane
tornado
blizzard
flash floods
earthquake
emergency survival kit

BIG IDEA Planning ahead and knowing what to expect can help you survive severe weather and natural disasters.

REAL LIFE ISSUES

Safe in a Storm. Dean is at home looking after his younger brother and sister when it begins to snow heavily. Turning on the radio, he hears that the storm is a blizzard and everyone is advised to stay indoors. However, Dean's younger siblings want to go out and play in the snow. Dean doesn't want to spoil their fun, but he knows he's responsible for keeping them safe. *Write a dialogue between Dean and his siblings in which he explains the need to stay indoors during the snowstorm and proposes an alternative activity for them to enjoy.*

After completing the lesson, review and analyze your response to the Real Life Issues question.

Storm Safety

MAIN IDEA It is important to pay attention to weather warnings and follow safety guidelines during a severe storm.

What's the worst storm you can remember? Was it a thunderstorm that knocked out the power, or a winter storm that dumped two feet of snow over your neighborhood? When a severe storm or any other type of harsh or dangerous weather conditions may occur, the National Weather Service (NWS) will issue a severe weather alert. A *watch* indicates that severe weather is possible during the next few hours. A *warning* means that severe weather has already been observed or is expected soon. Watches and warnings go out over radio, television, and the Internet to let the public know about the dangers and take steps to protect themselves.

Severe Thunderstorms

Thunderstorms produce heavy rain accompanied by lightning, strong winds, and sometimes hail or tornadoes. If you see lightning or hear thunder, use the 30/30 rule for lightning safety. Get or stay inside if you hear thunder within 30 seconds of seeing lightning. Stay inside for 30 minutes after hearing the last peal of thunder. Avoid bathing or showering, since plumbing and bathroom fixtures can conduct electricity. Unplug all electrical appliances. Avoid using a corded telephone, except in an emergency. Cordless and cellular phones are safe to use.

If you are in a car when a thunderstorm strikes and cannot reach secure shelter, stay in the car and avoid touching anything made of metal. If you are on open water, return to shore. If you are in a forest, seek shelter under shorter trees. If you are trapped in an open area, try to get into a low-lying spot such as a valley; however, be on the alert for flash floods.

Hurricanes

A **hurricane** is a powerful storm that generally forms in tropical areas, producing winds of at least 74 miles per hour, heavy rains, and sometimes tornadoes. In the United States, hurricanes strike mainly along the eastern and southern coasts. Hurricanes can cause **major** flooding, and flying debris can injure or kill people or cause property damage. High winds can topple trees, power lines, and even buildings. The deadliest part of a hurricane is the storm surge, a massive wave that sweeps in from the ocean, occasionally advancing up to hundreds of miles inland.

If a hurricane is predicted in your area, take steps to secure your property. Listen to radio or TV reports for information on the progress of the storm. Follow their instructions, and be prepared to evacuate the area if local authorities order you to do so.

Tornadoes

A **tornado** is a whirling, funnel-shaped windstorm that causes destruction as it advances along the ground in a narrow path. Hurricanes and severe thunderstorms can produce a tornado. Tornadoes are more common east of the Rocky Mountains. The whirling winds of a tornado can reach speeds of 300 miles per hour and leave a trail of damage a mile wide.

Although tornadoes can strike without warning, they often follow danger signs such as:

- darkened or greenish-looking skies.
- a hailstorm that produces large hailstones.
- a large, dark, low-lying cloud that may be rotating.
- a loud roar like that of a freight train.

Reading Check

Compare and Contrast What is the difference between a storm watch and a storm warning?

ACADEMIC VOCABULARY

major *(adjective)*: notable in effect or scope

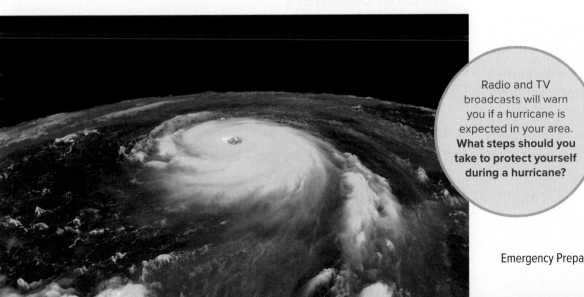

Radio and TV broadcasts will warn you if a hurricane is expected in your area. **What steps should you take to protect yourself during a hurricane?**

NOAA

If you see any of these signs, or if you see a tornado cloud in the distance, take shelter immediately. Safe places to go include the lowest level of a house or building, or the center of an interior room, such as a bathroom or closet. Stay as far away as you can from windows, doors, and outer walls. To protect yourself, crouch down as close to the floor as possible and use your arms and hands to shield your head. If possible, cover yourself with a mattress or blankets to protect yourself from falling debris.

If you are in a car or a mobile home when a tornado strikes, leave the vehicle and get into a secure shelter as quickly as possible. Never try to outrun a tornado in your car. If you are caught out in the open, lie flat in a ditch or other low-lying area and cover your head with your hands.

Winter Storms

Severe winter storms can block roads, knock down power lines, and cause floods. One type of hazardous winter storm is a **blizzard**. A blizzard is a snowstorm with winds that reach 35 miles an hour or more. To protect yourself during a winter storm, follow these guidelines:

- Stay indoors if at all possible. It's the safest place to be.

- If you must go outdoors, wear layers of loose-fitting, lightweight clothing. Choose an outermost layer that will repel wind and water. Wear a hat, a scarf to protect your mouth and neck, and mittens or gloves. Wear insulated, water-resistant boots to keep your feet warm and dry.

- Whenever you are outside in a winter storm, watch out for signs of frostbite and hypothermia.

- Avoid driving during a severe winter storm unless it is absolutely necessary. If you must go out, use main roads.

- If you are caught in a blizzard while driving, pull off the road and turn on your flashers. Stay in the car until help arrives or the storm ends. Turn on the engine and run the heater for about ten minutes each hour to help you stay warm. Roll down a window slightly to avoid carbon monoxide poisoning.

Natural Disasters

MAIN IDEA Knowing what to expect can protect you in a natural disaster.

Natural disasters include floods, earthquakes, and wildfires. All natural disasters have one thing in common: knowing what to expect is your best defense.

Floods

Some floods develop slowly, as heavy rain raises the level of rivers and lakes. However, **flash floods**, as their name suggests, occur suddenly and involve a dangerous surge of water in a short time. If flooding is expected, listen to radio and TV broadcasts for instructions.

Reading Check

Explain What is the best defense against all natural disasters?

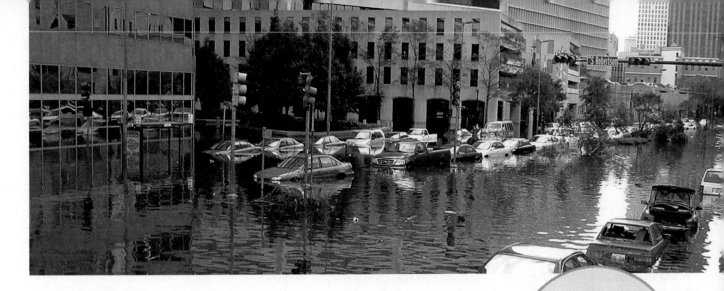

Marty Bahamonde/FEMA

If you are ordered to evacuate, secure your home and move essential items to an upper floor. Shut off utilities and disconnect electrical appliances. Avoid walking through moving water or driving into a flooded area. If floodwaters surround your car, leave the car and flee to higher ground.

After a flood, return home only when authorities tell you it is safe to do so. Clean and disinfect everything in your home that got wet. Floods can contaminate the water supply, so drink bottled water until the news tells you that the water in your area is safe to drink.

Floods are one of the most common natural disasters in the United States. **Why should you avoid drinking tap water after a flood?**

Earthquakes

An **earthquake** is a series of vibrations in the earth caused by a sudden movement of Earth's crust. Earthquakes are most common in western states. In the event of an earthquake, take the following precautions:

- **If you are indoors:** Drop to the ground. Take cover under a sturdy table or desk and hold on until the shaking stops. If there is no nearby table, crouch in a corner and cover your head with your arms.

- **If you are outdoors:** Stay clear of buildings, trees, streetlights, and power lines.

- **If you are in a car:** Stop the car and stay inside. Avoid stopping near or under trees, buildings, freeway overpasses, and power lines.

After an earthquake, be prepared for *aftershocks*—smaller tremors that occur after the main quake. Use caution when opening overhead cabinets. Be aware that utilities (such as gas, power, and sewer lines) may be damaged.

Wildfires

Wildfires are most likely to occur in especially dry regions. People who live in areas where wildfires are common can create a "safety zone" around their homes that is free of most vegetation and other flammable materials. If you spot a wildfire, call 911 to report it, then evacuate before the fire reaches your home. Before you leave, shut off gas and oil supplies at their source and clear away any flammable materials near the house. Close all doors and windows, but avoid locking the house, since firefighters may need to get inside.

Being Prepared for Emergencies

MAIN IDEA The right supplies can help you survive in an emergency.

In an emergency, you may need to evacuate your home in a hurry. Alternatively, you may need to "shelter in place"—stay in a secure location in your home until the crisis has passed. In either case, you'll need supplies to get you through the disaster. A set of items you will need in an emergency situation is called an **emergency survival kit.** A kit should include:

- a three-day supply of food and water for your family. Choose shelf-stable, ready-to-eat foods. Store at least three gallons of water per person (one gallon per person per day).

- a battery-powered radio or television (with extra batteries).

- a change of clothing for each family member.

- sleeping bags or bedrolls for each family member.

- first-aid supplies, including any necessary medications.

- duct tape and plastic sheeting, in case you need to seal off the windows in your home.

- money and copies of important documents, such as passports and birth certificates (in case you need to leave your home).

Keep a list of phone numbers and e-mail addresses for each member of your family so that you can reach each other in an emergency. Identify an out-of-town contact person to call if you can't get through to one another. Choose a meeting place for family members to go if you have to evacuate your area.

Reading Check

Classify Which two items would you need in your emergency survival kit if you had to evacuate your home?

Myths & Reality

Have you ever seen a show on television about storm chasers? What do you think about this myth?

Myth: You can outrun a tornado in a car.

Reality: Although tornadoes typically travel around 30 mph, they can go faster than 250 mph. Tornadoes are unpredictable and can change their direction in an instant. They are also capable of picking up a car and moving it through the air.

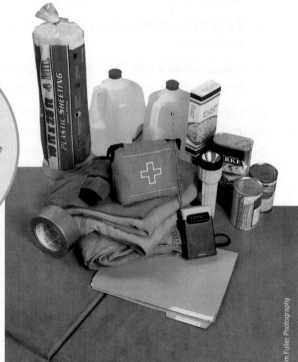

An emergency survival kit can help you wait out a disaster at home or travel with you if you must evacuate your area. **Why might you need each of the items shown here?**

Sheltering in Place

During certain disasters, including terrorist attacks, people in the area may need to "shelter in place" until it's safe to go outside. Select a small, interior room with as few windows as possible for your shelter in place. A room at or above ground level is best, and it should contain a landline phone, since cell phone systems can be overwhelmed in an emergency.

Follow these steps when taking shelter:

- Close and lock all windows and exterior doors. Also close window shades or blinds if there is a risk of explosions.

- Turn off all fans and heating and air-conditioning systems. Close fireplace dampers.

- Gather all family members and pets in your safe room. Bring your emergency survival kit with you. You should also have a plastic bucket with a tight lid to use for personal waste, along with soap, toilet paper, and disinfectant.

- Use duct tape and plastic sheeting to seal off the room you are in, including all vents and cracks around the door.

- Keep listening to your radio or television until you hear that it is safe to leave.

Activity

Role-play a scene involving a family sheltering in place. Show the steps the family takes to stay safe during the crisis.

Lesson 4 Review

Facts and Vocabulary

1. Explain the 30/30 rule for lightning safety.

2. Identify two warning signs of an approaching tornado.

3. Describe what you should do if traveling in a car during an earthquake.

Thinking Critically

4. **Synthesize.** Suppose you hear on the radio that a tornado watch has been issued for your area. How would you respond?

5. **Evaluate.** What are some of the possible consequences of not having an emergency survival kit?

Applying Health Skills

6. **Goal Setting.** Develop an emergency plan for your family. Make a list of the items you will gather for your emergency kit and the steps you will take in case of an emergency. Then set a deadline for completing your emergency preparedness goal.

Writing Critically

7. **Expository.** Choose one of the emergencies discussed in this lesson. Write an informational handout for families about what steps to take in this emergency.

Vocabulary Review

Use the correct vocabulary term to complete the following statements.

1. During an emergency, _____ can mean the difference between life and death.

2. Statutes that protect rescuers from being sued for giving emergency care are called _____.

3. You can protect yourself from disease by following _____.

Understanding Key Concepts

After reading the question or statement, select the correct answer.

4. Universal precautions require you to wear sterile gloves whenever you
   a. encounter an emergency.
   b. treat a burn.
   c. perform rescue breathing.
   d. come into contact with someone's blood.

5. When treating a minor burn, you should *not*
   a. cool the burned area with running water.
   b. apply ice to the burned area.
   c. cover the burn with a sterile gauze bandage.
   d. give the victim pain relievers.

Thinking Critically

After reading the question or statement, write a short answer using complete sentences.

6. **Predict.** What are the possible consequences of treating a wound without following universal precautions?

7. **Summarize.** Describe the procedure for treating an open wound.

8. **Evaluate.** How can you tell if a burn is minor enough to be treated at home?

Vocabulary Review

Correct the sentences below by replacing the italicized term with the correct vocabulary term.

9. A *shock machine* is a device that delivers an electric shock to the heart to restore its normal rhythm.

10. *First aid* is a lifesaving procedure that can replace a patient's normal heartbeat and breathing when these body functions have stopped.

11. *Fainting* is a life-threatening condition in which the heart is not delivering an adequate supply of blood to the body.

Understanding Key Concepts

After reading the question or statement, select the correct answer.

12. Before beginning rescue breathing, you should check to see
    a. whether the victim is breathing.
    b. whether the victim has a pulse.
    c. whether there is something in the victim's mouth.
    d. whether the victim has any open wounds.

13. A person who clutches his or her throat is most likely experiencing
    a. a heart attack.
    b. a stroke.
    c. choking.
    d. shock.

14. You should wrap your arms around the rib cage, rather than the abdomen, when assisting a choking victim who is
    a. an infant.
    b. seated.
    c. unconscious.
    d. pregnant.

Thinking Critically

After reading the question or statement, write a short answer using complete sentences.

15. Cause and Effect. What is the likely consequence of keeping automated external defibrillators in public places?

16. Describe. What is the correct position in which to place your hands for performing chest compressions?

17. Identify. List three symptoms of shock.

LESSON 3

Vocabulary Review

Choose the correct term in the sentences below.

18. A *fracture/dislocation* is a separation of a bone from its normal position in a joint.

19. Fainting is a form of temporary *concussion/ unconsciousness.*

20. *Poison/Venom* is a harmful substance secreted by some types of snakes, spiders, and insects.

Understanding Key Concepts

After reading the question or statement, select the correct answer.

21. You should always seek professional medical care for
   a. strains.
   b. sprains.
   c. fractures.
   d. animal bites.

22. When treating a nosebleed, you should *not*
   a. squeeze your nostrils shut.
   b. breathe through your mouth.
   c. try to swallow the blood.
   d. apply a cold compress to the nose.

23. The first step in any case of suspected poisoning is to
   a. find out what poison has been taken.
   b. call a poison control center.
   c. induce vomiting.
   d. see if the victim develops symptoms.

Thinking Critically

After reading the question or statement, write a short answer using complete sentences.

24. Explain. How can you tell if someone is unconscious?

25. Describe. When should you suspect that a victim has a concussion?

26. Evaluate. Under what circumstances are insect bites and stings medical emergencies?

LESSON 4

Vocabulary Review

Choose the correct term in the sentences below.

27. A *hurricane/tornado* is a powerful storm that generally forms in tropical areas, producing strong winds and heavy rains.

28. In a *blizzard/hurricane,* falling and blowing snow reduces visibility to less than a quarter mile, making it very easy to lose your way.

29. You should stay indoors and take cover under a sturdy table or desk during a(n) *earthquake/ flash flood.*

Understanding Key Concepts

After reading the question or statement, select the correct answer.

30. You should *not* stay in your car if you are out on the road during
   a. a severe thunderstorm that includes hail and sleet.
   b. a tornado.
   c. an earthquake.
   d. a wildfire.

31. If you are caught in a blizzard while driving, you should
   a. keep driving at a slow speed.
   b. pull off the road and turn on your emergency flashers.
   c. leave your car and attempt to find your way on foot.
   d. have the heater turned on the entire time and keep the windows tightly closed.

32. Earthquakes are most common in
   a. western states.
   b. eastern states.
   c. summer.
   d. winter.

Thinking Critically

After reading the question or statement, write a short answer using complete sentences.

33. **Compare and Contrast.** How are hurricanes and tornadoes alike? How are they different?

34. **Describe.** How should you respond to a wildfire?

35. **Explain.** Why is it necessary to clean and disinfect items that have been through a flood?

PROJECT-BASED ASSESSMENT

Administering First Aid

BACKGROUND

First aid is the immediate care given to someone who is injured or ill. First aid is provided until professional medical care can be reached. Proper first-aid procedures can help reduce further injury or even prevent death. Always remember: if immediate care is needed, please call 911.

TASK

Create a video that effectively demonstrates proper first-aid procedures.

AUDIENCE

Fellow students and adults in the community.

PURPOSE

Show the steps in first-aid procedures for specific injuries and medical conditions.

PROCEDURE

1. Choose several of the first-aid procedures discussed in the module to demonstrate in the video. Review the steps that are required in the procedures.

2. Collaborate as a group to write a script to accompany each first-aid procedure that you will demonstrate.

3. Make a storyboard of your video, in which you show what will happen in each scene in the video.

4. Work on special features that will appear in the video, such as props and titles.

5. Assign roles in the video to the members of your group, finalize the script, and rehearse the scenes.

6. Record your video, and present it to the class.

Math Practice

Solve Word Problems. Use the passage below to answer Questions 1–3.

While hiking, Antonio and his younger brother saw that a young woman had collapsed on the hiking trail. The woman was unconscious, not breathing, and had no heartbeat. "Here, take my cell phone," he told his brother. "Go back to the beginning of the trail entrance and call 911. Tell them that I'm starting CPR." As his brother ran for help, Antonio, who had been trained to perform CPR, began the procedure. Antonio began by doing 30 chest compressions followed by two rescue breaths. He repeated these two steps for four continuous cycles until paramedics arrived to take over.

1. Imagine that *x* represents the total number of chest compressions Antonio had to do until the paramedics arrived. Which expression below represents how many total minutes Antonio had to perform CPR on the woman?
   a. $x(4 \times 30)$
   b. $4x/30$
   c. $30x/4$
   d. $x/(4 \times 30)$

2. If Antonio performed CPR steadily as described, how much time has passed in three cycles of compressions and breaths?
   a. 45 seconds
   b. About 1 minute
   c. 3 minutes
   d. 3 minutes 45 seconds

3. How many total chest compressions did Antonio have to perform if the paramedics took 15 minutes to arrive?

Reading/Writing Practice

Understand and Apply. Read the passage below, and then answer the questions.

BROWNWOOD, TEXAS—At South Elementary today, a tornado touched down, injuring a teacher. Tyrone Rasco, a third-grade teacher who was standing outside the building, suffered minor injuries from the storm. Thirty children under the supervision of Ann Katz, a physical education teacher, were outside on a playground adjacent to the building. Because the playground was next to the building, Mrs. Katz rushed the children into the building as soon as she heard the tornado alarm. The kids hurried to hallways in the center of the building before the tornado hit. The storm broke the school's front door and most of its windows. "We are thankful that no students were injured in the storm," said Principal Jennifer Rodriguez.

1. What is the purpose of this article?
   a. To describe the damage that a tornado caused at a school
   b. To report about Mrs. Katz's actions
   c. To explain why people should stay inside during tornadoes
   d. To promote tornado warning systems

2. Which word or phrase has the same meaning as the words *adjacent to* in the second paragraph?
   a. next to
   b. nearby
   c. far from
   d. underneath

3. Write an article about how to stay safe during a tornado.

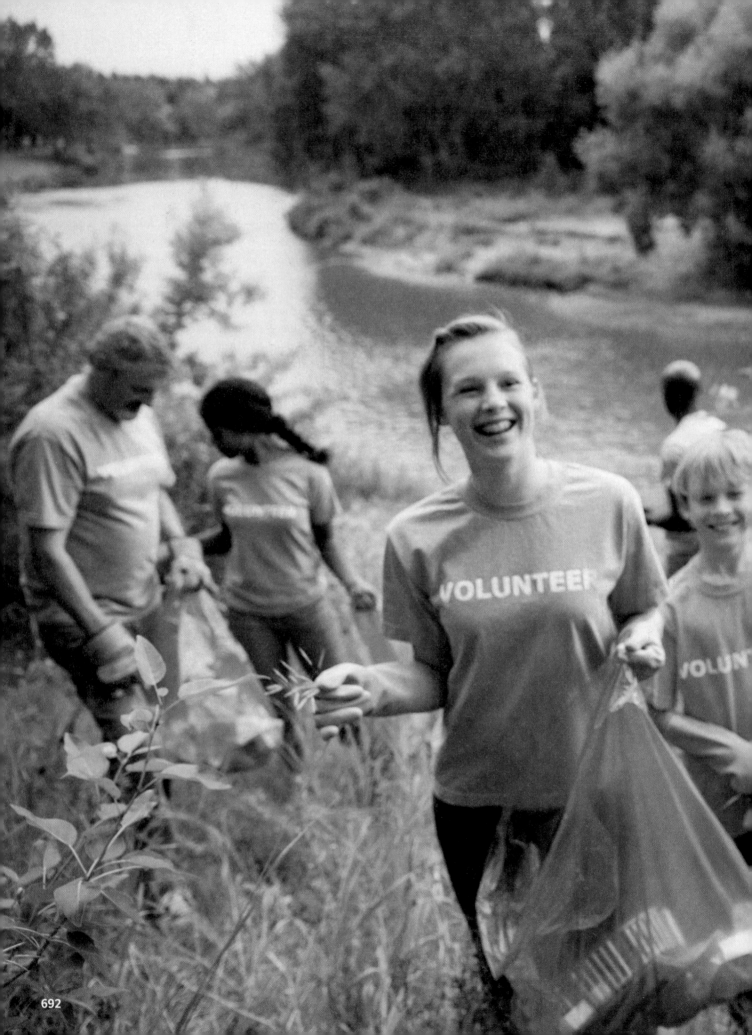

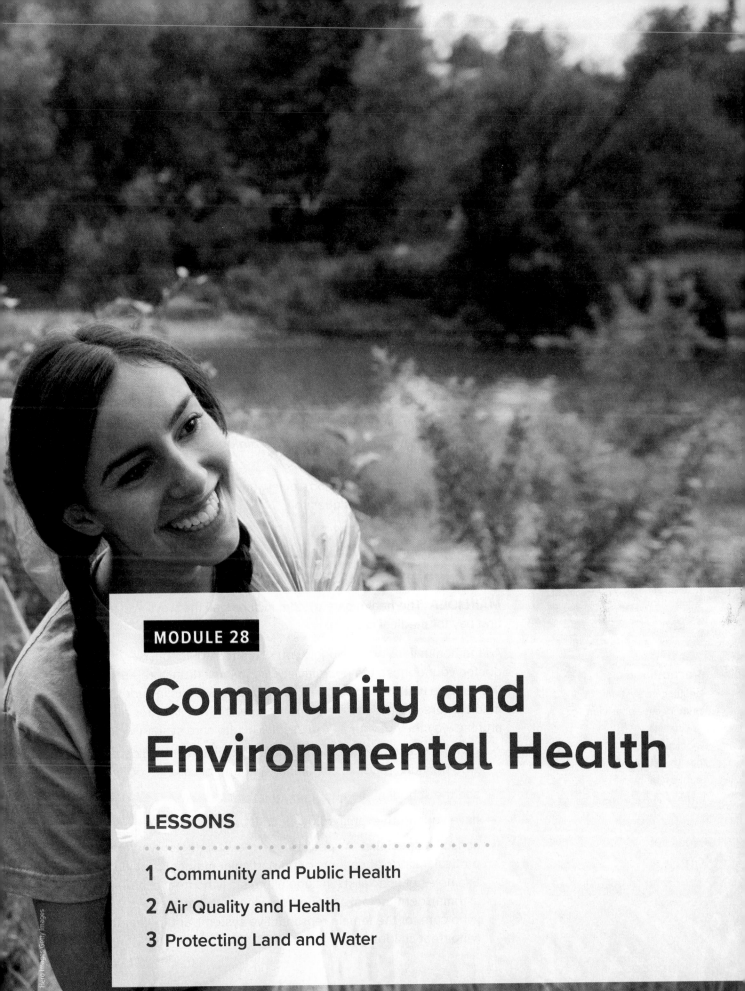

MODULE 28

Community and Environmental Health

LESSONS

1 Community and Public Health

2 Air Quality and Health

3 Protecting Land and Water

Community and Public Health

Create a Cluster Chart. Write "Health Care System" and circle it. Surround it with circles labeled "Health Care Professionals," "Health Care Facilities," "Health Insurance," and "Health Agencies." As you read, add details for each topic.

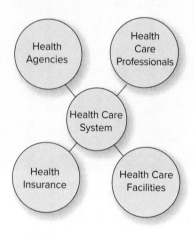

Vocabulary

health care system
primary care physician
specialists
medical history
health insurance
public health

BIG IDEA Many people and organizations work together to promote individual and public health.

REAL LIFE ISSUES

Choosing a New Doctor. Caleb's family is moving to a new town, so they need to choose a new family doctor. Their health insurer's website offers a "physician search" feature that looks for doctors within a given area. However, Caleb wants more from his new doctor than a convenient location. He wants someone who is easy to talk to, like his previous doctor. He isn't sure how he can find a new doctor he'll be comfortable with. *Brainstorm a list of questions Caleb could ask to help him choose a new doctor. Then write a dialogue between Caleb and a doctor he's considering.*

After completing the lesson, review and analyze your response to the Real Life Issues question.

The Health Care System

MAIN IDEA The health care system includes all the ways you receive and pay for medical care.

All the health care professionals you see on a regular basis—your doctor, your dentist, the pharmacist at your local drugstore—are part of the nation's **health care system**. A health care system includes all the medical care available to a nation's people, the way they receive care, and the way they pay for it. You use the health care system when you:

- go for a checkup with a **primary care physician**, a medical doctor who provides physical checkups and general care.

- see the school nurse about an injury.

- have your teeth examined by a dentist.

- consult a **specialist**. A specialist is a medical doctor who focuses on particular kinds of patients or on particular medical conditions. Examples of specialists include allergists (who treat allergies and asthma), dermatologists (who treat skin problems), gynecologists (who care for the female reproductive system), and pediatricians (who treat children).

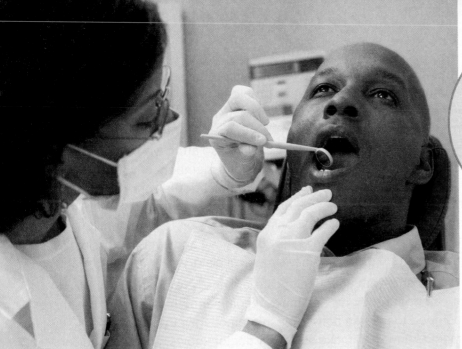

Your dentist is just one of the people who may provide health care to you. **Who are other members of your health care "team"?**

Types of Health Care Facilities

You can receive health care in a variety of settings. For instance, if you become ill or injured at school, you might see a school nurse. If you need a checkup, you might visit a doctor's office or a clinic. A clinic is a community health facility where patients can receive *outpatient care,* which means being treated and returning home the same day.

Hospitals provide both outpatient care and *inpatient care.* Inpatient care involves an overnight stay. Most hospitals have an emergency room where they handle urgent injuries or illnesses. Problems that are not life threatening may be treated at a facility called an *urgent care center.* Unlike ordinary doctor's offices, urgent care centers typically are open evenings and weekends. They usually will see patients without an appointment.

Other types of health care facilities deal with specific problems or situations. Here are some examples:

- Birthing centers deliver babies in a homelike setting staffed by nurse-midwives.

- Drug treatment centers help people recover from drug and alcohol abuse.

- Assisted-living facilities provide care for people who need some help with everyday activities but do not need extended medical care.

- Hospices provide care for people who are terminally ill.

You and Your Health Care

A doctor shouldn't be just someone you call when you're sick or injured, the way you'd call a plumber if you had a stopped-up drain. Ideally, you should have an ongoing relationship with your health care provider to keep track of your health. Seeing a primary care physician regularly allows you to build up a relationship of trust. To help your doctor, you can take a role in managing your health. Providing your doctor with information on your family history can help him or her identify health issues.

Your **medical history** is complete and comprehensive information about your immunizations and any health problems you have had to date. A family medical history is a biological record of the diseases that have occurred in your family. Because you and your relatives share genetics, diseases that occur in your relatives might also affect you. You can collect your family medical history by asking members of your family what illnesses they have had. However, some people consider medical information private, and may be unwilling to share this information. If this is the case, accept that response and move on to other family members. If you are adopted, it may be difficult and even impossible to obtain information on your family's medical history.

Your relationship with your health care provider is a partnership. Your doctor can treat problems and make recommendations for your health, but you need to take an active role in promoting your own wellness. You should know, and make sure your doctor knows, your full medical history. This includes:

- any health conditions you have now.

- major physical or psychological problems you've had in the past.

- all medicines you are taking.

- any allergies you have to food or medication.

- any health problems that run in your family.

- your lifestyle and habits (for example, diet and exercise).

Your doctor should keep a record of your medical treatment on file. It will include information about health conditions, medications, and results of lab tests. A current trend in health care is to store these records in electronic form. This makes it easier for doctors to share information with each other and check for such problems as drug interactions.

Whenever you have a doctor's appointment, note the reasons for your visit and list any questions you'd like to ask. During the visit, feel free to ask questions about the doctor's diagnosis or anything else you don't understand. Ask the doctor to write down any instructions so you won't forget them. If you have to fill a prescription at the pharmacy, you can also ask the pharmacist any questions you have about your medication.

Paying Health Care Costs

Modern health care can be very expensive. Most people need **health insurance** to help pay their medical bills. Health insurance includes private and government programs that pay for part or all of a person's medical costs. People typically pay for health insurance with a monthly fee, known as a *premium*. There are two main forms of health insurance:

- **Fee for service.** Under these plans, patients must pay for all their medical expenses up to a certain minimum amount, known as the *deductible*. After that, the insurance company covers a percentage of their costs. The portion that patients must still pay for is called *coinsurance*. In many cases, patients must pay medical bills up front and then send a form to the insurance company to be reimbursed.

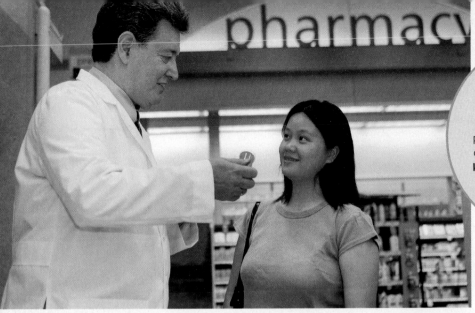

Your pharmacist can be a good source of information about both prescription and over-the counter medicines. **What kinds of questions might you ask a pharmacist?**

- **Managed care.** These plans hold down costs by limiting patients' choices and encouraging preventive care. Some plans, such as health maintenance organizations (HMOs), require patients to choose their doctors from among a limited pool of physicians. Managed-care plans also may not cover certain types of medical care. However, they require less paperwork than fee-for-service plans. Rather than paying medical costs up front and applying for reimbursement, the patient typically pays only a small fixed fee, known as a *co-payment,* for each visit.

Most Americans receive insurance through their jobs (or through a family member's job). This is called *group insurance.* The employer may pay for part of the employee's premiums. People who do not have insurance through their work may buy individual policies. People who cannot afford insurance may be covered under a government plan called *Medicaid.* All Americans over age 65 can receive coverage through a separate government program called *Medicare.*

Before selling a health policy to an individual, insurers generally require a medical exam. People who are found to be at a higher risk of developing health problems will be charged higher rates for insurance. A current **trend** in health insurance is for group health plans to follow this practice as well. This reduces the chance that a plan will end up with more high-risk employees in its pool than it can afford.

The 2010 Patient Protection and Affordable Care Act (PPACA) included a number of significant health care reforms. This law requires nearly all U.S. citizens to obtain health insurance and expands eligibility for Medicaid. The PPACA also offers incentives for businesses to provide health care benefits. In addition, in 2014 the act prohibited insurers from using *pre-existing conditions* (health problems a person had before joining the insurance plan) as reasons to deny coverage or refuse claims.

ACADEMIC VOCABULARY

trend *(noun)*: a line of general direction or movement

Reading Check

Explain What costs must patients pay out of pocket with a fee-for-service plan? With a managed care plan?

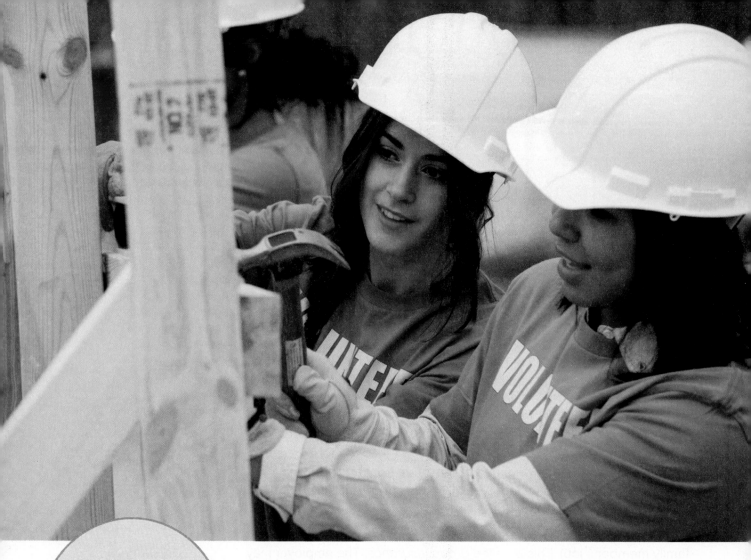

Ariel Skelley/Blend Images/Getty Images

Nonprofit organizations such as Americares promote community health in various ways. **What other groups contribute to public health?**

Public Health Services

MAIN IDEA Agencies at all levels of government promote public health.

Your physician and other health care professionals help you take care of your personal health. However, you are also part of a community, and some health issues affect the community as a whole. To help deal with these issues, various agencies exist to promote **public health**. Public health includes all efforts to monitor, protect, and promote the health of the population as a whole. Public health agencies operate on all levels—local, state, national, and even worldwide. They work to make communities healthier by:

- researching health problems.

- providing health services.

- educating the public.

- developing and enforcing policies that promote health.

Local Health Agencies

Local health departments are government agencies that operate at the state, county, or city level. They promote public health in various ways, including:

- investigating threats to public health, such as outbreaks of disease.

- helping to plan responses to public health emergencies.

- enforcing local health regulations.

- providing information about health issues.

Local health departments can tailor their programs to the specific needs of a particular community. For example, in some areas, cultural factors may make people resistant to the idea of vaccinating their children. Local health agencies can help spread the word about why childhood vaccination is important for public health.

REAL WORLD CONNECTION

Evaluating Health Care Services

Many communities offer a wide variety of health care options. People who live in these communities can choose from several different primary care physicians, dentists, and medical specialists. They may be able to receive care at a local hospital, an urgent care center, or a walk-in clinic.

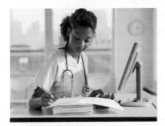

Activity: Mathematics

Conduct an Internet search for physicians using any online directories and hospital websites. Choose a physician near your home, and visit or call the office. Find out the answers to the following questions:

- When is the facility open?

- How much does an office visit cost? Which types of insurance are accepted?

- How soon can one get an appointment for a check-up? For a medical problem?

- Is the facility accepting new patients?

Write a brief report that evaluates this health care provider in terms of accessibility and cost.

National Health Agencies

Nonprofit agencies, such as the American Cancer Society and the American Heart Association, work at the national level, but they may also have local chapters. These groups focus on specific health problems or goals. They may provide health services or help educate the public about specific health issues. They may also fund research into new treatments to fight disease. Several departments of the U.S. government also promote public health at the national level.

- **Environmental Protection Agency (EPA).** The EPA protects the country's land, air, and water. A major part of its job is enforcing environmental laws. The agency also works to research issues related to the health of the environment and educate the public about these issues.

- **Occupational Safety and Health Administration (OSHA).** OSHA is part of the U.S. Department of Labor. It works to prevent injuries and other health problems in the workplace. OSHA sets safety standards for workplaces and helps train and educate workers.

- **United States Department of Agriculture (USDA).** The USDA has several offices that promote public health. For example, the **Food Safety and Inspection Service** ensures the safety of meat, poultry, and eggs. The **Food and Nutrition Service** provides food to needy families.

- **United Network for Organ Sharing (UNOS).** This agency maintains data on potential organ recipients and donors. In many states, people can indicate their choice to become an organ donor on a driver's license. When that person dies, his or her organs will be donated to save someone else's life.

- **The Department of Health and Human Services (HHS).** HHS includes ten agencies that promote public health in various ways.

The agencies in HHS oversee more than 300 health-related programs. **How does the FDA contribute to public health?**

HEALTH AND HUMAN SERVICES AGENCIES	
Administration for Children and Families (ACF)	Oversees programs to aid low-income families
Administration for Community Living (ACL)	Provides independent living support to people with disabilities and older adults
Agency for Healthcare Research and Quality (AHRQ)	Supports research on the health care system
Agency for Toxic Substances and Disease Registry (ATSDR)	Protects communities from hazardous waste exposure
Centers for Disease Control and Prevention (CDC)	Works to track, prevent, and control outbreaks of disease
Centers for Medicare and Medicaid Services (CMS)	Administers federal health insurance programs for elderly and low-income Americans
Food and Drug Administration (FDA)	Ensures the safety of foods and cosmetics and the safety and effectiveness of medicines
Health Resources and Services Administration (HRSA)	Provides access to health care for low-income and uninsured people
Indian Health Services (IHS)	Provides health care to Native Americans
National Institutes of Health (NIH)	Conducts and funds medical research
Substance Abuse and Mental Health Services Administration (SAMHSA)	Funds programs to prevent and treat substance abuse and mental disorders

Global Health Organizations

Many countries don't have the same access to health care that the United States and other developed nations have. Disasters such as war, drought, flooding, or economic collapse can harm the public health of a nation. Government agencies and private organizations from around the world work to help countries in crises like these.

- The **World Health Organization (WHO).** WHO is the health agency of the United Nations. Its goals include improving health care systems and fighting diseases such as AIDS and malaria.

- The **United Nations Children's Fund (UNICEF).** UNICEF works to promote children's health and well-being. Its services include immunization, disaster relief, and education.

- The **International Committee of the Red Cross.** This organization aids victims of war and other forms of violence. It also works to promote and strengthen humanitarian laws.

- The **U.S. Agency for International Development (USAID).** USAID provides aid to foreign countries to promote health, economic growth, and democratic reforms.

- The **Peace Corps.** The Peace Corps is a U.S. government agency that sends volunteers to developing nations to promote such goals as health, education, and economic development.

- **Cooperative for Assistance and Relief Everywhere (CARE).** CARE's goal is to fight global poverty. CARE works to promote education, improve sanitation, and fight HIV/AIDS.

Reading Check

Identify Which U.S. government agency sets safety standards for workplaces?

Fitness Zone

When I made the lacrosse team, I had to get a physical to show that I was healthy enough to play. I've had the same doctor since I was a kid, so she knew all about my medical history. She gave me a checkup, signed the permission form, and said she'd try to make it to one of my games. It's nice to have a doctor who really cares about you.

Lesson 1 Review

Facts and Vocabulary

1. Explain the difference between a primary care physician and a specialist.

2. List three types of health care facilities.

3. Identify two organizations that work to promote global health.

Thinking Critically

4. **Synthesize.** Why is it important for your doctor to know your medical history?

5. **Compare and Contrast.** Compare the advantages of fee-for-service insurance and managed care.

Applying Health Skills

6. **Accessing Information.** Use reliable print and online resources to learn more about one of the public health agencies listed in this lesson. Write a report explaining how the agency promotes public health and prevents disease.

Writing Critically

7. **Expository.** Write a newspaper-style article advising other teens about how they can take an active role in their own health care. Include tips on how to get the most out of a visit to the doctor.

Air Quality and Health

. . . .

BEFORE YOU READ

Create a Comparison Chart. Make a three-column chart. Label the columns "Outdoor Air Pollution," "Indoor Air Pollution," and "Noise Pollution." As you read, use the chart to define each term, list causes and effects, and identify solutions.

Outdoor Air Pollution	Indoor Air Pollution	Noise Pollution

Vocabulary

air pollution
smog
Air Quality Index (AQI)
greenhouse effect
climate change
noise pollution
decibel

. . . .

ACADEMIC VOCABULARY

component *(noun)*: a constituent part or ingredient

BIG IDEA Both outdoor and indoor air quality can affect your health.

REAL LIFE ISSUES

Saving Energy. Rachel has always been in the habit of turning on the television as soon as she comes home from school. Even if she's not really watching it, she likes having it on in the background. Lately, though, she's started to wonder about just how much electricity she's wasting by doing this—and how much air pollution she might be causing. This makes her wonder about what other habits she might have that waste energy and what she could do to cut back. ***Evaluate your own energy usage. How might you reduce the amount of energy you use? Write your thoughts in a paragraph.***

After completing the lesson, review and analyze your response to the Real Life Issues question.

Understanding Air Pollution

MAIN IDEA Indoor and outdoor air pollutants can harm human health and damage the natural environment.

You normally can't see it, but air is all around you. The quality of the air you breathe has a significant impact on your health. **Air pollution**, the contamination of Earth's atmosphere by harmful substances, poses serious health concerns. In fact, numerous studies have linked it to a wide variety of health problems, including lung disease, cardiovascular disease, and cancer.

Air Quality

In the United States, the Environmental Protection Agency (EPA) sets air quality standards to prevent and correct problems related to environmental air pollution. It has placed limits on the levels of six pollutants that harm human health and the environment.

- **Ozone (O3).** Ozone forms at ground level when certain other pollutants react chemically in the presence of sunlight. Ground-level ozone is a major **component** of **smog**, a brownish haze that sometimes forms in urban areas. Ozone irritates the lungs and makes breathing difficult. It can worsen respiratory problems such as asthma, bronchitis, and emphysema. (Ozone high up in the atmosphere, by contrast, helps prevent harmful solar rays from reach ground level. These harmful rays may cause skin cancer or eye disorders.)

- **Particulate matter (PM).** Particulate matter is a general term for small particles found in the air, such as dust, soil, soot, smoke, mold, and droplets of liquid. PM can cause difficulty breathing, various types of lung disease, and even heart attacks.

- **Carbon monoxide (CO).** Carbon monoxide is a colorless, odorless gas that forms when carbon in fuel is not burned completely. Outdoor sources of CO include auto exhaust and industrial processes. CO harms the body by preventing oxygen from reaching body tissues. At high enough levels, CO can be deadly.

- **Sulfur dioxide (SO2).** Sulfur dioxide comes chiefly from power plants, especially those that burn coal. In addition to harming respiratory health, SO2 can combine with water to form acid rain, which is harmful to plants and animals.

- **Nitrogen oxides (NOX).** Nitrogen oxides are highly reactive gases that form when fuel is burned at high temperatures, as in motor vehicles and power plants. NOX contributes to the formation of ground-level ozone, acid rain, PM, and a wide variety of toxic chemicals.

- **Lead.** This metal is found naturally in the environment as well as in manufactured products. Exposure to lead can damage the kidneys, liver, brain, and nerves and can cause cardiovascular disease and anemia.

To track the levels of pollutants in the air, the EPA has created the **Air Quality Index (AQI)**. The AQI is an index for reporting daily air quality. The AQI informs the public about local air quality and whether pollution levels pose health risks.

Greenhouse Gases

Air pollutants can also affect the environment on a global scale. Certain gases allow sunlight to enter the atmosphere but block radiation from escaping to outer space—much like the glass roof of a greenhouse. This process, the trapping of heat by gases in Earth's atmosphere, is called the **greenhouse effect**.

The EPA created this index to inform the public about daily air quality. **How can you use the AQI in your community to help protect your health?**

AIR QUALITY INDEX (AQI)		
Range	Air Quality	Color Code
0 to 50	Good: There is little or no health risk.	Green
51 to 100	Moderate: Some pollutants may pose a moderate health concern for a very small number of people	Yellow
101 to 150	Unhealthy for Sensitive Groups: Members of sensitive groups, such as people with lung disease, may experience health effects.	Orange
151 to 200	Unhealthy: Everyone may begin to experience health effects.	Red
201 to 300	Very Unhealthy: Everyone may experience more serious health effects.	Purple
301 to 500	Hazardous: Emergency conditions. The entire population is at risk.	Maroon

The chief greenhouse gas produced by human activity is carbon dioxide (CO_2). It comes mainly from the burning of fossil fuels in power plants and motor vehicles.

The greenhouse effect is actually normal and necessary. Without it, the planet would be too cold to support life. However, in the past 200 years, the concentration of greenhouse gases in Earth's atmosphere has risen. This has contributed to **climate change**. Since 1900, Earth's average surface temperature has risen by 1.2° to 1.4°F. If levels of greenhouse gas continue to rise, average temperatures could increase by anywhere from 2.0° to 11.5°F by the end of this century.

The exact effects of climate change are hard to predict. Already, though, glaciers are beginning to melt, causing sea levels to rise. In the future, global weather patterns may shift. Some areas might receive much less or much more rainfall than they do now. Plants and animals that cannot adapt to the new conditions could become extinct. The world's food supply could also be at risk if crop-growing areas are struck by drought.

Indoor Air Pollution

Research has found that in many cases, the air inside buildings contains more pollutants than the outdoor air in even the biggest cities. Common sources of indoor air pollution include household chemicals, such as cleaning fluids and pesticides, and chemicals used in building and furnishing materials. Lack of ventilation makes the problem worse by trapping air pollutants inside. Specific problems with indoor air quality include:

- **carbon monoxide,** produced by fuel-burning equipment such as stoves, furnaces, and fireplaces.

- **asbestos,** a mineral fiber. In the past, asbestos was often used as a fire retardant in insulation and building materials. Cutting or sanding these materials can release particles of asbestos into the air. Inhaling these particles can lead to lung cancer and other forms of lung damage.

- **radon,** an odorless, radioactive gas produced during the natural breakdown of the element uranium in soil and rocks. It can enter homes through dirt floors, cracks in concrete floors and walls, or floor drains. Exposure to high levels of radon can cause lung cancer.

Reducing Air Pollution

MAIN IDEA Your choices can fight air pollution.

You can make many choices to help reduce air pollution. Since power plants and home heating systems are sources of air pollution, reducing your use of energy is a good place to start. Here are some tips for saving energy:

- Switch off lights when you leave a room. Consider replacing incandescent light bulbs with compact fluorescent bulbs, which use less energy and last longer.

Reading Check

Cause and Effect How do human actions contribute to climate change?

- Turn off radios, computers, televisions, and other such appliances when they are not in use.

- In the winter, wear extra layers of clothing to stay warm so you can keep the thermostat at around 68°F. Turn the thermostat down even lower at night. In the summer, set the thermostat at around 78°F to keep the air conditioner from coming on too often. Instead, use a fan to stay cool.

- Insulate your home to reduce your need for heating and cooling. Seal leaks around doors, windows, and electrical sockets to prevent heated or cooled air from escaping.

- Wash clothes in warm or cold water rather than hot water.

- When cooking, don't preheat the oven longer than necessary. Try cooking small amounts of food in a toaster oven or microwave rather than a full-size oven, which uses more energy.

Cars are another major source of air pollution. Whenever you can, try walking, riding a bicycle, using public transportation, or carpooling to save gas. Another way to conserve gasoline is to reduce your use of motorized equipment, such as power mowers, chain saws, and leaf blowers. Use hand tools to get the job done.

Managing Indoor Air Pollution

One way to improve indoor air quality is to identify sources of pollution and get rid of them. Home test kits and detectors can help you measure the levels of radon and carbon monoxide in your home. Depending on what you find, you may be able to eliminate the pollution sources yourself, or you may need the help of a professional.

If you can't get rid of all the sources completely, you may be able to reduce the pollutant levels in the air by increasing the ventilation in your home. Opening windows and turning on window or attic fans can help get rid of pollutants that build up in the short term. You can also try using air cleaners to filter out particle pollution. However, these devices cannot eliminate most gaseous pollutants.

Noise Pollution

MAIN IDEA Exposure to loud noises can harm your health.

Traffic, loud music, construction equipment, and power tools such as lawnmowers are all sources of **noise pollution**. Noise pollution is harmful, unwanted sound that can be loud enough to damage hearing. All noises can be measured in **decibel** levels. A decibel is a unit that measures the intensity of sound. A level of 0 decibels represents the lowest level of sound the human ear can detect. Noise levels of 130 decibels or higher can cause short-term pain and long-term hearing damage.

Reading Check

Identify List three actions you and your family can take to reduce air pollution.

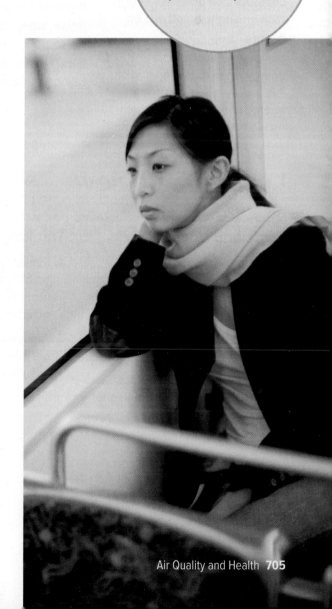

Riding mass transit is one way to reduce the air pollution associated with car use. **What are other transportation options that help reduce air pollution?**

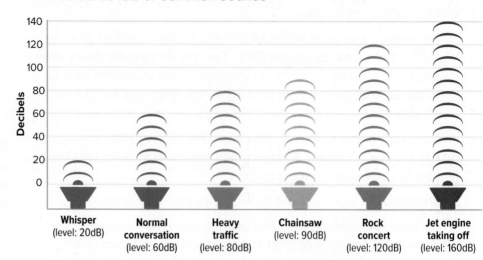

Decibel Levels of Common Sounds

| Whisper (level: 20dB) | Normal conversation (level: 60dB) | Heavy traffic (level: 80dB) | Chainsaw (level: 90dB) | Rock concert (level: 120dB) | Jet engine taking off (level: 160dB) |

A decibel is not a fixed unit of sound. Instead, each 10-decibel increase roughly doubles the loudness of a sound.

Reading Check

Define What is noise pollution?

Myths & Reality

Do you do things in your life to be more energy efficient? Consider this fact about saving energy.

Myth: Leaving lights and computers on uses less energy than turning them off and on.

Reality: Although some devices use a little extra energy when turned on and off, it is usually much less than the energy used by keeping them on when they are not needed.

If you are exposed to loud noise, you may experience a temporary hearing loss. This may be accompanied by ringing in the ears. In most cases, you will recover your normal hearing shortly after the noise stops. However, repeated exposure to noise at levels around 90 decibels or higher can lead to permanent hearing loss.

If you are going someplace where you are likely to be exposed to loud noise, wear earplugs or earmuffs. You can also avoid contributing to noise pollution by keeping the volume down on your stereos and TV sets. Use manual tools instead of power tools when you can, and avoid using your car horn unnecessarily.

Lesson 2 Review

Facts and Vocabulary

1. Name the six outdoor air pollutants for which the EPA sets limits.

2. Describe how radon is harmful to human health.

3. Describe what might result from repeated, prolonged exposure to sounds of 90 decibels or higher.

Thinking Critically

4. **Evaluate.** How might your health be affected if the EPA stopped regulating common air pollutants?

5. **Analyze.** Explain the connection between the greenhouse effect and climate change.

Applying Health Skills

6. **Decision Making.** The morning news has reported an AQI of 145. Paul, who has asthma, was planning to go in-line skating with his friends. Use the decision-making process to determine what you would do in Paul's place.

Writing Critically

7. **Persuasive.** Write a script for a public service announcement urging teens and others to take steps to reduce air pollution. List specific steps in your announcement and show how each is tied to the goal of reducing air pollution.

Protecting Land and Water

BIG IDEA Human actions can either damage or protect land and water.

REAL LIFE ISSUES

Reducing Waste. Carlos has started to notice just how much trash his family throws out every day. A lot of it seems to be packaging, like empty juice boxes and snack wrappers. He wonders whether making a few changes to their buying habits could make a big dent in the amount of waste they create. However, he's not sure how to convince his family it's worth the effort. ***Brainstorm a list of strategies to reduce waste. Then write a dialogue in which Carlos persuades his family to try some of these ideas.***

After completing the lesson, review and analyze your response to the Real Life Issues question.

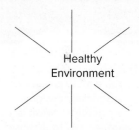

Healthy Environment

Waste Disposal

MAIN IDEA Wastes need to be disposed of safely.

When you throw a plastic fork or a banana peel into the trash, do you ever wonder where it's going to end up? Getting rid of the waste we produce is a big problem for society. If wastes aren't properly contained or destroyed, they can end up polluting the land and water we rely on to live. This pollution can harm human health by making water supplies unsafe to drink or contributing to the spread of pathogens.

Many types of waste are **biodegradable**, or able to be broken down by microorganisms in the environment. However, even biodegradable wastes will not break down if they are disposed of in ways that do not expose them to the environment. Many other wastes are not biodegradable. They need to be disposed of in ways that will do the least possible damage to the environment.

Solid Waste

Municipal solid waste (MSW) is another term for trash or garbage. There are two ways to dispose of MSW:

- **Landfills.** A landfill is a specially engineered area where waste can be buried safely. Modern landfills have a variety of safeguards in place to prevent wastes from damaging the nearby land and water. For example, they must be sited away from sensitive natural areas and operated in ways that control odor and pests. They also must use special liners to prevent leakage that could contaminate groundwater.

Vocabulary

biodegradable
landfill
hazardous wastes
deforestation
urban sprawl
wastewater
conservation
precycling
recycling

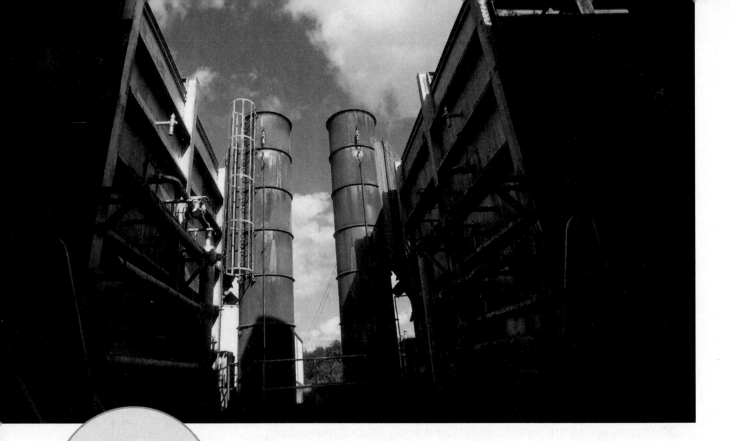

Barry Barker/McGraw-Hill Education

Some MSW is burned in specially designed incinerators. **What is another way to dispose of solid waste?**

- **Incineration.** Burning wastes in specially designed incinerators reduces the volume of trash that would otherwise to go into landfills. Waste incinerators use "scrubbers" and filters on their smokestacks to reduce air pollution. Some incinerators use the energy from burning waste to produce electricity, reducing the need for fuel.

Hazardous Wastes

Hazardous wastes are waste materials with properties that make them dangerous to human health or the environment. Hazardous wastes may be corrosive, chemically unstable, highly flammable, or toxic. Most hazardous wastes must be treated to make them less harmful before being discarded in special disposal sites. The types of hazardous waste are listed below.

- **Industrial wastes.** These include solvents used for cleaning and degreasing, as well as sludge and wastewater from certain industries, such as oil refining.

- **Household wastes.** Products such as pesticides, paints, cleaning fluids, and batteries may be hazardous when discarded. Some household wastes are banned from landfills and must be disposed of at special collection sites.

- **Radioactive wastes.** Sources such as nuclear power plants produce wastes that give off radiation. Exposure to radiation can increase the risk of cancer. It can also cause mutations—harmful changes in the body's DNA—which may be passed on to offspring. Extremely high levels of radiation can cause burns and radiation sickness. Because of these risks, such wastes must be isolated in secure storage sites until the radioactive materials decay, or cease to be radioactive.

- **Mercury.** This naturally occurring substance is highly toxic to humans and other animals. It is found in some medical and dental wastes and in certain parts of cars.

Problems of Development

MAIN IDEA Urban development has an impact on the environment.

Throughout human history, the number of people on the planet has been growing at a faster and faster rate. As the world population grows, so does our use of resources, including water and land. Wilderness areas give way to new urban developments, with drastic impacts on the environment.

Disappearing Forests

In many parts of the world, forests are being cleared away to make room for new developments, or agriculture. Timber from these forests is also used for fuel and manufacturing. This **deforestation**, or destruction of forests, causes a variety of problems.

- It destroys the habitats of plant and animal species.

- The loss of trees puts these areas at risk for soil erosion and flooding.

- It alters the local climate, making it hotter and drier over time.

- It contributes to climate change because trees absorb carbon dioxide, a greenhouse gas, from the atmosphere.

Urban Sprawl

The spreading of city development (houses, shopping centers, businesses, and schools) onto undeveloped land is called **urban sprawl**. Urban sprawl contributes to several environmental problems. For example, paved areas do not filter rainwater the way soil does. As a result, runoff can carry pollutants into the water supply. Sprawl also destroys wildlife habitats and reduces air quality.

To combat these problems, some city planners have embraced a concept called *smart growth*. It involves planning communities in ways that use fewer resources and create less pollution. One type of smart growth is *mixed-use development*. This means locating businesses, homes, and schools close together to make it easier for people to walk from place to place instead of driving. Smart growth also involves building more compactly to preserve open land and give people access to more **transit** choices.

Water: A Limited Resource

MAIN IDEA Pollution threatens our limited water supply.

Less than one percent of the planet's water is in a form humans can use. This limited supply makes water a precious resource. The EPA is responsible for protecting the water supply in the United States. It sets standards for the quality of drinking water and seeks to protect the health of oceans, rivers, and other water systems.

· · · · · · · · · · · ·

Reading Check

Explain What properties make certain wastes hazardous?

· · · · · · · · · · · ·

· · · · · · · · · · · ·

ACADEMIC VOCABULARY

transit *(noun)*: Conveyance of persons or things from one place to another.

· · · · · · · · · · · ·

....

Reading Check

Cause and Effect How does deforestation contribute to climate change?

. . . .

Sources of Water Pollution

Rivers, lakes, and aquifers (bodies of groundwater) provide much of our water supply. Pollutants can enter the supply in several different ways:

- **Runoff.** As rainwater or melting snow flows over the ground and into the water supply, it can pick up pollutants such as pesticides, fertilizers, salt, and animal wastes.

- **Wastewater.** This is used water from homes, communities, farms, and businesses. Wastewater can contain pollutants such as human and animal wastes, metals, and pathogens. The EPA requires that wastewater be treated to remove pollutants before it is released back into the environment. Consuming water that has not been properly sanitized can cause illness due to the presence of bacteria and viruses. Diseases such as cholera and giardia, which both cause intestinal discomfort and diarrhea, can be spread through water that has not been sanitized. Drinking water that contains lead can result in decreased kidney function and reproductive issues in both males and females.

- **Sediment.** Runoff can carry soil and other sediments into the water supply. This sediment can clog lakes and rivers, choking off plant and animal life.

- **Oil.** Spills from oil tankers and offshore drilling rigs can pollute the water. Oil poured down drains or onto the ground can also enter the water supply through runoff.

Water Scarcity

Not only is the world's water supply limited, but it is also unevenly distributed. An estimated 500 million people around the world have trouble getting the water they need to live. As the world population continues to grow, the demand for water increases. Disputes over water resources could lead to major conflict between nations.

Protecting the Environment

MAIN IDEA Conservation helps protect the environment.

People can help protect the environment by practicing **conservation**. This means avoiding waste through careful management of natural resources, such as energy, water, and materials. You can also conserve water and land by reducing water use and minimizing pollution.

For example:

- Repair leaky faucets, and never leave water running unnecessarily.

- Wait until you have a full load before doing laundry or running the dishwasher.

- Consider installing low-flow showerheads, faucet aerators, and low-flush toilets.

- Avoid over-watering your lawn and garden. Consider landscaping your yard with plants that require less water.

- Check with your local authorities to find out how to discard hazardous wastes such as motor oil, paint, and batteries safely.

Reduce, Reuse, Recycle. You can also conserve resources and reduce pollution by reducing the amount of waste you produce. There are three ways to do this, sometimes called *the three Rs.*

- **Reduce.** Source reduction is sometimes called **precycling.** This means reducing waste before it is generated. Examples include choosing products with less packaging and reusable products (such as cloth napkins) rather than disposable ones.

- **Reuse.** Next to precycling, the most efficient way to reduce waste is to reuse items. If you have an item that you no longer need, you can sell it, give it to a friend, or donate it to a charity instead of throwing it away. You can also repair broken items instead of buying new ones.

- **Recycle.** **Recycling** is the processing of waste materials so that they can be used again. It conserves materials and energy and reduces the need for new landfills and incinerators.

Reading Check

List What are three steps you can take to help conserve natural resources?

Character Check

When you dispose of hazardous household materials properly, you are demonstrating good citizenship and respect for the environment. Make a pledge to always dispose of hazardous materials in a responsible manner. Share your knowledge about the dangers of hazardous materials with others, and encourage them to make responsible decisions.

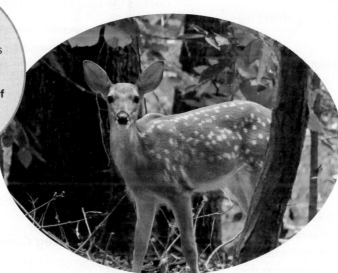

Forests play a vital role in the environment, providing oxygen, homes for a variety of living organisms, and natural beauty. **What are some of the consequences of destroying forests?**

Lesson 3 Review

Facts and Vocabulary

1. Name four types of hazardous wastes.

2. Describe how wastewater can harm the environment.

3. Describe the difference between the terms *reuse* and *recycle.*

Thinking Critically

4. **Analyze.** What rights do individuals and groups have when it comes to the environment?

5. **Explain.** How does population growth contribute to environmental problems?

Applying Health Skills

6. **Advocacy.** Create a comic book for elementary school students about a superhero who fights pollution. The comic book should contain a strong message encouraging young people to reduce land and water pollution.

Writing Critically

7. **Descriptive.** Write a description of a real or imaginary town that is built according to the principles of smart growth.

LESSON 1

Vocabulary Review

Use the correct vocabulary term to complete the following statements.

1. All the health care professionals you see are part of the nation's _____.

2. The two main forms of _____ are fee-for-service and managed care.

3. _____ includes all efforts to monitor, protect, and promote the health of the population as a whole.

Understanding Key Concepts

After reading the question or statement, select the correct answer.

4. You would likely see a specialist for
   a. an annual checkup.
   b. a flu shot.
   c. a minor injury.
   d. a condition that does not respond to normal treatment.

5. How are urgent care centers different from ordinary doctor's offices?
   a. They handle only medical emergencies.
   b. They can provide inpatient care.
   c. They see patients without appointments.
   d. They have several doctors working in the same place.

6. Which of the following is not a duty of local health departments?
   a. Investigating threats to public health
   b. Enforcing local health regulations
   c. Educating the public about health issues
   d. Funding research for new treatments

Thinking Critically

After reading the question or statement, write a short answer using complete sentences.

7. **Evaluate.** What are the benefits of seeing a primary care physician on a regular basis?

8. **Describe.** What does your medical history include?

9. **Evaluate.** What are the advantages of receiving group insurance through your employer over buying an individual policy?

10. **Explain.** What is the distinction between *health care* and *public health*?

11. **Explain.** What role does the Federal Trade Commission play in promoting public health?

LESSON 2

Vocabulary Review

Choose the correct term in the sentences below.

12. Particulate matter, carbon monoxide, and sulfur dioxide are all components of *air pollution/smog.*

13. *The greenhouse effect/climate change* is natural and is necessary to support life on earth.

14. The EPA created the *Air Quality Index/decibels* to track the levels of pollutants in the air.

15. Traffic, loud music, construction equipment, and power tools such as lawn mowers can all be sources of *air pollution/noise pollution.*

Understanding Key Concepts

After reading the question or statement, select the correct answer.

16. The pollutant that makes up the largest component of urban smog is
    a. ozone.
    b. carbon monoxide.
    c. sulfur dioxide.
    d. nitrogen oxides.

17. An AQI of 76 falls into the "moderate" range. This means that the quality of the air poses
    a. little or no health risk for anyone.
    b. a moderate concern for a very small number of people.
    c. a threat to members of sensitive groups, such as those with lung disease.
    d. a serious threat to everyone.

18. Which of the following is *not* a common indoor air pollutant?
    a. Asbestos
    b. Carbon monoxide
    c. Ozone
    d. Radon

19. Which of the following noises is loud enough to cause hearing damage?
    a. Whispered conversation
    b. Normal conversation
    c. Heavy traffic
    d. Rock concert

Thinking Critically

After reading the question or statement, write a short answer using complete sentences.

20. **Analyze.** How does reducing your use of energy combat climate change?

21. **Evaluate.** Suppose your school has old asbestos insulation in its walls. Is it a good idea to cut into the walls and remove it? Why or why not?

22. **Identify.** Give two examples of specific steps you can take to reduce air pollution.

23. **Synthesize.** Suppose your family wants to find out whether there is an unsafe level of carbon monoxide in your home, and fix the problem if there is. What steps would you take?

LESSON 3

Vocabulary Review

Correct the sentences below by replacing the italicized term with the correct vocabulary term.

24. Many types of waste are *recyclable,* or able to be broken down by microorganisms in the environment.

25. Waste materials with properties that make them dangerous to human health or the environment are known as *municipal solid waste.*

26. Soil erosion, flooding, and an increase in global temperatures are all problems associated with *urban sprawl.*

Understanding Key Concepts

After reading the question or statement, select the correct answer.

27. Which of the following is an example of smart growth?
    a. Zoning regulations that require homes and businesses to be in separate parts of a city or town
    b. Buying farmland to build new housing developments and shopping malls
    c. Buildings that have shops on the bottom level and apartments on the upper levels
    d. Widening streets to make more room for parking

28. Which of the following is *not* a problem associated with deforestation?
    a. Loss of habitat for plants and animals
    b. Increased soil erosion
    c. Changes in the local climate
    d. Destruction of old farms and ranches

29. The best way to dispose of used motor oil is to
    a. dump it down a storm drain.
    b. pour it out onto the ground.
    c. put it out with your regular trash.
    d. take it to a service station for recycling.

30. Which of the following is an example of precycling?
    a. Using cloth shopping bags
    b. Giving your old computer to a friend
    c. Repairing your broken radio instead of throwing it out and buying another
    d. Returning empty bottles to the manufacturer to be sterilized and refilled

Thinking Critically

After reading the question or statement, write a short answer using complete sentences.

31. **Explain.** Why do radioactive wastes need to be isolated in secure storage sites for a long time?

32. **Identify.** List three problems associated with urban sprawl.

33. **Analyze.** If 70 percent of Earth's surface is covered with water, why do 500 million people around the world have trouble getting the water they need?

34. **Evaluate.** Rank the strategies of precycling, reuse, and recycling in terms of their effectiveness in reducing waste. Give reasons for your answer.

PROJECT-BASED ASSESSMENT

Promoting Precycling

BACKGROUND

Precycling is a strategy for reducing waste before it is generated. It is an effective and important way to conserve natural resources, but it is not as widely understood or as widely promoted as recycling.

TASK

Create a blog that promotes two methods of precycling.

AUDIENCE

Students in your school.

PURPOSE

Show one strategy for precycling, and show the benefits of precycling.

PROCEDURE

1. Review the concept of precycling (covered in Lesson 3 of this module). Conduct an Internet search to explore the benefits of precycling. Investigate effective strategies for precycling that could be practiced by students.

2. In a group, brainstorm specific ways that the students at your school could practice precycling.

3. Select one of these precycling strategies to be the focus of your blog.

4. Present your blog to your teacher for consideration for the school's website.

Math Practice

Calculating Costs. Read the paragraph below, and then answer the questions.

Two families have medical insurance policies through different employers. The Lopez family pays $250 a month, and the insurance company will pay 85 percent of the cost of hospital stays. Family members pay $20 for each doctor visit. This insurance plan does not cover any vision costs. The Perez family's plan costs $410 a month, and hospital stays are completely covered. Family members pay $15 for each doctor visit. This plan pays the entire cost of an eye exam and $100 toward a pair of glasses or contact lenses.

1. Pedro Lopez had a hospital stay that cost $4,000. Before that, he had three doctor's appointments, each of which cost $93. Which function describes what Pedro has to pay? (Hint: C is Pedro's cost, H is the cost of the hospital stay, and D is the cost of each doctor visit.)
   a. $C = H + D$
   b. $C = H + 3D$
   c. $C = 0.15H + 20D$
   d. $C = 0.15H + 3D$

2. Melissa Perez has an eye exam and finds out she needs glasses. The glasses cost $395, and the exam is $95. How much does she have to pay?
   a. $295
   b. $300
   c. $395
   d. $490

3. In one year, both families had the following medical expenses: a hospital stay that cost $12,000, 14 trips to the doctor, four eye exams at $100 each, and two pairs of glasses at $300 each. Which policy would be the best to have under these circumstances? Why?

Reading/Writing Practice

Understand and Apply. Read the passage below, and then answer the questions.

Did you know that Americans throw away more than 245 million tons of trash each year? Much of that garbage ends up in landfills. Before these landfills fill up, we need to come up with new ways to get rid of our garbage. One way to do it is recycling. Some people worry that recycling costs too much, but it actually saves money because it uses less energy than manufacturing new items. Others say that people are too lazy to separate trash and wash out cans and bottles. This is not true. The best thing about recycling is that it is something everyone can do to help our planet. No matter what our age or our economic or education level, we can all take part. Earth is where we all are living and so we should care.

1. Which sentence should be added at the end of paragraph 2 to support the topic?
   a. It's hard to peel the labels off jars.
   b. It's better to precycle instead.
   c. Across the country, recycling rates have risen steadily over the years.
   d. My school started a recycling program.

2. What is the most effective way to rewrite the last sentence?
   a. We should all care about where we live.
   b. Why don't people care about recycling?
   c. Earth is our home, and we should keep it safe and healthy.
   d. Our planet is beautiful from space.

3. Write a persuasive paragraph urging sports arenas to recycle bottles and cans.

GLOSSARY/GLOSARIO

English

(A)

Abstinence A deliberate decision to avoid high-risk behaviors, including sexual activity and the use of tobacco, alcohol, and other drugs.

Abuse The physical, mental, emotional, or sexual mistreatment of one person by another.

Accident chain A sequence of events that leads to an unintentional injury.

Acquired Immune Deficiency Syndrome (AIDS) The final stage of the HIV infection.

Action plan A multi-step strategy to identify and achieve your goals.

Active listening Paying close attention to what someone is saying and communicating.

Addiction A physiological or psychological dependence on a drug.

Addictive drug A substance that causes physiological or psychological dependence.

Additive interaction Occurs when medicines work together in a positive way.

Adjust To bring to a more satisfactory state.

Adolescence The period between childhood and adulthood.

Adoption The legal process of taking a child of other parents as one's own.

Adoptive family A family consisting of a parent or parents and one or more adopted children.

Adrenal glands Glands that help the body deal with stress and respond to emergencies.

Advertising A written or spoken media message designed to interest consumers in purchasing a product or service.

Advocacy Taking action to influence others to address a health-related concern or to support a health-related belief.

Aerobic exercise All rhythmic activities that use large muscle groups for an extended period of time.

Affect To produce an effect upon.

Affirmation Positive feedback that helps others feel appreciated and supported.

Español

Abstinencia Decisión deliberada de evitar conductas de alto riesgo, como la actividad sexual, el consumo de tabaco, alcohol y otras drogas.

Abuso Maltrato físico, mental, emocional o sexual que una persona le provoca a otra.

Cadena de accidentes Serie de sucesos que generan una lesión no intencional.

Síndrome de inmunodeficiencia adquirida (SIDA) Etapa final de la infección por VIH.

Plan de acción Estrategia de varios pasos para identificar y lograr metas.

Escucha activa Escuchar atentamente lo que alguien dice o comunica.

Adicción Dependencia fisiológica o psicológica a una droga.

Droga adictiva Sustancia que causa dependencia fisiológica o psicológica.

Interacción aditiva Situación en la cual los medicamentos interactúan de una manera positiva.

Ajustar Traer a un estado más satisfactorio.

Adolescencia Etapa entre la infancia y la edad adulta.

Adopción Proceso legal para tener como hijo a un niño de otros padres.

Familia adoptiva Una familia compuesta por un padre o padres y uno o más hijos adoptados.

Glándulas suprarrenales Glándulas que ayudan al cuerpo a lidiar con el estrés y a reaccionar ante emergencias.

Publicidad Mensaje oral o escrito en los medios de comunicación, diseñado para incentivar a los consumidores a adquirir un producto o servicio.

Promoción Tomar medidas para influir en otras personas, con el propósito de abordar preocupaciones o apoyar creencias en relación con la salud.

Ejercicio aeróbico Toda actividad rítmica que use los grupos musculares grandes por un periodo prolongado.

Afectar Producir un efecto en algo o en alguien.

Afirmación Retroalimentación positiva que ayuda a que otras personas se sientan apreciadas y respaldadas.

GLOSSARY/GLOSARIO

English

Aggressive Overly forceful, pushy, or hostile.

Air pollution The contamination of Earth's atmosphere by harmful substances.

Air Quality Index (AQI) An index for reporting daily air quality.

Alcohol abuse The excessive use of alcohol.

Alcohol poisoning A severe and potentially fatal physical reaction to an alcohol overdose.

Alcoholic An addict who is dependent on alcohol.

Alcoholism A disease in which a person has a physical or psychological dependence on drinks that contain alcohol.

Alienation Feeling isolated and separated from everyone else.

Allergy A specific reaction of the immune system to a foreign and frequently harmless substance.

Alter To make different

Americans with Disabilities Act (ADA) A law prohibiting discrimination against people with physical or mental disabilities in the workplace, transportation, public accommodation, and telecommunications.

Amniocentesis A procedure in which a syringe is inserted through a pregnant female's abdominal wall to remove a sample of the amniotic fluid surrounding the developing fetus.

Anabolic-androgenic steroids Synthetic substances that are similar to male sex hormones.

Anaerobic exercise Intense, short bursts of activity in which the muscles work so hard that they produce energy without using oxygen.

Angina pectoris Chest pain that results when the heart does not get enough oxygen.

Anorexia nervosa An eating disorder in which an irrational fear of weight gain leads people to starve themselves.

Antagonistic interaction Occurs when the effect of one medicine is canceled or reduced when taken with another medicine.

Antibiotics A class of chemical agents that destroy disease-causing microorganisms while leaving the patient unharmed.

Antibody A protein that acts against a specific antigen.

Antibody screening test The first test to be run to detect HIV antibodies.

Español

Agresivo Excesivamente enérgico, insistente u hostil.

Contaminación atmosférica Contaminación de la atmósfera de la Tierra producto de sustancias peligrosas.

Índice de calidad del aire Indicador para informar sobre la calidad diaria del aire.

Abuso de alcohol Consumo excesivo de alcohol.

Intoxicación alcohólica Reacción física grave y potencialmente fatal a una sobredosis de alcohol.

Alcohólico Persona adicta al alcohol.

Alcoholismo Enfermedad en que la persona es adicta física o psicológicamente a las bebidas alcohólicas.

Alienación Sentirse solo y aislado de todo el mundo.

Alergia Reacción específica del sistema inmunológico a una sustancia extraña que usualmente es inofensiva.

Alterar Hacer diferente.

Ley para estadounidenses discapacitados (ADA) Ley que prohíbe la discriminación de personas con discapacidades físicas o mentales en los lugares de trabajo, transporte, lugares públicos y telecomunicaciones.

Amniocentesis Procedimiento en el cual se inserta una jeringa a través de la pared abdominal de una embarazada hasta llegar al líquido amniótico que rodea al embrión en desarrollo.

Esteroides anabolizantes-androgénicos Sustancias sintéticas semejantes a las hormonas masculinas.

Ejercicio anaeróbico Periodos cortos de actividad física intensiva, en los cuales los músculos trabajan tan arduamente que producen energía sin usar oxígeno.

Angina de pecho Dolor en el pecho causado porque el corazón no está recibiendo suficiente oxígeno.

Anorexia nerviosa Trastorno de la alimentación en la cual el miedo irracional a aumentar de peso provoca que las personas sigan una dieta de hambre.

Interacción antagónica Situación en la cual el efecto de un medicamento se elimina o reduce al interactuar con otro.

Antibióticos Tipo de agentes químicos que destruye los microorganismos que provocan enfermedades sin dañar al paciente.

Anticuerpo Proteína que ataca antígenos específicos.

Prueba de detección de anticuerpos Primera prueba realizada para detectar los anticuerpos del VIH.

GLOSSARY/GLOSARIO

English

Anticipate To expect.

Antigens Substances that are capable of triggering an immune response.

Anxiety The condition of feeling uneasy or worried about what may happen.

Anxiety disorder A condition in which real or imagined fears are difficult to control.

Apathy A lack of strong feeling, interest, or concern.

Appendicitis The inflammation of the appendix.

Appetite The psychological desire for food.

Approach A particular manner of taking steps.

Appropriate Proper or fitting.

Arrhythmias Irregular heartbeats.

Arteriosclerosis Hardened arteries with reduced elasticity.

Arthritis A group of more than 100 different diseases that causes pain and loss of movement in the joints.

Aspect A feature or phase of something.

Assault An unlawful physical attack or threat of attack.

Assertive Expressing your views clearly and respectfully.

Asthma An inflammatory condition in which the trachea, the bronchi, and bronchioles become narrowed, causing difficulty breathing.

Asymptomatic People who are infected show no symptoms, or the infections produce mild symptoms that disappear.

Atherosclerosis A disease characterized by the accumulation of plaque on artery walls.

Attribute A quality or characteristic.

Auditory ossicles Three small bones linked together that connect the eardrum to the inner ear.

Authority The right to make decisions and give commands.

Autoimmune disease A condition in which the immune system mistakenly attacks itself, targeting the cells, tissues, and organs of a person's own body.

Autonomy The confidence that a person can control his or her own body, impulses, and environment.

Available Present or ready for immediate use

Español

Anticipar Esperar.

Antígenos Sustancias capaces de provocar una respuesta inmune.

Ansiedad Estado en el cual una persona se siente abrumada o preocupada acerca de lo que le pueda pasar.

Trastorno de ansiedad Estado en el cual el miedo, ya sea real o imaginario, es difícil de controlar.

Apatía Falta de sentimientos intensos, interés o preocupación.

Apendicitis Inflamación del apéndice.

Apetito Deseo psicológico de comer.

Acceso Una manera particular de tomar medidas.

Apropiado Apropiado o quedando bien.

Arritmia Palpitaciones irregulares del corazón.

Ateroesclerosis Arterias endurecidas con elasticidad reducida.

Artritis Grupo de más de 100 enfermedades que causan dolor y pérdida de movimiento en las articulaciones.

Aspecto Característica o fase de algo.

Asalto Ataque o amenaza de ataque físico ilegal.

Asertivo Persona que expresa sus puntos de vista clara y respetuosamente.

Asma Condición inflamatoria en que la tráquea, los bronquios y los bronquiolos se estrechan provocando dificultad para respirar.

Asintomático Persona infectada que no presenta síntomas o infecciones que producen síntomas leves que desaparecen.

Ateroesclerosis Enfermedad caracterizada por la acumulación de depósitos en las paredes de las arterias.

Atributo Cualidad o característica.

Osículos auditivas Tres huesos pequeños conectados juntos que unen el tímpano con el oido interno.

Autoridad Derecho para tomar decisiones y dar órdenes.

Enfermedad autoinmune Condición en la cual el sistema inmune se ataca a sí mismo por error, afectando las células, los tejidos y los órganos del cuerpo de una persona.

Autonomía Capacidad que tiene una persona para controlar su propio cuerpo, impulsos y medio ambiente.

Disponible Presente o listo para su uso inmediato.

English

B

Bacteria Single-celled microorganisms.

Behavior therapy A treatment process that focuses on changing unwanted behavior through rewards and reinforcement.

Benign Noncancerous.

Bile A yellow-green, bitter fluid important in the breakdown and absorption of fats.

Binge drinking Drinking five or more alcoholic drinks at one sitting.

Binge eating disorder An eating disorder in which people overeat compulsively.

Biodegradable Able to be broken down by microorganisms in the environment.

Biopsy The removal of a small piece of tissue for examination.

Blended family A married couple and their children from previous marriages.

Blizzard A snowstorm with winds that reach 35 miles an hour or more.

Blood alcohol concentration (BAC) The amount of alcohol in a person's blood expressed as a percentage.

Blood pressure A measure of the amount of force that the blood places on the walls of blood vessels, particularly large arteries, as it is pumped through the body.

Body image The way you see your body.

Body language Nonverbal communication through gestures, facial expressions, behaviors, and posture.

Body mass index (BMI) A measure of body weight relative to height.

Brain stem A three-inch-long stalk of nerve cells and fibers that connects the spinal cord to the rest of the brain.

Bronchi The main airways that reach into each lung.

Bulimia nervosa An eating disorder that involves cycles of overeating and purging, or attempts to rid the body of food.

Bullying Deliberately harming or threatening another person who cannot easily defend himself or herself.

Español

Bacteria Microorganismos compuestos de una sola célula.

Terapia del conducta Terapia que se enfoca en cambiar las conductas no deseadas a través de recompensas y refuerzos.

Benigno No canceroso.

Bilis Líquido amargo de color amarillo verdoso que es importante para la descomposición y absorción de las grasas.

Borrachera Consumo de cinco o más bebidas alcohólicas consecutivas.

Trastorno de atracones compulsivos Trastorno de la alimentación caracterizada por comer demasiado y de manera compulsiva.

Biodegradable Algo que los microorganismos del medio ambiente pueden descomponer.

Biopsia La extirpación diagnóstica de una pequeña muestra de tejido.

Familia mixta Pareja casada y sus hijos de matrimonios anteriores.

Ventisca Tormenta de nieve con vientos que superan las 35 millas por hora.

Concentración de alcohol en la sangre Cantidad de alcohol en la sangre de una persona expresada como porcentaje.

Presión arterial Medida de la presión que ejerce la sangre sobre las paredes de los vasos sanguíneos, especialmente en las arterias grandes, a medida que es bombeada por el cuerpo

Imagen corporal Forma en que uno ve su propio cuerpo.

Lenguaje corporal Comunicación no verbal a través de gestos, expresiones faciales, comportamientos y postura.

Índice de masa corporal (IMC) Medida de peso corporal en relación con la estatura.

Vástago cerebral Ramificación de neuronas y fibras de tres pulgadas de largo que conecta la médula espinal con el resto del cerebro.

Bronquios Vías aéreas principales que llegan a los pulmones.

Bulimia nerviosa Trastorno de la alimentación que implica ciclos en que la persona come en exceso y purga o intenta eliminar la comida del cuerpo.

Intimidación Daño o amenazas deliberadas hacia una persona que no se puede defender fácilmente.

GLOSSARY/GLOSARIO

English

Español

C

Calorie A unit of heat used to measure the energy your body uses and the energy it receives from food.

Caloría Unidad de calor que mide la energía que usa el cuerpo y la energía que la comida proporciona al cuerpo.

Cancer Uncontrollable growth of abnormal cells.

Cáncer Crecimiento incontrolable de células anormales.

Capillaries Small vessels that carry blood from arterioles to small vessels called venules, which empty into veins.

Capilares Vasos sanguíneos delicados que transportan sangre desde las arteriolas hasta vasos pequeños conocidos como vénulas, las cuales terminan en las venas.

Carbohydrates Starches and sugars found in foods which provide your body's main source of energy.

Carbohidratos Almidones y azúcares que se encuentran en los alimentos, los cuales proporcionan al cuerpo la fuente principal de energía.

Carbon monoxide A colorless, odorless, and poisonous gas.

Monóxido de carbono Gas incoloro, inodoro y venenoso.

Carcinogen A cancer-causing substance.

Cancerígeno Sustancia que produce cáncer.

Cardiac muscles A type of striated muscle that forms the wall of the heart.

Músculo cardiaco Tipo de músculo estriado que forma las paredes del corazón.

Cardiopulmonary resuscitation (CPR) A first-aid procedure that combines rescue breathing and chest compressions to supply oxygen to the body until normal body functions can resume.

Resucitación cardiopulmonar (RCP) Procedimiento de primeros auxilios que combina la respiración artificial con compresiones en el pecho a fin de proporcionar oxígeno hasta que las funciones vitales puedan reanudarse.

Cardiorespiratory endurance The ability of your heart, lungs, and blood vessels to send fuel and oxygen to your tissues during long periods of moderate to vigorous activity.

Resistencia cardiorrespiratoria Capacidad que tienen el corazón, los pulmones y los vasos sanguíneos de enviar energía y oxígeno a los tejidos durante largos periodos de tiempo con actividad moderada a enérgica.

Cardiovascular disease A disease that affects the heart or blood vessels.

Enfermedad cardiovascular Enfermedad que afecta el corazón o los vasos sanguíneos.

Cartilage A strong, flexible connective tissue.

Cartílago Tejido conjuntivo fuerte y flexible.

Cerebellum The second largest part of the brain.

Cerebelo La segunda parte más grande del cerebro.

Cerebral palsy A group of neurological disorders that are the result of damage to the brain before, during, or just after birth or in early childhood.

Parálisis cerebral Grupo de trastornos neurológicos que son el resultado de daños al cerebro antes, durante o inmediatamente después del nacimiento o durante la niñez temprana.

Cerebrum The largest and most complex part of the brain.

Corteza cerebral La parte más grande y compleja del cerebro.

Cervix The opening to the uterus.

Cuello del útero La entrada del útero.

Chain of survival A sequence of actions that maximize the victim's chances of survival.

Cadena de supervivencia Secuencia de acciones que tiene como objetivo maximizar las posibilidades de supervivencia de una víctima.

Character The distinctive qualities that describe how a person thinks, feels, and behaves.

Carácter Características distintivas que describen cómo una persona piensa, siente y actúa.

Child abuse Domestic abuse directed at a child.

Maltrato infantil Abuso doméstico dirigido hacia los niños.

Cholesterol A waxy, fatlike substance.

Colesterol Sustancia cerosa de apariencia grasa.

Chorionic villi sampling (CVS) A procedure in which a small piece of membrane is removed from the chorion, a layer of tissue that develops into the placenta.

Biopsia de vellosidades coriónicas Procedimiento en el cual se saca una pequeña muestra de membrana del corion, una capa de tejido que se desarrolla en la placenta.

GLOSSARY/GLOSARIO

English

Chromosomes Threadlike structures found within the nucleus of a cell that carry the codes for inherited traits.

Chronic disease An ongoing condition or illness.

Chronic stress Stress associated with long-term problems that are beyond a person's control.

Circumstances An event that influences another event.

Cirrhosis Scarring of the liver tissue.

Citizenship The way you conduct yourself as a member of the community.

Climate change An overall increase in Earth's temperature.

Clique A small circle of friends, usually with similar backgrounds or tastes, who exclude people viewed as outsiders.

Closure Acceptance of a loss.

Cluster suicides A series of suicides occurring within a short period of time and involving several people in the same school or community.

Coercion Using force or threats to persuade another person to do something.

Cognition The ability to reason and think out abstract solutions.

Cognitive therapy A treatment method designed to identify and correct distorted thinking patterns that can lead to feelings and behaviors that may be troublesome, self-defeating, or self-destructive.

Commitment A promise or a pledge.

Communicable disease A disease that is spread from one living organism to another or through the environment.

Community A population of individuals in a common location.

Comparison shopping Judging the benefits of different products by comparing several factors, such as quality, features, and cost.

Competence Having enough skills to do something.

Component A constituent part or ingredient.

Español

Cromosomas Estructuras parecidas a hilos que se encuentran dentro del núcleo de una célula y que tienen los códigos de los rasgos heredados.

Enfermedad crónica Afección o enfermedad permanente.

Estrés crónico Estrés relacionado con problemas de largo plazo y fuera del control de una persona.

Circunstancia Acontecimiento que influye en otro acontecimiento.

Cirrosis Lesiones en el tejido del hígado.

Ciudadanía Manera de comportarse como miembro de la comunidad.

Cambio climático Aumento general de la temperatura de la Tierra.

Pandilla Grupo pequeño de amigos, generalmente con gustos y experiencias similares, que excluyen a otras personas consideradas ajenas a ellos.

Resignación Aceptación de una pérdida.

Serie de suicidios Varios suicidios que ocurren en un periodo de tiempo corto y que involucran a personas de un mismo colegio o comunidad.

Coerción Utilizar la fuerza o las amenazas para persuadir a otra persona a hacer algo.

Cognición Capacidad de razonar y generar soluciones abstractas.

Terapia cognoscitiva Terapia diseñada para identificar y corregir patrones de pensamiento distorsionados, los cuales pueden generar sentimientos y comportamientos problemáticos, contraproducentes o autodestructivos.

Compromiso Una promesa.

Enfermedad contagiosa Enfermedad que se quede transmitir de un ser vivo a otro o a través del medio ambiente.

Comunidad Población de personas que viven en el mismo lugar.

Compras informadas Evaluar los beneficios de diferentes productos comparando diversos factores, como calidad, características y precio.

Competencia Capacidad suficiente para realizar algo.

Componente Parete o ingrediente constitutivo.

GLOSSARY/GLOSARIO

English

Compromise A problem-solving method in which each participant gives up something to reach a solution that satisfies everyone.

Computer A device that can store, retrieve, and process data.

Concussion A jarring injury to the brain that can cause unconsciousness.

Conduct disorder Patterns of behavior in which the rights of others or basic social rules are violated.

Confidentiality Respecting the privacy of both parties and keeping details secret.

Confine To keep within limits.

Conflict Any disagreement, struggle, or fight.

Conflict resolution The process of ending a conflict through cooperation and problem solving.

Conservation Avoiding waste through careful management of natural resources.

Consistent Free from variation or contradiction.

Constructive Promoting improvement or development.

Constructive criticism Nonhostile comments that point out problems and encourage improvement.

Consumer advocates People or groups whose sole purpose is to take on regional, national, and even international consumer issues.

Contact Union or junction of surfaces.

Contract To draw together.

Contradict To imply the opposite of.

Cool-down Low-level activity that prepares your body to return to a resting state.

Cooperation Working together for the good of all.

Coping Dealing successfully with difficult changes in your life.

Cornea A transparent tissue in the eye that bends and focuses light before it enters the lens.

Crisis center A facility that offers advice and support to people dealing with personal emergencies.

Cross-contamination The spreading of pathogens from one food to another.

Crucial Important or essential.

Español

Acuerdo Método para resolver problemas en que cada participante debe sacrificar algo para llegar a una solución satisfactoria para todos.

Computadora Recuperar datos.

Conmoción cerebral Lesión violenta en el cerebro que puede conducir a la pérdida de conocimiento.

Trastorno de conducta Patrón de comportamiento en el cual se infringen los derechos de los demás o las reglas sociales básicas.

Confidencialidad Respetar la vida privada de ambas partes y mantener en secreto los detalles.

Confinar Encerrar en un lugar.

Conflicto Cualquier desacuerdo, pelea o enojo.

Resolución de conflictos Proceso de resolver un conflicto a través de métodos de cooperación y solución de problemas.

Conservación Evitar el desperdicio de recursos a través de un manejo correcto de los recursos naturales.

Coherente Sin variaciones ni contradicciones.

Constructivo Que promeuve mejoras o progresos.

Crítica constructiva Comentarios no hostiles que señalan los problemas y fomentan su mejoramiento.

Defensores del consumidor Gente o grupos cuyo único propósito es confrontar los problemas regionales, nacionales y hasta internacionales del consumidor.

Contacto Unión o conexión de superficies.

Contraer Reducirse, disminuir.

Contradecir Decir o hacer lo contrario.

Recuperación Actividad liviana que prepara al cuerpo para volver a un estado de descanso.

Cooperación Trabajar juntos para el beneficio de todos.

Sobrellevar Encargarse exitosamente de los cambios difíciles de la vida.

Córnea Tejido transparente que refracta y enfoca la luz antes de pasar al cristalino.

Centro para crisis Plantel que maneja emergencias y envía a un individuo que necesita ayuda a especialistas.

Contaminación cruzada Transmisión de agentes patógenos de una comida a otra.

Crucial Importante o esencial.

English

Culture The collective beliefs, customs, and behaviors of a group.

Cumulative risks Related risks that increase in effect with each added risk.

Custody The legal right to make decisions affecting children and the responsibility for their care.

Cyberbullying Cruel or hurtful online contact.

Cycle of violence Pattern of repeating violent or abusive behaviors from one generation to the next.

Cystitis An inflammation of the bladder.

D

Date rape One person in a dating relationship forces the other person to take part in sexual intercourse.

Dating violence When a person uses violence in a dating relationship to control his or her partner.

Decade A group or set of ten

Decibel A unit that measures the intensity of sound.

Decision-making skills Steps that enable you to make a healthful decision.

Defense mechanisms Mental processes that protect individuals from strong or stressful emotions and situations.

Defensive driving Being aware of potential hazards on the road and taking action to avoid them.

Defibrillator A device that delivers an electric shock to the heart to restore its normal rhythm.

Deforestation Destruction of forests.

Deoxyribonucleic acid (DNA) The chemical unit that makes up chromosomes.

Depressant A drug that slows the central nervous system.

Depression Prolonged feeling of helplessness, hopelessness, and sadness.

Dermis The thicker layer of skin beneath the epidermis that is made up of connective tissue and contains blood vessels and nerves.

Español

Cultura Las creencias, costumbres y comportamientos colectivos de un grupo de personas.

Riesgos acumulativos Riesgos relacionados que aumentan en efecto con cada nuevo peligro.

Custodia Derecho legal de tomar decisiones que afecten a los niños y la responsabilidad de cuidarlos.

Intimidación cibernético Contacto cruel o dañino que se produce en línea.

Ciclo de violencia Patrón de comportamiento violento o abusivo que se repite de una generación a la siguiente.

Cistitis Inflamación de la vejiga.

Violación durante una cita (violación por un conocido, violación a escondidas) Una persona que se encuentra en una cita obliga a la otra a participar en una actividad sexual.

Relacion violenta Cuando una persona usa violencia en una relación amorosa para poder controlar a su pareja.

Década Grupo o conjunto de diez.

Decibelios (Decibeles) Medida que se usa para expresar la intensidad del sonido.

Habilidades para tomar decisiones Pasos necesarios para tomar una decisión correcta.

Mecanismos de defensa Procesos mentales que protegen a los individuos de emociones y situaciones intensas o estresantes.

Conducción a la defensiva Estar consciente de posibles peligros en la carretera y tomar medidas para evitarlos.

Máquina de desfibrilación Un aparato que proporciona choques eléctricos al corazón para recuperar su ritmo normal.

Deforestación Destrucción de los bosques.

Ácido desoxirribonucleico (ADN) Unidad química que compone los cromosomas.

Depresor Sustancia que tiende a disminuir el funcionamiento (actividad) del sistema nervioso central.

Depresión Sentimiento prolongado de soledad, desesperación y tristeza.

Dermis La capa más gruesa de la piel que se encuentra debajo de la epidermis que está compuesta de tejidos conectivos y contiene vasos sanguíneos y nervios.

GLOSSARY/GLOSARIO

English

Designer drug A synthetic drug that is made to imitate the effects of hallucinogens and other drugs.

Developmental tasks Events that need to happen in order for a person to continue growing toward becoming a healthy, mature adult.

Devote To give time or effort to an activity.

Diabetes A chronic disease that affects the way cells convert sugar into energy.

Diaphragm A muscle that separates the chest from the abdominal cavity.

Dietary guidelines for Americans A set of recommendation about smart eating and physical activity for all Americans.

Dietary supplements Products that supply one or more nutrients as a supplement to, not as a substitute for, healthful foods.

Disability Any physical or mental impairment that limits normal activities, including seeing, hearing, walking, or speaking.

Dislocation A separation of a bone from its normal position in a joint.

Display To make evident.

Distracted driving Driving a motor vehicle while engaged in another activity, such as joking or talking with friends who are in the car, or using a mobile phone or other electronic device.

Distress Negative stress.

Divorce A legal end to a marriage contract.

Domestic Relating to the household or family.

Domestic violence Act of violence involving family members.

Drug overdose Taking more of a drug than the body can tolerate.

Drug therapy The use of certain medications to treat or reduce the symptoms of a mental disorder.

Drug watches Organized community efforts by neighborhood residents to patrol, monitor, report, and otherwise stop drug deals and drug abuse.

Español

Droga de diseño Sustancias sintéticas que tratan de imitar los efectos de los alucinógenos y otras drogas peligrosas.

Tareas requeridas para el desarrollo Sucesos necesarios para que una persona continúe creciendo y se convierta en un adulto saludable y maduro.

Dedicar Destinar tiempo o esfuerzo a una actividad.

Diabetes Una enfermedad crónica que afecta el modo en que las células del cuerpo convierten los alimentos en energía.

Diafragma El músculo que separa la cavidad toráxico de la cavidad abdominal.

Guías alimentarías para los estadounidenses Conjunto de recomendaciones acerca de alimentarse inteligentemente y de la actividad física para todos los estadounidenses.

Suplementos alimentarios Productos que suministran uno o más nutrientes en forma de suplementos, no de sustitutos, a los alimentos saludables.

Discapacidad Cualquier impedimento físico o mental que limita el desarrollo de actividades normales tales como ver, oír, caminar o dormir.

Dislocación Separación del hueso de su posición normal en una articulación.

Exponer Hacer evidente.

Conducción distraida Conducir un vehículo de motor mientras realiza otra actividad, como bromear o hablar con amigos que están en el automóvil, o usar un teléfono móvil u otro dispositivo electrónico.

Aflicción Estrés negative.

Divorcio Fin legal de un contrato de matrimonio.

Doméstico Relativo al hogar o a la familia.

Violencia doméstica (intrafamiliar) Acto de violencia que incluya a los miembros de una familia.

sobredosis Tomar una cantidad de droga que supera lo que el cuerpo puede tolerar.

Terapia farmacológica Uso de ciertos medicamentos para tratar o reducir los síntomas de una enfermedad mental.

Vigilantes de la droga Un grupo de personas de un vecindario organizadas para supervisar, controlar, denunciar o directamente frenar el abuso y la venta de drogas.

English

Drug-free school zone Areas within 1,000 feet of schools and designated by signs, within which people caught selling drugs receive especially severe penalties.

Drugs Substances other than food that change the structure or function of the body or mind.

Earthquake A series of vibrations in the earth caused by sudden movements of Earth's crust.

Eating disorders Extreme, harmful eating behaviors that can cause serious illness or even death.

Eggs Female gametes.

Elder abuse The abuse or neglect of older family members.

Embryo A cluster of cells that develops between the third and eighth week of pregnancy.

Emergency survival kit A set of items you will need in an emergency.

Emerging infection Communicable diseases whose occurrence in humans has increased within the past two decades or threatens to increase in the near future.

Emotional abuse A pattern of attacking another person's emotional development and sense of worth.

Emotional maturity The state at which the mental and emotional capabilities of an individual are fully developed.

Emotions Signals that tell your mind and body how to react.

Empathy The ability to imagine and understand how someone else feels.

Emphysema A disease that progressively destroys the walls of the alveoli.

Empty-nest syndrome The feeling of sadness or loneliness that accompanies seeing children leave home and enter adulthood.

Enable To make possible.

Encounter To experience.

Español

Zona de escuela libre de drogas Un área que comprende 1,000 pies alrededor de una escuela y se encuentra señalizada, en la cual las personas que son atrapadas vendiendo drogas son gravemente penalizadas o castigadas.

Drogas Sustancias distintas de los alimentos, que cambian la estructura o el funcionamiento del cuerpo o la mente de las personas.

Terremoto Serie de vibraciones en la tierra provocada por movimientos repentinos de la superficie de la tierra.

Trastorno alimentario Un comportamiento que se caracteriza por comer en forma extrema y dañina lo que causa que la persona se pueda enfermar o morir.

Óvulos Gametos femeninos.

Abuso de mayores El abuso o la negligencia de miembras ancianos de la familia.

Embrión Grupo de células que se desarrolla entre la tercera y la octava semana del embarazo.

Botiquín de emergencia Conjunto de elementos necesarios para una situación de emergencia.

Infección emergente Una enfermedad infecciosa cuya incidencia en humanos ha aumentado durante las últimas dos décadas o que amenaza con aumentar en el futuro cercano.

Abuso emocional Patrón de ataque al desarrollo emocional y al sentido de estima de otra persona.

Madurez emocional Un estado en el cual las capacidades mentales y emocionales de una persona se encuentran totalmente desarrolladas.

Emociones Señales que le comunican a la mente y al cuerpo cómo actuar.

Empatía La habilidad para imaginar y entender cómo siente otra persona.

Enfisema Una enfermedad que destruye progresivamente las paredes de los alvéolos.

Síndrome del nido vacío Sentimiento de tristeza y soledad que ocurre cuando los hijos, quienes ya se convirtieron en adultos, se van de la casa de sus padres.

Permitir Hacer posible.

Encuentro Expriencias.

GLOSSARY/GLOSARIO

English

Endocrine glands Ductless or tubeless organs or groups of cells that secrete hormones directly into the bloodstream.

Environment The sum of your surroundings.

Environmental tobacco smoke (ETS) Air that has been contaminated by tobacco smoke.

Epidemic An occurrence of a disease in which many people in the same place at the same time are affected.

Epidermis The outer, thinner layer of the skin that is composed of living and dead cells.

Epilepsy A disorder of the nervous system that is characterized by recurrent seizures–sudden episodes of uncontrolled electric activity in the brain.

Escalate Become more serious.

Estimate To determine roughly the size or extent of.

Ethanol The type of alcohol in alcoholic beverages.

Euphoria A feeling of intense well-being or elation.

Eventually At an unspecified later time.

Exclude To prevent or restrict the entrance of.

Exercise Purposeful physical activity that is planned, structured, and repetitive, and that improves or maintains physical fitness.

Expand To open up.

Exposure The condition of being unprotected.

Extended family A family that includes additional relatives beyond parents and children.

Extensor The muscle that opens a joint.

Factor An element that contributes to a particular result.

Fad diet Weight-loss plans that tend to be popular for only a short time.

Fallopian tubes A pair of tubes with fingerlike projections that draw in the ovum.

Family therapy Helping the family function in more positive and constructive ways by exploring the patterns in communication and providing support and education.

Español

Glándulas endocrinas Órganos o grupos de células sin conductos o tubos que secretan hormonas directamente al torrente sanguíneo.

Medio ambiente Todo lo que nos rodea.

Ambiente con humo de cigarro Aire que ha sido contaminado por el humo de cigarrillos.

Epidemia Una situación en la cual mucha gente contrae una enfermedad al mismo tiempo y en el mismo lugar.

Epidermis La capa más fina y externa de la piel la cual se encuentra compuesta de células vivas y muertas.

Epilepsia Trastorno del sistema nervioso caracterizado por convulsiones continuas–repentinos episodios de actividad eléctrica incontrolable en el cerebro.

Intensificar Situación que se hace más grave.

Estimar Determinar aproximadamente el tamaño o la extension de algo.

Etanol Tipo de alcohol que se encuentra en las bebidas alcohólicas.

Euforia Sentimiento de un intenso bienestar o alegría.

Eventual Sin especificar un rato más después.

Excluir Para prevenir o restringir la entrada de.

Ejercicio Actividad física dirigida que es planeada, estructurada y repetitiva y que tiene como objetivo el mantenimiento o el mejoramiento del estado físico de una persona.

Expandir Ampliar.

Exposición Falta de protección.

Familia extendida Familia que incluye a otros parientes, distintos a padres e hijos.

Extensor Músculo que abre una articulación.

F

Factor Elemento que contribuye a un resultado en particular.

Dietas de moda Planes para perder peso que son populares por poco tiempo.

Trompas de falopio Un par de conductos con terminaciones en forma de dedos que atrae el ovario.

Terapia familiar Ayudar a que la familia funcione de maneras más constructivas y positivas mediante la exploración de los patrones de comunicación y en proporcionar apoyo y educación.

English

Fermentation The chemical action of yeast on sugars.

Fertilization The union of a male sperm cell and a female egg.

Fetal alcohol syndrome A group of alcohol-related birth defects that includes both physical and mental problems.

Fetus Group of developing cells after about the eighth week of pregnancy.

Fiber A tough, complex, carbohydrate that the body cannot digest.

Fire extinguisher A portable device for putting out small fires.

First aid The immediate, temporary care given to an ill or injured person until professional care can be provided.

Flash floods Floods in which a dangerous volume of water builds up in a short time.

Flexibility The ability to move your body parts through their full range of motion.

Flexor The muscle that closes a joint.

Food additives Substances added to a food to produce a desired effect.

Food allergy A condition in which the body's immune system reacts to substances in some foods.

Foodborne illness Food poisoning.

Food desert An urban area where it is difficult to buy affordable or high-quality foods.

Food intolerance A negative reaction to food that does not involve the immune system.

Foster care The temporary placement of children in the homes of adults who are not related to them.

Fracture A break in a bone.

Friendship A significant relationship between two people that is based on trust, caring, and consideration.

Frostbite Damage to the skin and tissues caused by extreme cold.

Español

Fermentación Reacción química de la levadura en los azúcares.

Fertilización La unión del espermatozoide y el óvulo.

Síndrome de alcoholismo fetal Un grupo de defectos de nacimiento causados por el alcohol y que incluyen problemas físicos y mentales.

Feto Grupo de células en desarrollo después de las ocho semanas de embarazo.

Fibra Un carbohidrato complejo y duro que el cuerpo no puede digerir.

Extintor de incendios Aparato portátil para apagar fuego.

Primeros auxilios La atención inmediata y temporal que se le proporciona a una persona hasta que se le puede otorgar atención profesional.

Inundaciones rápidas Inundaciones en las cuales se acumula un volumen peligroso de agua en poco tiempo.

Flexibilidad La capacidad de mover una parte del cuerpo fácilmente y en muchas direcciones.

Músculo flexor Músculo que abre una articulación.

Aditivos alimentarios Sustancias que son adicionadas a los alimentos en forma intencional para generar un efecto deseado.

Alergia alimentaria Una condición en la cuál el sistema inmunológico del cuerpo reacciona a sustancias contenidas en algunos alimentos.

Enfermedad producida por alimentos Intoxicación alimentaria.

Desierto de comida Un área urbana donde es difícil comprar alimentos asequibles o de alta calidad

Intolerancia alimentaria Reacción negativa a los alimentos (o un elemento particular del alimento) en la cual no participa el sistema inmunológico.

Cuidados temporales Colocación provisoria de niños en hogares de adultos que no son sus parientes.

Fractura Ruptura de un hueso.

Amistad Una relación importante entre dos personas que está basada en solidaridad, confianza y consideración.

Congelación Daño a la piel y a los tejidos provocados por frío extremo.

GLOSSARY/GLOSARIO

English

Español

G

Gastric juices Secretions from the stomach lining that contain hydrochloric acid and pepsin, an enzyme that digests protein.

Gene therapy The process of inserting normal genes into human cells to correct genetic disorders.

Genes The basic units of heredity.

Genetic disorders Disorders caused partly or completely by a defect in genes.

Giardia A microorganism that infects the digestive system.

Goals Those things you aim for that take planning and work.

Good samaritan laws Statutes that protect rescuers from being sued for giving emergency care.

Graduated licensing A system that gradually increases driving privileges over time.

Greenhouse effect The trapping of heat by gases in Earth's atmosphere.

Group therapy Treating a group of people who have similar problems and who meet regularly with a trained counselor.

Guideline An outline of conduct.

Jugos gástricos La secreciones que provienen del revestimiento del estómago y que contienen ácido clorhídrico y pepsina, una enzima que digiere la proteína.

Terapia genética Un proceso que consiste en introducir genes normales en las células humanas para corregir trastornos genéticos.

Genes Unidades básicas de la herencia.

Trastorno genético Trastorno causado parcial o completamente por defectos en los genes.

Giardia Microorganismo que infecta el sistema digestivo.

Metas Las cosas de que te esfuerzas que necesita planificación y trabajo.

Leyes del buen samaritano Estatutos que protegen a los rescatistas de ser demandados por otorgar atención de urgencia.

Licencia graduada Sistema que gradualmente aumenta los privilegios de conducción en el transcurso del tiempo.

Efecto invernadero Calor atrapado por gases en la atmósfera de la Tierra.

Terapia de grupo Tratamiento de un grupo de personas que tienen problemas similares.

Pauta Un modelo de conducta.

H

Hair follicles Sacs or cavities that surround the roots of hairs.

Halitosis Bad breath.

Hallucinogens Drugs that alter moods, thoughts, and sense perceptions including vision, hearing, smell, and touch.

Harassment Persistently annoying others.

Hazardous wastes Waste materials with properties that make them dangerous to human health or the environment.

Hazing Making others perform certain tasks in order to join the group.

Health The combination of physical, mental/emotional, and social well-being.

Folículos pilosos Sacos o cavidades que rodean las raíces de los pelos.

Halitosis Mal aliento.

Alucinógenos Drogas que alteran el estado de ánimo, el pensamiento y la percepción, lo que incluye vista, oído, olfato y tacto.

Acoso Molestar continuamente a otra persona.

Desechos peligrosos Materiales de desecho que se caracterizan por ser peligrosos para la salud humana o el medio ambiente.

Acoso personal Forzando otras a complir ciertas tareas para formar parte del grupo.

Salud Combinación de bienestar físico, mental-emocional y social.

English

Health care system All the medical care available to a nation's people, the way they receive care, and the way they pay for it.

Health consumer Someone who purchases or uses health products or services.

Health disparities Differences in health outcomes among groups.

Health education Providing accurate health information and health skills teaching to help people make healthy decisions.

Health fraud The sale of worthless products or services that claim to prevent diseases or cure other health problems.

Health insurance Private and government programs that pay for part or all of a person's medical costs.

Health literacy A person's capacity to learn about and understand basic health information and services and to use these resources to promote one's health and wellness.

Health skills Specific tools and strategies to maintain, protect, and improve all aspects of your health.

Healthy People A nationwide health promotion and disease prevention plan designed to serve as a guide for improving the health of all people in the United States.

Heat exhaustion A form of physical stress on the body caused by overheating.

Heatstroke A dangerous condition in which the body loses its ability to cool itself through perspiration.

Hemodialysis A technique in which an artificial kidney machine removes waste products from the blood.

Hemoglobin The oxygen-carrying protein in blood.

Herbal supplements Dietary supplements containing plant extracts.

Heredity All the traits that were biologically passed on to you from your parents.

Español

Sistema de atención de salud Toda atención médica disponible para los habitantes de un país, la forma en que la reciben y el sistema de pago.

Consumidor de salud Cualquier persona que adquiere o consume productos o servicios de salud.

Desigualdades de salud Diferencias de los resultados de salud entre distintos grupos.

Educación en salud Proveer a las personas información adecuada y enseñar destrezas de salud para que puedan tomar decisiones saludables.

Fraude de salud Venta de productos o servicios inútiles que supuestamente sirven para prevenir enfermedades o mejorar otros problemas de la salud.

Seguro de salud Programas privados y gubernamentales que financian total o parcialmente los costos médicos de una persona.

Conocimientos de salud Capacidad que tiene una persona para aprender y comprender información básica de salud y los servicios relacionados, y usar esos conocimientos para mejorar su propia salud y bienestar.

Habilidades de salud Herramientas y estrategias específicas que ayudan a mantener, proteger y mejorar todos los aspectos de la salud.

Healthy People Plan de promoción de la salud y prevención de enfermedades diseñado para que sirva como guía en el mejoramiento de la salud de todos los habitantes de Estados Unidos.

Agotamiento debido al calor Forma de estrés físico provocado por el sobrecalentamiento del cuerpo.

Insolación Estado peligroso en el cual el cuerpo pierde su capacidad de enfriarse mediante la transpiración.

Hemodiálisis Técnica en la cual una máquina de diálisis limpia los desechos de la sangre.

Hemoglobina Proteína que lleva el oxígeno en la sangre.

Suplementos hierbas Suplementos alimentarios que contienen extractos vegetales.

Herencia Todo rasgo biológicamente transmitido de padres a hijos.

GLOSSARY/GLOSARIO

English

Hierarchy of needs A ranked list of those needs essential to human growth and development, presented in ascending order, starting with basic needs and building toward the need for reaching your highest potential.

Histamines Chemicals that can stimulate mucus and fluid production.

Homicide The willful killing of one human being by another.

Hormones Chemicals produced by your glands that regulate the activities of different body cells.

Hostility The intentional use of unfriendly or offensive behavior.

Human Immunodeficiency Virus (HIV) The virus that causes Acquired Immune Deficiency Syndrome (AIDS).

Hunger The natural physical drive to eat, prompted by the body's need for food.

Hurricane A powerful storm that generally forms in tropical areas, producing winds of at least 74 miles per hour, heavy rains, and sometimes tornadoes.

Hypertension High blood pressure.

Hypothermia Dangerously low body temperature.

"I" message A statement that focuses on your feelings rather than on someone else's behavior.

Illegal drugs Chemical substances that people of any age may not lawfully manufacture, possess, buy, or sell.

Illicit drug use The use or sale of any substance that is illegal or otherwise not permitted.

Immune system A network of cells, tissues, organs, and chemicals that fight off pathogens.

Immunity The state of being protected against a particular disease.

Implantation The process by which the zygote attaches to the uterine wall.

Español

Jerarquización de necesidades Lista priorizada de aquellas necesidades esenciales para el desarrollo óptimo del ser humano, presentada en orden ascendente, comenzando con las necesidades básicas y ascendiendo hacia la necesidad de alcanzar los potenciales máximos.

Estaminas Sustancias químicas que pueden estimular la producción de mucosidades y líquidos corporales.

Homicidio Cuando una persona mata intencionalmente a otra.

Hormonas Producciónes químicas secretadas por las glándulas que regulan las actividades de diferentes células corporales.

Hostilidad Comportamiento intencional que es antipático, desagradable u ofensivo.

Virus de la Inmunodeficiencia Humana (VIH) Virus que provoca el Síndrome de Inmunodeficiencia Adquirida (SIDA).

Hambre Impulso físico natural de comer, provocado por la necesidad del cuerpo de obtener alimento.

Huracán Una tormenta muy fuerte que se origina en áreas tropicales y que se caracteriza por vientos de al menos 74 millas por hora, fuertes lluvias, inundaciones y, algunas veces, tornados.

Hipertensión Presión arterial alta.

Hipotermia Descenso peligroso de la temperatura corporal.

Mensaje en primera persona Una declaracion enfocada en sus propias sensaciones mas bien que en el comportamiento de alguien mas.

Drogas ilegales Sustancias químicas que ninguna persona, cualquiera sea su edad, puede legalmente producir, poseer, comprar o vender.

Uso ilegal de drogas El uso o venta de cualquier sustancia que es ilegal o no permitida.

Sistema de defensas (inmunológico) Una combinación de células, tejidos, órganos y sustancias químicas que combaten a los agentes patógenos.

Inmunidad Estado de protección contra una enfermedad en particular.

Implantación El proceso en que el cigoto se adhiere a la pared uterina.

English

Incest Sexual contact between family members who cannot marry by law.

Infatuation Exaggerated feelings of passion.

Infection A condition that occurs when pathogens in the body multiply and damage body cells.

Inflammatory response A reaction to tissue damage caused by injury or infection.

Inguinal hernia Occurs when an organ or tissue protrudes through an area of weak muscle.

Inhalants Substances whose fumes are sniffed or inhaled to give a mind-altering effect.

Insecure Not confident or sure.

Instance To mention as a case or example.

Integrity A firm observance of core ethical values.

Intellectual disability A below-average intellectual ability present from birth or early childhood and associated with difficulties in learning and social adaptation.

Intense Existing in an extreme degree.

Intermediate Being at the middle place or stage.

Interpersonal communication The exchange of thoughts, feelings, and beliefs between two or more people.

Interpersonal conflict Conflicts between people or groups of people.

Intimacy Closeness between two people that develops over time.

Intoxication The state in which the body is poisoned by alcohol or another substance and the person's physical and mental control is significantly reduced.

Involve To require as a necessary accompaniment.

Isolation The act of being withdrawn or separated.

Item An object of concern or interest.

Español

Incesto Contacto sexual entre miembros de una familia que no pueden casarse por ley.

Enamoramiento Sentimientos exagerados de pasión.

Infección Una condición que ocurre cuando agentes patógenos entran al cuerpo, se multiplican y dañan las células.

Respuesta inflamatoria Reacción al daño de tejidos causada por una lesión o infección.

Hernia Cuando un órgano o tejido sobresale en un área de músculos débiles.

Inhalantes Sustancias cuyos gases se aspiran o inhalan para alcanzar un estado que altera la mente.

Inseguro Que no tiene confianza o seguridad.

Caso Para mencionar como un caso o ejemplo.

Integridad Adherencia firme a los valores éticos fundamentales.

Discapacidad intelectual Capacidad intelectual inferior al promedio que se presenta desde el nacimiento o la niñez temprana y que se relaciona con dificultades de aprendizaje y adaptación social.

Intenso Que existe en grado extremo.

Intermedio Que está en medio de un lugar o de una etapa.

Comunicación interpersonal Intercambio de pensamientos, sentimientos y creencias entre dos o más personas.

Conflicto interpersonal Desacuerdo entre personas o grupos de personas.

Intimidad Cercanía entre dos personas que se desarrolla en el transcurso del tiempo.

Intoxicación Estado en el cual el cuerpo se encuentra envenenado por el alcohol u otra sustancia, y el control físico y mental de la persona se encuentra reducido significativamente.

Implicar Que incluye algo.

Aislamiento Acción de retirar o separar.

Artículo Un objeto de atención o interés.

J

Jaundice A yellowing of the skin and eyes.

Ictericia Estado en el cual la piel y los ojos se ponen de color amarillo.

GLOSSARY/GLOSARIO

English

L

Labyrinth The inner ear.

Landfill A specially engineered area where waste can be buried safely.

Layer One thickness or fold spread over or under another.

Legal Permitted by law.

Leukoplakia Thickened, white, leathery-looking spots on the inside of the mouth that can develop into oral cancer.

Lifestyle factors The personal habits or behaviors related to the way a person lives.

Ligament A band of fibrous, slightly elastic connective tissue that attaches one bone to another.

Link A connecting element or factor.

Long-term goal A goal that you plan to reach over an extended period.

Lymph The clear fluid that fills the spaces around body cells.

Lymphocyte Specialized white blood cell that coordinates and performs many of the functions of specific immunity.

M

Mainstream smoke The smoke exhaled from the lungs of a smoker.

Major Notable in effect or scope.

Malignant Cancerous.

Malocclusion A misalignment of the upper and lower teeth.

Malpractice Failure by a health professional to meet accepted standards.

Manipulation An indirect, dishonest way to control or influence others.

Marijuana A plant whose leaves, buds, and flowers are usually smoked for their intoxicating effects.

Mastication The process of chewing.

Media Various methods for communicating information.

Mediation Bringing in a neutral third party to help others resolve their conflicts peacefully.

Español

Laberinto Oído interno.

Vertedero Área diseñada especialmente para enterrar los desechos en forma segura.

Capa Un espesor o pliegue extendido sobre o debajo de otro.

Legal Permitido por la ley.

Leucoplaquia Granos con apariencia de piel blanca dura y espesa que se encuentran dentro de la boca y que pueden llegar a producir un cáncer oral.

Factores del estilo de vida Hábitos o conductas personales relativos a la forma de vivir de las personas.

Ligamento Tejido conjuntivo fibroso y levemente elástico que une dos huesos.

Enlace Elemento o factor de conexión.

Meta a largo plazo Meta que planeas alcanzar en un periodo prolongado.

Linfa Líquido transparente que llena los espacios entre las células del cuerpo.

Linfocito Glóbulo blanco especializado que coordina y realiza muchas de las funciones de inmunidad específica

Humo directo Humo exhalado por los pulmones de un fumador.

Principal Notable en efecto o alcance.

Maligno Canceroso.

Oclusión defectuosa Alineación defectuosa de los dientes superiores e inferiores.

Mala práctica médica (mala praxis) Condición en la que un profesional de la salud no cumple con los estándares aceptados.

Manipulación Controlar o influenciar a otros de manera indirecta y deshonesta.

Marihuana Una planta cuyas hojas, brotes y flores son generalmente fumados por su efecto intoxicante.

Masticación Proceso de masticar.

Medios de comunicación Diversos métodos para comunicar información.

Mediación Proceso en el cual una tercera parte neutra ayuda a otros a resolver sus conflictos pacíficamente.

English

Medical history Complete and comprehensive information about your immunizations and any health problems you have had to date.

Medicine abuse Intentionally taking medications for nonmedical reasons.

Medicine misuse Using a medicine in ways other than the intended use.

Medicines Drugs that are used to treat or prevent diseases or other conditions.

Megadoses Very large amounts.

Melanin A pigment that gives the skin, hair, and iris of the eyes their color.

Melanoma The most serious form of skin cancer.

Menstruation The shedding of the uterine lining.

Mental Of or relating to the mind.

Mental disorder An illness of the mind that can affect the thoughts, feelings, and behaviors of a person, preventing him or her from leading a happy, healthful, and productive life.

Mental/emotional health The ability to accept yourself and others, express and manage emotions, and deal with the demands and challenges you meet in your life.

Metabolism The processes by which the body breaks down substances and gets energy from food.

Metastasis The spread of cancer from the point where it originated to other parts of the body.

Minerals Elements found in food that are used by the body.

Minor Not serious or involving risk to life.

Misinterpret To understand wrongly.

Monitor To watch or keep track of.

Mood disorders Illness that involves mood extremes that interfere with everyday living.

Mourning The act of showing sorrow or grief.

Mucous membrane The lining of various body cavities, including the nose, ears, and mouth.

Muscle cramps Sudden and sometimes painful contractions of the muscles.

Español

Historial médico Información completa acerca de las vacunas recibidas y los problemas de salud que una persona ha teido hasta la fecha.

Abuso de medicamentos Tomar medicamentos intencionalmente por razones no médicas.

Mal uso de medicamentos Uso de medicamentos de manera distinta del uso previsto.

Medicamentos Fármacos para tratar o prevenir una enfermedad u otro problema de salud.

Megadosises Gran cantidad.

Melanina Pigmento que da el color a la piel, el cabello y el iris del ojo.

Melanoma El cáncer de la piel más grave de todos.

Menstruación El eliminación del revestimiento del útero.

Mental Relativo a la mente.

Trastorno mental Enfermedad mental que puede afectar la manera de pensar, los sentimientos y el comportamiento de una persona, y que le impide tener una vida feliz, saludable y productiva.

Salud mental-emocional Habilidad para aceptarse a sí mismo y a otras personas, expresar, manejar las emociones y hacer frente a las exigencias y desafíos de la vida.

Metabolismo Proceso mediante el cual el cuerpo procesa las sustancias y obtiene energía de los alimentos.

Metástasis Extensión del cáncer desde el punto de origen a otras partes del cuerpo.

Minerales Elementos que se encuentran en los alimentos y son utilizados por el cuerpo.

Menor Que no es grave ni representa riesgo vital.

Malinterpretar Entender equivocadamente.

Controlar Vigilar o comprobar.

Trastornos del ánimo Enfermedad que involucran estados de ánimo extremos, los cuales interfieren con la vida diaria.

Luto Acto de mostrar pena o dolor.

Membrana mucosa Revestimiento de diferentes cavidades corporales que incluyen la nariz, los oídos y la boca.

Calambres musculares Contracciones repentinas y, algunas veces, dolorosas de los músculos.

GLOSSARY/GLOSARIO

English

Muscular endurance The ability of your muscles to perform physical tasks over a period without tiring.

Muscular strength The amount of force your muscles can exert.

MyPlate A visual reminder to help consumers make healthier food choices.

N

Neglect The failure to provide for a child's basic needs.

Negotiation The use of communication and, in many cases, compromise to settle a disagreement.

Nephrons The functional units of the kidneys.

Neurons Nerve cells.

Neutralize To counteract the effect of.

Nicotine The addictive drug found in tobacco.

Nicotine substitute A product that delivers small amounts of nicotine into the user's system while he or she is trying to give up the tobacco habit.

Nicotine withdrawal The process that occurs in the body when nicotine, an addictive drug, is no longer used.

Noise pollution Harmful, unwanted sound loud enough to damage hearing.

Noncommunicable disease A disease that is not transmitted by another person, a vector, or the environment.

Nuclear family Two parents and one or more children living in the same space.

Nutrient-dense Having a high ratio of nutrients to calories.

Nutrients Substances in food that your body needs to grow, to repair itself, and to supply you with energy.

Nutrition The process by which your body takes in and uses food.

Español

Resistencia muscular Capacidad de los músculos para hacer actividades físicas durante un periodo de tiempo sin fatigarse.

Fuerza muscular Fuerza que puedan ejercer los músculos.

MiPlato Un recuerdo visual para ayudar a los consumidoreselegir alimentos más saludables.

Abandono No satisfacer las necesidades básicas de un niño.

Negociación Uso de la comunicación y, frecuentemente, el compromiso para resolver un desacuerdo.

Nefronas Unidades funcionales de los riñones.

Neuronas Células nerviosas.

Neutralizar Contrarrestar el efecto de algo.

Nicotina Droga adictiva que se encuentra en el tabaco.

Sustituto de la nicotina Producto que libera pequeñas cantidades de nicotina en el cuerpo de una persona que está tratando de dejar de fumar.

Reacción al retiro de la nicotina Proceso que ocurre en el cuerpo cuando la nicotina, una droga adictiva, deja de ser consumida.

Contaminación acústica Nivel de ruido perjudicial y no deseado que es lo suficientemente alto como para dañar la audición de las personas.

Enfermedad no contagiosa Enfermedad que no se transmite entre las personas o por un vector, y que tampoco proviene del medio ambiente.

Familia nuclear Ambos padres y uno o más hijos que viven en el mismo espacio.

Rico en nutrientes Que tiene una relación alta de nutrientes a calorías.

Nutrientes Sustancias presentes en los alimentos que el cuerpo necesita para crecer, regenerarse y producir energía.

Nutrición Proceso mediante el cual el cuerpo absorbe y usa los alimentos.

English

O

Obese Having an excess of body fat.

Occupational Safety and Health Administration (OSHA) The agency within the federal government that is responsible for promoting safe and healthful conditions in the workplace.

Opiates Drugs like those derived from the opium plant that are obtainable only by prescription and are used to relieve pain.

Ossification The process by which bone is formed, renewed, and repaired.

Osteoarthritis A disease of the joints in which cartilage breaks down.

Osteoporosis A condition in which the bones become fragile and break easily.

Ovaries The female sex glands that store the ova, eggs, and produce female sex hormones.

Overdose A strong, sometimes fatal reaction to taking a large amount of a drug.

Overexertion Overworking the body.

Overload Exercising at a level that's beyond your regular daily activities.

Over-the-counter (OTC) Medicines you can buy without a prescription.

Overweight Heavier than the standard weight range for your height.

Ovulation The process of releasing a mature ovum into the fallopian tube each month.

P

Pancreas A gland that serves both the digestive and endocrine systems.

Pandemic A global outbreak of an infectious disease.

Paranoia An irrational suspiciousness or distrust of others.

Parathyroid glands Glands that produce a hormone that regulates the body's balance of calcium and phosphorus.

Partner A member of a couple.

Obeso Que tiene exceso de grasa corporal.

Administración de Seguridad y Salud Ocupacional (OSHA) Agencia del gobierno federal que es responsable de promover condiciones de trabajo seguras y saludables.

Opiáceos Drogas, como aquellas derivadas del opio, que sólo se obtienen con prescripción médica y se utilizan para aliviar el dolor.

Osificación Proceso mediante el cual el hueso se forma, renueva y repara.

Osteoartritis Enfermedad de las articulaciones en la cual el cartílago se deteriora.

Osteoporosis Enfermedad en la cual los huesos se vuelven frágiles y se rompen con facilidad.

Ovarios Glándulas sexuales femeninas que contienen los óvulos y producen hormonas sexuales.

Sobredosis Reacción fuerte, y algunas veces fatal, al consumir una droga en grandes cantidades.

Esfuerzo excesivo Cuando el cuerpo trabaja demasiado.

Sobrecarga Ejercitarse a un nivel que sobrepasa las actividades diarias normales.

Medicamentos de venta libre (OTC) Medicamentos que se pueden comprar sin prescripción médica.

Sobrepeso Peso superior al rango normal según la estatura.

Ovulacion El proceso de saltar un ovario maduro cada mes en las trompas de falopio.

Páncreas Glándula utilizada tanto por el sistema digestivo como el endocrino.

Pandemia Brote global de una enfermedad infecciosa.

Paranoia Sospecha o desconfianza irracionales hacia otras personas.

Glándulas paratiroides Glándulas que producen una hormona que regula el equilibrio de calcio y fósforo en el cuerpo.

Socio Persona asociada con otra.

GLOSSARY/GLOSARIO

English

Passive Unwilling or unable to express thoughts and feelings in a direct or firm manner.

Pasteurization Treating a substance with heat to kill or slow the growth of pathogens.

Pathogen A microorganism that causes disease.

Peer mediation Processes in which specially trained students help other students resolve conflicts peacefully.

Peer pressure The influence that people your age may have on you.

Peers People of the same age who share similar interests.

Penis A tube-shaped organ that extends from the trunk of the body just above the testes.

Peptic ulcer A sore in the lining of the digestive tract.

Percent One part in a hundred.

Perception The act of becoming aware through the senses.

Performance enhancers Substitutes that boost athletic ability.

Period The completion of a cycle.

Periodontal disease An inflammation of the periodontal structures.

Periodontium The area immediately around the tooth.

Peristalsis A series of involuntary muscle contractions that move food through the digestive tract.

Personal flotation device Life jacket.

Personal identity Your sense of yourself as a unique individual.

Personal safety The steps you take to prevent yourself from becoming the victim of crime.

Personality A complex set of characteristics that make you unique.

Phagocyte White blood cells that attack invading pathogens.

Español

Pasivo Persona que no está dispuesto o no es capaz de expresar sus pensamientos y sentimientos.

Pasteurización Tratamiento de una sustancia con calor para matar organismos patógenos o para hacer más lento su desarrollo.

Patógeno Microorganismo que causa enfermedades.

Mediación entre compañeros Proceso en el cual estudiantes especialmente entrenados ayudan a otros a resolver sus conflictos pacíficamente.

Presión de los compañeros La influencia que gente de tu misma edad puede tener en ti.

Compañeros Personas cuya edad e intereses son similares a los tuyos.

Pene Órgano con forma de tubo que se extiende desde el tronco del cuerpo, justo arriba de los testículos.

Úlcera péptica Herida en el revestimiento del tracto digestivo.

Porcentaje Una parte de cada cien.

Percepción Acto de tomar conciencia de algo a través de los sentidos.

Potenciadores del rendimiento Sustitutos que mejoran las capacidades atléticas.

Periodo Ciclo de tiempo.

Enfermedad periodontal Inflamación de la estructura de soporte dental.

Periodontio Área que rodea los dientes.

Movimientos peristálticos Serie de contracciones musculares involuntarias que mueven la comida a través del tracto digestivo.

Dispositivo de flotación personal Chaqueta salvavidas.

Identidad personal Sentirse como un individuo único.

Seguridad personal Medidas que se toman para evitar ser víctima de un delito.

Personalidad Conjunto complejo de características que hacen que una persona sea única.

Fagocito Glóbulo blanco que combate la invasión de patógenos.

English

Physical abuse A pattern of intentionally causing bodily harm or injury to another person.

Physical activity Any form of movement that causes your body to use energy.

Physical fitness The ability to carry out daily tasks easily and have enough reserve energy to respond to unexpected demands.

Physical maturity The state at which the physical body and all its organs are fully developed.

Physiological dependence A condition in which the user has a chemical need for the drug.

Pituitary gland A gland that regulates and controls the activities of all other endocrine systems.

Plaque A combination of bacteria and other particles, such as small bits of food, which adheres to the outside of a tooth.

Plasma The fluid in which other parts of the blood are suspended.

Platelets Types of cells in the blood that cause blood clots to form.

Platonic friendship A friendship with a member of the opposite gender in which there is affection but the two people are not considered a couple.

Pneumonia An infection of the lungs in which the air sacs fill with pus and other liquids.

Poison Any substance–solid, liquid, or gas–that causes injury, illness, or death when it enters the body.

Poison control center A round-the-clock service that provides emergency medical advice on how to treat poisoning victims.

Portion A part set off from the whole.

Pose To put or set forth.

Precycling Reducing waste before it is generated.

Prejudice An unfair opinion or judgment of a particular group of people.

Prenatal care Steps that a pregnant female can take to provide for her own health and the health of her baby.

Español

Abuso físico Patrón intencionalmente de causar daño o lesión corporal a otra persona.

Actividad física Cualquier forma de movimiento que provoque que el cuerpo consuma energía.

Buen estado Capacidad de realizar fácilmente las tareas diarias y tener suficiente energía para responder a exigencias inesperadas.

Madurez física Estado en el cual el cuerpo y todos sus órganos se encuentran totalmente desarrollados.

Dependencia fisiológica Enfermedad en la cual el usuario tiene una necesidad física de consumir una droga.

Glándula pituitaria Glándula que regula o controla las actividades de todas las glándulas endocrinas.

Placa Combinación de bacterias y otras partículas, tales como pequeños trozos de alimentos, que se adhieren a la parte externa de los dientes.

Plasma Líquido en el cual están suspendidos los componentes de la sangre.

Plaquetas Tipos de células sanguíneas que provocan la formación de coágulos.

Amistad platónica Amistad con una persona del sexo opuesto en la cual hay sentimientos mutuos de afecto, pero que no se consideran una pareja.

Neumonía Infección de los pulmones en la cual los alvéolos se llenan de pus y otros líquidos.

Veneno Cualquier sustancia, sea sólida, líquida o gaseosa, que al entrar en el cuerpo causa una herida, una enfermedad o la muerte.

Centro para el control de envenenamientos Servicio que funciona las 24 horas del día para dar consejos médicos de emergencia sobre el tratamiento de víctimas de intoxicaciones.

Porcíon Parte separada de un todo.

Plantear Exponer o presentar.

Reciclaje previo Reducir la basura antes de generarla.

Prejuicio Opinión o juicio injusto acerca de un grupo específico de personas.

Cuidado prenatal Todas las medidas que una mujer embarazada puede tomar para cuidar su propia salud y la de su bebé.

GLOSSARY/GLOSARIO

English

Prescription medicines Medicines that cannot be used without the written approval of a licensed physician or nurse practitioner.

Prevention Taking steps to keep something from happening or getting worse.

Primary care physician A medical doctor who provides physical check-ups and general care.

Priorities The goals, tasks, values, and activities that you judge to be more important than others.

Process A series of actions geared toward an end result.

Profound deafness Hearing loss so severe that a person affected cannot benefit from mechanical amplification such as a hearing aid.

Progression Gradually increasing the demands on your body.

Promote To contribute to the growth of.

Proteins Nutrients the body uses to build and maintain its cells and tissues.

Psychoactive drugs Chemicals that affect the central nervous system and alter activity in the brain.

Psychological Directed toward the mind.

Psychological dependence A condition in which a person believes that a drug is needed in order to feel good or to function normally.

Psychosomatic response A physical reaction, which results from stress rather than from an injury or illness.

Psychotherapy An ongoing dialogue between a patient and a mental health professional.

Puberty The time when a person begins to develop certain traits of adults of his or her gender.

Public health All efforts to monitor, protect, and promote the health of the population as a whole.

Pulp The tissue that contains the blood vessels and nerves of a tooth.

Español

Medicamentos con prescripción Medicamentos que no se pueden utilizar sin la aprobación escrita de un médico o enfermera profesionales.

Prevención Tomar medidas para evitar que algo ocurra o empeore.

Médico de atención primaria Médico que realiza chequeos físicos y se encarga del cuidado general de los pacientes.

Prioridades Metas, tareas, valores y actividades que se consideran más importantes que otras.

Proceso Serie de acciones para obtener un resultado final.

Sordera profunda Pérdida de la audición tan grave que no se beneficia con la amplificación mecánica (por ejemplo, los audífonos).

Progresión Aumento gradual de las exigencias corporales.

Promover Contribuir al crecimiento de algo.

Proteínas Nutrientes que el cuerpo utiliza para generar y mantener las células y los tejidos.

Drogas psicoactivas Sustancias químicas que afectan el sistema nervioso central y alteran la actividad del cerebro.

Psicológico Relativo a la mente.

Dependencia psicológica Enfermedad en la cual una persona cree que una droga es necesaria para sentirse bien o para funcionar normalmente.

Respuesta psicosomática Reacción física producida por el estrés en lugar de corresponder a una lesión o una enfermedad.

Psicoterapia Diálogo continúo entre un paciente y un profesional de la salud mental.

Pubertad Periodo en el cual una persona comienza a desarrollar ciertos rasgos de adultez que son característicos de su sexo.

Salud pública Todo esfuerzo para supervisar, proteger y promover la salud de la población como una unidad.

Pulpa Tejido que contiene los vasos sanguíneos y los nervios de un diente.

English

Español

R

Random violence Violence committed for no particular reason.

Range The distance between possible extremes.

Rape Any form of sexual intercourse that takes place against a person's will.

Rapid test Used in situations where the infected person might not come back to learn the results to the test. A blood sample is collected and analyzed immediately.

Reaction A response to a stimulus or influence.

Recovery The process of learning to live an alcohol-free life.

Recycling The processing of waste materials so that they can be used again.

Refusal skills Communication strategies that can help you say no when you are urged to take part in behaviors that are unsafe or unhealthful, or that go against your values.

Regulate To fix the time, amount, degree, or rate of.

Rehabilitation Process of medical and psychological treatment for physiological or psychological dependence on a drug or alcohol.

Relationship A bond or connection you have with other people.

Relaxation response A state of calm.

Remission A period of time when symptoms disappear.

Remove To get rid of.

Require To demand as necessary.

Rescue breathing Breathing for a person who is not breathing on his or her own.

Resilient The ability to adapt effectively and recover from disappointment, difficulty, or crisis.

Resolve To deal with successfully.

Resource A source of supply or support.

Respiratory tract The passageway that makes breathing possible.

Respond To react in response.

Violencia de azar Violencia infringida sin una razón en especial.

Rango Distancia entre posibles extremos.

Violación Cualquier tipo de acto sexual que ocurre contra la voluntad de una persona.

Prueba rápida Prueba que se realiza cuando la persona infectada podría no regresar para conocer los resultados. Se toma y analiza una muestra de sangre en forma inmediata.

Reacción Respuesta a un estimulo o influencia.

Recuperación Proceso de aprender a vivir sin consumir alcohol.

Reciclaje Proceso en el cual los desechos se pueden utilizar nuevamente.

Habilidades de negación Estrategias de comunicación que ayudan a decir no cuando te presionan a participar en actividades peligrosas, no saludables o que van en contra de tus valores.

Regular Organizar el tiempo, la cantidad, el grado o el rtimo de algo.

Rehabilitación Proceso de tratamiento médico y psicológico para la dependencia fisiológica o psicológica de una droga o del alcohol.

Relación Lazo que una persona tiene con los demás.

Respuesta de relajación Estado de calma.

Remisión Periodo en el cual desaparecen los síntomas.

Eliminar Deshacerse de algo o de alguien.

Requerir Solicitar como necesario.

Respiración de rescate Respiración artificial para una persona que no está respirando por sí misma.

Resiliencia Capacidad de adaptarse eficazmente y recuperarse después de una decepción, dificultad o crisis.

Resolver Manejar algo con éxito.

Recurso Fuente de suministro o apoyo.

Tracto respiratorio Vías que hacen posible la respiración.

Reaccionar Actuar en respuesta a algo o alguien.

GLOSSARY/GLOSARIO

English

Resting heart rate The number of times your heart beats per minute when you are not active.

Retina The inner layer of the eye wall.

Rheumatoid arthritis A disease characterized by the debilitating destruction of the joints due to inflammation.

Risk behaviors Actions that can potentially threaten your health or the health of others.

Road rage Responding to a driving incident with violence.

Role The parts you play in your relationships.

Role model Someone whose success or behavior serves as an example for you.

S

Sclera The white part of the eye.

Scoliosis A lateral, or side-to-side, curvature of the spine.

Scrotum An external skin sac, which holds the testes.

Sebaceous glands Structures within the skin that produce an oily secretion called sebum.

Secure To fasten or seal.

Sedentary Involving little physical activity.

Seek To go in search of.

Self-actualization To strive to become the best you can be.

Self-control A person's ability to use responsibility to override emotions.

Self-defense Any strategy for protecting yourself from harm.

Self-directed Able to make correct decisions about behavior when adults are not present to enforce rules.

Self-esteem How much you value, respect, and feel confident about yourself.

Semen A thick fluid containing sperm and other secretions from the male reproductive system.

Español

Frecuencia cardiaco en reposo Número de latidos por minuto que se producen cuando la persona se encuentra en estado pasivo.

Retina Capa interna de la pared ocular.

Artritis reumatoide Enfermedad caracterizada por la destrucción debilitadora de las articulaciones debido a la inflamación.

Comportamiento riesgoso Acciones que pueden poner en peligro tu salud o la de otras personas.

Agresividad al volante Reaccionar de manera violenta a un incidente de conducción.

Función Papel que desempeña una persona en una relación.

Modelo de conducta Alguien cuyo éxito o comportamiento sirve de ejemplo para otros

Esclerótica Parte blanca del ojo.

Escoliosis Desviación lateral, o de lado a lado, de la columna.

Escroto Saco de piel externa que sostiene los testículos.

Glándulas sebáceas Estructuras dentro de la piel que producen una secreción aceitosa llamada sebo.

Asegurar Dejar firme y seguro.

Sedentar Poca actividad física.

Buscar Hacer algo para encontrar a alguien o algo.

Realización personal Esfuerzo para lograr lo mejor de uno mismo.

Dominio de sí mismo Capacidad de una persona para controlar sus emociones por medio de la responsabilidad.

Defensa propia Cualquier estrategia para protegerse de un daño.

Auto-dirigido Capaz de tomar decisiones correctas acerca de su comportamiento en la ausencia de adultos que impongan las reglas.

Autoestima Valor, respeto y sentimiento de confianza que uno tiene de sí mismo.

Semen Líquido espeso que contiene los espermatozoides y otras secreciones del aparato reproductor masculino.

English

Separation A decision by two married people to live apart from each other.

Sexual abuse A pattern of sexual contact that is forced upon a person against his or her will.

Sexual assault Any intentional sexual attack against another person.

Sexual violence Any form of unwelcome sexual contact directed at an individual.

Sexually transmitted diseases (STDs) Infectious diseases spread from person to person through sexual contact.

Sexually transmitted infections (STIs) Infections spread from person to person through sexual contact.

Shock A life-threatening condition in which the heart is not delivering an adequate supply of blood to the body.

Short-term goal A goal that you can reach in a short period of time.

Siblings Brothers or sisters.

Side effects Reactions to medicine other than the one intended.

Sidestream smoke The smoke from the burning end of a cigarette, pipe, or cigar.

Significant Having meaning.

Single-parent family A family that consists of only one parent and one or more children.

Skeletal muscles Muscles attached to bone that cause body movements.

Smog A brownish haze that sometimes forms in urban areas.

Smoke alarm A device that produces a loud warning noise in the presence of smoke.

Smokeless tobacco Ground tobacco that is chewed or inhaled through the nose.

Smooth muscles Muscles that act on the lining of the body's passageways and hollow internal organs.

Sobriety Living without alcohol.

Español

Separación Cuando una pareja casada decide vivir aparte uno del otro.

Abuso sexual Patrón de contacto sexual realizado a la fuerza o contra la voluntad de una persona.

Agresión sexual Cualquier ataque sexual intencional en contra de otra persona.

Violencia sexual Cualquier forma de contacto sexual no deseado dirigido a una persona.

Enfermedades de transmisión sexual (ETS) Enfermedades que se transmiten a través del contacto sexual entre dos personas.

Infecciones de transmisión sexual Infecciones que se transmiten a través del contacto sexual entre dos personas.

Shock Enfermedad que puede ser fatal en la cual el corazón no envía suficiente sangre al cuerpo.

Meta a corto plazo Meta que se puede lograr en un periodo breve.

Hermanos Hermanos o hermanas.

Efectos secundarios Reacciones inesperadas a un medicamento.

Humo indirecto Humo que proviene de una colilla de cigarrillo, pipa o cigarro.

Significativo Que es importante.

Familias de un solo padre Una familia compuesta por un sólo padre y uno o más niños.

Músculos del esqueleto Músculos unidos a los huesos y que producen el movimiento del cuerpo.

Smog Bruma de color café que se forma algunas veces en las áreas urbanas.

Alarma de humo Dispositivo que emite un sonido de advertencia que se activa en presencia del humo.

Rapé Tabaco molido que es masticado o inhalado a través de la

Músculo liso Tipo de músculo que se encuentra en los órganos, los vasos sanguíneos y las glándulas

Sobriedad Vivir sin consumir alcohol.

GLOSSARY/GLOSARIO

English

Specialists Medical doctors who focus on particular kinds of patients or particular medical conditions.

Specificity Choosing the right types of activities to improve a given element of fitness.

Sperm Male gametes.

Spiritual health A deep-seated sense of meaning and purpose in life.

Spousal abuse Domestic violence or any other form of abuse directed at a spouse.

Sprains Injuries to the ligaments around a joint.

Stages of grief A variety of reactions that may surface as an individual makes sense of how a loss affects him or her.

Stalking Repeatedly following, harassing, or threatening an individual.

Stereotype Exaggerated or oversimplified beliefs about people who belong to a certain group.

Sterility The inability to reproduce.

Stigma A mark of shame or disapproval that results in an individual being shunned or rejected by others.

Stimulant A drug that increases the action of the central nervous system, the heart, and other organs.

Strains Overstretching and tearing a muscle.

Stress The reaction of the body and mind to everyday challenges and demands.

Stress management skills Skills that help you reduce and manage your stress.

Stressor Anything that causes stress.

Stroke An acute injury in which blood flow to the brain is interrupted.

Substance abuse Any unnecessary or improper use of chemical substances for non-medical purposes.

Suicide The act of intentionally taking one's own life.

Survival The continuation of life or existence.

Suspend To block temporarily.

Synergistic effect The interaction of two or more medicines that results in a greater effect than when the medicines are taken alone.

Español

Especialistas Médicos que se dedican a un tipo particular de pacientes o condiciones medicas particulares.

Especificar Elegir el tipo correcto de actividades que mejoren un elemento específico del bienestar fisico.

Espermatozoides Gametos masculinos.

Salud espiritual Un sentido profundo de significado y proposito en vida.

Abuso conyugal Violencia doméstica o cualquier forma de abuso dirigida hacia el esposo o la esposa.

Esguince Daño a los ligamentos que rodean una articulación.

Etapas del duelo Variedad de reacciones que pueden aparecer a medida que una persona entiende cómo le afecta una pérdida.

Acecho Seguimiento, acoso o amenaza repetidos que una persona hace a otra.

Estereotipo Creencias exageradas o demasiado simplificadas acerca de las personas que pertenecen a un grupo específico.

Esterilidad Incapacidad de reproducirse.

Estigma Señal de vergüenza o desaprobación que da como resultado el rechazo de una persona por parte de los demás.

Estimulante Droga que acelera el funcionamiento del sistema nervioso central, el corazón y otros órganos.

Distensión muscular Estirar en exceso y rasgar un músculo.

Estrés Reacción del cuerpo y la mente a las exigencias y desafíos de la vida diaria.

Habilidades para controlar el estrés Habilidades que le ayudan a reducir y manejar el estrés.

Estresante Cualquier cosa que produce estrés.

Accidente cerebrovascular Lesión aguda que interrumpe el flujo de sangre al cerebro.

Abuso de sustancias Cualquier uso inapropiado o excesivo de sustancias químicas con propósitos no médicos.

Suicidio Acto de quitarse la vida intencionalmente

Supervivencia Continuación de la vida o de la existencia.

Suspender Prohibir temporalmente.

Efecto sinérgico Interacción entre dos o más medicamentos que produce un efecto más fuerte que si se toman por separado.

English

Tar A thick, sticky, dark fluid produced when tobacco burns.

Technique A method of accomplishing a desired aim.

Technology Radio, television, and the Internet.

Tendon A fibrous cord that attaches muscle to the bone.

Tendonitis The inflammation of a tendon.

Testes Two small glands that secrete testosterone and produce sperm.

Testosterone The male sex hormone.

Thyroid gland Produces hormones that regulate metabolism, body heat, and bone growth.

Tinnitus A condition in which a ringing, buzzing, whistling, roaring, hissing, or other sound is heard in the ear in the absence of external sound.

Tolerance The ability to accept others' differences.

Tornado A whirling, funnel-shaped windstorm that extends from a storm to the ground and advances along the ground.

Toxin A substance that kills cells or interferes with their functions.

Trachea The windpipe.

Transit Conveyance of persons or things from one place to another.

Transitions Critical changes that occur in all stages of life.

Transmit To send from one person or place to another.

Traumatic event Any event that has a stressful impact sufficient to overwhelm your normal coping strategies.

Trend A line of general direction or movement.

Trigger To initiate or set off.

Tuberculosis A contagious bacterial infection that usually affects the lungs.

Tumor An abnormal mass of tissue that has no natural role in the body.

Español

Alquitrán Líquido espeso, pegajoso y oscuro que se forma al quemarse el tabaco.

Técnica Método para lograr el propósito deseado.

Tecnología Radio, televisión e internet.

Tendón Tejido fibroso que une los músculos a los huesos.

Tendinitis Inflamación de un tendón.

Testículos Par de pequeñas glándulas que secretan testosterona y producen espermatozoides.

Testosterona Hormona sexual masculina.

Tiroides Glándula que produce las hormonas que regulan el metabolismo, el calor del cuerpo y el crecimiento de los huesos.

Tinnitus Enfermedad en la cual se oye un timbre, zumbido, silbido, siseo, rugido u otro sonido en ausencia de ruidos externos.

Tolerancia Capacidad para aceptar las diferencias de los demás.

Tornado Tormenta de viento en forma de embudo giratorio que se extiende desde una tormenta hasta el suelo y avanza por la tierra.

Toxina Sustancia que mata células o que interfiere con su funcionamiento.

Tráquea Vía respiratoria principal.

Tránsito Desplazamiento de personas o cosas de un lugar a otra.

Transiciones Cambios críticos que ocurren en todas las etapas de la vida.

Transmitir Trasladar desde una persona o lugar a otro.

Suceso traumático Todo suceso que tiene un efecto estresante suficiente como para sobrepasar las estrategias normales para lidiar con un hecho.

Tendencia Linea general de dirección o movimiento.

Desencadenar Comenzar o iniciar algo.

Tuberculosis Infección bacteriana contagiosa que comúnmente afecta los pulmones.

Tumor Masa de tejido anormal que no cumple ninguna función natural en el cuerpo.

GLOSSARY/GLOSARIO

English

Español

Unconditional love Love without limitation or quantification.

Amor incondicional Amor sin límite ni cuantificación.

Unconsciousness The condition of not being alert or aware of your surroundings.

Inconciencia Condición en la cual una persona no está alerta o consciente de lo que lo rodea.

Underweight Below the standard weight range for your height.

Bajo peso Peso inferior al rango normal según la estatura.

Unintentional injury An injury resulting from an unexpected event.

Lesión no intencional Lesión resultante de un suceso inesperado.

Universal precautions Steps taken to prevent the spread of disease through blood and other body fluids when providing first aid or health care.

Precauciones universales Medidas que se toman para evitar el contagio de enfermedades a través de la sangre y otros fluidos corporales cuando se proporcionan primeros auxilios o atención médica.

Urban sprawl The spreading of city development (houses, shopping centers, businesses, and schools) onto undeveloped land.

Expansión urbana Crecimiento del desarrollo de una ciudad (casas, centros comerciales, negocios y escuelas) hacia zonas no desarrolladas.

Ureters Tubes that connect the kidneys to the bladder.

Uréter Cada uno de los dos canales que conectan los riñones y la vejiga.

Urethra The tube that leads from the bladder to the outside of the body.

Uretra Canal que nace en la vejiga y se extiende hacia el exterior del cuerpo.

Urethritis The inflammation of the urethra.

Uretritis Inflamación de la uretra.

Uterus The hollow, muscular, pear-shaped organ that nourishes and protects a fertilized ovum until birth.

Útero El órgano baso, muscular, en forma de pera que alimienta y protege el ovario hasta nacimiento

Vaccine A preparation of dead or weakened pathogens that are introduced into the body to stimulate an immune response.

Vacuna Preparación de agentes patógenos muertos o debilitados que se introducen en el cuerpo para estimular el sistema inmune.

Vagina A muscular, elastic passageway that extends from the uterus to the outside of the body.

Vagina Conducto muscular y elástico que va desde el útero hasta la parte externa del cuerpo de una mujer.

Valid Well-grounded or justifiable.

Válido Correctamente fundamentado o justificable.

Values The ideas, beliefs, and attitudes about what is important, that help guide the way you live.

Valores Ideas, creencias y actitudes sobre lo que es importante que guíen la vida de una persona.

Vector An organism that carries and transmits pathogens to humans or other animals.

Vector Organismo que lleva y transmite agentes patógenos a personas y otros animales.

Vegetarian A person who eats mostly, or only, plant-based foods.

Vegetariano Persona que come principal o exclusivamente alimentos que provienen de las plantas.

Vehicular safety Obeying the rules of the road and exercising common sense and good judgment while driving.

Seguridad vehicular Usar el sentido común, un buen criterio y obedecer las reglas de tránsito mientras se conduce.

English

Venom A poisonous secretion.

Verbal abuse The use of words to mistreat or injure another person.

Violence The threatened or actual use of physical force or power to harm another person and to damage property.

Virus A piece of genetic material surrounded by a protein coat.

Visualize To form a mental image of.

Vitamins Compounds found in food that help regulate many body processes.

Volume The degree of loudness.

W

Warm-up Gentle cardiovascular activity that prepares the muscles for work.

Warranty A company's or a store's written agreement to repair a product or refund your money if the product does not function properly.

Wastewater Used water from homes, communities, farms, and businesses.

Weight cycling A repeated pattern of losing and regaining body weight.

Wellness An overall sense of well-being or total health.

Workout The part of an exercise session when you are exercising at your highest peak.

Z

Zero tolerance policy A policy that makes no exceptions for anybody for any reason.

Español

Veneno Secreción venenosa.

Abuso verbal El uso de palabras para maltratar o dañar a otras personas.

Violencia Amenaza o uso de la fuerza física o el poder para maltratar a una persona o dañar una propiedad.

Virus Partícula de material genético rodeada de una capa proteica.

Visualizar Formarse una imagen mental.

Vitaminas Compuestos que se encuentran en los alimentos y que ayudan a regular muchos procesos corporales.

Volumen Intensidad del sonido.

Precalentamiento Actividad cardiovascular liviana que prepara los músculos para el ejercicio.

Garantía Acuerdo escrito en el cual una empresa o tienda se compromete a reparar un producto o a devolver el dinero si el producto no funciona correctamente.

Aguas residuales Agua ya utilizada que proviene de casas, comunidades, granjas e industrias.

Ciclo de peso Patrón repetido de subir y bajar de peso.

Bienestar Sensación general de gozar de buena salud.

Entrenamiento Parte de un programa de actividad física en la que los ejercicios se realizan en el nivel más alto de rendimiento.

Política de cero tolerancia Normativa en que no hay excepciones para nadie por ninguna razón.

INDEX

Page numbers in italics refer to pictures or features.

A

Abrasions, 665
Abstinence
    avoiding risk situations, 183–184
    committing to, 186–187
    consent, 182
    consequences, 184–186
    definition of, 16
    from high-risk behaviors, 16
    recommitting to, 187
    sexual activity, 182
    sexual content on TV, 183
Abuse, 156, 209
    child, 157
    definition of, 156
    domestic, 158–159
    effects of, 158
    elder, 158
    forms of, 211–212
    overcoming, 214–215
    protecting yourself from, 212
    in relationships, 210
    sexual, 158
Abusers, help for, 215
Acceptance
    healthy friendship, 171
    as stage of grief, 89
Accessing information, 11, 30
Accident chain, 636, 637
Accidents. *See* Unintentional injuries
Acetaminophen, 460
Achievement, need for, 59
Acquaintance rape, 212
Acquired immune deficiency syndrome (AIDS), 584
ACTH. *See* Adrenocorticotropic hormone
Action plan
    definition of, 38
    for reaching goals, 38–39
Active immunity, 560
Active listening, 29, 135
Addiction, 483, 520
Addictive drug, 474
Additive interaction, 462
Additives, food, 241
ADH. *See* Antidiuretic hormone
Adipose tissue, 230
Adjustment disorder, 100
Adolescence, 436, 438, 439–441
Adoption, 152, 445

Adoptive families, 145
Adrenal glands, 81, 391
Adrenal medulla, 391
Adrenaline, 81
Adrenocorticotropic hormone (ACTH), 391
Adulthood, 442–443
Advertising
    definition of, 40
    hidden messages/techniques used in, 40, *41*
    techniques, 501
Advocacy
    definition of, 32
    as health skill, 32
AEDs. *See* Automated external defibrillators
Aerobic activities, 295
Aerobic exercise, 290, 291
Affection
    set limits for, 182
Affirmation, 148
Aggressive communication, 133
Aggressive response, 178–179
Agreement, in peer mediation, 202
AIDS. *See* Acquired immune deficiency syndrome
AIDS Awareness Campaign, 593
AIDS-opportunistic infections, 587
Air pollution
    indoor, 704–705
    reducing, 704–705
    understanding, 702–704
Air quality, 702–703
Air Quality Index (AQI), 703
Airborne transmission, 551
Alarm, as stress response, 80, 81
Alcohol, 416
    avoiding, 504–505
    benefits, 504
    binge drinking and poisoning, 499
    definition, 494
    and driving, 506–507
    drug interactions, 497
    factors, 495–496, 500
    and family, 503
    health risks, 501–503
    and law, 501
    long-term effects, 497–498
    and pregnancy, 508–509
    refusing, 505
    and school, 503
    sexual activity, 502
    short-term effects, 494–497, *496*
    treatment, 510–511
    violence, 502

INDEX

mental health, 519
other consequences, 521
physical health, 519
social health, 520
society consequences, 522
trends, 523
Illnesses
changes in family related to, 154
foodborne, 244
Immune deficiency, 365
Immune response, 559
Immune system, 586–587
definition, 557
inflammatory response, 558
lymphocytes, 559
memory, 560
specific defenses, 559
Immunity, 560
Immunization, 562
Immunotherapy, 461
Impairment
hearing, 620–621
motor, 621
sight, 619–620
Implantation, 412, *413*
Impulse control disorders, 104
Incest, 211
Incineration, 708
Indigestion, 376
Individual decisions, 37
Indoor air pollution, 704–705
Industrial wastes, 708
Infancy, 426–427, *428*
Infatuation, 182
Infertility, 404
Inflammation, 460
Inflammatory response, 558
Influence teens, 519
Influenza, 553–554
Information support groups, 65
Ingredient list, 241
Inguinal hernia, 398
Inhalants, 527
Injuries
coping with, 303–305
major, 304–305
minor, 303–304
muscle/joint/bone, 675–676
Insecure teens, 204
Insulin, 616
Integrity, 62

Intellectual disability, 621
Internal conflicts, 194
Internal reproductive organs, 396
International Committee of the Red Cross, 701
Internet
health information from, 11
Internet predators, 635
Internet service provider (ISP), 634
Interpersonal communication skills, 29
active listening, 29
for healthy relationships, 123
"I" messages, 29, 137
with respect and caring, 29
Interpersonal conflicts, 194
Intimacy, 182
Intoxication, 495, 506
Introductions, in peer mediation, 202
Intruders, guarding against, 641–642
ISP. *see* Internet service provider

J

Jaundice, 555
Jealousy
as cause of conflict, 195
managing feelings, 172
Joint injuries, 675–676
Jordan, Michael, 59

K

Keratin, 318
Ketamine, 531
Kidney transplant, 383
Killed-virus vaccines, 561
Kleptomania, 103
Kübler-Ross, Elisabeth, 89

L

Labels
nutrition, 240–243
product, 41
Labyrinth, 326
Lacerations, 665
Lacrimal gland, 323
Lactose intolerance, 270, 377
Landfills, 707
Late adulthood
health concerns, 450
public health policies and programs, 451
Late childhood, 427
Lead, 417, 703

INDEX

INDEX